Pg 40

NUTRITION
AND DIET THERAPY

April 5   intro to Nutrition   Module 1
- Purpose of Food + Fluid
- RDA's & USRDA's
- Essential Nutrients   module 4+5

April 6   Essential Nutrients (con) Module 2+3
other Nutritional considurations   Module 6+7
- Convenience food + Combo foods.
- Nutritional Enrichment + fortification
- Desirable weight.

April 7   PP 60-62
        P 84
      Module 13

April 8   Module 15

April 12   Module 18
        Module 4,5,6,7

April 13   GUEST SPEAKERS.

April 14   N/C

April 15 REVIEW for Exam.

April

April 19   TEST

The Jones and Bartlett Series in Health Sciences

Biological Bases of Human Aging and Disease
Kart/Metress/Metress

Aquatics
Sova

Aquatic Student's Handbook
Sova

Basic Law for the Allied Health Professions
Cowdrey

Basic Nutrition: Self-Instructional Modules, Second Edition
Stanfield

The Biology of AIDS, Third Edition
Fan/Conner/Villarreal

The Birth Control Book
Belcastro

Children's Nutrition
Lifshitz

Contemporary Health Issues
Banister/Allen/Fadl/Bhakthan/Howard

Drugs and Society, Third Edition
Witters/Venturelli/Hanson

Essential Medical Terminology
Stanfield

First Aid and CPR
National Safety Council

First Aid and Emergency Care Workbook
Thygerson

Fitness and Health: Life-Style Strategies
Thygerson

Golf: Your Turn for Success
Fisher/Geertsen

Health and Wellness, Fourth Edition
Edlin/Golanty

Healthy People 2000
U.S. Department of Health and Human Services

Healthy People 2000-- Summary Report
U.S. Department of Health and Human Services

Human Anatomy and Physiology Coloring Workbook and Study Guide
Anderson

Interviewing and Helping Skills for Health Professionals
Cormier/Cormier/Weisser

Introduction to Human Disease, Third Edition
Crowley

Introduction to Human Immunology
Huffer/Kanapa/Stevenson

Introduction to the Health Professions
Stanfield

Medical Terminology (with Self-Instructional Modules)
Stanfield/Hui

The Nation's Health, Third Edition
Lee/Estes

Personal Health Choices
Smith/Smith

Principles and Issues in Nutrition
Hui

Sexuality Today
Nass/Fisher

Step Aerobics
Brown

Stress Management: A College Text
Sorenson

Teaching Elementary Health Science, Third Edition
Bender/Sorochan

Weight Management the Fitness Way
Dusek

Weight Training for Strength and Fitness
Silvester

Writing a Successful Grant Application
Reif-Lehrer

SECOND EDITION

NUTRITION AND DIET THERAPY

Self-Instructional Modules

Peggy S. Stanfield, M.S., RD

College of Southern Idaho

with the special assistance of
Y. H. Hui, Ph.D.

JONES AND BARTLETT PUBLISHERS
BOSTON   LONDON

Editorial, Sales, and Customer Service Offices
Jones and Bartlett Publishers
20 Park Plaza
Boston, MA 02116

Jones and Bartlett Publishers International
PO Box 1498
London W6 7RS
England

Library of Congress Cataloging-in-Publication Data

Stanfield, Peggy.
    Nutrition and diet therapy / Peggy S. Stanfield. — 2nd ed.
        p. cm.
    Includes index.
    ISBN 0-86720-336-6
    1. Diet therapy—Programmed instruction.   2. Nutrition—Programmed
instruction.   I. Title.
    [DNLM: 1. Diet Therapy—programmed instruction.   2. Nutrition—
programmed instruction. QU 18 S785n]
    RM216.S7251992
    615.8' 54' 077—dc20
    DNLM/DLC
    for Library of Congress   92-2885
                                                                CIP

Artwork for the opening pages of Modules 5, 9, 11, 12, 13, 16, 18, 21 is provided courtesy of Dr. Y. H. Hui. Artwork for the following modules is from the issue of *FDA Consumer* listed:

Module 1	September 1987, p. 16	Module 19	July/August 1982, p. 18
Module 2	September 1986, p. 6	Module 20	September 1987, cover
Module 3	April 1990, p. 11	Module 22	October 1986, p. 17
Module 4	June 1990, p. 5	Module 23	June 1991, p. 16
Module 6	July/August 1984	Module 24	September 1985, cover
Module 7	1983, p. 28	Module 25	March 1986, p. 6
Module 8	May 1982, p. 20	Module 26	April 1980, p. 19
Module 10	April 1980, p. 14	Module 27	September 1985, p. 12
Module 14	November 1987, p. 26		
Module 15	May 1982, p. 4		
Module 17	May 1991, p. 12		

Cover art: *Flowers and Fruit on a Table*, 1865
                Fantin-Latour, Ignace Henri Jean Théodore
                France, 1836–1904
                Oil on canvas
                Bequest of John T. Spaulding
                Courtesy, Museum of Fine Arts, Boston

Printed in the United States of America
96 95 94 93 92   10 9 8 7 6 5 4 3 2 1

Guidance and patience
made the first edition a reality.

Expertise and commitment
made the second edition possible.

A touch of "Chinese magic" made it all worthwhile.
Thank you again, Y. H.

Contents

MODULE 3
Meeting Energy Needs   29

MODULE 4
Carbohydrates and Fats: Implications for Health   44

MODULE 15
Diet and Disorders of Ingestion, Digestion, and Absorption   215

MODULE 16
Diet Therapy for Diabetes Mellitus   232

Preface

When this second edition of *Nutrition and Diet Therapy* is released in 1992, it will be exactly six years since the first edition appeared. I am grateful to all of you who have continued to use my book in spite of the volumes of recent textbooks on the subject.

This second edition is similar to the first one in two major respects. First, the format, style, and structure of each module remain the same. And, second, the content of 16 of the 27 modules is essentially the same, with appropriate updates. These chapters cover food habits, proteins, vitamins, minerals, life cycle, gastrointestinal diseases, liver disorders, and other topics.

The major differences between this and the previous edition are the inclusion of the 1989 Recommended Dietary Allowances, the 1990 dietary guidelines, a discussion of modified food groups, and the 1986 food exchange lists. Major changes in the chapters deal with normal and therapeutic nutrition. Normal nutrition encompasses carbohydrates and fats, life cycle, drugs, nutrition assessment, nutrition, and ecology. Therapeutic nutrition relates to the principles of diet therapy, surgical care, heart disorders, diabetes, renal diseases, acquired immune deficiency syndrome (AIDS), food allergy, burns, cancer, anorexia nervosa, and various childhood disorders. Also new in this edition is the recommendation of several commercial software programs applicable to nutrition and diet therapy. Finally, a food composition table is included in Appendix F.

In any revision process, there is a tendency to add new materials in addition to updating old ones. Unfortunately, two insurmountable factors are always present. The period of time designed for a course on the subject remains the same for the students. No matter how much new material is included, instructors can cover only so much information within the time allotment. And, as the size of a book increases, the cost to the student increases.

Although the publisher has given me a free hand in revising the first edition in view of the large adoption by instructors, I have worked long hours to keep the book to a reasonable length while including as much new and relevant information as possible. I believe I have succeeded. Space limitation does not permit me to discuss all the changes in detail. However, certain items deserve a brief note.

The new dietary guidelines are emphasized throughout the book, using many public messages developed by federal health agencies. The objective: each American should learn to eat better to prevent *illness* and *disease*.

New topics such as AIDS, food allergy, burns, cancer, anorexia nervosa, and total parenteral nutrition are presented in brief discussions in the book. These discussions serve to introduce students to these important clinical disorders within the time slot designed for a one-quarter or one-semester course in many nursing programs.

The new chapter on drugs is a timely topic. Most hospitalized patients are taking drugs in some form. In the last decade, there has been an explosion of information on the relationship among drugs, nutrition, and diet. This new chapter provides a good summary of the basic and latest developments in the field.

Although I have written more than six books, this is the first one in which I endorse commercial products. The beginning of each of two parts of the book contains an announcement of the availability of computer software on nutrition and/or diet therapy. I have given much thought and time to selecting these pieces of software. They are appropriate for the competency of the students using this book.

In return for our endorsement, the companies distributing the software have agreed to allow a large discount on the retail price of their products. They have also permitted us to reproduce their 1991 data bank on food compositions. Appendix F contains the latest information up to the time of printing this book. This will give the students an unusual opportunity to use recent data instead of using standard food composition tables, which can pose two problems: they may be several years old, or the latest ones containing many volumes of food items may not be available at the library. The first edition of this book was not accompanied by a food composition table.

I am excited about this new edition and I hope my readers share my enthusiasm. Your feedback on the coverage and other aspects of this book has always been an important guide for me. It gives me direction in preparing future editions of this book and other related books.

P. S. S.

Acknowledgments

Many thanks are extended to those of you who used the first edition and provided insight and information that helped improve the second edition.

I would like especially to acknowledge those individuals who have contributed in so many ways to move this edition from manuscript to publication. From Jones and Bartlett: Mr. Joseph Burns, Vice President; Ms. Heather Stratton, Editorial Assistant; and Ms. Helyn Pultz, Production Coordinator. From WordCrafters Editorial Services: Ms. Linda Zuk, Production Editor; and Ms. Fran Anderson, Copy Editor. My appreciation to Book 1 Desktop Packagers for a quality production.

Special thanks to my friends and colleagues at C.S.I., in particular the mailroom and library staffs for their efficiency and assistance in all respects. To all of my friends too numerous to name individually who support and encourage my efforts: You are very highly valued.

I would also like to express my gratitude to my family for their enduring patience and support.

P. S. S.

NUTRITION
AND DIET THERAPY

Part I

NUTRITION BASICS AND APPLICATIONS

1

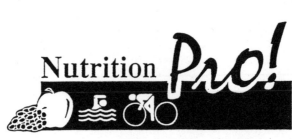

Nutrition and Exercise Software

SAVE !! 20%

Total the nutrients !
Analyze foods, menus & recipes.
Track fat, cholesterol, fiber,
calories, saturated fat...
18 nutrients in all !!

Compare to recommended nutrient amounts

Calculate exchanges. And, % calories from energy nutrients

```
---------------------ANALYSIS: Untitled----------------------
Weight: 1041 g  (36.7 oz.)
                 NUTRIENT VALUES (plus % GOAL for A Great Lady)
   NUTRIENT      AMT    GOAL% |---------25--------50--------75------100----->
  Calories       1461    75%
  Protein        44.7 g  98%
  Carbohydrates  199 g   70%
  Dietary Fiber  7.57 g  39%
  Fat-Total      60.6 g  93%
  Fat-Saturated  23.7 g  109%
  Fat-Mono       23.3 g  107%
  Fat-Poly       11 g    51%
  Cholesterol    75.6 mg 25%
  Vit A-Total    614 RE  77%
  Thiamin-B1     .822 mg 82%
  Riboflavin-B2  1.43 mg 119%
         EXCHANGES                         CALORIE BREAKDOWN
  Bread 5.55   Veg.          Prot. 12%
  Meat   2     Milk    2     Carb. 52%
  Fruit  5     Fat   9.65    Fat   36%
                             Alc.   0%
```

```
Name: A Great Lady          Age: 30       Female
Height: 5 ft. 6 in.         Wgt: 125 lb.  Lightly Active

EXERCISE LIST - DAY 1   Mins  Cals   DAILY ENERGY SUMMARY        Cals

Swimming - vigorous      30   175    BMR: Base energy needs      1368
Calisthenics             15    43    Lightly Active               588
Dancing - rock           60   259
                                     Recommended Daily calories  1957

                                     Exercise adjustment          477
                                     (average calories/day)

                                     Dieting adjustment             0
                                     (to LOSE 0.0 lb/week)

                                     Adjusted Daily Calories     2434

              Totals    1:45   477
```

Track calories used in exercise/activity. Lose or gain weight.

```
         Calories
         Protein
         Carbohydrates    Fresh Whole Mango
         Dietary Fiber    Boiled Sweet Potato
High     Fat-Total        Boiled Winter Squash-Avg
         Fat-Saturated    Canned Peas+Carrots w/Liq
         Fat-Mono         Ckd Winter Squash Cubes
         Fat-Poly         CndPeas+Carrots+Liq-LoSod
Low      Cholesterol      Cnd Tomato Paste w/Salt
High     Vit A-Total      Mixed Vegetables-frzn pkg
         Thiamin-B1       Turnip Greens Ckd f/Frzn
         Riboflavin-B2    Turnip Greens Ckd f/Raw
         Vitamin B6       Winter Squash Ckd f/Frzn
         Vitamin C        40% Bran Flakes Cereal
         Calcium          All-Bran Cereal
         Iron             Bran Buds Cereal
                          Cracklin'Oat Bran cereal
                          Fruit&FiberCereal ApplePS
```

Search for foods high or low in selected nutrients.

You get all this information and much more to keep you on the fitness fast-track!!
Includes 2000 food database & 110 exercises/activities. Add your favorites!!
Very Easy to Use -- gives new meaning to the words "user-friendly".
Keep Fit -- Order Yours Today!! For IBM/compatibles. Only $79.00. *your price $63*

(Ask about Macintosh availability)

☐ **YES! I want to keep fit !**

Please send me_____Nutrition Pro! programs. I've enclosed $79.00 each. *$63.00*
(Shipping/insurance: add $5.00)

My disk size:_____ (3.5 inch or 5.25 inch)

Name _____
Address_____
City/State/Zip_____
Signature: _____

SEND TO:

PAYMENT INFORMATION

☐ Check enclosed

☐ Visa or MasterCard
  #_____
  Expiration Date_____
  Phone_____

ESHA RESEARCH

PO Box 13028
Salem, OR 97309-1028 USA
Phone: (503) 585 - 6242   Fax: (503) 585 - 5543

Introduction to Nutrition

Time for completion
Activities: _____1½_____ hours
Optional examination: _½_ hour

Academic credit
Semester units: ³⁄₁₀
Quarter units: ⁴⁄₁₀

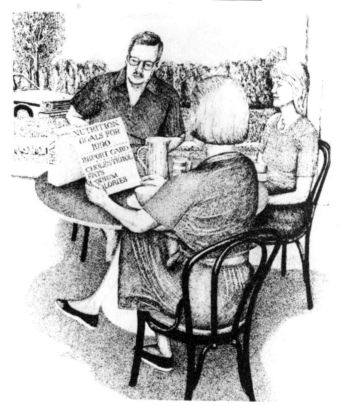

Outline

Objectives
Glossary
Background Information

ACTIVITY 1: Nutrition Definitions and Concepts
The Six Concepts
Responsibilities of Health Personnel
Progress Check on Activity 1

ACTIVITY 2: Food Selections
Recommended [Daily] Dietary Allowances (RDAs)
The Daily Food Guides
The Dietary Guidelines
The Exchange System

The Nutritional Labeling Laws
The National Cholesterol Education Program (NCEP)
Responsibilities of Health Personnel
Progress Check on Activity 2

ACTIVITY 3: Reliable Nutrition Sources and Services
Food Regulatory Agencies
Government and Private Resources
Food Laws
Summary
Responsibilities of Health Personnel
Progress Check on Activity 3
References

Objectives

Upon completion of this module the student should be able to:

1. Define major concepts and terms used in nutritional science.
2. Identify guidelines and rationale used for planning and evaluating food intake.
3. Describe some major concerns about diets of the American people.
4. Use appropriate sources and services to obtain reliable nutrition information.

Glossary

Adequate diet: one that provides all the essential nutrients and calories adequate to maintain good health and acceptable body weight.

Calorie (Cal): unit of energy; often used for the term *kilocalorie* (see also *kilocalorie*). Common usage indicating the release of energy from food.

Culture: the beliefs, arts, and customs that make up a way of life for a group of people.

Diet: (a) the foods that a person eats most frequently; (b) food considered in terms of its qualities and effects on health; (c) a particular selection of food, usually prescribed to cure a disease or to gain or lose weight.

Energy: capacity to do work; also refers to calories—that is, the "fuel" provided by certain nutrients (carbohydrates, fats, proteins).

Food: any substance taken into the body that will help to meet the body's needs for energy, maintenance, and growth.

Gram: a unit of weight in the metric system. 1 g = .036 oz. There are 28.385 grams to an ounce. This figure is usually rounded to 30 g for ease in calculation.

Health: the state of complete physical, mental, and social well-being; not merely the absence of disease and infirmity.

Kilocalorie: technically correct term for unit of energy in nutrition, equal to the amount of heat required to raise the temperature of one kilogram of water one degree centigrade.

Malnutrition: state of impaired health due to undernutrition, overnutrition, an imbalance of nutrients, or the body's inability to utilize the nutrients ingested.

Microgram: a unit of weight in the metric system equal to 1/1,000,000 of a gram.

Milligram: a unit of weight in the metric system equal to 1/1,000 of a gram.

Monitor: to watch over or observe something for a period of time.

Nutrient: a chemical substance obtained from food and needed by the body for growth, maintenance, or repair of tissues. Many nutrients are considered essential. The body cannot make them; they must be obtained from food.

Nutrition: the sum of the processes by which food is selected and becomes part of the body.

Nutritional status: state of the body resulting from the intake and use of nutrients.

Good nutritional status: the intake of a balanced diet containing all the essential nutrients to meet the body's requirements for energy, maintenance, and growth.

Poor nutritional status: an inadequate intake (or utilization) of nutrients to meet the body's requirements for energy, maintenance, and growth.

Optimum nutrition: the state of receiving and utilizing essential nutrients to maintain health and well-being at the highest possible level. It provides a reserve for the body.

Overnutrition: an excessive intake of one or more nutrients, frequently referring to nutrients providing energy (calories).

Recommended [Daily] Dietary Allowances (RDAs): levels of nutrients recommended by the Food and Nutrition Board of the National Academy of Sciences for daily consumption by healthy individuals, scaled according to sex and age.

Undernutrition: a deficiency of one or more nutrients, including nutrients providing energy (calories).

Background Information

The subject of nutrition is both exciting and confusing to the beginning student. Nutrition has become a major topic of conversation at places of work, at social gatherings, and in the media. We are living at a time when the focus of attention is on prevention of disease and responsibility for one's own health. The newest trends in health care stress the importance of nutrition education.

Throughout history, food and its effects on the body have been studied and written about, but most of the information gathered was based on trial and error findings. Many superstitions regarding the magical powers and healing capabilities of food also evolved.

The study of nutrition as a science is relatively new, developing in the last 70 years only after chemistry and physiology became established sciences. The study of nutrition is now a highly regarded discipline, and its technology and research advance yearly as human beings attempt to control their destiny by preventing or delaying the onset of a number of chronic diseases that are related to nutrition and lifestyle.

Every specialized field has a language of its own. A beginning student in nutrition needs to comprehend the language used in this discipline and to understand some basic concepts upon which the science is based. The activities in this module should assist you in gaining the knowledge and vocabulary necessary to understand the science of nutrition.

ACTIVITY 1: Nutrition Definitions and Concepts

The Six Concepts

The following list delineates major concepts and related generalizations for food and nutrition education. The U.S.D.A. (United States Department of Agriculture) formed the Interagency Committee on Nutrition Education in 1964. This committee developed the basic concepts that have become the framework for use in planning curriculi and nutrition education programs. This supports and substantiates the statements discussed in other modules in this book (Hui 1983, 408).

Concepts:

1. Nutrition defined
    Nutrition is the process by which food is selected and becomes part of the human body. This fundamental knowledge covers the basic facts upon which nutrition is founded.

2. Food and its handling
    a. Food contains nutrients that work together and interact with body chemicals to serve the needs of the body.
    b. No one food by itself contains all the nutrients in the appropriate amounts and combinations for optimal growth and health.
    c. Many different combinations of foods can provide the needed nutrients in appropriate amounts.
    d. Food contains important nonnutritive components, such as dietary fiber, which are also needed for healthy functioning of the body.
    e. Toxicants, additives, contaminants, and other nonnutritive factors in food affect its safety and quality.
    f. The way food is grown, processed, stored, and prepared for eating influences the amount of nutrients in the food, its safety, appearance, taste, cost, and waste.
    g. Food requires varying amounts of energy and other resources to produce, process, package, and deliver to the consumer.

3. Nutrients and dietary components
    a. Nutrients in the food we eat enable us to live, grow, keep healthy and well, and remain active.
    b. Each nutrient (carbohydrates, proteins, fats, vitamins, minerals, and water) has a specific function in the body.
    c. Nutrients must be obtained from outside the body on a regular basis because the body cannot produce them in sufficient amounts.
    d. Most healthy people can obtain all the nutrients in amounts needed from a variety of foods.
    e. Nutrients are distributed to and used by all parts of the body.
    f. Nutrient interactions may affect the amounts of nutrients needed and their functioning.
    g. The body stores some nutrients and withdraws them for use as needed.
    h. Nutrients are found in varying amounts, proportions, and combinations in the plant and animal sources that serve as food.
    i. Ongoing scientific research determines nutrients, their functions, and the amounts needed.
    j. Both dietary excesses and nutrient deficiencies affect health.
    k. Optimal intakes of nutrients and dietary components have both upper and lower limits.
    l. All persons throughout life have need of the same nutrients, but the amounts needed are influenced by age, sex, size, level of activity, specific activity, specific conditions of growth, state of health, pregnancy, lactation, and environmental stress.

4. Nutrition and physical activity
    a. Balancing energy intake and energy expenditure is important for achieving and maintaining desirable body weight.
    b. There is a relationship between nutrition and physical activity which affects health and well-being.

5. Food selection
    a. Food, or what people consider to be edible, is culturally defined.
    b. Physiological, cultural, social, economic, psychological, and geographic factors influence food selection.
    c. Knowledge, attitudes, and beliefs about food and nutrition affect food selection.
    d. Food availability and merchandising influence food choices.

6. National and international food policy
    a. Food plays an important role in the physical, psychological, and economic health of a society.
    b. Food production, distribution, and merchandising systems have economic, social, political, and ecological consequences.
    c. Effective utilization of individual and community resources is beneficial for the economic and nutritional well-being of the individual, family, and society.
    d. The availability of food and maintenance of nutritional well-being is a matter of public policy.
    e. Knowledge of food and nutrition combined with social consciousness enable citizens to understand and participate in the development and adoption of public policy affecting the nutritional well-being of societies.

Responsibilities of Health Personnel _____

1. Become familiar with terminology used in nutritional science.
2. Recognize that the basic concepts of nutrition, once they are learned, provide the needed background for nutritional education.
3. Practice and teach basic principles of nutrition.
4. Provide accurate nutrition education.

PROGRESS CHECK ON ACTIVITY 1

Questions

True/False

Circle T for True and F for False.

1. T (F) The science of nutrition was one of the first of the natural sciences to be developed.
2. (T) F The old superstitions about foods and their curative powers have been replaced by modern day science.
3. (T) F Most healthy people can obtain all the nutrients in amounts needed from a variety of foods.
4. T (F) Nutrients and food are different terms for the same thing.
5. (T) F No one food by itself contains all the nutrients in the appropriate amounts and combinations for optimal growth and health.

Multiple Choice

Circle the letter of the correct answer.

6. Food contains an essential nonnutritive substance known as
   (a.) fiber.
   b. additive.
   c. starch.
   d. energy.

7. All persons throughout life have need for the same nutrients
   a. in the same amounts.
   (b.) in varying amounts.
   c. in supplemental form.
   d. in specific combinations.

8. Malnutrition is a state of impaired health that may be due to all of these except
   a. excessive intake.
   b. inadequate intake.
   c. imbalance of nutrients.
   (d.) the body's inability to digest fiber.

Fill-in

9. Define: *nutrition* process of by which food becomes part of body

   culture Set of Beliefs, Arts + Custom that make up a way of life for a Group of people

   health A State of complete physical + mental well being.

ACTIVITY 2: Food Selections

Several food guides help us to determine nutrition needs and to plan and evaluate food intake. Nutrition scientists determine the essential components of an adequate diet and acceptable methods for selection. The appropriate diet in any stage of life is one that supplies sufficient energy and all the essential nutrients in adequate amounts for health. The Recommended [Daily] Dietary Allowances (RDAs), the United States Dietary Guidelines (based on U.S. Senate Dietary Goals), the daily food guides, and the Exchange System are the primary guidelines used to plan and evaluate food intake. An explanation of each of these follows.

Recommended [Daily] Dietary Allowances (RDAs) _____

According to the National Research Council of the National Academy of Sciences, "Recommended Dietary Allowances (RDAs) are the levels of intake of essential nutrients considered, in the judgment of the Committee on Dietary Allowances of the Food and Nutrition Board of the National Academy of Sciences, to be adequate to meet the known nutritional needs of practically all healthy persons." The 1989 RDAs are presented in Table 1-1.

Such recommendations are for the average daily amounts of nutrients that healthy population groups should consume over a period of time. They should not be confused with requirements for a specific individual, which vary considerably. Nutrition-related health problems such as premature birth, metabolic disorders, infections, chronic diseases, and the use of medications require special dietary and therapeutic measures.

Since nutritional requirements differ with age, sex, body size, and physiological state, the RDAs are presented for males and females in different age and weight groups. The allowances refer to the amount of nutrients that must

TABLE 1-1
Recommended Dietary Allowances.[a] Revised 1989

Category	Age (years) or Condition	Weight[b] (kg)	Weight[b] (lb)	Height[b] (cm)	Height[b] (in)	Protein (g)	Fat-Soluble Vitamins Vitamin A (µg RE)[c]	Vitamin D (µg)[d]	Vitamin E (mg α–TE)[e]	Vitamin K (µg)
Infants	0.0–0.5	6	13	60	24	13	375	7.5	3	5
	0.5–1.0	9	20	71	28	14	375	10	4	10
Children	1–3	13	29	90	35	16	400	10	6	15
	4–6	20	44	112	44	24	500	10	7	20
	7–10	28	62	132	52	28	700	10	7	30
Males	11–14	45	99	157	62	45	1,000	10	10	45
	15–18	66	145	176	69	59	1,000	10	10	65
	19–24	72	160	177	70	58	1,000	10	10	70
	25–50	79	174	176	70	63	1,000	5	10	80
	51+	77	170	173	68	63	1,000	5	10	80
Females	11–14	46	101	157	62	46	800	10	8	45
	15–18	55	120	163	64	44	800	10	8	55
	19–24	58	128	164	65	46	800	10	8	60
	25–50	63	138	163	64	50	800	5	8	65
	51+	65	143	160	63	50	800	5	8	65
Pregnant						60	800	10	10	65
Lactating	1st 6 Months					65	1,300	10	12	65
	2nd 6 Months					62	1,200	10	11	65

(continues)

Source: Adapted from National Research Council, National Academy of Sciences, 1989 *Recommended Dietary Allowances,* 10th Edition, Washington, DC, National Academy of Sciences.
[a]The allowances, expressed as average daily intakes over time, are intended to provide for individual variations among normal persons as they live in the United States under usual environmental stresses. Diets should be based on a variety of common foods in order to provide other nutrients for which human requirements have been less well defined.
[b]Weights and heights are actual medians for the U.S. population of the designated age. The use of these figures does not imply that the height-to-weight ratios are ideal.
[c]Retinol equivalents.
[d]As cholecalciferol.
[e]α-Tocopherol equivalents.
[f]Niacin equivalents.

be consumed daily in order to ensure that the nutritional requirements of most people are met. The amount by which the allowance is set above the average requirement, determined through scientific research, varies from nutrient to nutrient. For some nutrients, there is limited information about individual requirements.

The RDAs are the basis for virtually all feeding programs. They are used to interpret food consumption records, to evaluate the adequacy of food supplies in meeting nutritional needs, to plan and procure food supplies for groups, to establish guides for public food assistance programs, to evaluate new food products developed by industry, to establish guidelines for nutritional labeling of foods, and to develop nutrition education programs. Other nations have also developed recommended dietary standards and each is different from the others. In general, however, moderation has been the key word in developing daily allowances.

The technical information supplied by RDAs must be interpreted in terms of a selection of foods to be eaten daily if it is to be valuable from a practical standpoint. The RDAs should be met by consuming a wide variety of acceptable, tasty, and affordable foods, and not solely through supplementation or use of fortified foods. Various basic diet patterns may be devised to serve as guides in food selection. The daily food groups, the U.S. Dietary Guidelines, and the Exchange System function very well in this capacity.

The Daily Food Guides

The food group system was originally developed by the Institute of Home Economics and the agricultural research service of the U.S. Department of Agriculture (USDA). It was intended for use in conjunction with the RDAs

TABLE 1-1 (Continued)

	Water-Soluble Vitamins						Minerals						
Vitamin C (mg)	Thiamin (mg)	Riboflavin (mg)	Niacin (mg NE)[f]	Vitamin B$_6$ (mg)	Folate (µg)	Vitamin B$_{12}$ (µg)	Calcium (mg)	Phosphorus (mg)	Magnesium (mg)	Iron (mg)	Zinc (mg)	Iodine (µg)	Selenium (µg)
30	0.3	0.4	5	0.3	25	0.3	400	300	40	6	5	40	10
35	0.4	0.5	6	0.6	35	0.5	600	500	60	10	5	50	15
40	0.7	0.8	9	1.0	50	0.7	800	800	80	10	10	70	20
45	0.9	1.1	12	1.1	75	1.0	800	800	120	10	10	90	20
45	1.0	1.2	13	1.4	100	1.4	800	800	170	10	10	120	30
50	1.3	1.5	17	1.7	150	2.0	1200	1200	270	12	15	150	40
60	1.5	1.8	20	2.0	200	2.0	1200	1200	400	12	15	150	50
60	1.5	1.7	19	2.0	200	2.0	1200	1200	350	10	15	150	70
60	1.5	1.7	19	2.0	200	2.0	800	800	350	10	15	150	70
60	1.2	1.4	15	2.0	200	2.0	800	800	350	10	15	150	70
50	1.1	1.3	15	1.4	150	2.0	1200	1200	280	15	12	150	45
60	1.1	1.3	15	1.5	180	2.0	1200	1200	300	15	12	150	50
60	1.1	1.3	15	1.6	180	2.0	1200	1200	280	15	12	150	55
60	1.1	1.3	15	1.6	180	2.0	800	800	280	15	12	150	55
60	1.0	1.2	13	1.6	180	2.0	800	800	280	10	12	150	55
70	1.5	1.6	17	2.2	400	2.2	1200	1200	320	30	15	175	65
95	1.6	1.8	20	2.1	280	2.6	1200	1200	355	15	19	200	75
90	1.6	1.7	20	2.1	260	2.6	1200	1200	340	15	16	200	75

because it was easier to understand and would meet the needs of the population groups for which it was intended.

Currently, the USDA has divided foods into five groups as shown in Table 1-2. They are

1. Milk and milk products
2. Meat and meat alternates
3. Fruits and vegetables
4. Grains (bread and cereal)
5. Fats, sweets, and alcoholic beverages

Use of the food groups in their recommended serving sizes and number of servings per day as shown in Table 1-2 is intended to provide a good foundation for a daily meal plan. Again, the focus is on healthy individuals. It does not apply to infant feeding. The basic food guide is not a perfect tool; it omits some important information that people need in order to make informed choices. Women and children will need to include several iron-rich foods per week or take a supplement. Children and pregnant and lactating women may need a vitamin D supplement if they get little exposure to sunlight or do not increase their intake of fortified milk. Those people living in "goiter" regions—the inland areas (the Rocky Mountain States, Ohio, Wisconsin, and Michigan) where the soil and water contain little or no iodine—should be aware of the need for iodized salt. Children up to age 18 benefit from fluoride

in their drinking water, and foods containing fiber should be encouraged for all age groups. If one chooses a diet from the first four food groups, omits the fifth one, and uses the recommended size and number of servings, the diet furnishes 1,200 to 1,300 calories. This makes a very reliable, balanced reduction diet. However, calories should always be adjusted to individual needs, taking into account growth, age, size, and activities.

One of the most helpful tools for selecting a balanced diet is the USDA's "A Pattern for Daily Food Choices" (Table 1-3). It assists the consumer in following the dietary guidelines (see next section) without having to count anything other than the size of a serving. This is a complete diet plan; the Daily Food Guide (Table 1-2) is a foundation diet.

If the Daily Food Guide is combined with the pattern for daily food choices (Tables 1-2 and 1-3), eating habits will improve for the population. These are only guides to healthy eating and, like any plan designed for population groups, will need to be individualized. For example, the elderly and the very young both require alterations, as do pregnant women and lactating women and anyone with a specific disorder such as hypertension or elevated blood cholesterol.

For reference purposes, the Canadian Food Guide is shown in Figure 1-1.

TABLE 1-2
Recommended Numbers of Servings from the Daily Food Groups

Food Group	Serving Size	No. of Daily Servings
Milk and milk products Fluid milk	1 c., 8 oz., ½ pt., ¼ qt.	Children under 9: 2–3 Children ages 9–24: 3 Adults 25 and over: 2 Pregnant women: ≥ 3 Nursing mothers: ≥ 4 Pregnant teenagers: 4
Calcium equivalent	1 c. milk 2 c. cottage cheese 1 c. pudding 1 ¾ c. ice cream 1 ½ oz. cheddar cheese	
Meat and meat equivalents	2–3 oz. cooked lean meat without bone 3–4 oz. raw meat without bone 2 oz. luncheon meat (e.g., bologna) ¾ c. canned baked beans 1 c. cooked dry beans, peas, lentils 2 eggs 2 oz. cheddar cheese ½ c. cottage cheese 4 T. peanut butter	≥ 2
Fruits and vegetables	Varies by item: ½ c. cooked spinach 1 potato 1 orange ½ grapefruit	≥ 4, including 1 of citrus fruit and another fruit or vegetable that is a good source of vitamin C and 2 of a fair source 1, at least every other day, of a dark green or deep yellow vegetable for vitamin C ≥ 2 or more of other vegetables and fruits, including potatoes
Bread and cereals	1 slice of bread, 1 oz. ready-to-eat cereal ½ to ¾ c. cooked cereal, cornmeal, grits, macaroni, noodles, rice, or spaghetti	≥ 4
Fats, sweets, and alcohol		Foods from this group should not replace any from the four groups. Amounts consumed should be determined by individual energy needs.

The Dietary Guidelines

Before 1960, the primary goal of guidelines was to ensure growth and development and to improve resistance to disease through adequate nutrition. Currently, the emphasis is on improving or maintaining health as portrayed in two major documents:

1. U.S. Senate Committee on Nutrition and Human Needs: *Dietary Goals for the United States*, 2nd ed., 1977.
2. USDA and U.S. Department of Health and Human Services: *Dietary Guidelines*, 3rd ed., 1990.

A summary of such dietary guidelines is presented in Tables 1-4 and 1-5. Organizations such as the National Academy of Sciences, the American Heart Association, the American Cancer Society, the American Medical Association, and others have also issued their dietary recommendations for the American public. For details on their suggestions, consult the references at the end of this module.

Another guide, the Exchange System, is a more precise instrument in designing a proper diet.

TABLE 1-3
A Pattern for Daily Food Choices

When shopping, planning, and preparing meals for yourself and others, use this guide for a varied and nutritious diet . . .
- Choose foods daily from each of the first five major groups shown below.
- Include different foods from within the groups. As a guide, you can use the subgroups listed below the major food group heading.
- Have at least the smaller number of servings suggested from each group. Limit total amount of food eaten to maintain desirable body weight.
- Most people should choose foods that are low in fat and sugars more often. (See the bulletins on fat and sugar in this series.)
- Go easy on fats, sweets, and alcoholic beverages.

FOOD GROUP	SUGGESTED DAILY SERVINGS*
Breads, cereals, and other grain products ■ Whole-grain ■ Enriched	6 to 11 (Include several servings a day of whole-grain products.)
Fruits ■ Citrus, melon, berries ■ Other fruits	2 to 4
Vegetables ■ Dark-green leafy ■ Deep-yellow ■ Dry beans and peas (legumes) ■ Starchy ■ Other vegetables	3 to 5 servings (Include all types regularly; use dark-green leafy vegetables and dry beans and peas several times a week.)
Meat, poultry, fish, and alternatives (eggs, dry beans and peas, nuts and seeds) Milk, cheese and yogurt	2 to 3 servings—total 5 to 7 ounces lean 2 servings (3 servings for teens and women who are pregnant or breastfeeding; 4 servings for teens who are pregnant or breastfeeding)
Fats, sweets, and alcoholic beverages	Avoid too many fats and sweets. If you drink alcoholic beverages, do so in moderation.

WHAT COUNTS AS A SERVING?

The examples listed below will give you an idea of the amounts of food to count as one serving when you use the guide. . . .
- **Breads, cereals, and other grain products:** 1 slice of bread; ½ hamburger bun or english muffin; a small roll, biscuit, or muffin; 3 to 4 small or 2 large crackers; ½ cup cooked cereal, rice, or pasta; or 1 ounce of ready-to-eat breakfast cereal.
- **Fruits:** A piece of whole fruit such as an apple, banana, orange; a grapefruit half; a melon wedge; ¾ cup of juice; ½ cup berries, or ½ cup cooked or canned fruit; or ¼ cup dried fruit.
- **Vegetables:** ½ cup of cooked or chopped raw vegetables or 1 cup of leafy raw vegetables, such as lettuce or spinach.
- **Meat, poultry, fish, and alternates:** Serving sizes will differ. Amounts should total 5 to 7 ounces of lean meat, fish, or poultry a day. A serving of meat the size and thickness of the palm of a woman's hand is about 3 to 5 ounces and a man's, 5 to 7 ounces. Count 1 egg, ½ cup cooked dry beans, or 2 tablespoons of peanut butter as 1 ounce of lean meat.
- **Milk, cheese, and yogurt:** 1 cup of milk, 8 ounces of yogurt, 1½ ounces natural cheese, or 2 ounces of process cheese.

*WHAT ABOUT THE NUMBER OF SERVINGS?

The amount of food you need depends on your age, sex, physical condition, and how active you are. Almost everyone should have at least the minimum number of servings from each food group daily. Many women, older children, and most teenagers and men need more. The top of the range is about right for an active man or teenage boy. Young children may not need as much food. They can have smaller servings from all groups except milk, which should total 2 servings per day. You can use the guide . . . to help plan for the variety and amounts of foods your family needs each day.

Note: The pattern for daily food choices described here was developed for Americans who regularly eat foods from all the major food groups listed. Some people, such as vegetarians and others, may not eat one or more of these types of foods. These people may wish to contact a nutritionist in their community for help in planning food choices.
Source: USDA, Home and Garden Bulletin Number 232-1, 1986.

Canada's Food Guide

Variety

Choose different kinds of foods from within each group in appropriate numbers of servings and portion sizes.

Energy Balance

Needs vary with age, sex, and activity. Balance energy intake from foods with energy output from physical activity to control weight. Foods selected according to the Guide can supply 4000 - 6000 kJ (kilojules) (1000 - 1400 kilocalories). For additional energy, increase the number and size of servings from the various food groups and/or add other foods.

Moderation

Select and prepare foods with limited amounts of fat, sugar and salt. If alcohol is consumed, use moderate amounts.

milk and milk products

Children up to 11 years	2-3 servings
Adolescents	3-4 servings
Pregnant and nursing women	3-4 servings
Adults	2 servings

Skim, 2%, whole, buttermilk, reconstituted dry or evaporated milk may be used as a beverage or as the main ingredient in other foods. Cheese may also be chosen.

Some examples of one serving

- 250 mL (1 cup) milk
- 175 mL (3/4 cup) yoghurt
- 45 g (1 1/2 ounces) cheddar or process cheese

In addition, a supplement of vitamin D is not recommended when milk is consumed which does not contain added vitamin D.

meat, fish, poultry and alternatives

2 servings

Some examples of one serving

- 60 to 90 g (2-3 ounces) cooked lean meat, fish, poultry or liver
- 60 mL (4 tablespoons) peanut butter
- 250 mL (1 cup) cooked dried peas, beans or lentils
- 125 mL (1/2 cup) nuts or seeds
- 60 g (2 ounces) cheddar cheese
- 125 mL (1/2 cup) cottage cheese
- 2 eggs

breads and cereals

3-5 servings

Whole grain or enriched whole grain products are recommended

Some examples of one serving

- 1 slice bread
- 125 mL (1/2 cup) cooked cereal
- 175 mL (3/4 cup) ready-to-eat cereal
- 1 roll or muffin
- 125 to 175 mL (1/2 to 3/4 cup) cooked rice, macaroni, spaghetti or noodles
- 1/2 hamburger or weiner bun

fruits and vegetables

4-5 servings

Include at least two vegetables

Choose a variety of both vegetables and fruits – cooked, raw or their juices. Include yellow, green or green leafy vegetables.

Some examples of one serving

- 125 mL (1/2 cup) vegetables or fruits – fresh, frozen or canned
- 125 mL (1/2 cup) juice – fresh, frozen or canned
- 1 medium-sized potato, carrot, tomato, peach, apple, orange or banana

Figure 1-1
The Canadian Food Guide
Source: Canadian Ministry of Supply and Services. Used with permission.

The Exchange System

The value of the Exchange System lies in its versatility. It encourages thinking of nutrients in terms of food rather than grams of nutrients. It allows for flexibility and variety in the diet and facilitates good meal planning. Choices from each group balance the meal. Health practitioners utilize the Exchange System because it is an easy tool to use and teaches food selection in a practical way. It also meets the guidelines for limiting saturated fat and cholesterol intake. The most common food exchange system is the one published by the American Diabetes Association and the American Dietetic Association. Their system contains six exchange groups: milk, meat, vegetables, fruits, breads, and fats. This exchange system is based on the five food groups, with these major differences:

1. The vegetables and fruits are listed separately rather than as one group as in the five food groups.
2. The bread exchange list includes those starchy vegetables with carbohydrate content approximating that of breads and cereals.
3. Cheeses are included in the meat list instead of in the milk group as in the five food groups.

Additional details are provided in Module 16 and the appendix reproduces the exchange system published by the two organizations.

TABLE 1-4
U.S. Dietary Goals, 2nd Edition, 1977

1. To avoid overweight, consume only as much energy (calories) as is expended; if overweight, decrease energy intake and increase energy expenditure.
2. Increase the consumption of complex carbohydrates and "naturally occurring" sugars from about 28% of energy intake to about 48% of energy intake.
3. Reduce the consumption of refined and processed sugars by about 45% to account for about 10% of total energy intake.
4. Reduce overall fat consumption from approximately 40% to about 30% of energy intake.
5. Reduce saturated fat consumption to account for about 10% of total energy intake; and balance that with polyunsaturated and monounsaturated fats, which should account for about 10% of energy intake.
6. Reduce cholesterol consumption to about 300 mg a day.
7. Limit the intake of sodium by reducing the intake of salt to about 5 g a day.

The Goals Suggest the Following Changes in Food Selection and Preparation:
1. Increase consumption of fruits and vegetables and whole grains.
2. Decrease consumption of refined and other processed sugars and foods high in such sugars.
3. Decrease consumption of foods high in total fat, and partially replace saturated fats, whether obtained from animal or vegetable sources, with polyunsaturated fats.
4. Decrease consumption of animal fat, and choose meats, poultry and fish which will reduce saturated fat intake.
5. Except for young children, substitute low-fat and non-fat milk for whole milk, and low-fat dairy products for high-fat dairy products.
6. Decrease consumption of butterfat, eggs and other high cholesterol sources. Some consideration should be given to easing the cholesterol goal for premenopausal women, young children and the elderly in order to obtain the nutritional benefits of eggs in the diet.
7. Decrease consumption of salt and foods high in salt content.

U.S. Senate Select Committee on Nutrition and Human Needs. *Dietary Goals for the United States*, ed 2, 1977.

TABLE 1-5
1990 Dietary Guidelines for Americans

1. Eat a variety of foods.
2. Maintain healthy weight.
3. Choose diet low in fat, saturated fat, and cholesterol.
4. Eat plenty of vegetables, fruits, and grain products.
5. Use sugar in moderation.
6. Use salt and sodium in moderation.
7. If you drink alcoholic beverages, do so in moderation.

USDA. *Nutrition and Your Health: Dietary Guidelines for Americans*, 1990, 3rd ed.

Nutritional Labeling

Two recent (1990–1991) enactments have occurred that will prove very valuable to health professionals and consumers. The first is nutritional labeling; the other is the National Cholesterol Education Program (NCEP).

The Nutrition and Labeling Act of 1990 is the first labeling legislation enacted since the 1970s. Prior to 1990, nutritional labeling was optional except in cases where the manufacturer either added a nutrient to its product or made nutritional claims on the label or in advertising. Labeling is now mandatory.

The new act calls for sweeping changes in labels on food products and health claims on food labels. Manufacturers have until 1993 to phase in the required changes. However, certain specifics will be required regardless of any final changes in legislation. It is hoped that with the new labeling, Americans will be able to reduce their risk of disease by making choices that conform to the dietary guidelines. Many authorities have worked with the committee on food labeling to draft recommendations that will help consumers follow healthy diets. Briefly, the major changes required are these:

1. Food manufacturers must use readable, uniform labeling in a simple format. They must use standard serving sizes and household measurements. The use of standard sizes will prevent some manufacturers from manipulating servings to make their products look more healthful to consumers.

2. Important information that will appear on the new labels includes calories per serving (in household measures); calories from fat, protein, and carbohydrate; total fat, saturated fat, and cholesterol; sodium, sugar, fiber; and the sources of all carbohydrates and proteins.

3. Food categories requiring nutritional labeling will be extended to most foods regulated by the Food and Drug Administration (FDA), including packaged foods, fresh foods, and seafoods. Labeling will be mandatory on all dairy products regardless of whether

they are fortified, or whether any health claims are made for them. The Institute of Medicine (IOM) goes even further, recommending that all fresh foods (poultry, meat, produce, seafood) be required to have nutritional labeling at the point of purchase; this applies to the 20 most commonly consumed items in each of the categories for produce and seafood.

4. Exemptions have been made for meat and poultry since they are under USDA jurisdiction. Small retail outlets will also be exempt, as will restaurants and group food services.

5. The law severely restricts health claims on product labels. Only when strong scientific evidence exists may the manufacturers suggest relationships between ingredients in their products and prevention of specific diseases. The act spells the end of ambiguous descriptive terms. So far a total of ten terms have been identified. These ten topics will have precise and consistent definitions. They include the terms "free," "low," "lite" or "light," "lean," "less," "reduced," "no" or "non-" calories (low or high), "low cholesterol" and "cholesterol-free." References so far are limited to fiber, fat, calcium, and sodium.

6. Reference Daily Intakes (RDIs) will replace the present USRDAs as standards for individual nutrients. Values will apply to persons ages four and older and to specific populations. FDA also proposes Daily Reference Values (DRVs) for the macronutrients—saturated and unsaturated fats, cholesterol, fiber, carbohydrates (both simple and complex), sodium, and potassium.

All health professionals need to keep abreast of the new legislation for any changes or updates. The effects will impact not only individual consumers, but all institutions as well. Adherence to the requirements will greatly affect the industries that provide food products, especially manufacturing and marketing.

National Cholesterol Education Program (NCEP) _____

Program Description.   The NCEP is one of three principal programs administered by the Office of Prevention, Education, and Control of the National Heart, Lung, and Blood Institute (NHLBI) of the National Institutes of Health (NIH). The program came about after years of trials and scientific evidence that linked blood cholesterol levels to coronary heart disease. These trials showed that levels could be lowered safely by both diet and drugs. Hence, the National Cholesterol Education Program, today known as the NCEP, came into being.

Guidelines have been established for health professionals, patients, public, and the community. Among these important guidelines are two of particular interest to students of nutrition:

1. To increase the knowledge of health professionals regarding the major role that diet plays in reducing blood cholesterol.
2. To improve the knowledge, skills, and attitudes of students in the health professions regarding high blood cholesterol and its management.

Implementing dietary guidance through the use of nutrition labeling and standards of identity is one example of steps being taken to help Americans implement the guidelines. The major objective for this sweeping revision is to increase the availability of health-promoting foods.

Responsibilities of Health Personnel _____

1. Assume responsibility for own health through changes in eating habits and lifestyle patterns.
2. Select, prepare, and consume an adequate diet.
3. Promote good eating habits for all age groups.
4. Use appropriate guidelines when teaching clients regarding food selection.
5. Facilitate healthy lifestyles by encouraging clients to expand their knowledge of nutrition.
6. Use approved food guides when assessing and evaluating a client's intake.

PROGRESS CHECK ON ACTIVITY 2

Questions

Self Studies

1. On the RDA scale (see Table 1-1), underline in red the figures that are requirements for each of the following nutrients for a person of your age and sex. Record them below.

   My RDA:

   Kilocalories _____

   Protein _____ 50 _____ g

   Vitamin A _____ 800 _____ μg

   Vitamin C _____ 60 _____ mg

   Vitamin D _____ 5 _____ μg

   Vitamin E _____ 8 _____ mg

   Vitamin K _____ 65 _____ μg

   Folacin _____ 180 _____ g

   Niacin _____ 13 _____ mg

   Riboflavin _____ 1.2 _____ mg

Thiamin ___1.0___ mg

Vitamin B$_6$ ___1.6___ mg

Vitamin B$_{12}$ ___2.0___ mg

Calcium ___800___ mg

Phosphorus ___800___ mg

Iodine ___150___ µg

Iron ___10___ mg

Magnesium ___280___ mg

Selenium ___55___ µg

Zinc ___12___ mg

2. Using the food composition tables in Appendix A, look up the kilocalorie, protein, calcium, iron, vitamin A, thiamin, riboflavin, niacin and vitamin C content of the foods you ate on the most typical of the three days you recorded. Compare total values to your RDAs. Are you low in any nutrients? Which requirements are you meeting? (Note: More information on these nutrients is presented in other modules.)

3. Evaluate your diet record for fat, salt, sugar, and fiber. Look back at your diet and see if you should make any substitutions to more closely follow the Dietary Guidelines. Make a list of changes that could be made.

Multiple Choice

Circle the letter of the correct answer.

4. All of the following describe the Dietary Guidelines for Americans except the claim that they
   a. are published by USDA and DHHS.
   b. establish sodium intake.
   c. suggest moderating fat and salt intake.
   d. are intended to reduce incidence of disease.

5. The dietary guide designed specifically for nutritional labeling is the
   a. daily food guide.
   b. Exchange System.
   c. RDIs.
   d. RDA.

True/False

Circle T for True and F for False.

6. T F The Exchange System is used mainly for ill people.

7. T F If individuals wish to find out what *foods* they should eat to be healthy, they should look at the RDA table.

8. T F Individuals have the responsibility to change their own eating patterns.

ACTIVITY 3: Reliable Nutrition Sources and Services

Many of the health concerns of Americans involve questions relating to nutrition, and so a primary responsibility of the health professional is to provide answers about nutrition and diet. The questions most asked by the consumer are:

Is the food safe to eat?

Can disease be prevented by changing the type of food eaten?

Can optimal body weight be maintained throughout life? What is one's optimal body weight?

Are nutrients left in a food after commercial processing?

Will substances added to the food during processing cause cancer?

Is regular exercise healthful for everyone?

How does one know what information about nutrition to believe, since there is so much of it?

Some of these questions can be answered by reviewing the work of government agencies assigned to improve and protect our health.

Food Regulatory Agencies _____

The three federal regulatory agencies responsible for most of the food and nutrition policies in the United States are the FDA (Food and Drug Administration), the Federal Trade Commission (FTC), and the USDA (United States Department of Agriculture). The U.S. Treasury Department sets the standards for alcoholic beverages.

The FTC helps protect the public by requiring fair advertising of food products. Although regulation exists for advertisements and promotional material of products, the First Amendment guarantees freedom of speech in regard to books, pamphlets, or speeches. Writers can make any claim they wish. Aggressive education of the public is one way to combat the public's acceptance of all advertising claims by providing information that helps in the evaluation of available information, especially printed materials.

Food safety is the responsibility of both the USDA and the FDA. The USDA regulates meat and poultry by inspecting the entire process from the selection of live animals to their slaughter and final processing. It also sets grading standards for quality of the products.

The FDA administers the Federal Food, Drug, and Cosmetic Act and all its amendments. A large portion of the food supply is regulated by this agency. It inspects plants, investigates consumer complaints, enforces the addition of food additives and coloring, and monitors pesticide residues.

Health programs and disease control have always been the responsibility of health departments—national, state, and local. However, we are witnessing advances in food technology and nutritional sciences and an emphasis on self-health care, especially nutritional needs. As a result, nutrition education has become an added responsibility of health departments and other agencies involved in providing health-related services.

Health authorities agree that extensive and more effective distribution of scientific information about nutrition is necessary to combat misinformation about food and nutrition. For the public to become better informed about nutrition, the basic concepts should be taught from kindergarten through grade 12. The implementation of such programs in many public schools today is evidence of the efforts of health professionals to educate the public at an early age about nutrition and diet.

Government and Private Resources

Many state and federal agencies exist to provide nutrition services and regulate and control the flow of food products.

Table 1-6 lists responsibilities of federal agencies concerned with nutrition. Table 1-7 lists state, local, and private agencies that provide nutrition services. These agencies develop and disseminate current and accurate information regarding our food supply. Some informational materials can be obtained at no cost, while others are priced nominally. Most health care facilities, extension services, schools, and clinics can obtain bulk supplies of the materials at reduced prices.

Food Laws

The U.S. government is extensively involved in food and nutrition policy. Much legislation promulgated by the executive and judicial branches of government is aimed at protecting the consumer. The public has been exposed to many food and nutrition issues over the years. New problems are identified as new products are added to the market. Table 1-8 lists many of the federal laws affecting food and nutrition policies.

Summary

The concerns of the public and the responsibilities of health professionals can be managed by the extensive nutrition-related research available today. Many of the

TABLE 1-6
Food- and Nutrition-Related Responsibilities of Federal Agencies

Consumer Product Safety Commission (CPSC)—safety of food handling equipment.

Department of Agriculture (USDA)
  Economics Research Service (ERS)—analyses and reporting of food situation and outlook.
  Food and Nutrition Service (FNS)—administration of food stamp, school lunch, women, infants and children, and donated food programs.
  Food Quality and Inspection Service (FQIS)—inspection and labeling of meat, poultry, and eggs; grading of all foods; nitrite in cured meats and poultry.
  Human Nutrition Information Service (HNIS)—standard food consumption tables for nutritive value of food and educational materials.
  Science and Education Administration (SEA)—extension services, agricultural research service, cooperative state research service, National Agricultural Library.

Department of Health and Human Services (DHHS)
  Centers for Disease Control (CDC)—analyses and reporting of incidence of foodborne diseases.
  Food and Drug Administration (FDA)—food labeling, safety of food and food additives, inspection of food processing plants, control of food contaminants, food standards.
  National Institutes of Health (NIH)—research related to diet and health.

Environmental Protection Agency (EPA)—standards for drinking water and water pollution, use of pesticides on food crops.

Federal Trade Commission (FTC)—food advertising, competition in food industry.

National Marine Fisheries Service (NMFS)—inspection, standards, and quality of seafood.

Occupational Safety and Health Administration (OSHA)—employee safety in food processing plants.

concerns have been addressed by legislation, and research is allowing us to make significant progress in answering others. At the same time these advances are being made, however, there is a proliferation of fraudulent, inaccurate, and therefore potentially harmful literature on the market. Such material cannot be regulated because it is protected by the First Amendment. Health practitioners must continue to teach the basic principles, help people to choose food wisely, and refer them to the appropriate services and information, to allow consumers to become more aware of sound nutrition concepts and practices.

TABLE 1-7
State and Local Agencies and Nongovernmental Organizations that Provide Nutrition Services

Governmental

State and Local Levels

    Department of Agriculture
    State extension services
    State experiment stations
    State universities—departments of food and nutrition
    Departments of Welfare
    Departments of Health
    Department of Education

Nongovernmental

National Level

    American Medical Association Council on Foods
    National Academy of Sciences, Food and Nutrition Board
    American Red Cross
    Professional Organizations
        American Medical Association
        American Dietetic Association
        American Home Economics Association
        American Dental Association
        American Public Health Association
        American Heart Association
        American Nurses' Association
        American Institute of Nutrition
    Funds and Foundations
        Milbank Memorial Fund
        Nutrition Foundation
        Ford and Rockefeller Foundations
    Metropolitan Life Insurance Company
    Society of Nutrition Education
    Industry-sponsored
        American Dry Milk Institute
        National Dairy Council
        Cereal Institute
        National Livestock and Meat Board

State and Local Levels

    Educational agencies
    Social agencies
    Civic groups
    United Community Services
    Industry sponsored
    American Red Cross
    Infant welfare organizations
    Church groups

Responsibilities of Health Personnel

1. Evaluate literature, products, and advertising that pertain to nutrition.
2. Locate reliable resources and services.
3. Be aware of regulatory agencies that protect the consumer and use them when necessary.

TABLE 1-8
Examples of Major Federal Laws Affecting U.S. Food and Nutrition Policy

Federal Food, Drug and Cosmetic Act (1938) authorizes the Food and Drug Administration to oversee processing and labeling of foods in terms of safety, quality, and standards.

Agriculture Marketing Act (1946) authorizes the Department of Agriculture to inspect, grade, and certify all agricultural products.

Delaney Amendment (1958) prohibits addition to food of any substance shown to cause cancer in humans or animals.

Fair Packaging and Labeling Act (1965) authorizes Food and Drug Administration to regulate certain aspects of food labeling.

Egg Products Inspection Act (1970) requires inspection of egg products and surveillance of egg shells.

Federal Meat Inspection Act (1970) requires inspection of all meats and meat products for wholesomeness.

Poultry Products Inspection Act (1971) requires inspection of all poultry and poultry products for wholesomeness.

Food and Agricultural Act (1977) sets policies related to price and income supports for farmers, grain reserves, food assistance programs, research, and extension.

Saccharin Study and Labeling Act (1977) prohibited the Food and Drug Administration's proposed ban on saccharin and required the National Academy of Sciences to study food safety issues.

Infant Formula Act (1980) requires the Food and Drug Administration to regulate the manufacture of infant formulas.

Nutrition and Labeling Act (1990) requires the FDA to issue new food labeling.

4. Direct others to appropriate resources and services when needed.

PROGRESS CHECK ON ACTIVITY 3

Questions

True/False

Circle T for True and F for False.

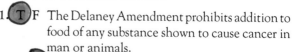

1. **T** F The Delaney Amendment prohibits addition to food of any substance shown to cause cancer in man or animals.
2. T **F** Health food stores are reliable sources of free and inexpensive literature about nutrition.
3. **T** F The *Journal of the American Dietetic Association*, the official publication of the American Dietetic Association, contains articles of interest to dietitians and nutritionists, news of legislative action on food and nutrition, and a useful

section summarizing articles from other journals of nutrition and related areas. Other professional journals widely subscribed to by nutritionists include the *Journal of Nutrition Education*, *Nutrition Reviews*, *The American Journal of Clinical Nutrition*, and *The CNI Report*.

Fill-in

4. Name five state or federal agencies that provide reliable nutrition information.

a. _F D A Food+Dug Admin._

b. _USDA US Department of Agricul._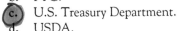

c. _FTC Federal trade Commission_

d. _FQIS Food Quality Inspection Service_

e. _DHHS Dep of Health Human Services_

Multiple Choice

Circle the letter of the correct answer.

5. Responsibilities of the Food and Drug Administration (FDA) include (circle the letter of as many as apply)
    a. food labeling.
    b. safety of food and food additives.
    c. inspection of food processing plants.
    d. control of food contaminants.
    e. food standards.

6. The agency which sets standards for alcoholic beverages is the
    a. FDA.
    b. FTC.
    c. U.S. Treasury Department.
    d. USDA.

7. Which agency is in charge of monitoring fair food advertising?
    a. FDA
    b. FTC
    c. U.S. Treasury Department
    d. USDA

References

American Institute for Cancer Research. 1991, Summer. New food labeling. *Newsletter*: No. 32.

An interpretive review of recent nutrition research. 1991, Sept./Oct. *Dairy Council Digest* 62(5). Rosemont, IL: National Dairy Council.

Anderson, J. V., and M. R. Van Nierop (eds.). 1989. *Basic nutrition facts: A nutrition reference*. East Lansing, MI: Michigan State University and the Michigan Department of Public Health.

Bakery, I. (ed.). 1982. *The psychobiology of human food selection*. New York: Van Nostrand Reinhold.

Banister, E. W. et al. 1988. *Contemporary health issues*. Boston: Jones and Bartlett.

Beaton, G. H. 1988. Criteria of an adequate diet. In M. E. Shils and V. R. Young (eds.). *Modern nutrition in health and disease* (7th ed.). Philadelphia: Lea & Febiger.

Berg, A. 1987. *Malnutrition: What can be done?* Baltimore: Johns Hopkins University Press.

Brown, J. L. 1987. Hunger in the U.S. *Scientific American* 256(2):37.

Connor, S. I., and W. E. Connor. 1986. *The new American diet*. New York: Simon and Schuster.

Draper, H. H. (ed.). 1985. *Advances in nutritional research*. New York: Plenum Press.

Ferguson, T. 1983. Type A behavior and the Type B solution. *Med. Self-Care* 12:36.

Food and Nutrition Board, National Research Council, National Academy of Sciences. 1989. *Recommended dietary allowances*. (10th ed.). Washington, DC: National Academy Press.

Food and Nutrition Board. 1989. *Diet and health*. Washington, DC: National Academy of Sciences.

Food and Nutrition Board. 1986. *What is America eating?* Washington, DC: National Academy Press.

Gussow, J. D., and P. R. Thomas. 1986. *The nutrition debate: Sorting out some answers*. Palo Alto, CA: Bull Publishing.

Halsted, C. H., and R. B. Rucker. 1989. *Nutrition and the origin of disease*. San Diego, CA: Academic Press.

Harper, A. E. 1988. Nutrition: From myth and magic to science. *Nutrition Today* 23(1): 8.

Haymes, E., and C. Wells. 1986. *Environment and human performance*. Champaign, IL: Human Kinetics.

Healthy people 2000. 1990, Nov./Dec. *Nutrition Today*, pp. 29–39.

Heiby, W. A. 1988. *The reverse effect: How vitamins and minerals promote health and CAUSE disease*. Deerfield, IL: Medi Science Publishers.

Katch, F. I., and W. D. McArdle. 1988. *Nutrition, weight control, and exercise* (3rd ed.). Philadelphia: Lea & Febiger.

Kittler, P. G., and K. Sucher. 1989. *Food and culture in America*. New York: Van Nostrand Reinhold.

Krebs-Smith, S. M. et al. 1987. The effects of variety in food choices on dietary quality. *Journal of the American Dietetic Association* 87:897.

Liebman, B. 1983. Too much of a good thing is toxic. *Nutrition Action* 10(4):6.

Logue, A. W. 1986. *The psychology of eating and drinking*. New York: W. H. Freeman.

Mayo Clinic. 1988. *Mayo Clinic diet manual*. Philadelphia: B. C. Dekker.

Miller, S. A., and M. G. Stephenson. 1987. The 1990 national nutrition objectives: Lessons for the future.

Journal of the American Dietetic Association 87:1665.

National cholesterol education program. 1991, May/June. *Nutrition Today*, pp. 36–41.

National Institute of Health. 1989. *Eating to lower your high blood cholesterol.* USDHS/PHS NIH Publication No. 89-2920. Baltimore: National Institute of Health.

National Research Council. 1986. *Nutrient adequacy.* Washington, DC: National Academy Press.

Nieman, D. C. et al. 1990. *Nutrition.* Dubuque, IA: William C. Brown.

Nutritional labeling: Comparison of proposals for regulatory reform. 1991, Jan. *Food Technology*, pp. 68–75. Chicago: Institute of Food Technologists.

Sanjur, D. 1982. *Social and cultural perspectives in nutrition.* Englewood Cliffs, NJ: Prentice-Hall, 1982.

Shils, M. E., and V. R. Young (eds.). 1988. *Modern nutrition in health and disease* (7th ed.). Philadelphia: Lea & Febiger.

USDA. 1986. *Dietary guidelines for Americans: Avoid too much fat, saturated fat and cholesterol.* Home and Garden Bulletin, No. 232-3. Washington, DC: United States Department of Agriculture, Human Nutrition Information Service.

USDA. 1986. *Eat a variety of foods.* Home and Garden Bulletin No. 232-1. Washington, DC: United States Department of Agriculture, Human Nutrition Information Service.

USDA. 1989. *Preparing foods and planning menus.* Home and Garden Bulletin No. 232-8. Washington, DC: United States Department of Agriculture.

USDA. 1985. *Thirty meals for two.* Home and Garden Bulletin No. 244. Washington, DC: United States Department of Agriculture.

Wardlaw, G. M., and P. M. Insel. 1990. *Perspectives in nutrition.* St. Louis: Mosby.

Williams, M. 1988. *Nutrition for fitness and sport* (2nd ed.). Dubuque, IA: William C. Brown.

Food Habits

Time for completion
Activities: _____1_____ hour
Optional examination: _½_ hour

Academic credit
Semester units: _²⁄₁₀_
Quarter units: _³⁄₁₀_

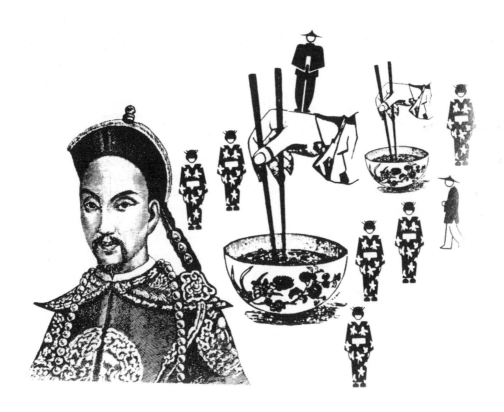

Outline

Objectives

Upon the completion of this module, the student should be able to:

1. Describe the cultural, social, and psychological factors that influence food behavior.
   a. Distinguish between biological necessity and cultural patterning.
   b. Identify the use of food in a culture.
   c. Explain the symbolism of food in a culture.
   d. Identify the social influences of food in a culture.
   e. Evaluate the psychological influence of food.
2. Determine the economic considerations that affect food intake.
3. Identify some common problems in the nutritional status of individuals in the United States.
4. Explain the ways that illness affects food acceptance.
5. Identify the dietary patterns of some ethnic, cultural, and religious groups in the United States.

Glossary

Culture (or acculturation):   traditions, values, or religions that comprise a way of life.
Foodways: way in which a distinct group selects, prepares, consumes, and uses food.
Food behaviors: result of the social, physiological, psychological, environmental, and sociocultural impact on a person's food preferences.
Heritage: that which is transmitted from preceding generations.

Physiological: physical development, state of health, mental attitudes.
Psychological: body image, perception of self, ways of coping.
Society (sociological):   interactions between people, governments, and so forth.
Suboptimal: below desirable, as in below desirable intake.

Background Information

Biologic necessity refers to the nutrient balance that the body requires in order to maintain life and health. Cultural patterning, on the other hand, establishes values, feelings, attitudes, and beliefs regarding food consumption. The required nutrient levels may or may not be met under influences of cultural patterning.

In recent years, because of improved research and interpretation of data regarding the nutritional status of individuals, scientists are sure that primary malnutrition exists in the United States. It is recognized that overnutrition, misinformation, ignorance, poor economic status, and poor eating habits are prevalent in this country. Malnutrition is difficult to manage in the United States because of the diverse cultures, subcultures, values, and experiences present in the country. Common nutritional problems are: obesity; iron-deficiency anemia, especially among low-income women of childbearing age and among infants; and suboptimal intakes of calcium, ascorbic acid, and vitamin A. Also, special nutritional problems affect the poor, the elderly, and the adolescent.

ACTIVITY 1: Factors Affecting Food Consumption

Eating behaviors develop from cultural, societal, and psychological patterns. These patterns, reflecting food habits that have been transmitted from preceding generations, are the heritage of any given ethnic group. They may be influenced by interactions with other groups, so that some intermingling of patterns is inevitable, but modifications are worked into the total structure over long periods of time and are acceptable only if they fit the existing customs.

According to one nutritionist, Corinne Robinson, food patterns reflect a people's social organization, including their economy, religion, beliefs about the health properties of foods, and attitudes about family. Great emotional significance is attached to the consumption of certain foods.

Food and Symbols

Eating behaviors are derived from many sources. In order to become part of a group's eating pattern, a food must be available and acceptable within the cultural context. The ways in which a food is determined to be acceptable vary greatly among societies and among individuals, and both conscious and unconscious criteria are applied. One such criterion is food symbolism, which is the meaning attached to food. Those foods symbolically designated as positive are acceptable, whereas a negative evaluation causes rejection.

Most food symbolism is related to security. This security can be emotional, biological, or sociological, or any combination of the three. For instance, foods believed to have safety and health benefits offer biological security. An example is food faddism—the belief that eating certain foods will bring special health benefits.

Great numbers of food taboos and superstitions are associated with biological symbolism. Food taboos are based on beliefs that certain foods or food combinations are bad or unsafe. Superstitions arise from beliefs about magical powers of foods. For example, certain herbs are believed to ward off old age. It does not matter that there may be little or no scientific basis for these beliefs; it is what the individual thinks that influences his or her choice.

Nowhere is food symbolism more pronounced than in the context of emotional security. A deep emotional attachment to food begins from the moment an infant receives his or her first food from a significant other. Eating is associated with love, caring, attention, and satisfaction. One of the causes of obesity may be a response to this emotional association. Food may also be used for discipline, punishment, reward for moral virtue, and bribery; hence, the response elicited by such uses of certain foods may be frustration, anger, and rejection.

Food is often used as a weapon or a crutch. A child learns the hidden meanings of food very quickly and will use this tool for power and manipulation—for example, refusing to eat, throwing a tantrum, or developing sudden whims. For teenagers, strenuous dieting, refusal to eat healthy foods, and voracious overeating are weapons that gain them attention, enable them to manipulate or avoid situations, and often give them a feeling of control over their bodies. Used this way, food becomes an emotional outlet for boredom, frustration, anxiety, and other stresses. Using food as a crutch is also a contributing factor in obesity.

Food and religion are linked symbolically with emotional security. In all religions, certain foods are used in ceremonial rites as a means of demonstrating faith and commemorating events. Prohibition of certain foods is also common practice. Examples of religious food symbolism include Holy Communion in Christian churches, the Jewish dietary laws, and the exclusion of animal flesh by Hindus and Buddhists. Fasting is common to most religions. Often the reasons for food prohibitions are obscure.

Sociological symbolism can include the use of food as status symbols—that is, certain foods are considered desirable because of high cost, difficulty in obtaining or preparing them, and superior quality. Examples include foods such as prime rib, imported wines, truffles, caviar, fancy and complicated desserts, and other such food choices.

Also of sociological significance is the use of foods as a means of communication. Eating together denotes acceptance. Almost all social occasions involve some sort of food or drink. Examples include refreshments at meetings, weddings, and feasts. Dinner parties and dinner dates are socially significant events. Foods communicate roles in life often as clearly as actions do.

Of the various kinds of security-related food symbolism, sociological symbolism is the one most likely to change. Social meanings attached to food are not as deeply imbedded in the psyche as are emotional and biological meanings. Social symbols change as situations and experiences change.

Illness modifies food acceptance. Anxiety, loneliness, lack of activity, and the disease process all contribute to an alteration of usual eating patterns. Appetite may diminish, and hostility and apathy about food may occur. Children may regress to an earlier developmental stage, and adults may regress to less mature states.

Some examples should help the student to understand the forces at work in the development of eating behaviors.

Examples of Food Behaviors

Example A

Mary W., age 65, states that she takes 2 tablespoons of lecithin, 1,200 mg of organic vitamin E, plus a cup of rose hips tea each day to "keep her arteries cleared out" and "prevent arthritis."

1. What eating behavior is being manifested by Mary?
2. Is this a superstition or a taboo?

Example B

Jane is your roommate. The night before the final exam in anatomy and physiology, the two of you go to the store and purchase six donuts, four candy bars, a bag of popcorn, a pound of peanuts, and a carton of cola beverages because you do not plan to take time out for dinner.

3. What eating behavior are you manifesting?
4. Was the choice of foods based on scientific evidence of the need for extra energy while studying strenuously?

Example C

Jesus Martinez, age 35, is admitted to your floor in the hospital for lab tests tomorrow. His lunch tray contains broiled fish, asparagus, baked potato, jello, and milk. It is an attractive tray. He does not touch the food. As he speaks no English and the nurse speaks no Spanish, there is a communication gap.

5. What may you assume is the cause of this rejection?

Example D

Ellen confides to you that her mother once made her sit at the breakfast table for three hours until she ate her bowl of oatmeal and that she will never touch another bite of oatmeal as long as she lives. "The thought of cold, sticky, nasty oatmeal makes me want to throw up," she says.

6. What factors are involved in Ellen's feelings about the oatmeal?

Example E

Mrs. Theo F. Jones III, wife of a prominent government official, is the guest of honor at a luncheon where hamburger casserole is the main entrée. She barely touches any of her food and leaves immediately afterward, even though she had planned to speak on a pet project.

7. Was Mrs. Jones ill, allergic to hamburger, or angry?
8. What type of food symbolism is manifested here?

Answers to Examples

1. Biological food symbolism. Food faddism—the belief that certain foods bring special health benefits—is very prevalent.
2. Superstition—a set of beliefs about the magical powers of food. There does not have to be a scientific basis for such beliefs.
3. Emotional food symbolism. Students' eating patterns change during exam time. They usually eat more, and the choices are usually high-calorie items. Such eating seems to help relieve strain.
4. There is no scientific evidence of need for extra calories while studying. One peanut would probably furnish enough energy for the entire study period.
5. There could be several causes, including anxiety, fear, unfamiliar surroundings, and strange people presenting the food, but the major cause is probably that these foods are not culturally acceptable.
6. Ellen is projecting an unpleasant memory associated with oatmeal. This frequently causes a food once eaten to become unacceptable. Psychotic patients often show great agitation by spitting on a food or dashing the tray to the floor when it brings back unpleasant memories. This is another example of emotional food symbolism.
7. Angry. Food is used as a status symbol, and hamburger is not included among status foods in our society. She felt rejected and humiliated by this menu because she felt it did not reflect her social standing.
8. Sociological food symbolism.

Poverty, Appetite, and Biological Food Needs

Economics is a very strong factor in the determination of food consumption. The costs of producing, transporting, and distributing food determine how much and what types of food are available. Lack of money affects not only the prices that people can pay for food but also the kinds of storage facilities they can afford to have within the household. Poor people often must buy cheap foods in small quantities and purchase items that do not require special storage facilities such as freezers or refrigerators. The cost of transportation may prohibit going to a large market, where volume purchases permit cheaper prices. Poverty is sometimes classified as a subculture in our society, and different attitudes and adaptations about foods emerge from this class than those found in the middle or upper

classes. Nurses should have an extensive knowledge of these differences.

Eating is generally prompted by hunger or appetite. Hunger is a physiological mechanism, controlled by the central nervous system. It is an unpleasant sensation. Appetite is a desire for food related to past experiences in response to stimuli such as smell, taste, and appearance. Appetite is not necessarily related to biological needs. People who are really hungry will eat many things not within their cultural frame of reference. They adapt physiologically and psychologically in order to survive. Appetite, on the other hand, can become uncontrolled behavior and can result in obesity. Obesity is a form of malnutrition, usually resulting in a deficiency of some essential nutrients in addition to excess fat in the body.

The biological food needs of a person throughout the life cycle have one requirement. The food consumed must provide essential chemical substances—nutrients—which the body can digest, absorb, and metabolize. In order to maintain life and health, the nutrients must reach the cells. Adequate nutrient intake depends on many factors, including age, sex, activity, size, and individual variations. The amounts of required nutrients may vary, but the types and kinds of nutrients established as being essential to life and health will remain the same throughout life. Research may add other, as yet unrecognized, essentials as scientific investigation progresses.

Summary

Feelings, attitudes, conditioning, and economics continually affect one's food consumption throughout life. Except for health professionals, who are very aware of the vital role that nutrition plays in the maintenance of health and the recovery from illness, most people give other aspects of food a priority over its importance for health.

Culture is a way of life. It is useful in adapting a person to his or her environment. Beginning with an infant's earliest experiences, individuals acquire customs and attitudes which they begin to internalize. Along with food, the child receives information that helps form his or her feelings and values; these remain on a subconscious level and are therefore very difficult to change. Eating habits, then, develop as a complex pattern of feelings, values, and customary behavior.

Abstract knowledge is rarely sufficient in itself to motivate someone to make a change. All the scientific knowledge and reasoning that can be brought to a person's attention will have little effect unless these facts can be related intimately to the individual's culture and eating habits. The person will respond more favorably if new knowledge is presented within the framework of the individual's culture, along with social and psychological conditioning, and situational dimensions. It is essential to encourage whatever good elements are found in the person's present eating pattern and to motivate the individual to change those elements that require alteration.

PROGRESS CHECK ON ACTIVITY 1

Questions

Self Studies

Analyze your eating patterns. Be as objective as possible. Answer the following questions about your behaviors.

1. What are the determining factors in the way you eat?
   likes, Dislikes, economih, Culture
   religion

2. What are the determining factors in the amount you eat? *Family Habits*

3. What determines your likes and dislikes? *Habits*
   Religion

True/False

Circle T for True and F for False.

4. T **F** Food habits result from human beings' instinctive behavior responses throughout life.

5. **T** F Social class structure in American society is largely determined by income, occupation, education, and residence.

6. **T** F Lifestyles change as society's values change.

7. T **F** From the time of birth, eating is a social act, building on social relationships.

8. T **F** High status foods usually become so because they have higher nutritional food values.

9. T **F** Food fads are usually long lasting and seldom change.

10. T **F** Special food combinations are effective as reducing diets and have special therapeutic effects.

11. T **F** Citrus fruits make the body acidic and produce "acid stomach."

12. **T** F Lean meat does not contribute to sexual potency or virility.

13. T **F** Gelatin builds strong fingernails.

Multiple Choice

Circle the letter of the correct answer.

14. Food fads are likely to develop in response to all of these except
    a. the striving of aging persons to regain their youth.
    b. different physiological requirements in certain individuals.
    c. peer group pressure on teenagers for social acceptance.
    d. the struggle of obese persons to lose weight.

15. The healthy body requires
    a. specific foods to control specific functions.
    b. certain food combinations to achieve specific physiological effects.
    c. "natural" foods to prevent disease.
    d. specific nutrients in a number of different foods to perform specific body functions.

16. Which of the following foods carries the most feminine symbolism?
    a. meat
    b. peaches
    c. cheese
    d. bread

17. Food habits in a given culture are largely based on all of these factors except
    a. food availability and agricultural development.
    b. genetic group differences in food tastes that lead to development of likes and dislikes.
    c. food economics, market practices, and food distribution.
    d. lifestyles and value systems.

18. Which principle(s) should guide the health worker in helping patients with different cultural food habits meet their nutritional needs? (Circle all that apply.)
    a. Learn as much as possible about the person's cultural habits related to nutrition and health.
    b. Encourage traditional practices that are beneficial.
    c. Do not interfere with practices that are harmless.
    d. Try to overcome harmful practices by persuasion and demonstration.

19. Common nutritional problems among the many cultures in the United States include
    a. obesity.
    b. iron-deficiency anemia.
    c. calcium deficiency.
    d. all of the above.

20. Ascorbic acid (vitamin C) deficiency among the lower economic classes is not due to

    a. dislike of citrus fruits.
    b. inability to digest foods containing vitamin C.
    c. ignorance of the daily need for vitamin C.
    d. lack of funds to purchase citrus fruits.
    e. any of the above.

21. Some diseases that are directly linked to eating patterns in the United States include (circle all that apply)

    a. heart disease.
    b. high blood pressure.
    c. cancer.
    d. diabetes.

ACTIVITY 2: Some Effects of Culture, Religion, and Geography on Food Behaviors

Basic Considerations

Large cultural groups are often subdivided into distinctive subcultures in the United States and each has an effect on the group's eating patterns. While many differences exist among small cultural groups, we will not attempt here to identify each separately. Religious group affiliations within cultural groups also change the patterns of eating as do occupation, income, and social class. Foodways can be changed as family units diversify, either perpetuating or modifying cultural practices. The influence of advertising, the tendency to move long distances, intermarriage, the employment of women, and the disruption of families often lead to more diversity within a group.

When first viewing cultural food practices, it may appear that nutrient intake is substandard. Closer examination, however, often reveals that this is not the case, and that, in fact, the culture has adapted certain practices peculiar to that group that make up for nutrients appearing to be missing or limited in the diet.

Reference Tables on Food Patterns

Table 2-1 describes the typical eating patterns of some prominent cultures in the United States and compares the foods used with the Basic Four food groups, with comments regarding certain adaptations. Regional differences are noted.

Table 2-2 describes some religious dietary practices.

Responsibilities of Health Personnel

Health care personnel have often treated clients with the assumption that they all share the same background and value systems. The influence of religion and culture on a client's attitude toward food is often overlooked.

It is not possible to be familiar with the dietary practices of all religions and cultures, and there remains a shortage of published information for the health practitioner on the subject. However, health practitioners need to be aware of dietary variations of groups and the diets most likely to be adhered to in order to give the best treatment. For example, an individual's refusal to eat a particular food or adhere to a particular diet may be due to restrictions imposed by the individual's religion or culture.

Some of the health problems of ethnic groups living in the United States are due to religious and cultural customs, as well as genetic differences. Measures for alleviating some of these problems are discussed below.

1. Those people whose diets may be low in calcium because they are lactose-intolerant can frequently tolerate buttermilk, yogurt, and fermented cheeses.

2. If changes in family eating patterns must be made, include the whole family when possible. In many cultures, children share in the preparation of food.

3. The diets of American Indians tend to be deficient in calories, calcium, riboflavin, vitamin C, and vitamin A. American Indians living on reservations show increased incidence of malnutrition, tuberculosis, and diabetes. Children often have kwashiorkor, a severe form of malnutrition. Because of religious as well as social requirements, American Indians seldom follow a modified diet. Adding hot spices such as chili peppers to the required foods sometimes helps in making foods more acceptable to them.

4. Yin and yang are somewhat complex concepts representing opposite conditions. In the Chinese culture, these conditions should balance each other. Pregnancy and birth are yin conditions for the Chinese. Therefore, the prescribed diet during this period balances out with yang foods. The yang foods given are rich in protein and calcium, which are beneficial. Pregnant women may refuse iron supplements for fear of hardening fetal bones.

5. The typical Chinese diet may be low in protein, calcium, and vitamin D. Many Orientals are vegetarians and when meat is used, it is used in limited quantity. Tofu (soybean curd) is a good source of protein and iron. If calcium salts are used to precipitate curd, tofu is also a good source of calcium. Some milk may be acceptable in custards.

6. Soy sauce is a favorite Oriental condiment and should be included in limited amounts instead of eliminated in a sodium-restricted diet. Rice and tea should also be in-

TABLE 2-1
Comparison of Eating Patterns of Certain U.S. Cultural Groups with the Basic Four Food Groups

Culture Group	Foods Widely Used	Foods Seldom Used	Comments
1. European American a. Western Region	*Meat Group:* beef, pork, poultry, fish, shellfish, eggs *Fruit/Vegetable Group:* all *Bread/Cereal Group:* bulgar, dark breads, wheat *Milk Group:* all cheeses, milk		Western European diet similar to U.S. pattern Rich desserts popular (strudel, kuchen [cake], butterhorns, pies, etc.) Diet tends to be high in fat, sugar
b. Central Region	*Meat Group:* sausages, pork, beef *Fruit/Vegetable Group:* sauerkraut, potatoes, onions, carrots, beans *Bread/Cereal Group:* all dark breads, especially rye *Milk Group:* cheeses more popular than milk		Seasonings include many highly salted items, garlic salt, celery salt, etc. Diet high in sodium
c. Italians	*Meat Group:* spiced sausages, meat sauces with peppers, cheeses, onions, tomato, fish *Fruit/Vegetable Group:* root vegetables, tomatoes *Bread/Cereal Group:* all pasta, yeast breads *Milk Group:* cheese *Other:* olive oil, spices	Milk	Calcium-rich diet Cheeses popular Diet high in sodium
2. Mexican American	*Meat Group:* meat, poultry, eggs (if income permits), dried beans *Fruit/Vegetable Group:* chili peppers, corn, tomatoes, potatoes, onions *Bread/Cereal Group:* tortillas *Milk Group:* cheeses (if income permits)	Milk	Foods are usually fried in animal fats. Green peppers, as well as tomatoes, good source of vitamin C; garlic used heavily. Lime-soaked corn tortillas supply a good source of calcium. Coffee used by children and adults. Diet is high in fat and sodium, low in calcium and folacin.
3. Southern Black	*Meat Group:* dried beans/peas, fish, pork *Fruit/Vegetable Group:* corn, yams, greens *Bread/Cereal Group:* cornbread, biscuits, white bread *Milk Group:* buttermilk occasionally *Other:* heavy seasonings (smoked foods, barbecue sauce, pickled, salt pork cured in brine)	Milk	Long cooking time for vegetables destroys some nutrients. Protein intake may be low if income is low. Common food preparation is frying in lard. All parts of the hog are used. Blacks have high incidence of lactose intolerance. Calcium-rich greens are popular. Diet contains excessive starch, sodium, and fat.
4. Oriental a. Cantonese (Southern Chinese)	*Meat Group:* beef, pork, poultry, seafood *Fruit/Vegetable Group:* mushrooms, bean sprouts, Chinese greens, bok choy *Bread/Cereal Group:* rice predominately *Milk Group:* limited quantity ice cream	Milk	All parts of the animal used, including blood. Vegetables are quickly cooked, conserving nutrients. Soy sauce used for seasoning; high salt content in the diet.
b. Northern Chinese	*Meat Group:* beef, poultry, seafood, pork, eggs, tofu *Fruit/Vegetable Group:* soybeans, Chinese greens, bamboo and alfalfa sprouts, bok choy *Bread/Cereal Group:* rice, noodles, bread, dumplings *Milk Group:*	Milk	Diet low in total fat. A high incidence of lactose intolerance is found among the Chinese people. Tea is a favorite beverage. Daily meals try to balance the yin (cold) and yang (hot) concepts. This is not related to the temperature of foods.

(continues)

TABLE 2-1 (Continued)

Culture Group	Foods Widely Used	Foods Seldom Used	Comments
c. Japanese Americans	*Meat Group:* salt and fresh-water fish, both steamed and eaten raw (sushi); beef, pork, eggs, poultry *Fruit/Vegetable Group:* all vegetables and fruits, soy bean products, sesame seeds *Bread/Cereal Group:* all complex carbohydrates, especially rice *Milk Group:*	Milk	The Issei retains the traditional food pattern: Nisei, Sansei, and especially Yansei likely to mix patterns or follow Western eating patterns. Traditional diet low in total fat, cholesterol, and animal protein (because only small amounts used mixed with other foods). Diet is low in sugar. Tea is a favorite beverage. Soy sauce and teriyaki sauce are used liberally. High incidence of lactose intolerance. The diet is high in sodium. Certain food combinations are thought harmful or healthful, i.e., *harmful:* cherries and milk; *helpful:* pickled plums and rice gruel.
5. American Indian a. Reservation and Rural	*Meat Group:* wild game, waterfowl, fish, beef *Fruit/Vegetable Group:* nuts, roots, berries, squash, beans, corn and blue cornmeal *Bread/Cereal Group:* mostly from cornmeal, but wheat products are also used. *Milk Group:*	Milk	Some tribes do not eat fish. Corn and blue cornmeal are used in childbirth and healing practices. Restrictions on normally acceptable foods are sometimes imposed by Shaman as a healing in pre and post natal periods. High incidence of lactose intolerance among the American Indian tribes.
b. City	Generally assimilated into the predominant culture: retains many traditional foods and food practices in home		

cluded whenever possible. Alternate seasonings to soy and teriyaki sauce should be encouraged.

7. Garlic, wine, and unsalted tomato puree can be suggested as ways of lowering the high sodium content of the Italian diet. Elimination of cold cuts and sausages may also be necessary.

8. The Jewish diet will usually be high in saturated fats and cholesterol. Jewish people have a high incidence of diabetes mellitus, obesity, and lactose intolerance. If feeding an orthodox Jewish client in a medical facility, a complete line of kosher frozen foods may have to be purchased. *Pareve* used on a food label means that the product contains no dairy, meat, or poultry products.

9. The diet of Mexican Americans tends to be high in fats and sodium and low in calcium and folacin. The practice of using the refined wheat tortilla instead of the lime-soaked corn tortilla should be discouraged. If spicy foods are limited or omitted from the Mexican diet, the health practitioner should be aware that this practice will decrease vitamins A and C in the diet, as the red and green peppers used are good sources of these vitamins.

10. Adaptations of diet for Muslims should not be difficult if kosher foods are available. Foods considered health-giving by Muslims include honey, dates, and sweets. These can be added to the modified diet unless contraindicated (as with diabetes, for example).

11. A hospitalized vegetarian should not have difficulty selecting from a hospital menu. Vegetarian diets, as practiced by religions such as the Seventh Day Adventist, tend to be low in saturated fats and cholesterol and high in fiber. Vegetarians are also taught how to combine plant proteins to get adequate essential amino acids. Between-meal feedings are discouraged by the Adventist faith and five- to six-hour meal intervals are practiced. This should be taken into consideration when hospital routine conflicts with their practice.

PROGRESS CHECK ON ACTIVITY 2

Questions

The following menu is an example of meeting a cultural variation when planning a nutritionally adequate diet for

TABLE 2-2
Some Religious Practices that Affect Dietary Habits in U.S.

Religion	Foods and Beverages Prohibited	Comments
Orthodox Jewish	All pork and pork products; all fish without scales or fins; improperly slaughtered meats; food containing blood; meats and poultry if combined with dairy products; all milk, cream and other dairy products with a meat meal or for 6 hrs. following	Kosher (Kashruth Laws) regulations are strict regarding slaughter and preparation of animal products and also regulate separation of milk and meat. Certain foods are designated pareve (neutral): fruits, uncooked vegetables, grains, tea, coffee. Two separate sets of dishes, utensils and cooking equipment maintained in kosher households. 24-hour fast on Yom Kippur.
Muslim	All pork and pork products; meat not slaughtered by a Muslim, Jew, or Christian; alcoholic beverages; stimulant beverages	Fast from dawn to dusk during the month of Ramadan (9th month of the Islamic calendar). Only kosher gelatin used: this eliminates marshmallow, gelatin desserts, and many candies. Only vegetable oils used in food preparation.
Seventh Day Adventist	Pork, pork products, shellfish, blood, all flesh foods (if strict), dairy products and eggs (if very strict), highly spiced foods, meat broths, stimulant and alcoholic beverages	Cereal-based beverages used. Children from strict vegetarian homes may be low in some nutrients.
Christian	Meats may be prohibited on certain religious occasions, alcohol and stimulant beverages prohibited by some denominations	Moderation in food and beverage intake is encouraged in most denominations.

an American Indian woman, age 25. Using it as a guide, plan a day's menu which meets the RDAs for any two cultural groups studied in this module. State the age, sex, and culture or religion of the group about which you are writing.

Breakfast	Lunch
1 c. cornmeal mush	1 slice fried Indian bread
1 tbsp. sugar	1 c. pinto beans
1 tsp. margarine	½ c. squash
*1 c. milk, fresh, or ½ c. evaporated	1 apple
1 c. orange juice	1½ oz. cheese
coffee, if desired	coffee, if desired

Dinner	Snacks (if desired)
3 oz. venison roast	any fruits
½ c. fried potatoes	oatmeal/raisin cookies
greens of choice	
blackberries	
yogurt or buttermilk	

*If tolerated

References

American Dietetic Association. 1989. Nutrition information on food labels. *Journal of the American Dietetic Association* 89:266.

Anderson, J. V., and M. R. Van Nierop (eds.). 1989. *Basic nutrition facts: A nutrition reference.* East Lansing, MI: Michigan State University and the Michigan Department of Public Health.

Aronson, V., and B. Fitzgerald. 1990. *Guidebook for nutrition counselors.* Englewood Cliffs, NJ: Prentice-Hall.

Aurand, L. W. et al. 1987. *Food composition and analysis.* New York: Van Nostrand Reinhold.

Bakery, L. (ed.). 1982. *The psychobiology of human food selection.* New York: Van Nostrand Reinhold.

Beare-Rogers, H. L. 1984. Dietary goals and recommendations in Canada. H. Canadian Diet. Assoc. 45:325.

Brown, L. K., and K. Mussell (eds.). 1987. Ethnic and regional foodways in the United States. *The performance of group identity.* Knoxville, TN: University of Tennessee Press.

Bryant, C. A. et al. 1985. *The cultural feast: An introduction to food and society.* St. Paul: West Publishing.

Copper, R. M. 1986. Health claims of foods—reflections on the food/drug distinction and on the law of misbranding. *American Journal of Clinical Nutrition* 44:325.

Farb, P., and G. Armelagos. 1980. *Consuming passions: The anthropology of eating.* Boston: Houghton Mifflin.

Fieldhouse, P. 1985. *Food and nutrition: Customs and culture.* New York: Methuen.

Food and Drug Administration. 1987. Food labeling: Public health messages in food labels and food labeling. *Rd. Reg.* 52:28843.

Food and Nutrition Board, National Research Council, National Academy of Sciences. 1989. *Recommended dietary allowances*. 10th ed. Washington, DC: National Academy Press.

Gussow, J. D., and P. R. Thomas. 1986. *The nutrition debate: Sorting out some answers*. Palo Alto, CA: Bull Publishing.

Harper, A. E. 1989. Scientific substantiation of health claims: How much is enough? *Nutrition Today* 24(2):17.

Harper, A. E. 1988. Nutrition: From myth and magic to science. *Nutrition Today* 23(1):8.

Hathcock, J. N. (ed.). 1987. *Nutritional toxicology*. Vol. 2. Orlando, FL: Academic Press.

Hegsted, D. M. 1986. Dietary Standards—Guidelines for prevention of deficiency or prescription for total health. *Journal of Nutrition* 116:478.

Herbert, V. 1987. Health claims in food labeling and advertising. *Nutrition Today* 22:25.

King, J. C. et al. 1978. Evaluation and modification of the basic four food guide. *Journal of Nutrition Education* 10:27.

Kittler, P. G., and K. Sucher. 1989. Food and culture in America. New York: Van Nostrand Reinhold.

Krebs-Smith, S. M. et al. 1987. The effects of variety in food choices on dietary quality. *Journal of the American Dietetic Association* 87:897.

Logue, A. W. 1986. *The psychology of eating and drinking*. New York: W. H. Freeman and Co.

Miller, S. A., and M. G. Stephenson. 1987. The 1990 national nutrition objectives: Lessons for the future. *Journal of the American Dietetic Association* 87:1665.

National Research Council. 1986. *Nutrient adequacy*. Washington, DC: National Academy Press.

Newman, J. M. 1986. *Melting pot: An annotated bibliography and guide to food and nutrition information for ethnic groups in America*. New York: Garland.

Obert, J. C. 1986. *Community nutrition*. New York: John Wiley & Sons.

Owen, A. Y., and R. T. Frankle. 1986. *Nutrition in the community: The art of delivering services*. St. Louis: Mosby.

Sanjur, D. 1982. *Social and cultural perspectives in nutrition*. Englewood Cliffs, NJ: Prentice-Hall.

Shils, M. E., and V. R. Young (eds.). 1988. *Modern nutrition in health and disease*. Philadelphia: Lea & Febiger.

Szilard, P. 1987. *Food and nutrition information guide*. Littleton, CO: Libraries Unlimited.

Wardlaw, G. M., and P. M. Insel. 1990. *Perspectives in nutrition*. St. Louis: Mosby.

Meeting Energy Needs

Time for completion
Activities: _____ 1½ _____ hours
Optional examination: ½ hour

Academic credit
Semester units: ⁴/₁₀
Quarter units: ⁵/₁₀

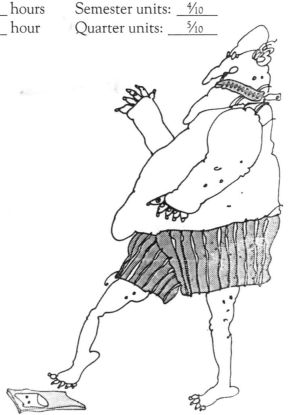

Outline

Objectives
Glossary
Background information

ACTIVITY 1: Energy Balance
Energy measurement
Basal metabolic rate
Energy and physical activity
Thermic effect of food
Energy intake and output
RDAs and body energy need
Calculating energy intake
Progress check on Activity 1

ACTIVITY 2: The Effects of Energy Imbalance
Definitions
Body composition
Undernutrition
Obesity
Progress check on Activity 2

ACTIVITY 3: Weight Control and Dieting
Calories, exercise, and eating habits
Guidelines for dieting
A multibillion dollar business
The basics of physical exercise
Summary
Responsibilities of health personnel
Progress check on Activity 3
References

Objectives

Upon completion of this module the student should be able to:

1. Describe how energy is measured.
2. Define energy balance.
3. Identify the energy producing nutrients and state their fuel value.
4. Calculate the calorie content of foods based on their carbohydrate, protein, fat, and/or alcohol content.
5. Relate food and activity to weight control.
6. List techniques for evaluating body weight.
7. Discuss methods for controlling body weight.
8. Evaluate the effects of under- and overnutrition.
9. State the health implications of being underweight.
10. Differentiate between overweight and obesity.
11. Analyze health problems associated with fad dieting and obesity.

Glossary

Anthropometric measurements: measurements of body size and composition, including height, weight, body circumference measurements (midarm, head, abdominal girth), and skinfold thickness (fat fold). In order to be valid, these measurements must be obtained in an accurate manner and compared to reference standards.

Basal metabolic rate (BMR): expression of the number of kilocalories used hourly in relation to the surface area of the body. The speed at which fuel is needed to maintain vital body processes at rest, or the amount of energy the body requires to carry out its involuntary maintenance work.

Basal metabolism: the amount of energy required to carry on vital body processes when the body is at rest.

Caloric density: the number of kilocalories in a unit of weight of a specific food.

Calorie (cal): unit of energy. The amount of heat necessary to raise one gram of water one degree centigrade. The energy released from food is too enormous to be described by these units, so nutritionists use the kilocalorie equivalent of 1,000 of these small calories (*see* kilocalorie).

Energy metabolism: all the chemical changes that result in the release of energy in the body.

Hyperplasia: increase in the total number of cells.

Hyperthyroidism: excessive secretion of the thyroid gland, increasing the basal metabolic rate.

Hypertrophy: enlargement of cells.

Hypothyroidism: deficiency of thyroid secretion resulting in a lowered basal metabolic rate.

Kilocalorie (kcal): unit of energy. The amount of heat needed to raise one kilogram of water one degree centigrade. Though not technically correct, most consumer and professional literature calls these units "calories." Nutritionists use a capital C when describing a kilocalorie.

Metabolism: the total of all the chemical and biological processes that take place in the body.

Synthesis: the process of building up; the formation of complex substances from simpler ones.

Thermic effect of food: the increase in metabolism caused by the digestion, absorption, and transportation of nutrients in the body.

Background Information

Weight control has become a twentieth century health problem. Before this century, excess weight was the mark of a healthy body, an affluent family, good mothering, and shapely beauty. Being underweight or what would now be considered normal weight was held in low esteem. These attitudes have since reversed. The terms "overweight," "overfat," and "obesity" are common to modern societies. In the United States, 35 percent of the population is overweight, 10 percent of whom are school children, and 33 percent of whom may be classified as obese. Another third of the population is struggling to keep a stable weight. It should not come as a surprise, then, that repercussions from obsessions about thinness occur.

Health professionals are witnessing cases of eating disorders such as anorexia nervosa and bulimia as a response to the pressures to be thin. At the same time, the opposite end of these disorders, obesity, is escalating. Due to psychogenic overtones, many scientists now believe that obesity and anorexia nervosa are conditions on a continuum of the same disorder. The manifestations of either appear to result in the same kinds of clinical disturbances.

Students in a health profession should be familiar with weight control in order to assist clients to achieve their optimal weight goals.

ACTIVITY 1: Energy Balance

Energy balance occurs when an individual's total caloric expenditure equals the individual's total caloric intake. Factors over which we have control are our intake and expenditure. There are some variables that influence our energy balance over which we have little or no control.

Energy Measurement

The energy value of a food is measured in kilocalories (kcals). Much work has been devoted to developing reference tables of foods' caloric values for use in estimating our energy intake. A food's caloric value is determined by its content of protein, fat, and carbohydrate. These are the only nutrients that produce energy; vitamins and minerals do not. Protein provides 4 kcal per gram (g), carbohydrate 4, and fat 9. For example, 1 teaspoon (tsp.) of sugar (carbohydrate) equals 5 g and 20 kcal and 1 tsp. salad oil equals 5 g and 45 kcal. Alcohol, while not a basic nutrient, provides 7 kcal/g and can create problems in weight control as well as other undesirable effects. Carbohydrates and fats are the preferred energy sources. Proteins will be used for energy if carbohydrates are not available in the diet. If carbohydrate supplies are limited, fat and protein stores will be used for energy and may result in a buildup of toxic byproducts (ketones) in the blood.

Total energy needs are measured in three major areas: the basal metabolic rate; activity or voluntary energy expenditure; and the thermic effect of food.

Basal Metabolic Rate

Basal metabolism, the energy required for the vital life processes, is measured in terms of basal metabolic rate (BMR) and is affected by several factors:

1. *Body composition and surface.* The BMR of a body is higher for a person with more muscle than fat. Also, the larger a person's amount of skin area is, the higher the BMR.
2. *Sex.* Women have lower BMR values than men do because of the difference in activity of sex hormones and women's generally smaller size.
3. *Age.* A person's BMR is highest during infancy. After adolescence, the BMR begins a gradual decline of about 2 percent each decade after the age of twenty.
4. *Body temperature.* A cold external temperature raises the BMR as the body tries to keep warm. However, a high internal temperature (fever) also significantly increases BMR.
5. *Physiological status.* Conditions such as malnutrition, elevated hormone production, and pregnancy influence the BMR. Growth increases BMR, while BMR decreases with arrested growth. Malnutrition decreases, hyperthyroidism increases, and hypothyroidism decreases BMR.

Energy and Physical Activity

Voluntary energy expenditure affects the energy balance. Muscular exercise burns calories, but mental or paperwork does not. The energy needed for various activities increases as the weight of the person increases, but overweight persons usually make up for this by becoming less active. Table 3-1 provides a partial listing of various activities and the amount of kilocalories needed for each.

TABLE 3-1

Approximate Energy Cost of Different Forms of Activities for a 70-kg (154 lb.) Man*

Activity	kcal/min
Basketball	9.0–10.0
Boxing	9.0–10.0
Cleaning	4.0–4.5
Coal mining	6.0–8.0
Cooking	3.0–3.5
Dancing	3.5–12.5
Eating	1.0–2.0
Fishing	4.0–5.0
Gardening	3.5–9.0
Horse riding	3.0–10.0
Painting	2.0–6.0
Piano playing	2.5–3.0
Running	9.0–21.0
Scrubbing floors	7.0–8.0
Standing	1.5–2.0
Swimming	4.0–12.0
Typing, electric	1.5–2.0
Walking	1.5–6.0
Writing	2.0–2.5

*The data in this table have been collected from many sources. Because of large variation among the results of different investigators, ranges of values are used so as to give a general idea of the relationship between types of activity and the energy cost.

Thermic Effect of Food

A person's BMR increases for about 12 hours after eating a meal. The digestion, absorption, transportation, and metabolism of nutrients all require energy. The production of heat following a meal is known as the thermic effect of food. This effect varies with the kind and amounts of food eaten and the person's metabolic needs. The use of nutrients to build new tissue requires more energy than the breakdown of nutrients to provide energy. The thermic effect of food varies from about 6 percent to 10 percent of total energy needs.

Energy Intake and Output

Energy balance results when the number of kilocalories consumed equals the number used for energy. The body weight is an index of this relationship of intake to output. Exercise is a valuable aid in achieving energy balance. If consistently more calories are consumed than used for energy, the result will be a weight gain. Excess calories are stored in the form of fat. If less is eaten than the body needs, the result will be weight loss. Energy must come from somewhere, so calories needed but not provided by food are withdrawn from body stores.

A pound of body fat represents 3,500 kcal. For every 3,500 kcal lacking in the diet, 1 pound (lb.) of body weight will be lost, and for every 3,500 kcal excess, 1 lb. of weight will be gained. It does not matter whether the excess or shortage occurs over a period of a week or a year.

Examples

Every calorie absorbed by the body must be used as energy or stored as fat. This principle is illustrated by the following examples:

1. Robert has an office job where he sits constantly programming a computer. He has been out of college for four years. Although he has tried to control his weight, his weight has still escalated. Let us compare his conditions during 1980 and 1984.

In 1980, Robert's daily kcal intake from food was 2,250. He played racquetball daily with his roommate. This, combined with other activities and his BMR, expended 2,250 kcal energy daily. He weighed 160 pounds when he graduated.

In 1984, Robert's food intake is still 2,250 kcal per day. He plays only one game of racquetball a week. This, combined with his other activities and BMR, expends 2,000 kcal of energy per day. All other variables have remained the same, including his eating habits. He now weighs 264 lb.

The equation is simple:

   a. 250 kcal/day excess = 1,750 kcal excess per week
   b. 1,750 kcal = 1/2 lb. body fat per week
   c. 1/2 lb. weight gain every week = 26 lb. per year
   d. 26 lb. per year × 4 years = 104 lb. weight gained

2. Jane is attending a wellness class at her local college and finds she is roughly 40 percent above her ideal body weight of 130 lb. Her average 24-hour food intake yields 1,800 kcal. Jane gets counseling from a health educator. They work out a program whereby Jane substitutes her daily late afternoon snack of 250 calories for a 2-1/2 mile brisk walk. The walk uses approximately 250 calories. At the end of a year Jane has reached her ideal weight of 130 lb. without "suffering" and feels much better physically and mentally. The equation is simple:

   a. 250 calorie deficit from food plus 250 calorie deficit from exercise = 500 calorie deficit per day
   b. 500 calories times 7 days a week = 3,500 calories or 1 lb. weight loss per week
   c. 1 × 52 weeks per year = 52 lb. weight loss per year
   d. 130 lb (ideal body weight) × 40 percent = 182 lb. (starting weight)
   e. 182 lb. – 52 lb. = 130 lb. (ideal body weight) at end of one year

Skinfold measurements following the successful loss of 52 lb. revealed that total percentage of body fat was 20 percent, well within the 18 to 25 percent normal range for females. This confirmed that body fat, not muscle and water, was lost. This pattern of weight loss is highly recommended for its value in maintaining a lower body weight once the goal is reached. It provides ample time to modify eating habits and lifestyles.

The difficulty people have balancing their intake and output of energy nutrients is clearly demonstrated by the fact that obesity is a major health problem in the United States. It is believed to cause or complicate many of the chronic disorders of later life.

RDAs and Body Energy Need

Table 3-2 shows the average energy needs for each sex and age group as set forth in the 1989 RDAs. Keep in mind that the RDAs are applicable to groups, not individuals.

Release of energy in the cells is a complex process requiring the activity of vitamins and minerals as well as enzymes and hormones. A person's total energy needs are based on basal metabolism, voluntary physical activity, and the thermic effect of food. The BMR is the speed at which fuel is spent to maintain the vital body processes at rest. It is influenced by body composition, sex, age, body temperature, and various other physical conditions. The effect of physical activity on total caloric need depends on the type of activity, the length of time over which it is performed, and the size of the person doing it.

Foods vary in energy value in proportion to the energy-producing nutrients they contain. Foods that contain fat or alcohol or have a low water content tend to have a relatively high energy value; lean meats, cereal foods, and starchy vegetables are intermediate in energy value; and fruits and vegetables are relatively low in energy value.

All essential nutrients should be provided within the calorie level required to maintain ideal weight. The more calories a person obtains from sugars, fats, and alcohol, the more likely he or she is to be poorly nourished.

Quick weight loss, usually obtained by extreme fad dieting, reflects loss of protein (muscle), tissue, and water rather than fat loss. In addition, very low-calorie diets decrease the BMR.

Calculating Energy Intake

There are several ways to calculate caloric intake. One is to use food value tables such as the one in Table 3-3. Caloric and nutrient values of foods are found in many publications. Perhaps the two most comprehensive and widely used food composition tables are USDA's Handbook #456, "Nutritive Value of American Foods in Common Units," and Bowes and Church's "Food Values of Portions Commonly Used." Also, familiarization with the foods and serving sizes contained in each of the groups in the Exchange System (see Appendix E) greatly facilitates

TABLE 3-2
Mean Heights and Weights and Recommended
Energy Intakes for the United States, 1989

Sex Group and Age (Years) or Condition	Weight		Height		REE[a]	Average Energy Allowance[b]		
	kg	lb	cm	in		Multiples of REE	per kg	per Day[c]
					(kcal/day)		—kcal—	
Infants								
0.0–0.5	6	13	60	24	320		108	650
0.5–1.0	9	20	71	28	500		98	850
Children								
1–3	13	29	90	35	740		102	1,300
4–6	20	44	112	44	950		90	1,800
7–10	28	62	132	52	1,130		70	2,000
Males								
11–14	45	99	157	62	1,440	1.70	55	2,500
15–18	66	145	176	69	1,760	1.67	45	3,000
19–24	72	160	177	70	1,780	1.67	40	2,900
25–50	79	174	176	70	1,800	1.60	37	2,900
51 +	77	170	173	68	1,530	1.50	30	2,300
Females								
11–14	46	101	157	62	1,310	1.67	47	2,200
15–18	55	120	163	64	1,370	1.60	40	2,200
19–24	58	128	164	65	1,350	1.60	38	2,200
25–50	63	138	163	64	1,380	1.55	36	2,200
51 +	65	143	160	63	1,280	1.50	30	1,900
Pregnant								
1st trimester								+0
2nd trimester								+300
3rd trimester								+300
Lactating								
1st 6 months								+500
2nd 6 months								+500

[a]REE = resting energy expenditure. Calculated based on FAO equations, then rounded.
[b]In the range of light to moderate activity, the coefficient of variation = 20%.
[c]Figure is rounded.
Source: Food and Nutrition Board, National Research Council, ©1989, National Academy of Sciences; reprinted with permission.

planning a diet within any given caloric allowance (see Module 15).

PROGRESS CHECK ON ACTIVITY 1

Questions

Fill-in

1. What are the three factors that determine a person's total energy needs? Describe each of these factors.

   a. basal metabolic RATE

   b. Activity a Voluntary energy expenditure

   c. thermic effect of foods

2. A ½ cup serving of New England clam chowder contains 4 g protein, 5 g fat, and 7 g carbohydrate. Using this information, calculate the energy value of this food serving:

EXAMPLE: ½ c. whole milk contains 4.2 g protein, 6 g carbohydrate, and 4.2 g fat. The calorie content of this milk is:

4.2 g protein × 4 kcal/g	= 16.8 kcal
6.0 g carbohydrate × 4 kcal/g	= 24.0 kcal
4.2 g fat × 9 kcal/g	= 37.8 kcal
	Total = 78.6 kcal

TABLE 3-3
Energy Value of Selected Foods Compared

Foods from Food Groups	Portion	Kcal
Meat and Alternates		
1. Beef (lean and fat)	3 oz.	245
(lean only)	3 oz.	140
2. Chicken, no skin, broiled	3 oz.	115
skin and flesh broiled	3 oz.	155
3. Fish, haddock, fried	3 oz.	135
shrimp, canned	3 oz.	100
tuna, in oil, drained	3 oz.	170
Vegetables and Fruits		
1. Beans, lima, cooked, drained	½ c.	95
green, snap	½ c.	15
2. Beets, cooked, diced	½ c.	25
3. Corn, canned	½ c.	85
4. Onions, cooked	½ c.	30
5. Carrots, grated	½ c.	20
6. Peas, green, cooked	½ c.	58
7. Grapes, raw	½ c.	32
8. Applesauce, unsweetened	½ c.	50
9. Apricots, unsweetened, cooked	½ c.	120
10. Orange juice	½ c.	55
11. Pineapple, canned, in juice	½ c.	40
Grains (Bread-Cereal)		
1. Bagel	1	165
2. Biscuit, baking powder, 2" diameter	1	90
3. Branflakes (40%)	1 c.	105
4. Bread, white or wheat	1 slice	70
5. Cake		
a. angel food, 1/12 of 10" diameter	1 piece	135
b. devils food, 1/16 of 9" diameter	1 piece	235
6. Cookies		
a. chocolate chip (small)	1	50
b. brownies (small)	1	85
7. Pies		
a. apple, 1/7 of 9" diameter	1 piece	350
b. pecan, 1/7 of 9" diameter	1 piece	490
8. Pizza (cheese), 5½"	1 piece	185
9. Popcorn, plain	1 c.	20
Milk and Alternates		
1. Milk, fluid, whole	1 c.	160
skim	1 c.	90
buttermilk from skim	1 c.	90
2. Cheese, cheddar	1 oz.	115
cottage, creamed	1/2 c	130
creamed	1 cu. inch	60
3. Ice cream, vanilla	1 c.	255
4. Ice milk, regular hardened	1 c.	200
soft serve	1 c.	265
5. Yogurt, whole milk	1 c.	150
low fat	1 c.	125

From nutritive value of edible parts of foods.

3. What is the guide for determining whether your caloric intake is in balance with your energy needs? Explain.

MAINTAINING BODY WT

What happens to excess calories?

STORED AS FAT IN ADIPOSE TISSUE

4. Explain the error in the statement: "Potatoes are fattening."

They are a bread—starch of the carbohydrate group + contain only 4cal/gram

5. A twenty-five-year-old woman who is 5'2" tall and weighs 125 lb. consumes 1,800 calories a day to maintain her weight. She wishes to lose 3 lb. of weight per week.

   a. In order to lose this 3 lb. of weight per week, how many calories per day could she eat?

   b. Is a weight loss of 3 lb. per week realistic for this woman? Explain.

6. Identify the exchange group to which the following energy values belong (values are rounded).

   a. 90 kcal

   b. 60 kcal

   c. 70 kcal

   d. 25 kcal

   e. 45 kcal

   f. 55 kcal

Matching

Match the phrases on the right to the items on the left which best describe them.

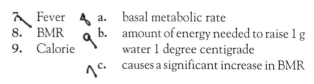

7. Fever
8. BMR
9. Calorie

a. basal metabolic rate
b. amount of energy needed to raise 1 g water 1 degree centigrade
c. causes a significant increase in BMR

ACTIVITY 2: The Effects of Energy Imbalance

Definitions

Malnutrition is a general term indicating an excess, deficit, or imbalance in one or more of the essential nutrients. It is also used to describe an excess or deficit of calories. Physical, psychosocial, and economic factors can contribute to the development of malnutrition.

Malnutrition is classified as either primary or secondary. Primary malnutrition is due to poor food choices or inadequate food supply. Secondary malnutrition refers to faulty body functioning, such as the inability to digest certain essential foods. It may also be a result of certain drug therapies.

Two other terms that are used to describe malnutrition are undernutrition and overnutrition. These terms are frequently identified in the underweight or overweight individual, indicating either inadequate or excessive caloric intake. Both types can interfere with body processes and affect health.

Underweight is generally accepted as being below 10 percent of ideal body weight, and overweight is defined as 10 to 20 percent above ideal body weight. Ideal weight is usually obtained from the height and weight charts published by the Metropolitan Life Insurance Company. They reflect average weights maintained throughout life that are related to the longest life expectancy. Although the tables take into account frame size, they give no criteria for its determination. The height and weight tables can indicate only gross estimates of ideal weight.

Body Composition

Body composition is a much more accurate indicator of ideal body weight than are weight and height tables in determining the fatness or leanness of a person. For survival, some fat is needed to insulate the body from environmental temperature fluctuation, regulate the body's internal temperature, and protect the body against shock. The ideal range of body fat varies with survival needs.

Ideally, adult males in Western society should have about 15 to 20 percent body fat, and adult females 20 to 25 percent. Based on percentages then, women and men who measure over 20 percent and 25 percent body fat, respectively, are considered obese.

Some accurate measurements of body composition used to determine body weight are:

1. Water displacement and determination of specific gravity. This method is accurate, but requires special equipment. Most medical centers and hospitals have the equipment and will charge a nominal fee for a standard measurement. Many persons participating in fitness and conditioning programs have this type of assessment performed prior to and at intervals during the program.
2. Skinfold thicknesses measured by calipers at specific body sites. These measurements should be taken by a skilled person, and assessed by comparing to reference standards.
3. Anthropometric measurements including skeletal, head, muscle, and body contour circumferences. These measurements are useful at any age, but especially for evaluating growth in children.
4. Radiological and laboratory studies to identify signs of malnutrition. Tests such as measuring an individual's radioactive potassium content are useful in determining lean body mass. A high potassium count indicates little fat tissue.

Undernutrition

When an individual is undernourished, nutrient reserves dwindle, tissues become deprived of essential nutrients, and medical disorders result. Protein stores are depleted as muscle tissue is used as a source of energy. Antibody production against invasions of bacteria and viruses becomes limited. Lack of nutrient reserves may lead to more severe forms of malnutrition such as marasmus and kwashiorkor or the mixed condition of protein energy malnutrition (PEM). These conditions are discussed further in Module 5.

A woman who is underweight during pregnancy is at high obstetric risk. Newborn infants of such women are also likely to have problems, such as being small for gestational age (SGA, underweight through full term) and/or premature.

The most severe form of undernutrition is anorexia nervosa, a condition due largely to psychological problems. It manifests as a physiological disorder where signs of starvation are evident. It requires psychiatric treatment before and during nutritional rehabilitation. This disorder is life-threatening and can recur after recovery.

Obesity

Overview

Being overweight may be more of a social than a medical problem. The overweight individual may develop a distorted body image manifested in low self-esteem, embarrassment, and social isolation. Counseling the obese individual toward a regular exercise routine and an accurate perception of body weight and composition is beneficial.

The average American who is overweight to mildly obese is likely to have gained the extra weight over a period of several years. The grossly obese individual usually gains several hundred pounds in the teens to early twenties. The term overweight usually refers to body weight in excess of some standard and does not indicate the degree of fatness.

Adopting a regular exercise program and a controlled diet will permit the overweight individual to reduce to a normal weight. There appears to be a significant difference between the overweight and the obese individual in terms of percentage of body fat and the appearance of body systems changes that accompany the deposition of adipose tissues.

Fat Cells

The fundamental characteristics of adipose tissue are determined in the last three months of gestation, the first three years of life, and during adolescence. The adipose cell is 72 percent lipid (fat), 23 percent water, and is very active. It recycles its lipids. The total amount of body fat depends on the size of the cells (hypertrophy) and the number of cells (hyperplasia). All obese people show enlargement of fat cells, but the obese individual who has three to five times the number of fat cells as the nonobese will be more resistant to weight loss. This is usually the case in juvenile onset obesity. These individuals remain resistant to significant weight loss throughout life, and constitute a population group with high health hazards.

Health Risks

Beyond the social, psychosocial, and aesthetic problems that must be dealt with by the obese, there are also a number of serious health problems caused by obesity. Among these problems are:

1. Hernias: abdominal and hiatal hernias are especially common. Hiatal hernias are displacement of part of the stomach into the chest cavity.
2. Varicose veins and osteoarthritis: extra load on the weight-bearing joints creates a high incidence of these two conditions.
3. Winter coughing and bronchitis: common because of fat surrounding the diaphragm.
4. Decreased tolerance for exercise: poor breathing ability lowers oxygen intake.
5. Cholelithiasis (gallbladder stones): 96 percent of these stones are composed of cholesterol derived from the saturated fats of the body.
6. High blood lipids: both triglyceride and cholesterol levels tend to rise in the obese, leading to a higher risk of heart disease.
7. Hypertension (high blood pressure) and kidney diseases: common conditions among the obese due to the increased work load, the building of additional capillary systems to nourish the fat cells and move the additional weight. Newest studies implicate obesity rather than excess sodium intake as the major contributor to high blood pressure.
8. Type II diabetes: common among the obese. Many scientists believe that this disorder is a result of long-term obesity.
9. Increased cancer risk: breast, uterine, pancreatic, and gallbladder carcinomas are being studied in regard to their relationship to obesity.
10. Sexuality and the obese:
    a. Sexual response diminishes due to both aesthetic reasons and physical barriers.
    b. Folds of fatty tissue around the scrotum raise local temperature and can led to infertility in the male.
    c. Skin infections and irritations, especially around the genital areas, occur because of heat and moisture and folds of fat make it difficult to clean the areas.
    d. Menstrual disorders are common in obese females.
    e. Obese women experience difficult pregnancies, and infants are likely to suffer fetal distress. There is also a higher stillborn rate among obese women.
11. Premature aging has been noted among the obese. It is estimated that the life span of an obese individual is reduced by fifteen years.

Questions to Ask

The health practitioner should consider a variety of factors that may make a client vulnerable to obesity. Some assessments the health practitioner should make are:

1. What are the cultural practices? The main staples of the diet may be calorie-dense with a small variety of other foods.
2. What is the income level? People in a low income level tend to eat filling and cheap foods (usually high in fats, sugars, and starches). Intake of protein foods, fruits, and vegetables may be low.

3. What does the client believe about weight in relation to health? In Western society, thinness is a fetish, and large amounts of time and money are spent attaining it. At the same time, obesity is rampant. This is a paradox. Among some ethnic groups living in the United States, overweight and obesity are acceptable and perhaps even desirable states.

4. What is the emotional status? For what reasons do clients eat? What is their general mood? Are they dependent or independent? How do food and activity fit their daily living patterns? How do they adapt to stress?

Summary

Obesity is a multifaceted problem involving physiological, psychological, and cultural factors, all of which are resistant to current therapeutic efforts. "Obesity" is the precise term to use in referring to a gain of excess fat. "Overweight" is a more general term referring to increased weight gain in all body parts (fat, water, cells). The obese person is overweight, but the overweight person is not necessarily obese, and being overweight is not always undesirable. However, the public usually does not distinguish between the two terms.

Obesity may occur in two ways: existing adipocytes (fat cells) may enlarge or "hypertrophy"; or the number of fat cells may increase in a process called "hyperplasia." All obese individuals experience hypertrophy, but not all have abnormal amounts of fat cells. Hyperplastic obesity is also called "juvenile onset" because development of extra adipocytes occurs during early or late childhood. Adult onset obesity is strictly hypertrophic. Once hyperplastic obesity has developed, weight can be lost from the cells, but the number of cells is not reduced.

The exact mechanism that causes obesity is not known, but the main factor appears to be overeating combined with inadequate levels of activity. Metabolic and glandular disorders account for only 2 to 5 percent of all obesity. Heredity, basal metabolic rate, and body type all influence the development of obesity.

Obesity has not been shown to cause disease, but it may predispose and complicate numerous serious health problems, including diabetes, digestive disease, arthritis, cerebral hemorrhage, difficulty in breathing, angina pectoris, circulatory collapse, varicose veins, hypertension, kidney disease, infertility, and dermatologic problems. Obesity lowers sexual drives and is connected with complications of pregnancy and premature aging. Obesity accounts for many psychological and social problems such as low self-esteem and discrimination in sports, school, and jobs.

PROGRESS CHECK ON ACTIVITY 2

Questions

True/False

Circle T for True and F for False.

1. T **F** The term "obesity" is used to indicate excess body weight of 15 percent or more above ideal body weight.
2. **T** F Increasing the amount of energy expended for physical activity is a means of weight control.
3. **T** F The energy value of a weight reduction diet usually ranges between 1,000 and 1,500 calories, depending on individual size and need.
4. T **F** In the Exchange System of dietary control, foods listed in one group may be exchanged freely with foods listed in another group.
5. T **F** Between-meal snacks should never be eaten on a weight reduction diet.

For someone giving practical suggestions for persons on reduction diets, which of the following statements are true and which are false?

6. T **F** Purchase special low calorie foods and eat separately from the rest of the family.
7. **T** F Eat only from the Basic Four food plan in the amounts recommended to lose weight for most young adults.
8. **T** F Even when the diet plan is followed carefully, some weeks you will not show any weight loss.
9. T **F** Do not eat more than three meals per day.
10. **T** F Avoid dependence on appetite suppressants.
11. **T** F Personal adaptation to the diet plan is mandatory.
12. **T** F When eating in a restaurant, order single items instead of combinations.
13. T **F** Eat as much meat as you wish, but never eat carbohydrates.

Multiple Choice

Circle the letter of the correct answer.

14. Obesity as a health hazard increases the risk in which of the following diseases or conditions? (Circle all that apply.)
    a. hypertension
    b. diabetes
    c. heart disease
    d. cancer

15. A reduction of 1,000 calories in an obese person's daily diet would enable the individual to lose weight at which of the following rates?
    a. 1 lb. per week
    b. 2 lb. per week

c.   3 lb. per week
d.   4 lb. per week

16. Which of the following food portions has the lowest caloric value?
    a.   4 oz. lean meat
    b.   1/2 c. orange juice
    c.   one slice bread
    d.   one 8 oz. glass whole milk

17. In the Exchange System of diet management, which of the following foods may be exchanged for one slice of bread?
    a.   one scoop cottage cheese
    b.   one medium orange
    c.   3 c. of popcorn (popped)
    d.   one egg

18. In the Exchange System, which one of the following food items is "free" and therefore can be eaten as desired?
    a.   mustard
    b.   carrots
    c.   catsup
    d.   lean meat
    e.   orange juice

19. Which of the following foods is not a member of the meat exchange group?
    a.   poultry
    b.   eggs
    c.   cheese
    d.   peanut butter
    e.   bacon

20. In order to maintain ideal body weight, the energy value of the daily diet should (circle all that apply)
    a.   be equal to the energy used by the body at rest.
    b.   include the energy used in activities of daily living.
    c.   be controlled by appetite.
    d.   be controlled by medication.

21. A pound of adipose tissue has an energy value of
    a.   1,750 calories.
    b.   3,500 calories.
    c.   4,000 calories.
    d.   9,000 calories.

22. Sue's intake for a 24-hour period contained 190 g carbohydrate, 75 g protein, and 50 g fat. The energy value of her diet (rounded to nearest number) is
    a.   2,000 calories.
    b.   1,750 calories.
    c.   1,500 calories.
    d.   1,200 calories.

23. Sue's basic metabolic rate used 1,350 calories in 24 hours and her daily activities used 400 calories. If her energy intake (from question 22 above) remained the same for a week, and her energy output remained the same for a week, Sue should:
    a.   lose 1/2 lb.
    b.   gain 1/2 lb.
    c.   maintain her present weight.
    d.   lose 2 lb.

24. John has an 8 oz. glass of cola (which contains 100 calories) each day, in excess of his energy needs. If he continues this practice for one year, how much weight will he gain (round to nearest whole number)?
    a.   2 lb.
    b.   6 lb.
    c.   10 lb.
    d.   none

Situation

25. On October 1 Joe decides that he must lose 20 lb. before the next tennis meet scheduled for December 7. He begins a diet of 700 kcal per day reduction and plays an hour of active tennis every day (count active tennis as using 300 kcal per hour). Answer the following questions regarding this situation.
    a.   How many pounds per week will Joe lose if he continues his diet and exercise program?

    _____

    _____

    b.   Will Joe lose 20 lb. in time for the tennis meet?

    _____

    c.   How many pounds a week would Joe lose if he only increased his exercise to one hour per day and did not diet? _____

    _____

    d.   Would Joe lose 20 lb. in time for the meet by exercise alone? _____

ACTIVITY 3: Weight Control and Dieting

The best advice that one can give clients regarding weight control is to prevent the excess accumulation. The recommended approach is a controlled, but not deficient, eating pattern, combined with a regular exercise program. Weight problems are easier to correct when they begin to develop.

Waiting until excess weight accumulates over the years presents great difficulties. Simple monitoring of one's body weight and attention to the fit of clothing through the years can assist with weight control. Weighing should be done on the same scale weekly at the same time of day, without clothing on, so that the variables, and therefore excuses, are minimized. The practice of keeping some clothing (such as a uniform or other correctly fitted garment) and trying it on for size twice each year is another monitoring device.

Calories, Exercise, and Eating Habits

If a person is more than 10 percent below or above normal weight, a sensible caloric adjustment and exercise program should be considered. Situations beyond this overweight/underweight standard should be undertaken only on the advice of a physician and with guidance from a dietitian or nutritionist.

Behavior modification can be a useful tool in achieving and maintaining weight control. Reasons for the weight fluctuation can be identified and measures taken to change the situations or alter the behaviors that cause the problems. Behavior modification is also useful in weight maintenance once the desired weight has been reached, since a change in eating behaviors and activity is achieved over a long period of time and gives the dieter a chance to gain permanent control. An exercise program that is enjoyable is more likely to remain a part of the individual's lifestyle. While rewarding oneself for satisfactory weight loss or gain is recommended (positive reinforcement) in behavioral programs, the satisfaction that comes from improved appearance and attitude about self can be sufficiently motivating to require no additional reinforcement. The habit of daily exercise may require encouragement, support, and coercion to get started, but if the exercise program is done long enough, it becomes self-enforcing.

Guidelines for Dieting

Portion control, balanced menus meeting the RDAs, and judicious food preparation are the keys to successful dieting. Weight loss is most satisfactorily achieved by planning meals around nutritionally sound food guides. One guide that contains all of the recommendations is the food exchange lists for meal planning. These were discussed in Module 1 and the complete exchange lists appear in Appendix E. Table 3-4 uses these lists to prepare menu plans at 12 different caloric levels. Table 3-5 provides a sample menu for a 1,200 kcal diet using the exchange lists in Appendix E and Table 3-4.

A Multibillion Dollar Business

While Americans are extremely diet conscious, they are also extremely unwilling to make the effort required to diet for longer than a few days. Despite the simple logic that excess calorie intake leads to excess body weight, most people prefer to believe that there is a magic formula and an easy shortcut to weight control. It would be nice to believe that some of these combinations and concoctions could increase longevity, improve sexual prowess, prevent aging, and promote glamorous body images, but they do not. Many entertainers have capitalized on these hopes by implying that purchasing and using their health and beauty books or aids will fulfill all one's fantasies about looking good. The quacks and charlatans of the past were the first to discover the gullibility of the public and prey upon their superstitions and susceptibility. Lack of education regarding actual body needs and the utilization of foods has created a fertile field for misinformation. Some of this information is misleading and costly. Some of it is dangerous for health. The amount of money (over $10 billion per year) spent on these books and products could be used to educate and purchase nutritious foods for many people, thereby helping to truly alleviate weight problems.

Few government standards require information to be scientifically sound to be published, and so it is left to the consumer to distinguish between valid diet advice and literature containing little truth, aimed at a gullible public. A review of the number of diet books on the best-seller list indicates that the current trend seems to be in favor of the fad diet.

Potential health hazards should be appraised whenever a diet is chosen that varies considerably from the pattern of the Basic Four or guidelines for healthy eating. These diets will range from mildly to severely imbalanced, and thereby create an imbalance in the body's nutriture. Some consequences include altered metabolism, fluid and electrolyte imbalance, and deficits in essential nutrients. The more imbalanced, limited, or restricted in nutrients and energy a diet regime is, the greater the potential harm. Fortunately, most fad diets are so restrictive that many people adhere to them for only a few days. Documented deaths from these diets are increasing as more and more people become obsessed with thinness and wish to attain their weight goals in the shortest possible time.

While most of the fad diets are rejuvenated old schemes, many are new and use more sophisticated but still invalid approaches. Some of these fad diets are listed in Table 3-6. Below is a list of books approved by nutritionists for weight reduction.

List of Books Approved by Nutritionists for Weight Reduction

Altschul, A. M., ed. 1987. *Weight Control: A Guide for Counselors and Therapists.* New York: Greenwood Press.

Bennett, W. et al. 1983. *The Dieter's Dilemma.* New York: Basic Books.

Brownell, K. D. 1985. *The LEARN Program for Weight Control.* Philadelphia: University of Pennsylvania.

Byerly, L. et al. 1987. *Popular Diets: How They Rate*, 2nd ed. Santa Monica, CA: California Dietetic Association.

TABLE 3-4
Using the Food Exchange Lists to Prepare Menu Plans at 12 Different Caloric Levels

Food Type	Food Exchange List	Number of Exchanges Assigned to the Daily Permitted Number of Kilocalories											
		600	800	900	1,000	1,100	1,200	1,300	1,400	1,500	1,600	1,700	1,800
Breakfast													
Meat (medium fat)	2	1	1	1	1	1	1	1	1	1	1	1	1
Vegetables	3	0	0	0	0	0	0	0	0	0	0	0	0
Fruits	4	1	1	1	1	1	1	1	1	1	1	1	1
Bread	1	½	1	1	1	1	1	1	1	1	1	1	1
Milk (nonfat)	5	½	½	½	1	1	1	1	1	1	1	1	1
Fats	6	0	0	0	0	0	1	1	1	1	1	1	1
Lunch													
Meat (medium fat)	2	2	2	2	2	2	2	2	2	2	2	2	2
Vegetables*	3	1	1	1	1	1	1	1	1	1	1	1	1
Fruits	4	1	1	1	1	2	2	2	1	2	2	2	1
Bread	1	½	0	1	1	1	2	1	2	2	2	2	2
Milk (nonfaat)	5	0	½	½	½	½	½	½	½	½	½	½	½
Fats	6	0	0	0	0	0	0	1	1	1	2	2	2
Dinner													
Meat (medium fat)	2	2	2	2	2	2	2	2	3	3	3	3	3
Vegetables*	3	1	1	1	1	1	1	1	1	1	1	1	1
Fruits	4	1	1	1	1	1	1	1	1	1	1	1	2
Bread	1	0	1	0	0	1	1	2	2	2	2	2	2
Milk (nonfat)	5	0	0	½	½	½	½	½	½	½	½	1	1
Fats	6	0	0	0	0	0	0	1	1	2	2	2	2

*One of the two daily servings of vegetables must be raw and have few calories (see the exchange lists in Appendix E).
Adapted from A. Dean, *Home and Family Circle*, ext. bulletin 782, Cooperative Extension Service, Michigan State University and the food exchange lists in Appendix E.

TABLE 3-5
Sample Menu for a 1,200-kcal Diet Using the Exchanges in Table 3-4

Breakfast	Lunch	Dinner
½ c. orange juice	1 small boiled frankfurters	2 oz. broiled hamburger
1 poached egg	½ c. cooked green beans	½ c. cooked summer squash
1 slice toast	1 slice whole wheat toast	Sliced tomato on lettuce
1 tsp. margarine	1 medium tangerine	½ c. cooked rice
1 c. skim milk	1 small banana	1 small apple
Salt, pepper	½ c. skim milk	12 grapes
Coffee or tea	Salt, pepper	½ c. skim milk
	Coffee or tea	Salt, pepper
		Coffee or tea

Frankle, R. T. and Yang, M. U. 1988. *Obesity and Weight Control*. Rockville, MD: Aspen.

Frankle, R. T., ed. 1985. *Dietary Treatment and Prevention of Obesity*. London: Libbey.

Ikeda, J. 1987. *Winning Weight Loss for Teens*. Palo Alto, CA: Bull.

Mellin, L. 1987. *Shapedown: Just for Teens*. Larkspur, CA: Balboa.

Schartz, H. 1986. *Never Satisfied: A Cultural History of Diets, Fantasies, and Fat*. New York: Free Press.

Stare, F. J. and Whelan, E. M. 1987. *The Harvard Square Diet*. Buffalo, NY: Prometheus Books.

Stunkard, A. J. et al., ed. 1984. *Eating and Its Disorders*. New York: Raven Press.

The Basics of Physical Exercise

Increasing physical exercise is a healthful means of promoting weight maintenance. Even small amounts of physical activity performed regularly have impressive effects over a long period of time. Spending an extra 100 kcal per day in activity will result in a ten-pound weight loss in one year without any dieting.

Certain types of exercise (aerobic) can produce dramatic changes in weight. Jogging, brisk walking, rope jumping, and bicycling are examples of this type of exercise. Also, aerobic exercise can increase cardiovascular fitness, raise body metabolic rate, and decrease appetite

TABLE 3-6
Examples of Fad Diets

A. Advocating one particular type of food
   1. The Rice Diet
   2. The Banana Diet
   3. Candy Diet
   4. Grapefruit Diet
   5. Ice Cream Diet
   6. "Nova Scotia" Diet
   7. Vegetable and fruit diets
   8. Eating with Wine
   9. Yogurt Diet

B. Advocating a large protein intake
   1. Dr. Stillman's Quick Weight Loss Diet
   2. Dr. Stillman's Inches Off Diet
   3. New Diet Does It
   4. Lazy Lady Diet
   5. Ratio Diet

C. Advocating a low carbohydrate intake
   1. Carbo-Calorie Diet
   2. Carbo-Cal Diet
   3. Dr. Yudkin's Diet
   4. Drinking Man's Diet
   5. Air Force Diet
   6. Airline Pilots' Diet (Astronauts' Diet)

D. Advocating a low-carbohydrate, high-fat diet
   1. Dr. Atkin's Diet Revolution
   2. Calories Don't Count
   3. Eat, Drink and Get Thin
   4. Eat and Become Slim

E. Miscellaneous
   1. The Miracle Diet
   2. No Will Power Diet
   3. McCall's Snack Diet
   4. Zen Macrobiotic Diet
   5. Nine-Day Wonder Diet
   6. Olympia Diet
   7. Magic Formula-Plus Diet
   8. Miraculous Eggnog Diet
   9. Fabulous Formula Diet
   10. Counterweight Diet
   11. Working Man's Diet
   12. Amazing "New You" Diet
   13. Hambletonian Wonder-Week Diet
   14. Editor's Diet
   15. North Pole Slenderizing Plan
   16. Melon-Berry Diet
   17. Vinegar/Lecithin/B_6/Kelp Diet

(contrary to popular belief). It may lower cholesterol levels, and provides a healthy way to release tension. Coping with stress through exercise rather than overeating is a major means of weight control. Additional benefits of exercise are improved appearance as muscles are firmed and enhanced confidence and self-esteem. People who exercise regularly suggest that their thought processes and overall efficiency are improved.

Exercise should be undertaken slowly and, for the older person, with medical supervision. Exercise should never hurt; the axiom "no pain, no gain" is inaccurate. If exercise hurts, it is too strenuous and may injure the person. Mild regular exercise at a steady pace can be as effective as strenuous exercise, which can be traumatic for some. The former may become enjoyable as well as therapeutic.

Summary

A sedentary lifestyle for most Americans has decreased energy needs to the point where, if weight is to remain stable, total caloric intake should not exceed the BMR by more than a few hundred calories. The continual consumption of more calories than are expended results in obesity. It is necessary for people to understand that obesity is not a problem of fattening foods, but of total overconsumption of foods that contain calories. Weight control can be achieved by maintaining a balance between total calories consumed and those expended.

Eating a balanced diet of moderate proportions and exercising regularly are valuable for maintaining energy balance, once the balance has been achieved. The consequences of either excess or deficit energy can be severe and create or complicate conditions and disorders that shorten the life span.

Diets to achieve weight control need to be varied; foods should meet acceptable criteria for essential nutrients as well as psychological and aesthetic criteria. They should be lifetime diets. For optimum health, weight control should be established from early childhood. Crash diets, fraudulent and fad diets may be hazardous to one's health and should be avoided, and regular exercise should become a part of the plan to control body weight.

Although the disease continuum of obesity–anorexia nervosa is a complex phenomenon, the measures for promoting a healthy, stable, normal weight throughout the life span are simple and practical, once these principles are understood and practiced.

Responsibilities of Health Personnel

1. Follow and teach the principle that a balanced diet contains adequate nutrients and calories and maintains a stable weight.
2. Make accurate assessments and judgments regarding appropriate use of food and diets used for weight loss.
3. Recognize that malnutrition, whether due to an excess or deficit in nutrients and calories, must be resolved.
   a. Substitute appropriate foods if malnutrition is due to poor food choices.
   b. Be prepared to find resources when an inadequate food supply is the problem.

c. Recognize the impact of faulty body function or intake of drugs on nutrient intake and recommend appropriate steps.

4. Recognize the differences among overweight, overfat, and obese and be prepared to explain to others. Use a variety of tools to determine body fat.

5. Know the health risks of being underweight and be prepared to teach others how to gain weight while maintaining a quality diet.

6. Recognize the symptoms of anorexia nervosa and bulimia and seek appropriate referrals. Nursing personnel may be specially trained in this area and can work with psychiatrists and psychologists in the treatment of severe eating disorders.

7. Use techniques from the behavioral sciences to assist clients in controlling weight.

8. Explain the use of exercise in promoting stable body weight and relaxing tensions. Demonstrate some helpful exercises for different age groups.

9. Use and teach acceptable diet control methods which include use of a balanced diet, proper food preparation, portion control, and sound food guides for selection.

10. Educate yourself and others to the dangers and health hazards of the fad diets on the market today.

11. Evaluate all literature regarding reduction diets and the actual diets using scientific criteria.

12. Teach and practice basic principles of weight maintenance.

13. Evaluate all reduction diets carefully. Realize that there are countless diets for weight loss, and that most popular diets promise weight loss without deprivation.

14. Educate yourself and others of approved diets that are balanced and provide optimum nutrients for maintenance of health.

15. Encourage individuals who wish to lose weight to increase exercise at the same time as they reduce the quantity of food intake.

16. Advise clients that successful diet plans require adaptation to a new lifestyle that includes altered food intake and exercise.

17. Be aware that the best prescription for obesity is diet modification. The use of drugs and surgical procedures is dangerous and a last resort.

18. Promote low calorie diets that contain the essential nutrients in proper proportions. Diets should
   a. be based on the daily food guide
   b. contain a minimum of 1,200 kcal for women and 1,500 kcal for men
   c. follow the dietary guidelines for distribution of nutrients: 50 percent of total calories as complex carbohydrate, 20 percent as protein, and 30 percent as fat, with approximately half of the fat being unsaturated
   d. provide weight loss of 1 to 2 lb. per week

19. Advise clients to weigh themselves once per week. If exercise is undertaken, measurements may be more accurate than weighing.

20. Encourage the attitude that clients are adopting a more healthful diet instead of giving up certain foods.

21. Recognize the plateau periods in weight reduction and encourage the dieter to stay with the diet until the body readjusts.

22. Become familiar with behavior modification techniques for changing eating habits and assist clients to use those that work for them.

PROGRESS CHECK ON ACTIVITY 3

Questions

Multiple Choice

Circle the letter of the correct answer.

1. Behavior modification is an educational tool used to
   a. change people's eating habits.
   b. achieve weight control.
   c. maintain desired weight.
   d. all of the above.

2. Mary lost 10 lb. in 6 weeks and rewarded herself with a new blouse. This is an example of
   a. pampering oneself.
   b. negative reinforcement.
   c. positive reinforcement.
   d. self-gratification.

3. Aerobic exercise is defined as
   a. exercise performed inside a building.
   b. exercise that causes sweating.
   c. exercise that increases oxygen intake.
   d. exercise that is strenuous.

Fill-in

4. List 3 potential health hazards of unbalanced diet regimes.
   a. Altered Metabolism
   b. Fluid & Electrolyte imbalance
   c. Nutritional Deficiet

True/False

5. T F Although the Grapefruit Diet is unbalanced, Dr. Stillman's "Inches Off" diet should be all right for weight reduction.

6. T F Entertainers cannot afford to offer poor nutrition advice for fear of lawsuits.

7. T F The major reason for misinformation is lack of education.

8. T F It is possible to lose weight without dieting if you exercise regularly.

References

Altshul, A. M. (ed.). 1987. *Weight control: A guide for counselors and therapists*. New York: Greenwood Press.

Anderson, G. H. 1988. Metabolic regulation of food intake. In *Modern nutrition in health and disease*, 7th ed. M. E. Shils and V. R. Young (eds.). Philadelphia: Lea & Febiger.

Atkinson, R. L. et al. 1984. A comprehensive approach to outpatient obesity management. *Journal of the American Dietetic Association* 84(4):4398.

Bender, A. E., and L. J. Brookes (eds.). 1987. *Body weight control: The physiology, clinical treatment and prevention of obesity*. New York: Basic Books.

Bennett, W. et al. 1983. *The dieter's dilemma*. New York: Basic Books.

Berry, E. M. et al. (eds.). 1987. Recent advances in obesity research: V. *Proceedings of the 5th International Congress on Obesity*. London: John Libbey.

Boakes, et al. 1987. *Eating habits, food, physiology, and learned behavior*. New York: Wiley.

Bourne, G. H. (ed.). 1987. *Energy, nutrition of women*. New York: Karger.

Brownwell, K. 1988. The yo-yo trap. *American Health* 7(2):78.

Brownwell, K. D., and J. P. Fore (eds.). 1986. *Handbook of eating disorders: Physiology, psychology, and treatment of obesity, anorexia, and bulimia*. New York: Basic Books.

Bursztein, S. et al. 1989. *Energy metabolism, indirect calorimetry, and nutrition*. Baltimore: Williams & Wilkins.

Byerly, L. et al. 1987. *Popular diets: How they rate*, 2nd ed. Santa Monica, CA: California Dietetic Association.

Fenhouse, D. 1987. The OPTIFAST Program: A viable treatment for obesity. *Topics in Clinical Nutrition* 2(2):69.

Fisher, M. C. et al. 1985. Nutrition evaluation of published weight-reducing diets. *Journal of the American Dietetic Association* 85(4):450.

Fomon, S. J., and W. C. Heird (eds.). 1986. Energy and protein needs during infancy. *Bristol-Myers Nutrition Symposia*. Vol. 4. Orlando, FL: Academic Press.

Food and Nutrition Board, National Research Council, National Academy of Sciences. 1989. *Recommended dietary allowances*, 10th ed. Washington, DC: National Academy Press.

Forbes, G. B. 1988. Body composition: Influence of nutrition, disease, growth, and aging. In *Modern nutrition in health and disease*, 7th ed. M. E. Shils and V. R. Young, eds. Philadelphia: Lea & Febiger.

Fox, S. I. 1987. *Human physiology*, 2nd ed. Dubuque, IA: W. C. Brown.

Frankle, R. T., and M. U. Yang. 1988. *Obesity and weight control*. Rockville, MD: Aspen.

Frankle, R. T. (ed.). 1985. *Dietary treatment and prevention of obesity*. London: Libbey.

Ikeda, J. 1987. *Winning weight loss for teens*. Palo Alto, CA: Bull.

Jequier, E. 1987. Energy, obesity, and body weight standards. *American Journal of Clinical Nutrition* 45(Supplement):1035.

Kinney, J. M. et al. (eds.). 1988. *Nutrition and metabolism in patient care*. Philadelphia: Saunders.

Konstat, D. A. 1988. USDA fat-measuring meter to be made commercially. *Journal of the American Dietetic Association* 88(4):486.

Lukaski, H. C. 1987. Methods for the assessment of human body composition: Traditional and new. *American Journal of Clinical Nutrition* 46:537.

Martin, R. J. et al. 1987. Control of food intake: Mechanisms and consequences. *Nutrition Today* 22(5):4.

McArdle, W. D. et al. 1986. *Exercise physiology: Energy, nutrition, and human performance*, 2nd ed. Philadelphia: Lea & Febiger.

Mellin, L. 1987. *Shapedown: Just for teens*. Larkspur, CA: Balboa.

Nash, J. D. 1987. Eating behavior and body weight: Physiologic influences. *American Journal of Health Promotion* 1:5.

Weighley, E. S. 1984. Average? Ideal? Desirable? A brief review of height-weight tables in the United States. *Journal of the American Dietetic Association* 84:417.

Woo, R. et al. 1985. Regulation of energy balance. *Annual Review of Nutrition* 5:411.

Wright, E. D. et al. 1988. Physical exercise and energy requirements. *Clinical Nutrition* 7(1):9.

Module 4

Carbohydrates and Fats: Implications for Health

Time for completion

Activities: _____1_____ hour

Optional examination: _½_ hour

Academic credit

Semester units: _²⁄₁₀_

Quarter units: _³⁄₁₀_

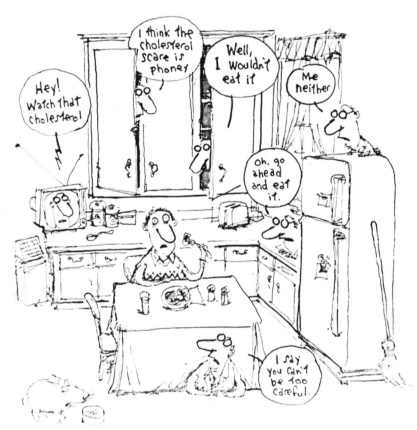

Outline

Objectives

Carbohydrates and Health

Upon completion of this module the student should be able to:

1. Identify the types of carbohydrates, their fuel value, and storage methods.
2. Summarize the major functions and food sources of carbohydrates.
3. Discuss nutritive and nonnutritive sweeteners.
4. Evaluate blood glucose level as an indicator of certain body conditions.
5. Define fiber and list its functions and food sources.
6. Discuss health problems associated with excess sugar or low fiber intake.
7. Describe the effects of carbohydrate consumption on athletic activity.

Fats and Health

Upon completion of this module the student should be able to:

1. Classify fats and state their fuel value.
2. List the major functions and food sources of fats.
3. Discuss body utilization of essential fatty acids and cholesterol.
4. Explain the difference between saturated and unsaturated fatty acids and identify their food sources.
5. Evaluate storage of fat in the body and the relationship of fat to normal body weight.
6. Relate a body's health to excess total fat intake and excess saturated fat intake.

Glossary

Carbohydrates

Cellulose: a fibrous form of carbohydrate that makes up the framework of a plant. A component of fiber.

Complex carbohydrates: a class of carbohydrates called polysaccharides; foods composed of starch and cellulose.

Diabetes mellitus: a condition characterized by an elevated level of sugar in blood and urine, increased urination, and increased intake of both fluid and food, with an absolute or relative insulin deficiency. Complications include heart disease, high blood pressure, and kidney disease. Diabetes can cause blindness and is frequently associated with severe infections.

Fiber: a group of compounds that make up the framework of plants. Fiber includes the carbohydrate substances (cellulose, hemicellulose, gums, and pectin) and a noncarbohydrate substance called lignin. These compounds are not digested by the human digestive tract.

Glycogen: the form in which carbohydrate is stored in humans and animals.

Insulin: a hormone secreted by the pancreas that is necessary for the proper metabolism of blood sugar.

Ketosis: an accumulation of ketone bodies from partly digested fats due to inadequate carbohydrate intake.

Lactose intolerance: a condition in which the body is deficient in lactase, the enzyme needed to digest lactose (the sugar in milk). Leads to abdominal bloating, gas, and watery diarrhea. Affects 70 to 75 percent of blacks, almost all Orientals, and 5 to 10 percent of whites.

"Naturally occurring" sugars: sugars found in foods in their natural state; for example, sugar occurs naturally in grapes and other fruits.

Refined food: food that undergoes many commercial processes resulting in the loss of nutrients in the food.

Fats

Atherosclerosis: thickening of the inside wall of the arteries by fatty deposits, resulting in plaques that narrow the arteries and hinder blood flow. Can lead to heart disease.

Bile salts: the substance from the gallbladder that breaks fats into small particles for digestion.

Cholesterol: a fatlike compound occurring in bile, blood, brain and nerve tissue, liver, and other parts of the body. Cholesterol comes from animal foods and is used by the body for the synthesis of necessary tissues and fluids. Cholesterol is also found in plaques that line the inner wall of the artery in atherosclerosis.

Fatty acids: the basic unit of all fats. Essential fatty acids are those that cannot be produced by the body and must be obtained in the diet. A saturated fatty acid is one in which the fatty acids contain all the hydrogen they can hold. A monounsaturated fatty acid is one into which hydrogen can be added at one double bond. Polyunsaturated fatty acids have two or more double bonds into which hydrogen can be added.

Hydrogenation: the addition of hydrogen to a liquid fat, changing it to a solid or semisolid state. Generally, the harder the product, the higher the degree of saturation with hydrogen.

Lipoproteins: transport form of fat (attached to a protein) in the bloodstream.

Satiety value: a food's ability to produce a feeling of fullness.

Background Information

Carbohydrates

Carbohydrates are the most abundant organic substances on earth, comprising approximately 70 percent of plant structure. They are the main source of the body's energy.

In the United States, about 50 percent of dietary energy comes from carbohydrates. This level of intake is considered acceptable, but the type of carbohydrates consumed has caused concern among health professionals. Although both starches and sugars are carbohydrates, they differ in food sources and nutrient values. Starches are mainly found in vegetables, breads, and cereals. They provide protein, vitamins, minerals, water, and calories. Sugars, on the other hand, furnish only calories and no nutrients. They are derived from sugar cane and sugar beets. The typical Western diet contains more carbohydrates from sugary foods than from starches. The government guidelines for healthy eating strongly recommend the reverse. Fiber, another plant component, is also an important carbohydrate. Although it neither furnishes energy nor is digestible, it is important for health. All plant foods contain fiber and we obtain it mainly from cereal grains, especially unrefined ones.

Fats

Fats, chemically termed lipids, are also organic compounds. They are insoluble in water. Most fat in the diet is in the form known as triglycerides. Fats differ in chemical structure from carbohydrates, though both contain carbon, hydrogen, and oxygen. Based on their chemical bonding arrangements, fats can be saturated, monounsaturated, or unsaturated. Many different properties of fats are determined by the degree of saturation.

The typical Western diet derives approximately 38 to 40 percent of its total daily calories from fats, mainly saturated fats. Ninety percent of fats in the American diet come from fats and oils, meat, poultry, fish, and dairy products. We are presently advised to eat about 30 percent of our total daily calories from fat, with at least 10 percent in unsaturated forms.

Dietary fats are important because they serve as stored energy reserves and as carriers of essential fatty acids and fat-soluble vitamins. Fats must combine with bile from the gallbladder to be digested. Since they are not soluble in water, they must attach themselves to proteins before they can travel through the intestinal walls, lymph system, and bloodstream. From the bloodstream they are delivered to body tissues.

Cholesterol, which is a cross between fat and alcohol, is derived both from foods and body synthesis. Though much maligned because of its implication in heart disease, cholesterol is an important body component and is transported by low-density or high-density lipoproteins in body circulation. Lipoproteins are discussed in Module 14 in relation to cardiovascular disease and will not be explored here.

ACTIVITY 1: Carbohydrates: Characteristics and Effects on Health

Definitions and Classification

Carbohydrates are composed of carbon, hydrogen, and oxygen. Sugars, starches, and fiber are the main forms in which carbohydrates occur in food. Starches and sugars are the major source of body energy. They are the cheapest and most easily used form of fuel for the body. Fibrous materials provide bulk and aid digestion. Although most carbohydrates occur in plant foods, a few are of animal origin. These include glycogen, which is stored in the liver and muscle as a small reserve supply, and lactose, a sugar found in milk.

Carbohydrates are classified as monosaccharides (simple sugars), disaccharides (double sugars), and polysaccharides (mainly starches). All carbohydrates must be reduced to simple sugars (monosaccharides) in the intestine before they can be absorbed into the bloodstream. Glucose, a simple sugar, is the form in which carbohydrates circulate in the bloodstream. Glucose is commonly referred to as blood sugar. Table 4-1 classifies carbohydrates according to their chemical structures.

The nutrients and calories contributed by different carbohydrates vary. For example, whole grains, enriched cereal products, fruits, and vegetables provide vitamins, minerals, fiber, and energy. Sugars, sweets, and unenriched refined cereals provide calories only.

TABLE 4-1
Classification of Carbohydrates

Carbohydrates	
Starches	Sugars
Kinds and Sources	Kinds and Sources
Polysaccharides	**Monosaccharides**
1. Starch—cereals grains vegetables	1. Glucose—blood sugar
	2. Fructose—sugar found in fruit
2. Dextrin—digestion product infant formula	3. Galactose—digestion product
3. Cellulose*—stems, leaves coverings seeds skins, hulls	**Disaccharides**
	1. Sucrose—table sugar
4. Pectin*—fruits	2. Lactose—sugar found in milk
5. Glycogen—muscle and liver	3. Maltose—germinating seed

*Nondigestible.

Functions

Energy Source

Carbohydrates are the most economical and efficient source of energy. They furnish 4 kcal/g of energy. The body requires a constant source of energy to support its vital functions.

Protein-Sparing Action

Carbohydrates prevent protein from being used as energy. Carbohydrate, protein, and fat can all be used to produce energy. However, the body utilizes carbohydrate first. When not enough carbohydrate is present, the body uses protein and fat for its energy needs. Thus, an adequate amount of carbohydrate can spare protein which can then be used for tissue building and repair rather than energy.

Special Functions

Under normal conditions, the tissues of the central nervous system (especially the brain) can use only glucose as an energy source. Muscles can use either glucose or fats as fuel. Body fat is used by the muscles only during exercise.

Some carbohydrate is needed for the proper utilization of fat. In the absence of carbohydrate, fats are not completely burned, and ketosis results (see later discussion). Severe restriction of carbohydrate in reducing diets can cause ketosis, which can produce adverse effects.

Carbohydrates are important components of certain substances needed for regulating body processes. They also encourage the growth of beneficial bacteria involved in the production of certain vitamins and in the absorption of calcium and phosphorus.

They also provide fiber, which promotes normal functioning of the lower intestinal tract. Lack of fiber is believed to contribute to many health problems.

Blood Glucose

The form of carbohydrate used by the body is a monosaccharide, glucose. All forms of carbohydrate except fiber eventually are broken down by the body to glucose. Glucose is the form of sugar found in the blood and its control at normal blood levels is important to health. Without sufficient glucose, the body will use its protein to make glucose, since the brain requires glucose to function. This diverts protein from its important functions of building and repairing tissues. When carbohydrate is insufficient, the body metabolizes fat differently to produce ketosis as described above. Ketosis is a condition in which unusual byproducts of fat breakdown (known as ketons) accumulate in the blood. Ketosis during pregnancy can result in brain damage and irreversible mental retardation in the infant. Some experts suggest that ketosis is potentially dangerous for all adults.

Blood glucose levels vary. Normal levels range between 70 to 120 mg per 100 ml of blood. When blood sugar is less than 70 mg, hunger occurs. After eating, blood sugar levels normally rise. The beta cells in the pancreas respond to the increase by secreting insulin. Insulin causes the liver, muscle, and fat cells to increase their uptake of sugar, which in turn reduces the blood sugar levels to normal. The glucose entering the cells is then converted to glycogen or fat or is used for energy if the body needs it. Insulin also assists in regulating the metabolism of fat by the body.

Insulin is the only hormone that directly lowers blood sugar levels. If there is insufficient production of insulin by the pancreas, or if it is unavailable, the blood cannot be cleared of excess glucose. This condition is hyperglycemia, the term used to describe blood glucose levels above the normal range. It occurs in diabetes mellitus. This abnormal response to glucose can sometimes be controlled by diet therapy and weight control, but in certain types of diabetes, insulin may have to be administered to help lower blood glucose levels.

When blood glucose drops below the normal limits, the condition is called hypoglycemia. Symptoms of hypoglycemia vary, depending on blood sugar level. Early symptoms produce weakness, dizziness, hunger, trembling, and mental confusion. If the levels drop very low, convulsions or unconsciousness may occur. Although it can occur, as a spontaneous reaction in some people, most often it happens when a diabetic uses excess insulin and/or has not eaten for a long period. A glucose tolerance test will determine true hypoglycemia. People who are not diabetic but are sensitive to changes in blood sugar levels should follow a calculated diet much the same as a diabetic, avoiding sweets and eating regular balanced meals.

Sources, Storage, Sweeteners, and Intake

The major food sources of carbohydrate are plants, which vary in the amounts of sugar and starches they provide. Milk and milk products containing lactose are the only significant animal sources of carbohydrates. Food sources of carbohydrate include cereal grains, fruits, vegetables, nuts, milk, and concentrated sweets. Table 4-2 compares the carbohydrate content (starch, sugar, and fiber content) of selected foods.

Nutritive sweeteners provide calories. Examples include sugar, honey, molasses, and syrup (corn, maple). The most common is table sugar, which comes from sugar beets or sugar cane. Table sugar is sucrose, two simple sugars chemically joined. Sugar can be white or brown. White sugar contains mainly sucrose. Brown sugar contains trace amounts of protein, minerals, vitamins, water, and pigment in addition to sucrose.

TABLE 4-2
Carbohydrate Content of Some Selected Foods

Food	Serving Size	Carbohydrate Content
Milk	1 c.	12 g
Cheddar cheese	1 oz.	Trace
Creamed cottage cheese	½ c.	3 g
Grapefruit	½ c.	15 g
Banana	1	30 g
Dried prunes	5 large	29 g
Bread	1 slice	15 g
Oatmeal, cooked	½ c.	15 g
Cornflakes	¾ c.	15 g
Macaroni	½ c.	15 g
Rice	½ c.	15 g
Asparagus	½ c.	3 g
Mashed potato	½ c.	15 g
Split peas	½ c.	21 g
Peanut butter	2 tbsp.	6 g
Walnuts	¼ c.	5 g
Sunflower seeds	¼ c.	7 g
Sugar	1 tbsp.	12 g
Yellow cake with icing	⅟₁₆th 8" cake	40 g
Apple pie	⅟₇th 9" pie	51 g

Source: Nutritive Value of Foods, USDA Home and Garden Bulletin No. 72, Washington, DC: U.S. Department of Agriculture, 1981.

Synthetic sweeteners are nonnutritive and furnish no calories. They have been used for many years by diabetics and dieters. Since 1969 saccharin was the only legal nonnutritive sweetener until the recent availability of aspartame. Cyclamates were used until 1969, when they were banned because they were shown to cause bladder cancer in rats. Since the consumption of artificially sweetened beverages and foods has increased drastically in recent years, the Food and Drug Administration (FDA) is studying saccharin and aspartame carefully. Aspartame is made from the amino acids aspartic acid and phenylalanine. Although it is on the GRAS (generally recognized as safe) list, precautions are advised about the use of aspartame by pregnant women and young children. Other people may be sensitive to aspartame and should avoid using it.

In general, carbohydrate stores in the body are small. Carbohydrate in excess of the body's energy needs is stored in limited amounts in the liver and muscle. Most excess is converted to fat and stored as such. Less than one pound is stored as glycogen. This amount can furnish energy for 12 to 24 hours. However, the excess converted to fat can be stored in unlimited amounts in the body.

A carbohydrate deficiency leads to a loss of muscle tissue as protein is burned to meet energy and glucose needs. In addition, fats are incompletely broken down and a condition of ketosis results. Prolonged carbohydrate deficiencies can cause damage to the liver. Low fiber diets are associated with constipation and are linked to colon cancer. Scientists now recommend that 50 to 60 percent of the daily caloric intake be from carbohydrate foods, especially the complex carbohydrates (starches).

Of the classes of carbohydrate, sugars and sweets are the least desirable. Overconsumption of sugar promotes dental caries and frequently leads to a poor nutritional quality diet. Table 4-3 shows the sugar content of some popular foods. Diabetes mellitus and lactose intolerance are examples of diseases in which carbohydrates are not utilized normally by the body.

Athletic Activities

Contrary to popular opinion, athletes do not need special diets, supplements, formulas, concoctions, or excess protein intakes. Except for an increased energy requirement, athletes require the same basic nutrients that all people require. The amount of energy expended in training and competition determines the amount of food needed.

The recommended distribution of nutrients for anyone is 50 to 60 percent of daily caloric intake from carbohydrate, 15 to 20 percent from protein, and 30 to 35 percent from fat. If energy needs increase, the distribution should remain the same, with the size of individual portions being increased to meet the requirements.

Since protein RDA for adults is 0.8 g per kg of body weight, athletes have the same RDA unless they are still growing with increasing muscle mass or are prone to repeated injuries. Examples include teenage athletes and football or hockey players. An increase of 1 to 1.5 g protein per kg body weight may be needed in these circumstances. Athletes have the same need for fats as nonathletes. Increasing protein (and fats) in the diet will not improve performance and may actually hinder it. The high protein, low carbohydrate diet frequently recommended to athletes can lead to ketosis, dehydration, diarrhea, and other unhealthy conditions.

Carbohydrates are the most efficient energy source for both athletes and nonathletes and, as such, should be used to meet their need for increased energy. Athletes' carbohydrate needs are better met through extensive use of grains, fruits, and vegetables instead of sugary foods. For the body to convert foods into energy, certain vitamins and minerals are necessary. These are found only in nutrient-dense foods, not in candies and other sweets. Athletes, including those playing in cold weather, do not require extra vitamins if their diet is balanced. Excess vitamins will be excreted if they are water-soluble and stored if fat-soluble. Stored fat-soluble vitamins can be toxic.

Athletes in general have less body fat than nonathletes, but if they consume more calories than they expend, they will be overweight. The low carbohydrate fad diets are not recommended for weight loss since they can cause de-

TABLE 4-3
Sugar Content of Selected Foods

Food	g/100 g Food		
	Glucose	Sucrose	Total
Bakery products			
Chocolate chip cookies	0.7	22.2	25.0
Beverages			
Cola	4.1	2.1	10.6
Dairy products			
Vanilla ice cream	–	–	22.4
Fast food			
Cheeseburger	1.9	0.1	5.1
Fruits and fruit juices			
Apples, raw	2.3	3.3	13.3
Orange juice, canned	5.3	0.7	10.6
Grains and cereals			
Cornflakes, ready-to-eat	1.4	2.6	6.8
Macaroni, cooked	0.3	0.3	1.3
Legumes			
Lentils, cooked	0.0	0.0	1.8
Meat and poultry products			
Beef, corned	0.1	0.6	0.7
Nuts and seeds			
Pistachios, dried, shelled	0.2	0.1	6.6
Sugar and sweets			
Chocolate, dark, sweet	0.1	48.5	48.7
Vegetables			
Broccoli, raw	0.6	No data	2.0
Squash, raw	0.9	No data	2.2
Miscellaneous			
Dressing, cole slaw	4.5	13.2	21.4

Source: Matthews, R. H. et al. 1987. Sugar content of selected foods: Individual and total sugars. USDA/HNIS Home Economics Research Report No. 48. Washington, DC: United States Department of Agriculture.

creased muscular strength and work performance. The body burns its protein tissues for energy when no carbohydrate is available. If an athlete needs to gain weight, he or she needs to eat large food portions and snacks that are high in all major nutrients. Fast weight gain is usually all water and fat, not muscle. Remember, 1 lb. of fat contains 3,500 calories, but 1 lb. of muscle contains less than 1,900 calories.

For athletes, water is the nutrient most often lost and most easily restored. During prolonged heavy exertion, water should be replaced. The practice of using high electrolyte solutions is unnecessary, since the lost electrolytes can be replaced with an adequate diet and regular fluids.

The practice of carbohydrate loading can be risky. It should not be used for the adolescent or preadolescent groups and is dangerous to those with diabetes or high blood fat levels.

Health Implications

Health risks are associated with excessive sugar consumption, but it is difficult to make positive correlations between sugar consumption and the development of many diseases that have been linked to it. Included among the associations of sugar and health problems are:

1. *Obesity.* Sugar is often named as being the cause of obesity. If persons are obese, they certainly have consumed excess calories. It is probably an overall excess intake rather than sugar alone. Sugar is usually curtailed in reduction diets along with fats and alcohol because such foods contribute mainly calories.

2. *Cardiovascular disease.* Except for certain types of lipid disorder, in which an individual exhibits abnormal glucose tolerance along with an elevation of blood triglycerides, research studies cannot prove any correlation between sugar intake and cardiovascular disorder. Obesity is probably more closely related to this disorder than a high sugar consumption.

3. *Diabetes.* The cause of the malfunction of the pancreas is not known, but heredity plays a role as well as obesity. The chance of becoming diabetic more than doubles for every 20 percent of excess weight, according to the U.S. National Diabetes Commission. While studies have shown that the incidence of diabetes rose in population groups that "westernized" and started consuming excess sugary foods, most researchers agree that individuals have become fat from excess calories, not just sugar.

4. *Dental caries.* Carbohydrates, especially sugar, play a role in tooth decay. Sucrose is especially implicated. The frequency of eating sugar, sweets, and similar snacks is more damaging than the amount eaten in one sitting. Good oral hygiene (brushing after meals) helps prevent dental caries. The general state of health also influences susceptibility to caries.

5. *Cancer.* Population group studies have not linked nonnutritive sweeteners to cancer. Certain groups with increased susceptibility to bladder cancer include some heavy saccharine users. This correlation is also associated with heavy cigarette smokers. At present, the use of saccharine is in a "suspended" status—that is, if new data show definitive hazards, the use of this substance will be banned.

6. *Fiber.* Low fiber diets are believed to play a major role in the onset of diverticulosis and may contribute to appendicitis. The added pressure in the colon caused by a low fiber intake may increase the occurrence of hemorrhoids, varicose veins, and hiatal hernia. Colon cancer has been linked to low fiber diets, but the relationship is not clear. There are several theories regarding the cause and effect relationships, but at the present time the general recommendation is to maintain a balanced diet with ample intake of fiber and fluids. No RDA has been set for fiber, but 15 g/day is recommended in "Healthy People 2000."

PROGRESS CHECK ON ACTIVITY 1

Questions

Fill-in

1. Using meal planning food exchange lists in the appendix, rank the following foods by carbohydrate content, beginning with the food that has the most carbohydrate. If two foods have the same value, give them the same number.

    _4_ a. 1 orange
    _2_ b. 1 c. whole kernel corn
    _1_ c. 1/10 of a devil's food cake with icing (from a mix)
    _3_ d. 1 slice wheat bread
    _5_ e. 1/2 c. zucchini squash
    _3_ f. 1/2 c. cooked oatmeal

2. Rank the following vegetables by carbohydrate content, beginning with the one that has the most carbohydrate. If two foods have the same value, give them the same number.

    _3_ a. 1/2 c. green beans, cooked
    _3_ b. 1/2 c. cooked carrots
    _2_ c. 1 baked potato
    _1_ d. 1 sweet potato
    _4_ e. 1 stalk broccoli
    _5_ f. 1/2 c. lettuce, chopped

3. If a person's carbohydrate intake is greater than his or her energy needs, what happens to the excess? ____
    STORED AS FAT

4. What is the function of fiber in the diet? _____
    PROMOTE good bowel elimination

5. Name three good food sources of fiber.
    a. Fruits, Veg.
    b. whole grain
    c. Bran.

6. Name two health problems related to overconsumption of sugar.
    a. Obesity
    b. cavities.

7. Why are diets that severely restrict carbohydrates dangerous? A RISK of ketosis dehydration, diarrhea + loss of muscle mass.

Multiple Choice

Circle the letter of the correct answer.

8. If a 2,000 kcal/day diet derives approximately 1,000 kcal from carbohydrates, how many grams of carbohydrate does that diet contain?
    a. 150 g
    b. 200 g
    c. 250 g
    d. 400 g

9. Identify the trend in food consumption in the United States that has occurred since the turn of the century.
    a. Potato consumption has continued to increase.
    b. Consumption of refined sugar and processed sugar products has increased.
    c. Fruit and vegetable consumption has greatly increased.
    d. Consumption of cereals has greatly increased.

10. Cellulose is a _____ carbohydrate.
    a. digestible
    b. nondigestible
    c. disaccharide
    d. processed

11. Which two of the following food groups contain the greatest amounts of cellulose and other food fiber?
    a. meat and dairy products
    b. whole grain cereals
    c. fruit juices
    d. raw fruits and vegetables

12. Which of the following represent blood sugar levels within the normal range?
    a. 30 to 60 mg per 100 ml
    b. 70 to 120 mg per 100 ml
    c. 140 to 160 mg per 100 ml
    d. 100 to 120 mg per 100 ml

13. Insulin is secreted by the
    a. alpha cells of the pancreas.
    b. beta cells of the pancreas.
    c. nephron of the kidney.
    d. digestive cells in the intestinal wall.

14. From the items below, choose the snack which is the least caries-producing.
    a. plain popcorn and an apple
    b. taffy and raisins
    c. noodles with butter
    d. sherbet and 7-Up float

15. Carbohydrates are the raw materials that we eat mainly as
    a. starches and sugars.
    b. proteins and fats.
    c. plants and animals.
    d. pectin and cellulose.

16. Carbohydrates provide one of the main fuel sources for energy. Which of the following carbohydrate foods provides the quickest source of energy?
    a. slice of bread
    b. glass of orange juice
    c. chocolate candy bar
    d. glass of milk

17. Chemical digestion of carbohydrates is completed in the small intestine by enzymes from the
    a. pancreas and gallbladder.
    b. gallbladder and liver.
    c. small intestine and pancreas.
    d. liver and small intestine.

18. The refined fuel glucose is delivered to the cells by the blood for production of energy. The hormone controlling use of glucose by the cells is

a. thyroxin.
b. growth hormone.
c. adrenal steroid.
d. insulin.

Matching

Match the phrases on the right with the terms on the left that they best describe.

19. Insulin
20. Hyperglycemia
21. Glycemia
22. Hypoglycemia
23. Glucagon

a. hormone which causes the release of glucose into the blood
b. means glucose in the blood
c. means low blood glucose levels
d. means high blood glucose levels
e. hormone that affects the uptake of glucose from the blood into various body cells

Match the carbohydrate in Column A to its type in Column B. Terms may be used more than once.

Column A	Column B
24. Sucrose	a. polysaccharide
25. Glucose	b. monosaccharide
26. Glycogen	c. disaccharide
27. Lactose	
28. Grains	
29. Fructose	
30. Cellulose	

ACTIVITY 2: Fats: Characteristics and Effects on Health

Dietary Fats and Health _____

In the last 10 years, many studies have improved our understanding of the role of nutrition in health promotion and disease prevention. Diet is associated with a number of chronic diseases, such as cardiovascular disease, diabetes, and cancer. The focus has changed to maintenance of health. As a result, the Public Health Service set national nutrition objectives for 1990, which included a segment on lowering fats and cholesterol in the diet. Major objectives were lowering of mean cholesterol levels of the adult population 18–74 years of age to levels at or below 200 mg/dl, and of children aged 1–14, to levels at or below 150 mg/dl. A second major objective included measures whereby 70 percent of adults could identify major foods that were low in fat content (as well as high in calories and sugars and good sources of fiber).

In addition, the U.S. Department of Health and Human Services has done a major study on high blood cholesterol in adults and has begun a national cholesterol education program. The general aim of this program is to reduce elevated cholesterol levels while maintaining a nutritionally adequate diet. The ultimate goal is lowering LDL-cholesterol, but the first priority is bringing the total cholesterol down to appropriate levels. If persons have normal levels, the goal is to keep them in their optimum range, since studies have shown that cholesterol levels tend to increase with age. Primarily, this is due to lifestyle, such as lack of exercise, smoking, eating high-fat diets, and gaining excess weight. Diet therapy for clinical management of high cholesterol is further discussed in the module on cardiovascular disease.

Definitions and Food Sources _____

Although both fats and carbohydrates contain carbon, hydrogen, and oxygen, fats are entirely different compounds from carbohydrates because of their chemical structures. Foods that contribute fat to the diet include whole milk and milk products containing whole milk or butterfat, such as butter, ice cream, and cheese; egg yolk;

meat, fish, and poultry; nuts and seeds; vegetable oils; and hydrogenated vegetable fats (shortenings and margarine).

A fat is classified as saturated, monounsaturated, or polyunsaturated according to the type of fatty acids it contains in greatest quantity. Saturated food fats are generally solid at room temperature and come from animal sources. Saturated fats are found in whole milk and products made from whole milk; egg yolk; meat; meat fat (bacon, lard); coconut oil and palm oil; chocolate; regular margarine; and hydrogenated vegetable shortenings. Unsaturated food fats are generally liquid at room temperature and come from plant sources. They can be monounsaturated or polyunsaturated. Sources of polyunsaturated fats are safflower, sunflower, corn, cottonseed, soybean, and sesame oil; salad dressings made from these oils; special margarines that contain a high percentage of such oils; and fatty fish such as mackerel, salmon, and herring. Sources of monounsaturated fats are olive oil and most nuts. Diets rich in saturated fat and/or cholesterol can lead to elevated blood cholesterol levels. Polyunsaturated and monounsaturated fats appear to lower blood cholesterol level.

Cholesterol is a fatlike substance (lipid) that is a key component of cell membranes and a precursor of bile acids and steroid hormones. Cholesterol travels in the circulation in spherical particles containing both lipids and proteins called lipoproteins. A lipoprotein is made up of fats (cholesterol, triglycerides, fatty acids, etc.), protein, and a small amount of other substances. The cholesterol level in blood plasma is determined partly by inheritance and partly by the fat and cholesterol content of the diet. Other factors, such as obesity and physical inactivity, may also play a role.

Organ meats and egg yolk are very rich sources of cholesterol; shrimp is a moderately rich source. Other sources include meat, fish, poultry, whole milk, and foods made from whole milk or butterfat. Table 4-4 describes the fat and cholesterol content of representative foods. Both saturated fats and cholesterol are believed to be important to our health. Consumers should not be misled by "low cholesterol" labels on food packages, which imply that cholesterol alone plays a role in our health.

Three major classes of lipoproteins can be measured in the serum of a fasting individual: very low density lipoproteins (VLDL), low density lipoproteins (LDL), and high density lipoproteins (HDL). The LDL are the major culprits in cardiovascular diseases (CVD) and typically contain 60–70 percent of the total serum cholesterol. The HDL usually contain 20–30 percent of the total cholesterol, and their levels are inversely correlated with risk for coronary heart disease (CHD). The VLDL, which are largely composed of triglycerides, contain 10–15 percent of the total serum cholesterol.

Functions, Storage, and Excess Intake

Fat functions in the body as

1. a source of essential fatty acids
2. the most concentrated source of energy (9 kcals/g)
3. a reserve energy supply in the body
4. a carrier for the fat-soluble vitamins (A, D, E, and K)
5. a cushion and an insulation for the body
6. a satiety factor (satisfaction from a fatty meal)

All fats that are not burned as energy are stored as adipose tissue. Most people have a large storage of fat in the body.

High fat intake in the United States is associated with a high incidence of obesity and disorders of heart and blood vessels. Persons with elevated levels of blood cholesterol are more prone to atherosclerosis. Dietary fats are usually restricted in diseases that interfere with their digestion or absorption, such as gallbladder disease and pancreatitis. A high fat diet is sometimes used in the treatment of epilepsy in children who do not respond to drug treatment.

United States dietary goals recommend a reduction in daily fat intake from the present 40 percent of total calories to 30 percent (Step 1) and eventually in the new Step 2 program to 20 percent, with only 10 percent from saturated fats. Clearly this requires a major change in eating patterns.

PROGRESS CHECK ON ACTIVITY 2

Questions

Fill-in

1. If 30 percent of a 1,500-calorie diet derives from fat, how many grams of fat per day will be consumed?

   50 grm

2. Classify the following foods as polyunsaturated, monounsaturated, or saturated by placing P, M, or S by them.
   S lamb chops
   S nondairy whipped topping
   S mayonnaise
   M olive oil
   S regular margarine
   P safflower oil

3. Rank the following foods according to fat content, listing the one with the highest fat content first. If two foods have the same value, give them the same number.
   ____ 1/2 c. ice cream
   ____ 1 c. whole milk
   ____ 3 oz. sirloin steak

_____ 20 potato chips
_____ 1 glazed doughnut
_____ 2 oz. white turkey meat

4. What is the function of cholesterol in the body?
Production of body cell, vit D c all of sunlight
AND hormones

Multiple Choice

Circle the letter of the correct answer.

5. According to U.S. dietary goals, the 30 percent fat intake in Question 1 is
   a. high for average consumption.
   b. low for average consumption.
   c. average consumption.
   d. used only for calculated diets.

6. What substance emulsifies fats in the intestines?
   a. bile salts
   b. fatty acids
   c. lipases
   d. hydrochloric acids

7. The fat-splitting enzymes are
   a. bile salts.
   b. fatty acids.
   c. lipases.
   d. hydrochloric acids.

8. How many kcal does 35 g of fat supply?
   a. 140
   b. 245
   c. 315
   d. 400

9. Which meal provides the _greatest_ satiety?
   a. apple juice, toast with jelly, two poached eggs, coffee
   b. cereal with skim milk and sliced bananas, grape juice
   c. orange juice, toast with peanut butter, two eggs scrambled in one tablespoon margarine
   d. English muffin, cantaloupe, 1 oz. cream cheese, jelly

10. A 2,000 kcal daily diet containing 42 percent fat provides how many g of fat?
    a. 42 g
    b. 93 g
    c. 500 g
    d. 840 g

Matching

Match the fat in Column A to its type in Column B. Terms may be used more than once.

Column A	Column B
A 11. Steak	a. saturated
B 12. Peanuts	b. unsaturated
A 13. Egg yolk	
A 14. Olives	
15. Coconut	

Optional exercise: List the fats you have eaten (both on and in foods) for three days and compare them to Table 4-4. This will emphasize the amount and kinds of fat you use in your diet.

References

Andon, S. A. 1987. Applications of soluble dietary fiber. _Food Techno._ 41:74.

Ballard-Barbash, R., and C. W. Callaway. 1987. Marine fish oils: Role in prevention of coronary artery disease. _Mayo Clinic Procedures_ 62:113.

Beare-Rogers, J. (ed.). 1988. _Dietary fat requirements in health and development._ Champaign, IL: American Oil Chemists' Society.

Bierman, E. L., and A. Chait. 1988. Nutrition and diet in relation to hyperlipidemia and atherosclerosis. In _Modern nutrition in health and disease,_ 7th ed. M. E. Shils and V. R. Young (eds.). Philadelphia: Lea & Febiger.

Binkley, R. W. 1988. _Modern carbohydrate chemistry._ New York: Marcel Dekker.

Bjoerntorp, P. et al. 1985. _Current topics in nutrition and disease. Vol. 14. Dietary fiber and obesity._ New York: Alan R. Liss.

Brewer, E. R. et al. 1987. Food group system of analysis with special attention to type and amount of fat—fat methodology. _Journal of the American Dietetic Association_ 87(5):584.

Connor, S. L., and W. E. Connor. 1986. _The new American diet._ New York: Simon and Schuster.

Council for Agricultural Science and Technology. 1986. Diet and coronary disease. _Nutrition Today_ 21:26.

Das, U. N. et al. 1988. Clinical significance of essential fatty acids. _Nutrition_ 5:337.

Dreher, M. L. 1987. _Handbook of dietary fiber: An applied approach._ New York: Marcel Dekker.

Fletcher, A. M. 1989. _Eat fish, live better._ New York: Harper & Row.

Food and Nutrition Board, National Research Council, National Academy of Sciences. 1989. _Recommended dietary allowances,_ 10th ed. Washington, DC: National Academy Press.

Fox, S. I. 1987. _Human physiology,_ 2nd ed. Dubuque, IA: William C. Brown.

Greenwald, P. et al. 1987. Dietary fiber in the reduction of colon cancer risk. _Journal of the American Dietetic Association_ 87(9):1178.

TABLE 4-4
Fat and Cholesterol Comparison Chart

Example of	Item	Saturated Fatty Acids (grams)	Total Fat (grams)	Cholesterol (milligrams)
Beef	Top round, lean only, broiled	2.2	6.2	84
100 grams	Ground lean, broiled medium	7.3	18.5	87
(3½ ounces)	Beef prime rib, meat, lean and fat, broiled	14.9	35.2	86
Processed Meats	Dutch loaf, pork and beef	6.4	17.8	47
100 grams	Sausage smoked, link, beef and pork	10.6	30.3	71
(3½ ounces)	Bologna, beef	11.7	28.4	56
	Frankfurter, beef	12.0	29.4	48
	Salami, dry or hard, pork, beef	12.2	34.4	79
Pork	Ham steak, extra lean	1.4	4.2	45
100 grams	Pork, center loin, lean only, braised	4.7	13.7	111
(3½ ounces)	Pork, spareribs, lean and fat, braised	11.8	30.3	121
Poultry	Chicken broilers or fryers, roasted:			
100 grams	• Light meat without skin	1.3	4.5	85
(3½ ounces)	• Light meat with skin	3.1	10.9	84
	• Dark meat without skin	2.7	9.7	93
	• Dark meat with skin	4.4	15.8	91
	• Chicken skin	11.4	40.7	83
Fin Fish	Cod, Atlantic, dry heat cooked	0.1	0.7	58
100 grams	Perch, mixed species, dry heat cooked	0.2	1.2	115
(3½ ounces)	Snapper, mixed species, dry heat cooked	0.4	1.7	47
	Rockfish, Pacific, mixed species, dry heat cooked	0.5	2.0	44
	Tuna, bluefin, dry heat cooked	1.6	6.3	49
	Mackerel, Atlantic, dry heat cooked	4.2	17.8	75
Mollusks	Clam, mixed species, moist heat cooked	0.2	2.0	67
100 grams	Mussel, blue, moist heat cooked	0.9	4.5	56
(3½ ounces)	Oyster, eastern, moist heat cooked	1.3	5.0	109
Crustaceans	Crab, blue, moist heat cooked	0.2	1.8	100
100 grams	Lobster, northern, moist heat cooked	0.1	0.6	72
(3½ ounces)	Shrimp, mixed species, moist heat cooked	0.3	1.1	195
Liver and Organ	Chicken liver, cooked, simmered	1.8	5.5	631
Meats	Beef liver, braised	1.9	4.9	389
100 grams	Pork brains, cooked	2.2	9.5	2,552
(3½ ounces)				
Eggs				
(1 yolk = 17 grams)	Egg yolk, chicken, raw	1.7	5.6	272
(1 white = 33 grams)	Egg white, chicken, raw	0	Trace	0
(1 whole = 50 grams)	Egg, whole, chicken, raw	1.7	5.6	272
Nuts and Seeds	Chestnuts, European, roasted	0.4	2.2	0
100 grams	Almonds, dry roasted	4.9	51.6	0
(3½ ounces)	Sunflower seed kernels, dry roasted	5.2	49.8	0
	Pecans, dry roasted	5.2	64.6	0
	Walnuts, English, dried	5.6	61.9	0
	Pistachio nuts, dried	6.1	48.4	0
	Peanut kernels, dried	6.8	49.2	0
	Cashew nuts, dry roasted	9.2	46.4	0
	Brazil nuts, dried	16.2	66.2	0
Fruits	Peaches, raw	0.010	0.09	0
100 grams	Oranges, raw	0.015	0.12	0
(3½ ounces)	Strawberries, raw	0.020	0.37	0
	Apples, with skin, raw	0.058	0.36	0
Vegetables	Cooked, boiled, drained:			
100 grams	• Potato, without skin	0.026	0.10	0
(3½ ounces)	• Carrots	0.034	0.18	0

(continues)

TABLE 4-4 (Continued)

Example of	Item	Saturated Fatty Acids (grams)	Total Fat (grams)	Cholesterol (milligrams)
	• Spinach	0.042	0.26	0
	• Broccoli	0.043	0.28	0
	• Beans, green and yellow	0.064	0.28	0
	• Squash, yellow, crookneck	0.064	0.31	0
	• Corn	0.197	1.28	0
	Avocado, raw, without skin or seed:			
	• Florida origin	1.74	8.86	0
	• California origin	2.60	17.34	0
Grains and Legumes 100 grams (3½ ounces)	Split peas, cooked, boiled	0.054	0.39	0
	Red kidney beans, cooked, boiled	0.07	0.5	0
	Oatmeal, cooked	0.19	1.0	0
Milk and Cream 1 cup (8 fluid ounces)	Skim milk	0.3	0.4	4
	Buttermilk (0.9% fat)	1.3	2.2	9
	Low fat milk (1% fat)	1.6	2.6	10
	Whole milk (3.7% fat)	5.6	8.9	35
	Light cream	28.8	46.3	159
	Heavy whipping cream	54.8	88.1	326
Yogurt and Sour Cream 1 cup (8 fluid ounces)	Plain yogurt, skim milk	0.3	0.4	4
	Plain yogurt, low fat (1.6%)	2.3	3.5	14
	Plain yogurt, whole milk	4.8	7.4	29
	Sour cream	30.0	48.2	102
Soft Cheeses 1 cup (8 fluid ounces)	Cottage cheese, low fat (1% fat)	1.5	2.3	10
	Cottage cheese, creamed	6.0	9.5	31
	Ricotta, part skim	12.1	19.5	76
	Ricotta, whole milk	18.8	29.5	116
	American processed spread	30.2	48.1	125
	Cream cheese	49.9	79.2	250
Hard Cheeses (8 ounces)	Mozzarella, part skim	22.9	36.1	132
	Mozzarella, whole milk	29.7	49.0	177
	Provolone	38.8	60.4	157
	Swiss	40.4	62.4	209
	Blue	42.4	65.1	170
	Brick	42.7	67.4	213
	Muenster	43.4	68.1	218
	American processed	44.7	71.1	213
	Cheddar	47.9	75.1	238
Vegetable Oils and Shortening 1 cup (8 fluid ounces)	Canola oil	14.8	218.0	0
	Safflower oil	19.8	218.0	0
	Sunflower oil	22.5	218.0	0
	Corn oil	27.7	218.0	0
	Olive oil	29.2	216.0	0
	Soybean oil	31.4	218.0	0
	Margarine, regular soft tub*	32.2	182.6	0
	Margarine, stick or brick*	34.2	182.6	0
	Peanut oil	36.4	216.0	0
	Household vegetable shortening*	51.2	205.0	0
	Cottonseed oil	56.4	218.0	0
	Palm oil	107.4	218.0	0
	Coconut oil	188.5	218.0	0
	Palm kernel oil	177.4	218.0	0
Animal Fats 1 cup (8 fluid ounces)	Chicken fat	61.2	205.0	174
	Lard	80.4	205.0	195
	Mutton fat	96.9	205.0	209
	Beef fat	102.1	205.0	223
	Butter	114.4	183.9	496

*Made with hydrogenated soybean oil and hydrogenated cottonseed oil.
Source: "Facts about blood cholesterol," USPHS/PHS/NIH, Publication number 88-2696, Rev. Nov. 1987.

Guyton, A. 1986. *Textbook of medical physiology*, 3rd ed. Philadelphia: Saunders.

Hepburn, F. N. et al. 1986. Provisional tables on the content of omega-3 fatty acids and other fat components of selected foods. *Journal of the American Dietetic Association* 86(6):788.

Jenkins, D. J. A. 1988. Carbohydrates (B): Dietary Fiber. In *Modern nutrition in health and disease,* 7th ed. M. E. Shils and V. R. Young (eds.). Philadelphia: Lea & Febiger.

Klurfeld, D. M. 1987. The role of dietary fiber in gastrointestinal disease. *Journal of the American Dietetic Association* 86(6):732.

Lands, W. E. M. 1986. *Fish and human health*. Orlando, FL: Academic Press.

Leaf, A., and P. C. Weber. 1988. Cardiovascular effects of n-3 fatty acid. *New England Journal of Medicine* 318:549.

MacDonald, I. 1988. Carbohydrates (A): General. In *Modern nutrition in health and disease,* M. E. Shils and V. R. Young (eds.), 7th ed. Philadelphia: Lea & Febiger.

Matthews, R. J. et al. 1987. *Sugar content of selected foods: Individual and total sugars*. USDA/HNIS Home Economics Research Report No. 48. Washington, DC: United States Department of Agriculture.

National Institute of Health. 1989. *National Cholesterol Education Program: Expert panel on detection, evaluation, and treatment of high blood cholesterol in adults*. USDHHS/PHS/National Institute of Health.

Reiser, S., and J. Hallfrisch. 1987. *Metabolic effects of dietary fructose*. Boca Raton, FL: CRC Press.

Simopulos, A. P. et al. (eds.). 1986. *Health effects of polyunsaturated fatty acids in seafoods*. Orlando, FL: Academic Press.

Skinner, S. et al. 1985. *The milk sugar dilemma: Living with lactose intolerance*. East Lansing, MI: Medi-Ed Press.

Slavin, J. L. 1987. Dietary fiber: Classification, chemical analyses and food sources. *Journal of the American Dietetic Association* 87(9):1164.

Trowell, H. et al. 1985. *Dietary fibre, fibre-depleted foods and disease*. London: Academic Press.

USDA. 1986. *Dietary guidelines for Americans: Avoid too much fat, saturated fat and cholesterol*. Home and Garden Bulletin, No. 232-3. United States Department of Agriculture, Human Nutrition Information Service.

Williams, G. M. (ed.). 1988. *Sweeteners: Health effects*. Princeton, NJ: Princeton Scientific Publishing Co.

Yetiv, J. Z. 1988. Clinical application of fish oils. *Journal of the American Medical Association* 260–265.

Proteins and Health

Time for completion
Activities: _____1_____ hour
Optional examination: ½ hour

Academic credit
Semester units: ²⁄₁₀
Quarter units: ³⁄₁₀

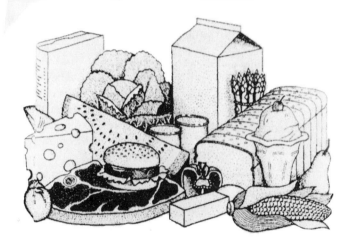

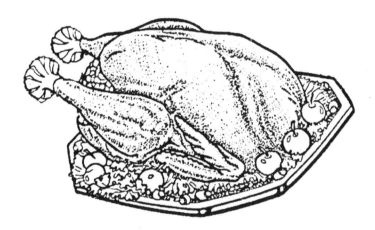

Outline

Objectives
Glossary
Background Information

ACTIVITY 1: Protein as a Nutrient
Definitions, Essentiality, and Requirement
Protein Sparing
Functions, Storage, Sources, and Utilization

ACTIVITY 2: Meeting Protein Needs and Vegetarianism
Requirements for Protein and Amino Acids
Vegetarianism: Rationale and Classification
Vegetarianism: Diet Evaluation
Vegetarianism: Diet Planning
Excessive and Deficient Protein Intake
Responsibilities of the Health Professional
Progress Check on Activity 2
References

Objectives

Upon completion of this module the student should be able to:

1. Identify the structure of proteins and their fuel value.
2. Define complete and incomplete protein and essential amino acids.
3. Discuss protein quality and the concept of limiting amino acids.
4. Describe the amino acid requirements of humans and their RDAs for protein.
5. Explain the method of measuring protein in the body.
6. Summarize the major functions and food sources of protein.
7. Analyze the all-or-none law in protein metabolism and the concept of protein sparing.
8. Recognize various vegetarian diet regimes and their relationship to adequate protein intake.
9. Compare the effects on health of inadequate or excessive protein intake.
10. Specify certain conditions where alteration in protein intake may be needed.

Glossary

Amino acids: compounds containing nitrogen which are the building blocks of the protein molecule.

Antibody: a protein substance produced within the body that destroys or weakens harmful bacteria.

Biologic value of protein (BV):   the ability of a protein to support the formation of body tissue.

Complementary proteins: two or more protein foods whose amino acid compositions complement each other so that one has what the other lacks.

Complete protein: a protein containing all the essential amino acids.

Essential amino acids: amino acids that cannot be synthesized by the body and must be provided by food.

Immobility: the condition of being inactive owing to disability, such as that experienced by the person confined to bed or a wheelchair.

Incomplete protein: a protein lacking one or more of the essential amino acids or containing some of the amino acids in only very small amounts.

Kwashiorkor: a severe protein deficiency disease that occurs in infancy or early childhood and in high-risk hospitalized patients.

Marasmus: a condition characterized by a loss of flesh and strength due to underfeeding; a lack of sufficient calories for a prolonged period of time.

Meat analogs: See *TVP*.

Nonessential amino acids: amino acids that can be synthesized by the body to meet its needs.

Synthesis: the process of building complex compounds from simple ones when they are furnished to the body.

Textured vegetable protein (TVP):   protein that is drawn from plant protein, spun into fibers, and manufactured into products that imitate animal protein foods. Also called meat analogs.

Vegetarianism: the practice of eating no animal flesh.

Background Information

Genetics involves the passing of characteristics from one generation to the next. These characteristics make a person unique. The entire genetic process creates one important substance: protein. Each protein molecule is made of many units called amino acids. There are twenty to twenty-five different amino acids in nature. The word protein comes from the Greek word *protos*, which means "primary."

All living substances, including plants and viruses, contain protein. Approximately 18 to 20 percent of the human body is protein. It is present in all body tissues and fluids except bile and urine. Protein is made up of about 16 percent nitrogen, in both body tissue and food. The quantity of protein in a given sample, therefore, is measured by the amount of nitrogen it contains. Nitrogen or protein balance of the body is an important factor in determining the body's health.

Protein is an important factor in the American diet. Individuals' use and abuse of protein due to misconceptions and inaccurate information about it have led to unusual and sometimes dangerous eating practices. Many athletes take powdered protein supplements in the hope of increasing their muscle size or strength. The liquid protein crash diets many people have tried have caused some deaths. Some type of protein foods are completely avoided by some religious sects. The use of protein foods to denote masculinity (meats) and femininity (eggs, milk), and for status symbols (lobster instead of sardines) is significant in learning about people's lifestyles and cultural patterns.

The role that protein plays in the healthy diet is an important one, but should not be exaggerated. Without an adequate supply of this essential compound, all growth, repair, and maintenance of the body cells cease and the body dies. On the other hand, excessive consumption of protein, or protein foods eaten to the exclusion of other types of food, is not healthy.

All proteins are not alike. The health practitioner needs a thorough knowledge of the functions, requirements, and sources of protein to counsel clients on how to meet their protein needs.

ACTIVITY 1: Protein as a Nutrient

Definitions, Essentiality, and Requirement

Proteins are composed of carbon, hydrogen, oxygen, and nitrogen; they provide the foundation of every body cell. Proteins are broken down to amino acids by the body.

Amino acids are classified as *essential*—that which cannot be produced by the body and must be obtained from food; and *nonessential*—that which can be produced by the body.

Proteins are also categorized as complete or incomplete. Whether a protein food can be used for the growth and repair of tissue depends upon its biological value. Proteins of high biological value are complete proteins and contain all essential amino acids in adequate amounts to promote growth. Those of low biological value are called incomplete proteins; they may not supply all the essential amino acids or may supply some of them in limited amounts.

The essential amino acid that provides the least adequate kind of protein in meeting human nutritional needs is termed the limiting amino acid. In a complete protein, the limiting amino acid poses no problem. In an incomplete protein, the limiting amino acid is responsible for the poor utilization of its fellow essential amino acids.

Individuals consuming this incomplete protein must be provided a source of the limiting amino acid. Animal proteins (except gelatin) are complete proteins; vegetable proteins (for example, dried beans and peas) are incomplete.

Protein of high biologic value can result from complementary mixtures of vegetable proteins, in which one vegetable protein supplies the amino acid that the other vegetable protein is lacking.

The all-or-none law of protein metabolism states quite simply that all of the essential amino acids must be present in the diet at the same meal or none of them can be utilized. Therefore, the complete proteins should be mixed with the incomplete ones in order to achieve adequate growth and repair. Vegetarians must be especially careful to consume complementary proteins in order to satisfy the all-or-none law. The recommended daily protein intake for adults is 0.8 g per kg of body weight, less than the amount ordinarily consumed by Americans. Daily protein intake should be in the form of complete good quality protein and/or complementary protein foods.

Protein Sparing

There are twenty to twenty-five amino acids, twenty of which are commonly found in food. When an amino acid is considered nonessential, it can be produced by the body, using available oxygen, carbon, hydrogen, and nitrogen. Essential amino acids must be supplied by the diet. Eight essential amino acids are required by adults; nine are required by infants.

The distinction between essential and nonessential requires further amplification. Individuals cannot survive without a dietary supply of the proper amounts of the essential amino acids. However, our bodies need the nonessential amino acids to achieve optimal protein metabolism. Biochemically, we need the carbon skeleton and amino-groups of the essential and nonessential amino acids, respectively.

It is of great importance, then, to have good sources of both essential and nonessential amino acids to provide sufficient nitrogen. The ratio of ingested amino acids, which is dependent on adequate food sources, must be present in proper proportion to permit efficient manufacture and repair of all the tissues in the body. In addition, there must be sufficient carbohydrate available to meet energy needs, otherwise body protein will be broken down for energy use. This is the protein-sparing action of carbohydrate that was discussed in Module 4. Since plant proteins contain large amounts of carbohydrate, but animal proteins contain little or none, a combination of both is desirable to meet daily requirements. The animal protein will complete the inadequate amino acids pattern of plants, and plant sources will provide the needed carbohydrate. Clinical evidence indicates that the human body can deteriorate when fed only essential amino acids.

Functions, Storage, Sources, and Utilization

Functions. The main function of protein is to provide the body with the amino acids necessary for growth and maintenance of body tissues. Cells, enzymes, hormones, antibodies, muscles, blood, and all tissues and fluid except bile and urine require protein.

Storage. Proteins in the form of amino acids are the building blocks of the body. Protein as such is not stored; therefore, a daily intake is required.

Sources. Animal sources of protein include milk and milk products, meat, fish, poultry, and eggs. Plant sources include breads and cereal products, legumes, nuts and seeds, and textured vegetable protein. Cereal grains are the primary source of protein for the majority of the world's population. The production of large animals for protein will become less practical as the world's population grows and space for humans must take precedence over space for raising large animals.

The health practitioner should be familiar with the complementary proteins in foods. Animal protein is relatively expensive. As the world's protein supply diminishes, an understanding of complementarity will become increasingly important. The proper mixing of ingested plant protein foods can provide nutritional value similar to that of animal protein.

Adequate amounts of high quality protein are not difficult to obtain in diets that contain dairy products and eggs. However, achieving nutritional balance in a strict vegetarian diet requires considerable knowledge of the contributions of various food to our dietary requirements. Activity 2 discusses the use of vegetarian diets.

Utilization.   To be absorbed, proteins must be broken down to individual amino acids or small peptides (byproducts of protein digestion composed of two to ten amino acids).

The products of protein digestion are absorbed into the bloodstream as amino acids and are transported via the portal vein to the liver and then to all the body cells. Some amino acids stay in the liver to form liver tissue itself or to produce a wide variety of blood proteins. The remaining amino acids circulate in the bloodstream, from which they are rapidly removed and utilized by the tissues.

When amino acids are broken down, the nitrogen-containing part is split off from the carbon chain. Most of the nitrogen is converted to urea in the liver and excreted via the kidneys. Then the carbon-containing portion that remains is utilized for energy. Proteins provide 4 kcal per g, the same as carbohydrates.

PROGRESS CHECK ON ACTIVITY 1

Fill-in

1. Keep a 24-hour food record.

    a. List all the complete proteins you consumed.

    _____

    _____

    _____

    b. List all the incomplete proteins you consumed.

    _____

    _____

    _____

    c. Identify which food(s) has the highest quality protein. _____

    _____

    _____

2. Why is it important to space consumption of good quality protein throughout the day? *All essential amino acids must be present at the time in the body or the body cant utilize them*

3. Is protein deficiency common in the United States?

    No except for many

Multiple Choice

Circle the letter of the correct answer.

4. Substances are classified as protein when they contain
    a. carbon, oxygen, and nitrogen.
    b. carbon, oxygen, hydrogen, and sulfur.
    c. carbon, hydrogen, oxygen, and nitrogen.
    d. carbon, calcium, phosphorus, and iron.

5. Adults require _____ essential amino acids and infants require _____ essential amino acids. (Circle the letter that fills in the blanks with the correct numbers.)
    a. 8, 7
    b. 8, 9
    c. 7, 8
    d. 6, 7

6. An amino acid is said to be essential if it
    a. is needed by the body.
    b. cannot be synthesized by the body.
    c. contains vitamins and minerals.
    d. combines with nonessential amino acids.

7. On days when a person exercises strenuously his or her protein intake should be
    a. increased greatly.
    b. reduced sharply.
    c. about the same as usual.
    d. reduced by half.

8. For protein synthesis to occur
    a. all the essential amino acids must be present.
    b. sufficient nitrogen to form nonessential amino acids is needed.
    c. the diet must have adequate calories from carbohydrate and fat.
    d. all of the above.

True/False

Circle T for True and F for False.

9. T F Foods of animal origin contain substantial quantities of high quality protein.
10. T F Malnutrition affects physical and mental development.

ACTIVITY 2: Meeting Protein Needs and Vegetarianism

Requirements for Protein and Amino Acids

Recommended protein intakes are based on the amount of nitrogen (quantity) and kind of amino acids (quality) consumed. The quantitative value of protein foods is made by comparing the amount of protein in a serving of food to the amount required by humans. Animal protein sources are highly concentrated, with the single exception of bacon, which is considered a fat in the exchange lists. Soybean products are quite concentrated in protein, although they contain a limiting amino acid, which reduces the quality of the product.

The protein content of some common foods is compared in Table 5-1. In general, if the exchange list is followed, each meat exchange provides 7 g of protein. The value of protein for 1 exchange of milk is 8 g and for bread or vegetables, 3 g of protein per each exchange. Serving sizes are as follows: 1 exchange meat = 1 oz.; milk = 1 c.; vegetable = 1/2 c.; and bread = 1 slice.

The quality of a protein is dependent on the essential amino acids it contains compared to the essential amino acid needs of the body. Quality is sometimes expressed as biological value (BV). This is a measure of the body's retention of the nitrogen contained in the ingested protein. Eggs, with a BV of 100, have the highest quality of any dietary proteins. Milk, at 93, follows a close second. Most meats, fish, and poultry have a BV of about 75. Any BV of 70 or above is considered sufficient for sustaining growth and maintenance of body tissue. Requirements for protein differ by age, sex, and physical state of the body. Factors influencing protein utilization can be modified by the digestibility of the protein and the overall composition of the diet as well as the source of the protein and its amino acid balance.

The RDA for protein is set by nitrogen balance studies. A healthy adult should be in nitrogen balance. When new tissue is being formed, the body retains more nitrogen than it excretes, creating a positive nitrogen balance. This is the case during periods of growth such as pregnancy and childhood. Negative nitrogen balance occurs when muscles are breaking down, such as with bedridden persons or when very low calorie reducing diets are used. More nitrogen is excreted than is taken in.

The 1989 RDAs recommend the following allowances for mixed (animal and vegetable) proteins:

Infants 0–5 months: 13 g	Males 19–24 years: 58 g
Infants 5 months–1 year: 14 g	Females 11–14 years: 46 g
Children 1–3 years: 16 g	Females 15–18 years: 44 g
Children 4–6 years: 24 g	Females 19–24 years: 46 g
Children 7–10 years: 28 g	Adult males 50–50+: 63 g
Males 11–14 years: 45 g	Adult females 25–50+: 50 g
Males 15–18 years: 59 g	

The values may be adapted to individual uses based on this formula for adult men and women: Multiply body weight in kg by 0.8 g. For children and adolescents, the amount of protein varies with the growth cycle, ranging from 2.0 g per kg body weight for infants to 0.8 g at adulthood. To convert body weight from pounds to kilograms, divide the pound weight by the factor 2.2.

The requirement for protein and each essential amino acid varies with age in absolute and relative quantities. Approximately 40 percent of an infant's protein must be from essential amino acids, but only 20 percent for an adult. A food that may be an adequate protein source for adults may be inadequate for the young child. Protein requirements increase in certain kinds of illnesses or malnutrition.

Protein consumption in the United States is quite high, ranging between 100 to 120 g per day. This exceeds the RDAs with their value of 50 g for women and 63 g for men, where respective body weights are 63 kg and 79 kg. Approximately two-thirds of the protein consumed in the United States is from animal sources. Excess protein intake has raised questions about health risks. These risks will be discussed later in this activity.

TABLE 5-1
Protein Content of Some Common American Foods

Food Product	Serving Size	Protein (g)
Cheese, natural, cheddar	1 oz.	7
Milk, whole, 3.3% fat	1 c.	8
Ice cream, regular, hardened	1 c.	5
Egg, cooked in any form	1	6
Butter	1 tbsp.	trace
Beef, ground, lean, broiled	3 oz.	18
Tuna, canned in oil, drained	3 oz.	24
Apple	1	trace
Grapefruit	1/2	1
Bread, white, enriched	1 slice	2
Breakfast cereal, hot, cooked (oatmeal or rolled oats)	1 c	5
Spaghetti, tomato sauce with cheese	1 c.	6
Beans, cooked, drained	1 c.	15
Peanut butter	1 tbsp.	4
Walnuts, English, chopped	1 c.	18
Cabbage, raw, shredded	1 c.	1
Corn, canned, cream style	1 c.	5
Potatoes, cooked, baked (2/lb)	1	4
Beer	12 fl. oz.	1
Gelatin, dry	7 oz.	6
Yeast, brewer's, dry	1 tbsp.	3

Source: Adapted from Nutritive Value of Foods, USDA Home and Garden Bulletin No. 72, Washington, DC: U.S. Department of Agriculture, 1981.

For optimal use of protein, intake should be spread throughout the day rather than being consumed at one meal. The servings do not need to be large, but the all-or-none law discussed earlier must be applied in this case.

Vegetarianism: Rationale and Classification

There are many reasons why individuals eliminate animal foods from their diets. The most common reasons are economic concerns, religious guidelines, health considerations, and concern for animal life.

When a vegetarian consumes no meat, fowl, or fish as food, the further restrictions on the remaining part of the diet can be classified as follows:

1. Fruitarians: individuals who eat only fruit.
2. Vegans: individuals who eat no animal flesh nor any food of animal origin. They are sometimes called strict vegetarians.
3. Lacto-vegetarians: individuals who eat plant proteins combined with milk.
4. Ovo-vegetarians: individuals who eat plant proteins combined with eggs.
5. Lacto-ovo-vegetarians: individuals who eat both milk and eggs along with plant proteins.

Semivegetarians restrict red meats only—that is, beef, pork, lamb, game animals. Fish, poultry, dairy foods, eggs, and plants furnish proteins for their diet.

Vegetarianism: Diet Evaluation

Generally, the more restrictive the vegetarian's diet is, the more likely it is to be deficient in one or more major nutrients. The simplest and easiest of the vegetarian diets to balance is the lacto-ovo-vegetarian, with its use of eggs and milk. This diet offers high quality protein for both children and adults, but may be low in iron if nonmeat sources of this mineral are not included. Both milk and eggs are poor sources of iron. A high intake of legumes, seeds, nuts, and enriched grains will increase iron intake substantially. Vegetarian diets may contain so much bulk that the stomachs of children are full before they get enough calories. If this happens, protein may be inefficiently used for energy instead of building. The semivegetarian diet presents no nutritional problems, if the iron intake is sufficient.

Those people who follow either lacto- or ovo-vegetarian diets must plan more carefully. While the protein content of either diet is adequate, the ovo-vegetarian may be low in calcium and phosphorus intake because of avoidance of milk. Cases of rickets (vitamin D deficiency disease) have been reported in vegetarian children who have no milk intake.

The strict vegetarian (vegan) diet presents several problems. It tends to be low in calcium, vitamin D, vitamin B_{12}, riboflavin, and zinc. None of the vegetable sources furnish adequate calcium. Calcium is poorly absorbed from vegetables because of the fiber content of the calcium-binding oxalic acid found in some greens. Also, a vegan may be lacking in vitamin D, since it is obtained from animal sources only. If the person does not receive adequate sunlight, which can help vitamin D synthesis under the skin, any existing calcium deficiency will be compounded by a dietary lack of vitamin D.

Problems with protein quality and quantity often occur among vegans. If vegetables and cereals are the only sources of protein, not only will they be of low quality but the digestibility factor is often low. Because of high fiber content, many nonmeat sources are not well digested. Beans are especially difficult for children. Soybeans contain a trypsin inhibitor that interferes with the function of trypsin, a major enzyme for digesting protein. Some vegetarian children tend to be smaller and show symptoms of undernutrition, but nutrient deficiencies vary with the number of dietary items restricted and the children's overall meal plans. Complementary protein mixes do not give an amino acid pattern fully usable by the body as animal protein does, but correct combinations can increase protein quality by up to 50 percent. Children should not be put on a vegan diet unless medical and nutritional expertise is available to monitor their health. When foods are chosen wisely, a vegetarian child can meet his or her nutritional needs. The Zen macrobiotic diet is the most restricting of all the vegetarian diets. It is approached in 10 stages (from −3 to +7), each becoming more restricted than the last. The +7 stage consists of only brown rice and limited amounts of water. People on this diet can suffer from scurvy, anemia, emaciation, osteoporosis, heart arrythmias, and loss of kidney function. Acute malnutrition and deaths have occurred from zealous pursuit of this diet. Highly touted as a spiritual or purifying diet used by Eastern religions, it actually bears little resemblance to these religions' dietary practices. It is totally inadequate in nutrients.

Vegetarianism, when properly managed, can be a healthy way to eat. Children are especially at high risk of failure to thrive if they are not supplemented with fortified foods containing essential nutrients missing from their diets. Vegetarians may be at lower risk for gastrointestinal disorders (such as constipation, diverticulosis) and colon cancer because of the high fiber content of the diet. On the other hand, osteoporosis, which affects three out of five women over the age of sixty, is a high risk factor among many vegetarians. The avoidance of animal products with their high saturated fat content may lower the risk of coronary heart disease. Because of less fat in the diet, vegetarians also tend to have a lower incidence of obesity.

Vegetarianism: Diet Planning

To assure adequate intake of nutrients, vegetarians must carefully follow certain guidelines:

1. Include 2 c. legumes daily to meet calcium and iron requirements.
2. Include 1 c. dark greens daily to meet iron requirements for women.
3. Include at least 1 tbsp. fat daily for proper absorption of vitamins.

Tables 5-2 and 5-3 indicate the food groups for lacto-ovo- and strict vegetarians. Table 5-4 provides sample menus.

Figure 5-1 shows some complementary protein combinations. Recommended cookbooks for vegetarian cooking which may be helpful in planning adequate meals are provided in the references for this module.

The health professional should be aware that some vegetarians believe that all medical problems can be prevented or cured by their diet and fail to seek help when they need it.

While some religious groups that are vegetarian or semivegetarian show a lower incidence of certain diseases that afflict the United States population (such as colon cancer, coronary heart disease), it must be remembered that these groups' general lifestyles also differ from others. They generally avoid tobacco and alcohol, suffer few stresses, and exercise regularly. These factors contribute to a lower risk for these diseases.

It is not possible to document that a vegetarian diet alone promotes better health, but this practice together with other lifestyle changes may lead to healthy habits.

Excessive and Deficient Protein Intake

Normal tissue growth in infancy and childhood and during pregnancy and lactation requires more amino acids than those needed for tissue maintenance. As has been demonstrated in many laboratory studies, in the absence of adequate protein, growth is slowed down or even stopped.

The feeding of infants in strict vegetarian families is of particular concern to the health professional. If breast

TABLE 5-2
Food Groups for Lacto-Ovo-Vegetarians

Food Groups	Major Products	Daily Servings
Meat equivalents	Legumes, pulses, nuts, textured vegetable proteins (soy meat analogs and other formulated plant protein products and spun soy isolates), eggs	2
Milk and dairy products	Milk, cheese, yogurt, many other milk products	2
Breads and cereals	All varieties	4–6
Fruits and vegetables	All varieties	Vegetables: 3 Fruits: 1–3

TABLE 5-3
Food Groups for Strict Vegetarians

Food Groups	Major Products	Daily Servings
Meat equivalents	Legumes, pulses, nuts, textured vegetable proteins (soy meat analogs and other formulated plant protein products and spun soy isolates)	*2
Milk equivalents	Soybean milk, preferably fortified with calcium, vitamins B_2 and B_{12} (if not fortified, supplements, especially vitamin B_{12}, may be necessary)*	*2
Breads and cereals	All varieties	4–6
Fruits and vegetables	All varieties	Vegetables: 4 Fruits: 1–4**

*Nut milks are nutritionally inadequate, especially for infants.
**Including a source of vitamin C.

feeding is not possible, a formula such as nutritionally fortified soybean milk should be provided. The soybean formula fortified with vitamin B_{12} should continue to be given by cup after the child is weaned. A wide variety of foods should be chosen, with emphasis on those that are high in iron and vitamins A, B complex, and C. In addition to soybean milk, mixtures of legumes and cereals are needed to supply sufficient protein.

Excesses

Questions raised about excessive protein intake of Americans include the following:

1. Excess nitrogen must be cleared by the kidneys. This may negatively affect kidneys that are malfunctioning, damaged, or underdeveloped.
2. High protein consumption has recently been cited as one factor in bone demineralization, especially if coupled with low calcium intake.
3. While inconclusive at this time, research indicates that high protein consumption may increase risks of colon cancer by changing the internal environment and altering the bacteria of the colon.
4. Large amounts of protein, especially of animal origin, also contain saturated fats. Most authorities are convinced that saturated fats contribute to a high incidence of heart disease.

TABLE 5-4
Sample Vegetarian Menus

Vegan	Lacto-Ovo-Vegetarian
Breakfast	
Orange juice	Orange juice
Oatmeal/honey	Cheese/mushroom omelet
Soy milk	Whole wheat toast
Toasted soy wheat bread	Tea
Tea	
Lunch	
Split pea soup	Split pea soup
Peanut butter sandwich on soy wheat bread	Peanut butter sandwich on wheat bread
Fruit salad with sunflower seeds	Fruit and cottage cheese
Almonds/raisins	Salad/mayonnaise
Tea	Milk
Dinner	
Vegetable soup	Vegetable soup
Green salad with nuts and seeds	Green salad with nuts and seeds
Soybean croquettes fried in oil	Whole wheat bread with margarine
Pears	Yogurt with oranges and strawberries
Soybean milk	Tea or milk

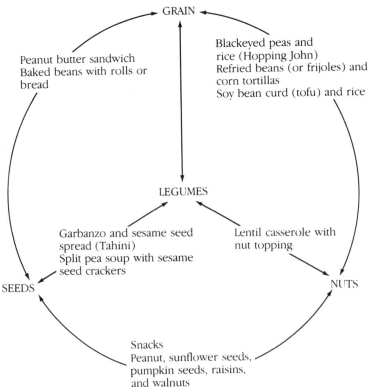

Figure 5-1
Complementary Vegetable Proteins

5. Since excess protein from any source is converted to fat and stored as adipose tissue, it can contribute to obesity.

Deficiencies

Large losses of protein may occur during illness or surgical procedures. These situations require substantial increases in protein consumption. Lack of increased protein intake during illness will result in delayed wound healing, slow convalescing, low resistance to infections, and inability to return to optimum health.

Protein-energy-malnutrition (PEM) is the most serious and widespread deficiency disease in developing countries. The two major types are nutritional marasmus, due primarily to caloric deficiency; and kwashiorkor, due primarily to a deficiency of protein.

The clinical features of kwashiorkor and marasmus are illustrated in Figure 5-2. Although they are treated as two separate diseases, they are closely related. Diets low in calories will almost always be low in protein. Even if there is adequate protein, the body will use it for energy instead of for growth and development.

While primarily considered a child's disease, PEM also develops in adults. Adults with PEM exhibit weight loss, fatigue, and other symptoms of acute malnutrition. A low intake of protein and calories also results in the deficiency of three nutrients: vitamin A, iron (causing anemia), and iodine (causing endemic goiter). Vitamin A, being a fat-soluble vitamin, will be low in a protein-restricted diet. Vitamin A deficiency negatively affects growth, skin, and vision, sometimes causing blindness. Many women die in childbirth from low iron levels. If there is an infection from parasites such as hookworm, even less iron is available. PEM will produce stunted growth and mental retardation. A malnourished woman is likely to give birth to a premature, often retarded infant with less resistance to infection and illness. Poorly nourished persons have a shortened life expectancy and common childhood diseases are often fatal to the malnourished child. Enzyme and hormone production is inadequate in these victims. Although they badly need extra nutrients, they are unable to digest and absorb them.

Some infants are born with an inability to metabolize phenylalanine, an essential amino acid. Mental retardation results if the disease is not treated. Phenylketonuria will be discussed in Part IV. The protein in specific foods is considered to be the cause of food allergies. In this case, careful addition of protein foods to an infant's diet must be practiced.

Responsibilities of the Health Professional

The health professional should

1. Recommend moderate amounts of animal protein. Excess protein is wasteful, since the excess is converted to energy and excess energy is converted to fat. Protein food is an expensive form of energy.

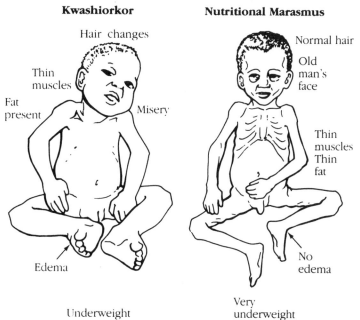

Kwashiorkor

Hair changes

Thin muscles

Fat present

Misery

Edema

Underweight

Nutritional Marasmus

Normal hair

Old man's face

Thin muscles
Thin fat

No edema

Very underweight

Figure 5-2
Comparison of Children with Kwashiorkor and Marasmus
Source: D. B. Jelliffe, Clinical Nutrition in Developing Countries, 1968. U. S. Department of Health, Education and Welfare, Public Health Service.

2. Be aware that protein foods are not low in calories. They provide the same number of calories per gram as carbohydrates. Furthermore, protein foods from animal sources (such as meats, cheese) frequently contain excessive calories from fat.

3. Advise clients to eat good quality protein at each meal to provide a consistent supply of essential amino acids. Protein cannot be stored in the body and is used constantly in its major functions.

4. Plan some meals for clients around complementary vegetable protein foods for variety, economy, and increased fiber.

5. Be aware that meals containing legumes and grains are very nourishing and less expensive than meals containing meat.

6. Be aware of the importance of eating extra protein during illnesses, which cause excessive breakdown of body tissue.

7. Recognize that certain illnesses require alterations in amounts and types of protein ingested.

PROGRESS CHECK ON ACTIVITY 2

Matching

Match the nutrient listed in Column A to the statement that best describes it in Column B. Terms may be used more than once.

	Column A		*Column B*
A	1. Calcium	a.	Strict vegetarian diets are at risk of being deficient in this nutrient.
B	2. Vitamin A		
A	3. Iron		
A	4. Vitamin B$_{12}$	b.	Strict vegetarian diets are generally adequate in this nutrient.
B	5. Thiamin		
A	6. Riboflavin		
A	7. Vitamin D		

Match the food item on the left to the statement on the right that best describes its protein content. Terms may be used more than once.

C	8. Legumes	a.	High quality, high quantity
A	9. Cheese	b.	Low quality, low quantity
B	10. Broccoli	c.	Low quality, high quantity
B	11. Potato		
A	12. Tuna		

Multiple Choice

Circle the letter of the correct answer.

13. An individual who will not eat meat, fish, poultry, or eggs but drinks milk with his or her plant foods is a(n)
    a. vegan.
    b. ovo-vegetarian.
    c. fruitarian.
    d. lacto-vegetarian.

True/False

Circle T for True and F for False.

14. T F Excessive protein intake may place a strain on the kidneys.

Case Study

Mary and Leon are married college students, both twenty-one years of age. They are living on a limited income and became vegetarians two years ago when they became involved in the ecological movement on campus. Mary, who at 5'9" weighs 110 lb., has just discovered that she is pregnant with her first child. She requests advice about an appropriate diet. From the information available, answer the following:

15. List other data you will need to gather about her diet habits before you can assist her. _____
_____
_____

16. What is the basic nutritional increase she will need during her pregnancy? How much increase? _____
_____

17. What is her general protein requirement according to her weight? _____
_____
_____

18. Is her weight appropriate for her height? Should she gain extra weight over the 24 to 30 lb. increase recommended for the normal pregnancy? _____
_____
_____

19. If she and Leon are vegans, will she be able to get the quality and quantity of protein she will need? List several food combinations that would help. _____
_____
_____

20. Why would adequate carbohydrate foods be important in her prenatal diet? _____
_____
_____

21. If she has an adequate diet during her pregnancy, will she be in positive or negative nitrogen balance? Explain your answer. _____

_____

_____

References _____

ADA Reports. 1988. Position of the American Dietetic Association: Vegetarian diets. *Journal of the American Dietetic Association* 88:351.

Braunwall, E. et al. 1987. *Harrison's principles of internal medicine*, 11th ed. New York: McGraw-Hill.

Carpenter, K. J. 1986. The history of enthusiasm for protein. *Journal of Nutrition* 116:1364.

Dwyer, J. T. 1988. Health aspects of vegetarian diets. *American Journal of Clinical Nutrition* 48:712.

Food and Nutrition Board, National Research Council, National Academy of Sciences. 1989. *Recommended dietary allowances*, 10th ed. Washington, DC: National Academy Press.

Fox, S. I. 1987. *Human physiology*, 2nd ed. Dubuque, IA: W. C. Brown.

Freeland-Graves, J. H. 1986. Health practices, attitudes, and beliefs of vegetarians and nonvegetarians. *Journal of the American Dietetic Association* 86:913.

Freeland-Graves, J. H. 1988. Mineral adequacy of vegetarian diets. *American Journal of Clinical Nutrition* 49:859.

Fukagawa, N. K., and B. R. Yong. 1987. Protein and amino acid metabolism and requirements in older persons.

Clinical Geriatric Medicine 3:329.

Guyton, A. 1986. *Textbook of medical physiology*, 3rd ed. Philadelphia: Saunders.

Hautvast, J. 1987. Proteins and selected vitamins. In Diet and health: Scientific concepts and principles. *American Journal of Clinical Nutrition* 45(supplement):1044.

Madison, D. et al. 1987. *The greens cookbook*. New York: Bantam Books.

Munro, H. N., and M. C. Crim. 1988. The proteins and amino acids. In *Modern nutrition in health and disease*, 7th ed. M. E. Shils and V. R. Young (eds.). Philadelphia: Lea & Febiger.

Murray, R. K. et al. 1988. *Harper's biochemistry*. Norwalk, CT: Appleton & Lange.

Pike, R., and M. Brown. 1985. *Nutrition: An integrated approach*, 3rd ed. New York: Wiley.

Ratto, T. 1986. Protein. *Medical Self-Care* 37:24.

Shulman, M. R. 1987. The vegetarian good life. *Health* 19(7):36.

Stryer, L. 1988. *Biochemistry*, 3rd ed. New York: W. H. Freeman.

Wurtman, R. J., and E. Ritter-Walker (eds.). 1988. *Dietary phenylalanine and brain function*. Cambridge, MA: Birkhauser Boston.

Young, V. R. 1987. Kinetics of amino acid metabolism: Nutritional implications and some lessons. 1987 McCollum Award Lecture. *American Journal of Clinical Nutrition* 46:709.

Young, V. R. et al. 1987. Amino acid requirements in the adult human: How well do we know them? *Journal of Nutrition* 117:1483.

Module 6

Vitamins and Health

Time for completion
Activities: _____1½_____ hours
Optional examination: ½ hour

Academic credit
Semester units: ³⁄₁₀
Quarter units: ⁴⁄₁₀

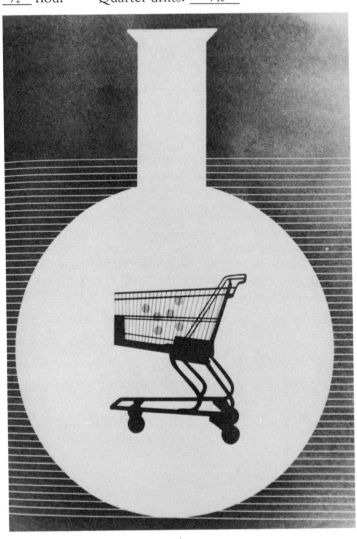

Outline

Objectives
Glossary
Background Information

ACTIVITY 1: The Water-Soluble Vitamins
Reference Tables
Progress Check on Activity 1

ACTIVITY 2: The Fat-Soluble Vitamins
Reference Tables
Progress Check on Activity 2
Responsibilities of Health Personnel
Summary
Progress Check on Module 6
References

Objectives

Upon completion of this module, the student should be able to:

1. Describe the general characteristics of vitamins.
2. Identify the fat-soluble vitamins and list
   a. their functions
   b. their food sources
   c. the results of a deficiency or excess
   d. the conditions requiring an increase
   e. the specific characteristics of each
3. Identify the water-soluble vitamins and list
   a. their functions
   b. their food sources
   c. the results of a deficiency or excess
   d. the conditions requiring an increase
   e. the specific characteristics of each
4. State RDAs for selected vitamins and discuss amounts of foods needed to meet the requirements.
5. Discuss health risks associated with massive intake of vitamins to prevent or treat disease.
6. Evaluate the effectiveness of megavitamin intake.
7. Indicate population groups for whom vitamin-mineral supplements may be necessary.

Glossary

Carotene: a yellow pigment in plants that can be converted to vitamin A in the intestinal wall.

Cheilosis: a condition in which lesions appear on the lips and the angles of the mouth (cracks).

Coenzyme: a substance such as a vitamin that can attach to the inactive form of an enzyme to make it an active compound or complete enzyme.

Collagen: a gelatin-like protein substance found in connective tissue and bones; a cementing material between body cells.

Dermatitis: inflammation of the skin.

Enzyme: a compound that speeds up the rate of a chemical reaction without itself being changed in the process.

Glossitis: inflammation of the tongue.

Hypervitaminosis: a toxic condition due to excessive accumulation of a vitamin in the body.

Megadose: a very large dose of a vitamin, 5 to 100 times or more the daily recommended allowance.

Organic: (1) containing carbon, a chemical definition; (2) free of chemical fertilizers, pesticides, and additives; a definition used by the lay public. In this module, organic refers to the first definition.

Osteomalacia: a disease occurring in adults in which bones become softened; caused by a deficiency of vitamin D and calcium. Adult rickets (see *Rickets*).

Osteoporosis: a disease in which calcium is lost from bones, causing them to fracture easily.

Provitamin or precursor: an ingested substance that is converted into a vitamin in the body. For example, carotene is the precursor of vitamin A, tryptophan the precursor of niacin.

Rickets: the vitamin D- and calcium-deficiency disease in children; results in bone malformation; equivalent to osteomalacia in adults.

Scurvy: the vitamin C-deficiency disease; characterized by loss of appetite and growth, anemia, weakness, bleeding gums, loose teeth, swollen ankles and wrists, and tiny hemorrhages in the skin.

Background Information

A. What are vitamins?
   1. Vitamins are essential organic substances needed daily in very small amounts to perform a specific function in the body. Although they are grouped under one term because they all contain carbon, the essentiality of vitamins for one species may not apply to another.
   2. Vitamins cannot be manufactured by the human body; they must be obtained from the diet. Monkeys and guinea pigs need the same outside sources of vitamins as humans do, whereas rabbits, rats, and dogs are able to manufacture some of them in the body.
   3. Vitamins are essential for growth and health. An absence or deficiency of vitamins creates specific disorders.
   4. The amount of vitamins needed is very small. The total daily requirement is less than 1 teaspoon.
   5. Currently, thirteen vitamins are identified as essential. Continued research may identify additional essential vitamins.
   6. Synthetic vitamins are nutritionally equivalent to naturally occurring vitamins.

B. What can vitamins do?
   1. In the digestive process, vitamins interact with other vitamins and/or nutrients to enhance absorption.
   2. Vitamins can function as coenzymes; that is, they can work with enzymes to speed up body chemical reactions. They are used up in the reactions, whereas the enzymes remain unchanged.
   3. Vitamins help release energy from biological reaction during metabolism. They do not provide energy.
   4. Vitamins are not a structural part of the body.

C. How are vitamins named?
   1. Vitamins are named by letters of the alphabet, sometimes with a number, such as vitamins A, B_1, B_2, C, D.

2. Vitamins are also given chemical names, for example, retinol, ascorbic acid, thiamin, and riboflavin refer to vitamins A, C, B_1, and B_2, respectively.

D. How are vitamins classified? Vitamins are classified into groups with regard to their solubility in either fat or water.
   1. The four fat-soluble vitamins
      a. vitamin A (retinol)
      b. vitamin D (cholecalciferol)
      c. vitamin E (tocopherol)
      d. vitamin K (menadione)
   2. The nine water-soluble vitamins
      a. vitamin C (ascorbic acid)
      b. vitamin B complex:
         vitamin B_1 (thiamin)
         vitamin B_2 (riboflavin)
         niacin
         vitamin B_6 (pyridoxine)
         vitamin B_{12} (cobalamin)
         folacin or folic acid
         pantothenic acid
         biotin

   Several vitamins exist in more than one chemical form.

E. How is food preparation related to the solubility of vitamins? The solubility of vitamins is directly related to their retention in foods during preparation.
   1. Water-soluble vitamins are lost into cooking water. For greater vitamin retention, the following general guidelines apply:
      a. Use only a small quantity of cooking water.
      b. Use leftover cooking water for making gravies, soups, and sauces. Do not discard it.
      c. Minimize cutting food into pieces.
      d. Use the shortest cooking time. Cooking with a lid helps to shorten cooking time.
   2. Fat-soluble vitamins are not affected by cooking and preparation in water, but may be destroyed by
      a. high cooking-heat, sun-drying or other forms of dehydration.
      b. oxidation that accompanies rancidity in fat. Fat-soluble vitamins are found in fat.

F. How are vitamins stored?
   1. Excess fat-soluble vitamins are stored in body fat and organs, especially the liver. This storage ability
      a. can delay deficiency for several months, even if the host does not receive such vitamins in the diet.
      b. means that the host needs a dietary supply every other day instead of daily.
      c. does not mean that the host is immune to large doses. Megadoses are toxic to the body.
   2. The body does not store excess water-soluble vitamins, but instead excretes them in the urine. As a result
      a. vitamin deficiency appears only a few weeks after dietary deprivation.
      b. the vitamins must be consumed daily.
      c. vitamin supplements do not have extra benefits if a person is consuming an adequate diet. Any excess is lost in the urine.
      d. some people assume that excess intake of water-soluble vitamins is harmless. However, there are reports documenting the ill effect of excess ingestion of these vitamins.

A summary of the characteristics of the two classes of vitamins is found in Table 6-1.

ACTIVITY 1: The Water-Soluble Vitamins

Reference Tables _____

The water-soluble vitamins, as discussed in the background information, are ascorbic acid (vitamin C) and the B vitamin complex. Tables 6-2 through 6-10 summarize the specific characteristics of each of these vitamins. Study them in preparation for the progress check below.

PROGRESS CHECK ON ACTIVITY 1

Multiple Choice

Circle the letter of the correct answer.

1. A person on a strict vegetarian diet is most likely to become deficient in which of the following vitamins?
   a. B_{12}
   b. folacin
   c. ascorbic acid
   d. B_6

2. Vitamin B_6 requirements are increased
   a. with increased energy intake.
   b. with increased protein intake.
   c. when on a reduction diet.
   d. with increased carbohydrate intake.

3. A deficiency of vitamin B_{12} produces
   a. pernicious anemia.
   b. cheilosis.
   c. microcytic anemia.
   d. sickle cell anemia.

TABLE 6-1
A General Comparison of Water- and Fat-Soluble Vitamins

Criteria	Vitamins	
	Water Soluble	Fat Soluble
1. Medium in which soluble	Aqueous, such as water	Nonpolar, organic, such as oil, fat, or ether
2. Number known to be essential to humans	9	4
3. Number human body can synthesize if precursors are provided.	1	2
4. Body storage capacity	Minimal	High
5. Body handling of excess intake	Mainly excreted; low toxicity to body	Optimal amount stored; rest excreted; toxicity to body high for two vitamins
6. Means of body disposal	Urine	Bile; if conjugated, urine
7. Urgency of dietary intake	At short intervals, e.g., daily	At longer intervals, e.g., weekly or monthly
8. Rapidity of symptom appearance if deficient	Fast	Slow
9. Chemical constituents	C, H, and O; S, N, and Co in some vitamins	C, H, and O only

4. Research studies have shown that a one-gram dose of vitamin C daily
   a. will reduce the total number of colds among adults.
   b. is no more effective against cold symptoms than is 75 mg daily.
   c. will lessen the effects of a hangover.
   d. will be stored in the body.

5. Which condition(s) may result in folic acid deficiency?
   a. a strict vegetarian diet
   b. use of contraceptive pills and/or pregnancy
   c. malabsorption syndromes
   d. all of the above

6. The 1989 RDA gives a safe and adequate intake for ascorbic acid as
   a. 400 IU per day.
   b. 60 mg per day.
   c. 2 to 3 mg per day.
   d. 40 g per day.

7. Risks associated with megadose ascorbic acid intake include all except
   a. bladder infections.
   b. possible increase in kidney stone formation.
   c. diarrhea.
   d. eye infections.

8. Ascorbic acid plays a major role in the formation of which protein?
   a. histidine
   b. keratin
   c. collagen
   d. mucus

9. All of the following refer to vitamin B_{12} except
   a. it requires an intrinsic factor for absorption.
   b. a deficiency results in pernicious anemia.
   c. food sources rich in vitamin B_{12} include asparagus and broccoli.
   d. vitamin B_{12} is necessary for normal red blood cell formation.

10. Riboflavin is
    a. added to white flour for enrichment.
    b. found abundantly in milk and cheese.
    c. an essential nutrient.
    d. all of the above.

11. Niacin
    a. can be made by the body from tryptophan, an essential amino acid.
    b. is found in abundance in meats, poultry, and fish.
    c. is fat soluble.
    d. is none of the above.

TABLE 6-2
Vitamin C (Ascorbic Acid)

Functions	Food Sources	Results of Deficiency or Excess	Conditions Requiring Increase	Specific Characteristics

Essential in formation of collagen, a protein that binds cells together.
 	
Needed to heal wounds, build new tissue, and provide strength to supporting tissue.
 	
Aids formation of bone matrix and tooth dentin.
 	
Absorbs iron which promotes prothrombin formation.
 	
Helps maintain elasticity of blood vessels and capillaries.
 	
Acts as an antioxidant, protecting the cells from oxidation.
 	
Has a sparing effect on several vitamins; especially A, B, and E.
	RDA: 60 mg adults
	
	Excellent Sources
	chili peppers, green peppers
	parsley
	broccoli
	kale
	cabbage
	strawberries
	papaya
	oranges (and juice)
	lemons
	grapefruit (and juice)
	guava
	tangerines
	cantaloupe
	watermelon
	
	Good Sources
	tomatoes (and juice)
	white potatoes (with skin on)
	sweet potatoes
	honeydew melon
	pineapple
	
	The only animal source of vitamin C is liver.
		Deficiency
		acute deficiency—scurvy*
		delayed wound healing
		failure to thrive (children)
		decayed and breaking teeth
		iron deficient gingivitis anemia (if iron intake also low)
		low resistance to infection (especially infants)
		small vessel hemorrhage seen under skin
		easy bruising
		
		Excess
		(specific effects depend on the individual's tolerance level)
		rebound scurvy
		interference with certain drugs
		gastrointestinal upsets and diarrhea
		bladder irritations
		kidney stones
		interference with anticoagulant drug therapy
			Pregnancy and lactation
			Malnutrition
			Alcoholism/drug addiction
			Infections, burns, injuries, fever
			Certain drug therapies, e.g., isoniazid,† OCAs**
			High stress conditions
				1. Vitamin C is easily destroyed by heat, storage, exposure to air, dehydration alkali (such as baking soda), and lengthy exposure to copper and iron utensils.
				2. Vitamin C deficiency is rare in developed countries, but can occur in any cases of serious neglect such as psychiatric problems, substance abuse, advanced age, and lack of knowledge about nutrition.
				3. Extra care must be taken in preparation of foods containing vitamin C to prevent excessive loss:
				  a. use small amount water
				  b. avoid prolonged cooking
				  c. cut up just before use
				  d. avoid leftovers
				  e. cook quickly, covered or steamed
				  f. use any cooking liquid (do not drain)

*See definition in glossary
†Drug used in treatment of tuberculosis
**Oral contraceptive agents

12. Pyridoxine
    a. is a coenzyme in protein metabolism and heme formation.
    b. is found in wheat, corn, meats, and liver.
    c. aids functioning of the nervous system.
    d. is all of the above.

13. Cobalamin
    a. requires intrinsic factor from the stomach for absorption.
    b. should be supplemented in the average person's diet.
    c. is toxic if taken in excess.
    d. is none of the above.

TABLE 6-3
Vitamin B₁ (Thiamin)

Functions	Food Sources	Results of Deficiency or Excess	Conditions Requiring Increase	Specific Characteristics
Releases energy from fat and carbohydrate. Helps transmit nerve impulses. Breaks down alcohol. Promotes better appetite and functioning of the digestive tract.	*RDA:* adult male 1.5 mg adult female 1.1 mg *Excellent Sources* sunflower seeds sesame seeds soybeans wheat germ peanuts animal sources: liver, kidney, pork *Good Sources* enriched cereals enriched pasta enriched or brown rice whole grains oatmeal animal sources: eggs, poultry	*Deficiency* acute: beri-beri* subacute: loss of appetite, vomiting, leg cramps, mental depression, edema, weight loss *Excess* no evidence of toxicity in excess amounts. May create a shortage of other B vitamins if taken exclusively	Any condition that increases metabolic rate Alcoholism Old age (whether elderly are on low-calorie diets or not) Pregnancy and lactation growth periods People on fad diets Illness/stress conditions Athletic training (whenever extra need for kcal)	The B vitamins have four common properties: 1. All of them function as coenzymes in biochemical reactions. 2. All are water soluble. 3. All are natural parts of yeast and liver. 4. All promote the growth of bacteria. If there is a deficiency in one of the B vitamins, there will be deficiencies in the others. The B vitamins function together— excess of one creates greater need for the others. Converted rice contains more thiamin than other types of rice.

*Beri-beri: means "I cannot." Major symptoms are paralysis, heart and vessel impairment.

14. Factors that may cause a deficiency of water-soluble vitamins include
    a. taking no vitamin supplement.
    b. fad diets.
    c. high fat diets.
    d. none of the above.

15. A deficiency of vitamin C
    a. causes delayed wound healing.
    b. decreases iron absorption.
    c. increases capillary bleeding.
    d. all of the above.

16. Water-soluble vitamins
    a. are generally stored by the body.
    b. are destroyed by fats and oils.

    c. are minimally excreted.
    d. none of the above.

17. B complex vitamins
    a. function as coenzymes.
    b. are best supplied by supplements.
    c. can be synthesized by the body.
    d. are excreted in feces.

18. Which of the following is the poorest source of ascorbic acid?
    a. cheddar cheese
    b. baked potato
    c. strawberries
    d. coleslaw

TABLE 6-4
Vitamin B$_2$ (Riboflavin)

Functions	Food Sources	Results of Deficiency or Excess	Conditions Requiring Increase	Specific Characteristics
Releases energy from fat, carbohydrate, and protein. Essential for healthy skin and growth. Promotes visual health. Functions in the production of corticosteroids* and red blood cells.	RDA: set according to age groups adult males: 1.7 mg adult females: 1.3 mg *Excellent Sources* milk cheese wheat germ yeast liver and kidney *Good Sources* meat, poultry, fish eggs dark green leafy vegetables dry beans and peas nuts	*Deficiency* lesions around the mouth and nose hair loss scaly skin failure to thrive (children) light sensitivity clouding of the cornea of the eye weight loss glossitis *Excess* no evidence yet that this nutrient is toxic in large amounts	Increase in body size, metabolic rate, or growth rate, such as pregnancy, lactation, and growth Alcoholism Poverty Old age Strict vegetarian diets that prohibit meat, eggs, and milk Stress and malabsorption of nutrients Any condition where there is loss of gastric secretions (achlorhydria) may precipitate a deficiency Following burns or any surgical procedure where there is extensive protein loss	1. No evidence that the requirement for B$_2$ goes up as kcal rise. 2. Few individuals in the U.S. show any deficiency. 3. Foods high in calcium are usually high in B$_2$. 4. Before riboflavin is absorbed it must be phosphorylated (combined with phosphorus). Both are found in milk and cheeses. 5. Is sensitive to light; should be kept in opaque containers. 6. Cooking and drying may enhance the availability. 7. Only partially water-soluble. 8. If a deficiency occurs, multiple B vitamins are given because of their interrelationships. 9. B$_2$ is destroyed by alkaline.

*Hormones of the adrenal cortex that influence or control key body functions.

ACTIVITY 2: The Fat-Soluble Vitamins

Reference Tables _____

The fat-soluble vitamins, as discussed earlier, are vitamins A, D, E, and K. Other than the general characteristics noted, these vitamins bear no resemblance to water-soluble vitamins nor to each other. In Tables 6-11 through 6-14, the specific characteristics of each fat-soluble vitamin are outlined for easy reference. Study them in preparation for the progress check below.

PROGRESS CHECK ON ACTIVITY 2 _____

Multiple Choice

Circle the letter of the correct answer.

1. All except _____ are good sources of vitamin A.
   a. egg yolks
   b. potatoes
   c. dark green and deep yellow vegetables
   d. beef liver

2. Toxicity symptoms of vitamin A include all except
   a. joint pain, loss of hair, jaundice.
   b. anorexia, fatigue, weight loss.
   c. vasodilation, decreased glucose tolerance.
   d. skin rash, edema.

TABLE 6-5
Vitamin B$_6$ (Pyridoxine)

Functions	Food Sources	Results of Deficiency or Excess	Conditions Requiring Increase	Specific Characteristics
Forms reactions that break down and rebuild amino acids. Produces antibodies and red blood cells. Aids functioning of the nervous system and regeneration of nerve tissue. Changes one fatty acid into another.	*RDA:* adult male 2.0 mg adult female 1.6 mg *Excellent Sources* yeast sunflower seeds wheat germ wheat bran avocado banana animal source: liver *Good Sources* meats poultry fish whole grains nuts	*Deficiency* decreased antibody production anemia vomiting failure to thrive (children) skin lesions liver and kidney problems central nervous system abnormalities: confusion irritability depression convulsions *Excess* no toxicity reported with megadoses, but dependency may be induced with large doses	Increased protein intake Pregnancy Use of oral contraceptive agents, isoniazid Advancing age	1. B$_6$ deficiencies occur almost entirely in wealthy, developed countries. 2. The essential fatty acid, linoleic, is converted to B$_6$ to arachidonic. 3. Converts tryptophan to niacin. 4. Involved in conversions and catabolism of all the amino acids.

3. Which of the following foods would you recommend in order to increase a person's vitamin A intake?
   a. grapefruit
   b. egg whites
   c. potatoes
   d. pumpkin

4. Vitamin D is needed by the body to
   a. digest protein.
   b. absorb amino acids.
   c. absorb calcium.
   d. make collagen.

5. Fat-soluble vitamins
   a. may be altered by exposure to alkali.
   b. are stable to ordinary cooking.
   c. can store in liver and tissues.
   d. all of the above.

6. Carotene, or provitamin A, is contained in significant amounts in all of these except
   a. corn, cauliflower.
   b. spinach, collard greens.
   c. apricots, pumpkin.
   d. green pepper, peaches.

7. Vitamin D functions to
   a. enhance calcium and phosphorus absorption.
   b. enhance mineralization of bones and cartilage.
   c. lower serum calcium levels.
   d. all of the above.

8. Excess vitamin D
   a. is stored in adipose tissue and the liver.
   b. can cause calcification of soft tissue such as blood vessels and renal tubules.
   c. is excreted in the urine.
   d. a and b.

9. The only demonstrated function of vitamin E in humans is to
   a. increase sexual prowess.
   b. increase fertility.
   c. act as an antioxidant.
   d. prevent heart disease.

10. The only known function of vitamin K is its
   a. use in forming blood-clotting factors.
   b. antioxidant property.
   c. antirachitic property.
   d. antibiotic property.

TABLE 6-6
Vitamin B$_{12}$ (Cobalamin)

Functions	Food Sources	Results of Deficiency or Excess	Conditions Requiring Increase	Specific Characteristics
Aids proper formation of red blood cells. Part of the RNA-DNA nucleic acids; is therefore essential for normal function of all body cells, especially gastrointestinal tract, nervous system. Bone marrow formation. Used in folacin metabolism. Prevention of pernicious anemia.	*RDA:* male and female adults 2.0 µg *Animal products are the main food sources:* clams/oysters organ meats eggs shrimp chicken pork	*Deficiency* glossitis anorexia weakness weight loss mental and nervous symptoms abdominal pain constipation/diarrhea macrocytic anemia and if intrinsic factor also missing: pernicious anemia (see #4 under characteristics) *Excess* no toxicity observed; but at high doses, vitamins are considered drugs and often create imbalances in the functioning of other nutrients.	Strict vegetarian diet (vegans) Malabsorption Stomach injury Total gastrectomy Pregnancy and lactation Old age	1. The normal liver will store enough B$_{12}$ to last for two to five years. 2. B$_{12}$ is made only by microorganisms in the intestines. 3. Only 30–70% of what is consumed is absorbed. 4. B$_{12}$ must bind to the *intrinsic factor* which is a protein secreted by stomach lining. 5. Calcium is also necessary in this reaction. 6. Absorption of B$_{12}$ is influenced by body levels of B$_6$. 7. The elderly are at highest risk of developing pernicious anemia. 8. Smooth, bland foods are indicated for megaloblastic and pernicious anemia (the mouth is sore). 9. All foods needed for blood cell production included.

*Folic acid deficiency is frequently associated with B$_{12}$ deficiency, creating a vicious cycle.

Matching

Match the following statements with the letter of their corresponding vitamin.

B 11. Inadequate intake causes osteomalacia and rickets.

A 12. Inadequate intake causes poor night vision and skin infection.

D 13. Promotes normal blood clotting.

C 14. Prevents destruction of unsaturated fatty acids.

    a. vitamin A
    b. vitamin D
    c. vitamin E
    d. vitamin K

Responsibilities of Health Personnel _____

1. Treat clients' vitamin deficiency diseases by supplying the missing vitamin(s) as drug therapy (through tablets, capsules, or intravenously) as an adjunct to a high protein, high calorie balanced diet.
2. Treat borderline vitamin deficiencies by supplying the appropriate diet and including rich sources of the missing vitamin(s).
3. Be aware that some patients may not be able to take food or medication by mouth. Nausea and anorexia, common among people suffering from vitamin-deficiency diseases, may require different forms of ingestion.

TABLE 6-7
Niacin

Functions	Food Sources	Results of Deficiency or Excess	Conditions Requiring Increase	Specific Characteristics
Releases energy from carbohydrates, protein, fat. Synthesizes proteins and nucleic acids. Synthesizes fatty acids from glucose.	*RDA:* adult males: 19 mg** adult females: 15 mg given in tryptophan equivalents (60 mg tryptophan equals 1 mg niacin) *Excellent Sources* yeast peanuts and peanut butter soybeans sesame seeds sunflower seeds animal sources: beef, poultry, fish, organ meats especially high *Good Sources* meats nuts wheat germ enriched cereals, bread, pasta	*Deficiency* acute: Pellagra* subacute: weakness, indigestion, anorexia, lack of energy, cracked skin, sore mouth and tongue, failure to thrive (children), insomnia, irritability, mental depression; damage to the skin, gastrointestinal tract, and central nervous system *Excess* (megadose treatment for certain conditions) severe flushing glucose intolerance gastrointestinal disorders irregular heartbeat vision disturbances liver damage	Whenever more kcal are consumed, e.g.: pregnancy/lactation illness stress chronic alcoholism intestinal disorders	1. Niacin is synthesized in the body from tryptophan, an essential amino acid. Diets adequate in protein are adequate in niacin. 2. Niacin is stable in foods; it can withstand reasonable periods of heat, cooling, and storage. 3. Niacin is water-soluble; use the cooking liquids (do not drain off).

*The 3 Ds of Pellagra symptoms: 1. Dermatitis (inflammation of the skin); 2. Diarrhea (inflammation in the gastrointestinal tract); 3. Dementia (mental confusion); (if untreated: add death).

4. Be aware that most outright deficiency diseases occur among alcoholics, drug abusers, psychiatric patients, the aged, low income groups, or people on extreme diets.
5. Be aware that borderline deficiencies cut across all socioeconomic lines, and are due to poor eating habits and ignorance of essential nutrients.
6. Be prepared to give multivitamin and mineral supplements to allow the metabolic interrelationships among the vitamins and their action as catalysts and coenzymes to occur.
7. Request extra vitamins for clients with conditions that increase the metabolic rate.
8. Be aware that very low-fat diets lead to decreased intake and absorption of the fat-soluble vitamins.
9. Be aware that the fat-soluble vitamins A and D are highly toxic in doses that greatly exceed the RDAs.
10. Request fat-soluble vitamin supplements in aqueous form any time there is a disease where fat malabsorption occurs, such as celiac disease or cystic fibrosis.

Summary

Vitamins are organic compounds that are required in the diet in very small amounts, but which perform very important functions. They are classified on the basis of solubility in either water or fat.

Fat-soluble vitamins are stored in the fats of foods and in the body. Because of this, humans may not need a daily source. Excess intakes of fat-soluble vitamins can be toxic, especially vitamins A and D. Fat-soluble vitamins can withstand factors such as heat and pressure.

Daily consumption of water-soluble vitamins is necessary because the body does not store them. These vitamins are easily lost from food not properly prepared, stored, or processed. While large doses of water-soluble vitamins are usually not considered toxic, an excess intake of certain vitamins results in adverse side effects.

No vitamin provides energy, but some vitamins are involved in releasing energy from the metabolism of carbohydrate, protein, and fat. Vitamins are considered as

TABLE 6-8
Folic Acid (Folacin, Folate)

Functions	Food Sources	Results of Deficiency or Excess	Conditions Requiring Increase	Specific Characteristics
Synthesizes the nucleic acids (RNA-DNA). Essential for breakdown of most of the amino acids. Necessary for proper formation of red blood cells.	*RDA:* adult males: 200 µg adult females: 180 µg *Excellent Sources* liver/kidney yeast oranges/orange juice* green leafy vegetables asparagus* broccoli wheat germ* nuts *Good Sources* melons sweet potato pumpkin	*Deficiency* slows growth, interferes with cell regeneration *Macrocytic Anemia* (red blood cells are large and too few and have less Hbg than normal) *Megoblastic Anemia* (young red blood cells fail to mature, reduction in white blood cells; also histidine, an amino acid, not utilized) *Excess* no toxic effect from megadose, but will mask pernicious anemias,† vitamin supplements may not contain more than 0.1 mg/folacin (by law)	Whenever the metabolic rate is high: pregnancy/ lactation** infections/fever growth of malignant tumors hyperthyroidism anemias Excess alcohol intake Use of oral contraceptive agents Malabsorptive disorders Certain other diseases, e.g.: leukemia Hodgkin's disease cancer Use of drugs in anticonvulsant therapy When chemotherapy is used for cancer	1. When there is a folic acid deficiency, the diet must include all the other nutrients needed to produce red blood cells, i.e.: protein copper iron B_{12}/vitamin C 2. Persons with macrocytic or megoblastic anemia have sore mouths and tongues; soft bland foods or liquids may be needed. 3. Prolonged cooking destroys most of the folacin. 4. Folic acid deficiency is common in the third trimester of pregnancy; the requirement is six times the normal amount.

*Highest in folacin
**400 µg required for pregnancy; 280 for lactation
†Pernicious anemia does not respond to iron and folacin; requires treatment with B_{12}.

coenzymes and therefore do not undergo changes during biological reactions.

Megavitamin therapy is a controversial topic. Promoters have linked massive doses of vitamins with the prevention and treatment of numerous human diseases, but most of these "cures" remain unproven or have been shown to be dangerous. Nutrients are considered drugs when they are used in large doses for treating any disease. At high doses, vitamins behave differently than at recommended doses. The Food and Drug Administration (FDA) has tried but failed to limit or prohibit the sale of megavitamins without a prescription.

Many people believe that "natural" vitamins are better than synthetic ones, and that natural vitamins are "pure" and contain no chemicals. Both beliefs are untrue. The chemical structure of a synthetic and a natural vitamin is exactly the same, and the body cannot distinguish between them. In addition, "natural" vitamins have synthetic substances holding them together. There is only one difference between a natural and a synthetic vitamin: the natural one costs two to three times more.

Supplementing the diet with vitamins has been another long-standing controversial issue. Most nutritionists are in agreement that you cannot compensate for a poor diet by taking a supplement; many foods contain necessary nutrients not included in commercial supplements. But some population groups are at high risk of vitamin deficiency and probably need a supplement. These groups include

1.   women during pregnancy and lactation
2.   infants
3.   anyone on a diet containing fewer than 1,000 calories per day

TABLE 6-9
Pantothenic Acid

Functions	Food Sources	Results of Deficiency or Excess	Conditions Requiring Increase	Specific Characteristics
Helps release energy from carbohydrate, fat, and protein. Aids in formation of cholesterol, hemoglobin, and other hormones. Assists in synthesizing certain fatty acids.	*RDA:* Estimated adequate intake: 5–10 mg/day approximate need *Richest Sources* liver, kidney fish whole grains Is found in every plant and animal food	*Deficiency* uncommon; not observed under normal conditions Induced deficiencies cause headaches, insomnia, nausea, vomiting, tingling of hands and feet poor coordination *Excess* no toxicity observed	*Rare Situations* severe malnutrition (e.g., prisoner-of-war, starving children)	1. Most commonly occurring of all the vitamins 2. Name taken from the Greek and means "everywhere"

4. strict vegetarians
5. many senior citizens
6. persons with certain illnesses or convalescing from surgery

Other than for the last group, nutrient supplements should not be taken in megadose quantities. They should be administered in quantities that assist the person to fulfill the FDA requirements.

TABLE 6-10
Biotin

Functions	Food Sources	Results of Deficiency or Excess	Conditions Requiring Increase	Specific Characteristics
Acts as a coenzyme in metabolism of fat and carbohydrate.	*RDA:* Estimated 30–100 µg/day considered adequate *Richest Sources* liver/kidney egg yolk milk yeast Is found in almost all foods	*Deficiency* uncommon; intestinal bacteria produces biotin. can be induced large scale use of raw eggs as in tube feedings, etc., may cause development of symptoms such as: nausea muscle pain dermatitis glossitis abnormal EKG (electrocardiogram) elevated cholesterol level	Anyone consuming raw eggs in quantity Some infants under age of 6 mo.	1. Biotin can be bound by *avidin*, a protein in raw egg, and becomes unavailable to the body.

TABLE 6-11
Vitamin A (Retinol)

Functions	Food Sources	Results of Deficiency or Excess	Conditions Requiring Increase	Specific Characteristics
Enables eye to adjust to changes in light (formation of rhodopsin in the retina). Helps maintain healthy skin and mucous membranes as well as the cornea of the eye. Develops healthy teeth and bones. Aids reproductive processes. Synthesizes glycogen in the liver. Regulates fat metabolism in formation of cholesterol. Aids formation of cortisone in the adrenal gland.	*RDA:* males 1,000 µg RE* females 800 µg RE* *Excellent Sources* liver carrots cantaloupe sweet potato winter squash pumpkin apricots broccoli green pepper dark green leafy vegetables *Good Sources* tomatoes (and juice) butter margarine peaches	*Deficiency** night blindness (inability to see in dim light) keratinization (formation of a horny layer of skin, cracking of skin) xerophthalmia (cornea of eye becomes opaque, causing blindness) faulty bone growth, defective tooth enamel, less resistance to decay decreased resistance to infection, impaired wound healing *Excess* highly toxic in excessive doses (1–3,000 µg RE/kg/ body weight) accumulates in liver, causing enlargement, vomiting, skin rashes, hair loss, diarrhea, cramps, joint pain, dry scaly skin, anorexia, abnormal bone growth, cerebral edema	Self-neglect due to psychiatric disturbances, old age, alcoholism, lack of nutritional knowledge Pregnancy and lactation Protein-deficient diets Any condition of fat malabsorption Infectious hepatitis Gallbladder diseases	1. Preformed vitamin A (retinol) is found only in animal sources. 2. Provitamin A (carotene) is found in plant sources and is a yellow-orange group of pigments. It is called a precursor. 3. Xerophthalmia is an important world health problem: more than 100,000 children go blind yearly, especially in underdeveloped countries. 4. Very low fat diets decrease absorption. 5. Vitamin A must be bound to protein for transport. 6. Bile salts must be in the intestine for absorption. 7. Is stable at usual cooking temperatures. Covered pan recommended. 8. Processing and advance preparation cause only minimal loss. 9. Hypervitaminosis is usually from megavitamin supplements. 10. Excess intake of foods with carotene may discolor skin but is not harmful. 11. Beta carotene is being considered for prevention of certain types of skin cancer.

*1 retinol equivalent equals 1 µg retinol or 6 µg beta carotene.
**Deficiencies more uncommon in Western countries because of dietary abundance.

TABLE 6-12
Vitamin D (Cholecalciferol)

Functions	Food Sources	Results of Deficiency or Excess	Conditions Requiring Increase	Specific Characteristics
Promotes the absorption of calcium and phosphorus in the intestine. Helps maintain blood calcium and phosphorus levels for normal bone calcification. Aids in formation of bone matrix.	RDA:* 10 µg *Sources:* irradiated fortified vitamin D milk minimal amounts present in fish, egg yolk, butter *Primary food source* fish, liver (cod liver, halibut liver) oils *Synthetic form* from irradiation of plants; used most in supplements and dairy products *Principal source* sunlight; ultraviolet rays penetrate a cholesterol-like substance in the skin which is converted to active vitamin D in the kidney	*Deficiency* *severe* rickets, serious decalcification of bones, osteomalacia (tender, painful bones in adults), tooth decay *Excess* high blood calcium levels kidney damage growth retardation vomiting, diarrhea, weight loss	Invalids (housebound) Individuals who are rarely exposed to sunlight Premature infants Children of strict vegetarians who drink no fortified milk Pregnancy and lactation Early childhood Breast-fed infants Any disease that interferes with fat absorption or vitamin D absorption Chronic renal failure Certain drug therapies that interfere with absorption Dark-skinned people	1. Ultraviolet light is filtered out by smog, fog, smoke, and window glass 2. Can be classified as a hormone since it can be made by the body. 3. Milk, unless fortified, is a poor source of vitamin D. 4. As much as 95% of ultraviolet rays for conversion to vitamin D may be prevented in dark-skinned races. 5. Vitamin D permits 30–35% absorption of ingested calcium: without it only 10% is absorbed.

*As cholecalciferol 10 µg = 400 IU of vitamin D.

PROGRESS CHECK ON MODULE 6

Matching

Match the vitamin to the letter of the phrase that best describes it.

C 1. Riboflavin
A 2. Thiamin
D 3. Vitamin B₆
E 4. Vitamin B₁₂
B 5. Niacin

a. requirement is based on the amount of carbohydrate in diet
b. may be synthesized from the amino acid tryptophan
c. deficiency causes cracked skin around the mouth, inflamed lips, and sore tongue
d. helps change one amino acid into another
e. a cobalt-containing vitamin needed for red blood cell formation

Match the nutrients listed in the left column with the major sources of those nutrients in the right column.

D 6. Vitamin B₁₂   a. orange juice
E 7. Riboflavin   b. dark green leafy vegetables
A 8. Vitamin C   c. sunshine
C 9. Vitamin D   d. meats
B 10. Beta-carotene   e. milk

True/False

Circle T for True and F for False.

11. T F Synthetic vitamins are nutritionally equivalent to naturally occurring vitamins.
12. T F Vitamin losses from fruits and vegetables can occur as a result of poor conditions of harvesting and storage.
13. T F Natural and synthetic vitamins are used by the body in the same way.

TABLE 6-13
Vitamin E (Tocopherol)

Functions	Food Sources	Results of Deficiency or Excess	Conditions Requiring Increase	Specific Characteristics
The only *demonstrated* function is as an antioxidant (protects vitamin A and unsaturated fats from destruction; protects red blood cells from destruction by preventing oxidation of cell membrane). Protects vitamin C and fatty acids. Believed to enter into biochemical changes which release energy. Assists in cellular respiration. Helps synthesize other body substances. Helps maintain intact cell membranes.	RDA: 8–10 mg T.E.* *Best Sources (plant)* vegetable oils margarines shortenings sunflower seeds wheat germ nuts whole grains *Good Sources (animal)* liver codfish butter human milk	*Deficiency* none observed except in premature infants or SGA** infants *Excess* headache nausea fatigue dizziness blurred vision skin changes thrombophlebitis†	Premature infants (or SGA)** Whenever greater amounts of polyunsaturated fats are ingested Possibly in disorders resulting in fat malabsorption	1. Does not travel well across placenta of pregnant women. 2. Is usually given with vitamin A when there is a vitamin A deficiency. 3. Vitamin E content of breast milk is adequate for the infant. 4. Many animal disorders have responded to vitamin E therapy but have not been effective for humans. For this reason, vitamin E is the most controversial of all vitamin therapies. 5. Contrary to popular opinion, excess intake creates side effects. 6. The role of vitamin E as an antioxidant is being linked to retardation of the aging process.

*Tocopherol equivalents
†Blood clots in veins.
**SGA = small for gestational age.

14. (T) F Vitamin K is required for the synthesis of blood-clotting factors.
15. (T) F B vitamins serve as coenzymes in metabolic reactions in the body.
16. (T) F There is no RDA for vitamin K because it is produced by the body.

Classification

Classify the following phrases as descriptive of either water-soluble or fat-soluble vitamins.

Water soluble = a   Fat-soluble = b

17. _b_   are stored in appreciable amounts in the body

18. _A_   are excreted in the urine
19. _A_   require regular consumption in the diet because storage in the body is minimal
20. _B_   deficiencies are slow to develop
21. _A_   B complex and vitamin C are examples of
22. _D_   vitamins A, D, E, and K are examples of

Multiple Choice

Circle the letter of the correct answer.

23. Which of the following food preparation methods is most likely to cause large losses of vitamins?
    a. cooking fruits and vegetables whole and unpared
    (b.) dicing fruits and vegetables into small pieces

TABLE 6-14
Vitamin K (Menadione)

Functions	Food Sources	Results of Deficiency or Excess	Conditions Requiring Increase	Specific Characteristics
Prothrombin formation (prothrombin is a protein which converts eventually to fibrin, the key substance in blood clotting) Blood coagulation	RDA: males 70–80 µg females 60–65 µg The two sources are: 1. intestinal bacteria and 2. food sources: dark green vegetables cauliflower tomatoes soybeans wheat bran small amounts in: egg yolk organ meats cheese	*Deficiency* hemorrhaging when blood does not clot *Excess* irritation of skin and respiratory tract with the synthetic form, menadione toxicity found only in newborns who are administered doses above 5 mg causes excessive breakdown of red blood cells	Newborn infants Persons on antibiotics Persons with diseases where there is chronic diarrhea or poor absorption Possibly prior to surgery	1. Deficiency is rare since it is synthesized by intestinal bacteria. Food sources not usually needed by healthy people. 2. The intestinal tract of the newborn may be free of bacteria for several days. 3. Antibiotics kill the natural bacteria in the intestine.

c. cutting fruits and vegetables into medium-size, chunky pieces

d. cutting just before serving time

24. When cooking vegetables to conserve vitamins, which is preferred?
   a. small amounts of water
   b. large amounts of water
   c. no water
   d. addition of baking soda

25. Which vegetable preparation method tends to conserve the most vitamins?
   a. boiling
   b. simmering
   c. stir-frying
   d. baking

26. Excessive vitamin intake has
   a. not been demonstrated to be beneficial in humans.
   b. been shown to cause toxicity by some vitamins.
   c. been shown to cause increased excretion of the water-soluble vitamins.
   d. all of the above.

27. An important role of the water-soluble vitamins is to serve as
   a. enzymes.
   b. hormones.
   c. electrolytes.
   d. coenzymes.

28. Vitamin/mineral supplements are generally recommended for _____ because they are at higher risk of developing deficiencies.
   a. infants
   b. pregnant and lactating women
   c. strict vegetarians
   d. persons with malabsorption diseases

29. One should avoid taking vitamin pills unless especially prescribed by one's doctor because
   a. they are too expensive.
   b. fat-soluble vitamins are stored in the body and can build up to toxic levels.
   c. water-soluble vitamins in excess of daily requirements may become toxic to the liver.
   d. edema can result from high blood levels of water-soluble vitamins.

30. Good food sources of thiamin include all except
   a. lean pork, beef, and liver.
   b. citrus fruits.
   c. green leafy vegetables.
   d. sunflower and sesame seeds.

References

Bauerfeind, J. C. 1988. Vitamin A deficiency: A staggering problem of health and sight. *Nutrition Today* 23(2):34.

Beck, W. S. 1988. Cobalamin and the nervous system. *New England Journal of Medicine* 318:752.

Carpenter, K. J. 1986. *The history of scurvy and vitamin C.* New York: Cambridge University Press.

Cohen, M., and A. Bendich. 1986. Safety of pyridoxin—A review of human and animal studies. *Toxicology Letters* 34:129.

Cooper, B. A., and D. S. Rosenblatt. 1987. Inherited defects of vitamin B_{12} metabolism. *Annual Review of Nutrition* 7:291.

DeLuca, H. F. 1988. Vitamin D and its metabolites. In *Modern nutrition in health and disease,* 7th ed. M. E. Shils and V. R. Young (eds.). Philadelphia: Lea & Febiger.

Farrell, P. M. 1988. Vitamin E. In *Modern nutrition in health and disease,* 7th ed. M. E. Shils and V. R. Young (eds.). Philadelphia: Lea & Febiger.

Food and Nutrition Board. 1989. *Diet and health.* Washington, DC: National Academy of Sciences.

Goodman, L. 1985. *Goodman and Gilman's the pharmacological basis of therapeutics.* New York: MacMillan.

Heiby, W. A. 1988. *The reverse effect: How vitamins and minerals promote health and disease.* Deerfield, IL: Medi Science Publishers.

Herbert, V. D. 1988. Pseudovitamins. In *Modern nutrition in health and disease,* 7th ed. M. E. Shils and V. R. Young (eds.). Philadelphia: Lea & Febiger.

Ink, S. L., and L. M. Henderson. 1984. Vitamin B-6 metabolism. *Annual Review of Nutrition* 4:455.

Isler, O. et al. 1988. *Vitamine II.* New York: Georg Thiem Verlag.

Liebman, B. 1983. Too much of a good thing is toxic. *Nutrition Action* 10(4):6.

Levine, M. 1986. New concepts in the biology and biochemistry of ascorbic acid. *New England Journal of Medicine* 314:892.

Machlin, L. J. (ed.). 1984. *Handbook of vitamins: Nutritional, biochemical, and clinical aspects.* New York: Marcel Dekker.

McLaren, D. S. 1988. Clinical manifestations of nutritional disorders. In *Modern nutrition in health and disease,* 7th ed. M. E. Shils and V. R. Young (eds.). Philadelphia: Lea & Febiger.

National Academy of Sciences, Subcommittee on Vitamin A Deficiency Prevention and Control, Committee on International Nutrition Programs, Food and Nutrition Board, Commission on Life Sciences, National Research Council. 1987. *Vitamin A supplementation: Methodologies for field trials.* Washington, DC: National Academy Press.

Olson, J. A. 1987. Recommended dietary intakes (RDI) of vitamin K in humans. *American Journal of Clinical Nutrition* 45:687.

Olson, J. A. 1988. Vitamin A, retinoids, and carotenoids. In *Modern nutrition in health and disease,* 7th ed. M. E. Shils and V. R. Young (eds.). Philadelphia: Lea & Febiger.

Olson, R. E. 1988. Vitamin K. In *Modern nutrition in health and disease,* 7th ed. M. E. Shils and V. R. Young (eds.). Philadelphia: Lea & Febiger.

Roe, D. A. (ed.). 1986. Nutrition and the skin. *Contemporary issues in clinical nutrition.* New York: Alan R. Liss.

Shils, M. E., and V. R. Young (eds.). 1988. *Modern nutrition in health and disease,* 7th ed. Philadelphia: Lea & Febiger.

Zeisel, S. H. 1988. Choline. In *Modern nutrition in health and disease,* 7th ed. M. E. Shils and V. R. Young (eds.). Philadelphia: Lea & Febiger.

Minerals, Water, and Body Processes

Time for completion

Activities: _____2_____ hours

Optional examination: ½ hour

Academic credit

Semester units: 3/10

Quarter units: 4/10

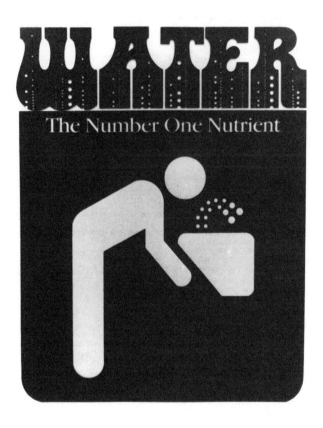

WATER
The Number One Nutrient

Outline

Objectives

Upon completion of this module, the student should be able to:

1. Explain the role of minerals in regulating body processes.
2. List the essential minerals and their major functions.
3. Describe the characteristics of the minerals and the difference between macro- and microminerals.
4. Identify major food sources of each mineral.
5. List the minerals for which there are RDAs and the amounts required to maintain health.
6. Discuss factors that affect the absorption of minerals.
7. Describe the clinical effects of a deficiency or excess of each mineral.
8. Summarize food handling procedures that minimize mineral loss.
9. Identify the major sources and functions of water in the body.
10. Evaluate the routes by which water is lost from the body.
11. Explain how fluid and electrolyte balance is maintained.
12. Analyze the recommended practices to maintain fluid and electrolyte balance during athletic activity.

Glossary

Minerals

Gram (g):   metric measure, 28.3 g = 1 oz.; usually rounded to 30 g for ease of calculation.

Hyper: excess of normal.

Hypo: less than normal.

Inorganic: a compound of inert elements such as minerals.

Macro: involving large quantities.

Micro: involving minute quantities.

Microgram (mcg):   1/1000 of a mg; 1/10,000 of a gram.

Milligram (mg):   1/1000 of a gram.

Organic: any compound containing carbon.

pH: degree of acidity or alkalinity of a solution: a pH of 7 is neutral; below 7 is acid; above 7 is alkaline.

Water

Electrolyte: an ionic (charged particle) form of a mineral.

Extracellular: fluids such as blood plasma and cerebrospinal fluid. Fluid around and between cells.

Fluid and electrolyte balance: maintenance of a stable internal environment by means of regulation of the water and minerals in solution within and around the cells.

Interstitial: fluid found between the cells. Blood plasma is often considered with it because of similarity in composition.

Intracellular: fluid contained within a cell.

Osmolarity: osmotic pressure difference between pressures across a membrane. Total number of dissolved particles per unit of fluid outside the cell equals the number of dissolved particles inside the cell.

Solute: solid matter in a solution.

Background Information

Mineral Occurrences

Only 4 percent of human body weight is composed of minerals. The other 96 percent is composed of water and the organic compounds of carbon, hydrogen, oxygen, and nitrogen that we know as carbohydrates, proteins, and fats. Minerals are inorganic elements. When plant or animal tissue is burned, the ash which remains is the mineral content. Minerals are present in the body in combination with organic compounds, as inorganic compounds, and alone.

Many minerals have been proven essential to human nutrition, and there are others with unknown essentiality. Still other minerals enter the body as pollutants through contamination of air, soil, and water.

Minerals vary widely in the amounts the body will absorb and excrete. Some minerals require the presence of other minerals in the body to function properly. Some minerals are transported by carriers in the body. Most minerals are toxic when ingested at just slightly higher than the safe and effective levels.

Mineral Classifications

Minerals are divided into two general categories—macrominerals and microminerals—based on the quantity in which they are found in the body.

The macrominerals are calcium (Ca), phosphorus (P), potassium (K), sodium (Na), sulfur (S), magnesium (Mg), and chlorine (Cl). The microminerals are iron (Fe), zinc (Zn), manganese (Mn), fluorine (F), copper (Cu), cobalt (Co), iodine (I), selenium (Se), chromium (Cr), and molybdenum (Mo). Microminerals are frequently referred to as "trace elements" because they are present in the body in such small quantities (less than .005 percent of body weight). These essential trace elements are required daily in the body in the milligram range.

Mineral Essentiality and Functions

Those microminerals with functions not yet known are not discussed here. The macro- and microminerals essential to human nutrition are the ones we will discuss. *Essential* refers to those substances the body is unable to manufacture; they must be available from an outside source. Essential minerals improve growth and development and regulate vital life processes.

Minerals are

1. A part of the structure of all body cells.
2. Components of enzymes, hormones, blood, and other vital body compounds.
3. Regulators of
   a. acid base balance of the body.
   b. response of nerves to stimuli.
   c. muscle contractions.
   d. cell membrane permeability.
   e. osmotic pressure and water balance.

Mineral Acidity and Alkalinity

Since the acid base balance (pH) of the body is regulated by acid and base (alkaline) forming minerals, we can group foods according to their predominant acid or base mineral content.

Sodium (Na), magnesium (Mg), potassium (K), iron (Fe), and calcium (Ca) are the minerals that produce an alkaline (base) residue (ash). The foods that are base-(alkaline) producing, with high levels of these minerals, include most fruits and vegetables. The exceptions are plums, prunes, and cranberries, which are acid-producing fruits.

The acid-forming elements are sulfur (S), phosphorus (P), and chlorine (Cl). The foods containing the largest amounts of these minerals are the grains and protein foods (milk, cheese, meats, and eggs).

Mineral Absorption and Solubility

Minerals are absorbed best by the body at a specific pH. For instance, neither calcium nor iron will be absorbed in an alkaline medium. They require an acid pH for absorption.

The acid and base properties of minerals, then, become an important consideration when planning for maximum absorption of the minerals and other nutrients.

Most of the minerals in foods occur as mineral salts, which are generally water-soluble. Minerals can be lost in cooking water in much the same way that water-soluble vitamins can. Therefore, foods should be cooked in the smallest amount of water possible for the shortest length of time and covered. Steam cooking and stir-frying methods conserve minerals. The water in which the foods have been cooked should be reused in cooking other foods; this recycles the minerals for the body.

Water: A Primer

A meaningful discussion of minerals is not possible without explaining the role of water. A major factor of the internal environment of the body is the fluid and electrolyte balance. The fluid involved is water, and most of the electrolytes are ionic forms of essential minerals. Specifically, these are sodium (Na^+), potassium (K^+), magnesium (Mg^{++}), calcium (Ca^{++}), chloride (Cl^-), sulfate (SO_4^-), and phosphates (HPO_4^- and $H_2PO_4^=$).

Muscle tissue is relatively high in water content, while adipose (fat) tissue is relatively low. Fifty to seventy percent of adult body weight is water, depending on the amount of fat tissue. The water content of the body falls with age, unrelated to body weight. An infant has a higher percent of body water than an adult. Water above immediate needs cannot be stored for future use.

In a normal person, daily water intake equals output; the balance is controlled. Thirst usually is a reliable guide to such regulation in a healthy person.

Since minerals and water are so interrelated, there is only one progress check for the two activities in this module. This approach permits the student to integrate the knowledge of minerals and water.

ACTIVITY 1: The Essential Minerals: Functions, Sources, and Characteristics

Reference Tables

Since each mineral has particular functions, food sources, and specific characteristics, the student should study Tables 7-1 to 7-15, which describe these factors in detail. In this activity, we will specifically discuss only calcium, potassium, sodium, and iron. The student should follow the information in the corresponding tables for these and the other minerals.

Calcium

Calcium is the mineral present in the largest amount in the human body. Ninety-nine percent of it is in the bones and

teeth. The remainder (1 percent) is in body fluids, soft tissue, and membranes. Refer to Table 7-1.

The 1989 Recommended Daily Allowance (RDA) for calcium for an adult is 800 mg to 1,200 mg daily, depending on age. The calcium equivalents for 1 cup (8 oz.) of milk are as follows: (1 c. milk = app. 300 mg calcium)

1. 8 oz. yogurt
2. 1½ oz. cheddar cheese
3. 2 cups cream cheese
4. 2 cups cottage cheese
5. 1¾ cups ice cream
6. 4 oz. canned salmon with bones
7. 15 to 24 medium oysters

TABLE 7-1
Calcium (Ca)

Functions	Food Sources	Results of Deficiency or Excess	Conditions Requiring Increase	Specific Characteristics
Aids bone and tooth formation. Maintains serum calcium levels. Aids blood clotting. Aids muscle contraction and relaxation. Aids transmission of nerve impulses. Maintains normal heart rhythm.	RDA = 1200 mg for a 24-year-old adult *Milk Group* milk and cheeses* yogurt *Meat Group* egg (yolk) sardines, salmon† *Vegetable Group* *green leafy vegetables** legumes nuts *Grain Group* whole grains	*Deficiency* rickets (childhood disorder of calcium metabolism from a vitamin D deficiency resulting in stunted growth, bowed legs, enlarged joints, especially legs, arms, and hollow chest) osteomalacia (adult form of rickets: a softening of the bones) osteoporosis (widespread disorder, especially in women, wherein bones become thin, brittle, diminish in size and break) slow blood clotting tetany (see Specific Characteristics) poor tooth formation *Excess* renal calculi (see Specific Characteristics) hypercalcemia (deposits in joints and soft tissue)	Low intake (any age) Low serum calcium due to: growth pregnancy lactation Any condition that causes excess withdrawal, such as: body casts immobility low estrogen levels	1. Body need is major factor governing the amount of calcium absorbed. Normally 30–40% of dietary calcium is absorbed. 2. Presence of vitamin D and lactose (milk sugar) enhance absorption. 3. An acid environment in the gastrointestinal tract enhances absorption (see acid base balance). 4. Calcium in the bones and teeth are constantly withdrawn and replaced to keep the serum level stable. 5. The parathyroid hormone controls regulation. 6. The intake of calcium and phosphorus should be 1:1 ratio for optimal absorption. 7. Tetany is a condition resulting from a deficiency of calcium that causes muscle spasms in legs, arms. 8. Renal calculi are kidney stones. Ninety-six percent of all stones consist of calcium. 9. Overdoses of vitamin D can cause hypercalcemia, as can prolonged intake of antacids and milk. 10. Acute calcium deficiency does not usually occur without a lack of vitamin D and phosphorus also.

*Best source
**Some contain binding agents
†With bones included

The absorption of calcium depends upon body need, vitamin D, the amount of calcium in the body fluids, ratio of calcium to phosphorus, and the acidity of the gastrointestinal tract. Calcium is stored in the bones and teeth, but is withdrawn and replaced as serum calcium fluctuates, maintaining a steady state. Calcium is excreted via feces and urine. It is prevented from intestinal absorption by a low vitamin D intake, by alkaline, and by finding agents such as oxalic and phytic acid, which are naturally occurring acids in certain vegetables. It is currently suspected that a high protein intake over extended periods of time can decrease the absorption and increase the excretion of calcium. It is believed that the phosphorus content of protein foods upsets the calcium-to-phosphorus ratio in the food, the intestinal system, and the body.

TABLE 7-2
Phosphorus (P)

Functions	Food Sources	Results of Deficiency or Excess	Conditions Requiring Increase	Specific Characteristics
Aids bone and tooth formation. Maintains metabolism of fat and carbohydrates. Part of the compounds that act as buffers to control pH of the blood.	*RDA:* 1200 mg for a 24-year-old adult *Meat Group** cheeses (especially cheddar), peanuts, beef, pork, poultry, fish, eggs *Milk Group* milk and milk products *Vegetable/Fruit Group*** all foods in this group *Grain*** wheat, oats, barley, rice *Other* carbonated drinks contain large amounts of phosphorus	*Deficiency* rickets osteomalacia osteoporosis slow blood clotting poor tooth formation disturbed acid base balance *Excess* same as calcium	Low intake, especially of protein foods, due to: growth pregnancy lactation illness	1. Approximately 80% of phosphorus is in bones and teeth in a ratio with calcium of 2:1. 2. Aids in producing energy by phosphorylation. 3. Phospholipids assist in transferring substances in and out of the cells. 4. Phosphorus is more efficiently absorbed than calcium; approximately 70% is absorbed. Some factors that enhance or decrease absorption of calcium affect phosphorus the same way. 5. Consumption of antacids lowers phosphorus absorption. 6. Both calcium and phosphorus are released from bone when serum levels are low. 7. Diets containing enough protein and calcium will be adequate in phosphorus.

*Best source
**Fair to poor source

One clinical disorder of calcium metabolism is osteoporosis, which is the thinning of bones through calcium loss. The person with osteoporosis has less bone substance. The bones become thin and brittle, prone to breaking easily. Compressed vertebra fractures are common. Osteoporosis is the most common bone disorder in the United States, affecting women about three times as often as men. Though the disorder is most often seen in older women, it starts in early adulthood without symptoms. The amount of bone an older woman has is influenced by the amount of calcium in her diet throughout her adulthood. Among the reasons women develop osteoporosis more often than men are

1. They have smaller body frames with less bone mass.
2. They eat many "nonfattening" foods that contribute little calcium.
3. Their bodies have reduced estrogen levels after menopause. The disappearance of this hormone upsets the balance between deposition and withdrawal of body calcium.

One cause of osteoporosis is reduced calcium intake and absorption. This absorption of calcium is controlled by

1. Heredity: osteoporosis tends to run in families.
2. Estrogen: less calcium will be absorbed and deposited when body estrogen decreases.
3. Dietary factors and exercise.

A low calcium intake after a person reaches adulthood leads to osteoporosis because the body will start "consuming" its own bones. For example, after 25 years on a low calcium diet, the body can theoretically use up one-third of the body skeleton. As a major body organ, the skeleton is not a static system. Minerals, especially calcium, are constantly removed from the bones and used for other body functions. The bones are an important reservoir for calcium. When there is a chronic shortage of calcium in

TABLE 7-3
Sodium (Na)

Functions	Food Sources	Results of Deficiency or Excess	Conditions Requiring Increase	Specific Characteristics
Maintains water balance. Normalizes osmotic pressure. Balances acid base. Regulates nerve impulses. Regulates muscle contraction. Aids in carbohydrate and protein absorption.	*Estimated minimum requirement:* 500 mg for a 24-year-old adult table salt (40% sodium) milk and dairy foods protein foods (fish, shellfish, meat, poultry, eggs) processed foods: any containing baking soda, baking powder, and preservative additives some drinking water is high in sodium some vegetables contain fair sources of sodium: spinach, celery, beets, carrots	*Deficiency* *hypo*natremia (low serum sodium): nausea headache anorexia muscle spasms mental confusion fluid and electrolyte imbalance *Excess* *hyper*natremia (high serum sodium) cardiovascular disturbances hypertension edema mental confusion	Excessive loss of body fluids: high use of diuretics vomiting/ diarrhea heavy perspiring burns Certain diseases: cystic fibrosis Addison's disease	1. More than half the body sodium is in the fluid surrounding the cells. It is the major *cation* of the extracellular fluid. Its functions are very similar to potassium. 2. Most Americans consume far more sodium than the RDA. 3. Extracellular fluids include fluid in the blood vessels, veins, arteries, and capillaries. 4. Sodium is well conserved by body. 5. Hyponatremia due to inadequate intake is uncommon. A condition causing excess fluid loss such as described in column 4 (Conditions Requiring Increase) would be necessary. 6. Hypernatremia is related to high incidence of hypertension in the U.S. 7. Dietary guidelines for Americans encourage less consumption of sodium, especially for those at high risk of developing high blood pressure. 8. Often a reduction in intake can be done simply by omitting salt added to food in preparation or at the table. Elimination of high salt snack foods and foods preserved in salt also is helpful.

the diet, it is withdrawn from bones so that the body maintains a normal level of this mineral in the blood.

Although osteoporosis cannot be "cured," its symptoms (such as pain) can be decreased by

1. a calcium-rich diet
2. exercise
3. avoidance of things that decrease the body's ability to absorb calcium

Further, it is believed that such practices can prevent osteoporosis or delay its onset.

Potassium

About 95 percent of ingested potassium is readily absorbed by the body. Potassium circulates in all body fluids, primarily located within the cell. Excesses are usually efficiently excreted. Aldosterone, a hormone secreted by the adrenal gland, signals the kidney to excrete what is not needed.

TABLE 7-4
Potassium (K)

Functions	Food Sources	Results of Deficiency or Excess	Conditions Requiring Increase	Specific Characteristics
Maintains protein and carbohydrate metabolism. Maintains water balance. Normalizes osmotic pressure. Balances acid base. Regulates muscle activity.	*Estimated minimum requirement*: 500 mg for a 24-year-old adult *Milk Group* all foods *Meat Group* all foods (best sources: red meats, dark meat, poultry) *Vegetable/Fruit Group* all foods (especially oranges, bananas, prunes) *Grain Group* especially whole grains *Other* coffee (especially instant)	*Deficiency* hypokalemia (see Specific Characteristics) fluid and electrolyte imbalances tissue breakdown *Excess* hyperkalemia (see Specific Characteristics) renal failure severe dehydration shock	Inadequate intake (starvation, imbalanced diets) Gastrointestinal disorders, especially diarrhea Burns, injuries Diabetic acidosis Chronic use of diuretics Adrenal gland tumors	1. The major cation in the *intra*cellular fluid. 2. Balances with sodium to maintain water balance and osmotic pressure. 3. When there are excess acid elements, potassium combines and neutralizes, thus maintaining acid base balance. 4. Potassium is poorly conserved by the body. 5. Hypokalemia is a condition where there is low serum potassium. It manifests itself in muscle weakness, loss of appetite, nausea, vomiting, and rapid heart beat (tachycardia). 6. Hyperkalemia is a condition that causes serum potassium to rise to toxic levels. It results in a weakened heart action which causes mental confusion, poor respiration, numbness of extremities, and heart failure.

The average U.S. diet supplies from two to six grams of potassium daily. Its deficiency is not a problem until certain abnormal conditions arise. Refer to Table 7-4.

Sodium

The kidneys, under the influence of aldosterone, normally control sodium excretion according to need and intake. It is excreted via the kidneys, with small amounts lost in the feces. Large amounts can be lost in perspiration during strenuous activity and in a hot environment. Severe vomiting in certain disorders and chronic use of diuretics increase sodium loss. Ninety-five percent of sodium is recirculated through the enterohepatic system by kidney reabsorption. If the serum sodium rises, water is retained and blood volume increases. This, in turn, increases blood pressure. Refer to Table 7-3.

Iron

While the total amount of iron needed daily in the human body is small, iron is one of the most important micronutrients. Iron intake, especially in the female, is low. Iron-deficiency anemia is a major problem in the United States, especially for those high risk groups noted under characteristics in Table 7-8. It occurs usually as a result of inadequate intake, impaired absorption, blood loss, or repeated pregnancies. Iron is poorly absorbed in the intes-

TABLE 7-5
Magnesium (Mg)

Functions	Food Sources	Results of Deficiency or Excess	Conditions Requiring Increase	Specific Characteristics
Assists in regulation of body fluids. Activates enzymes. Regulates metabolism of carbohydrate, fat, and protein. Necessary for formation of ATP (energy production). Component of chlorophyll. Works with Ca, P, and vitamin D in bone formation.	*RDA for a 24-year-old:* 350 mg (male), 280 mg (female) grains, green vegetables, soybeans, milk, meat, poultry	*Deficiency* fluid and electrolyte imbalance skin breakdown *Excess* magnesemia	Alcoholism Inadequate intake of Ca, P, or any disease affecting their use Growth Pregnancy Lactation Prolonged use of diuretics	1. Magnesium deficiencies occur most often in disease states such as cirrhosis of the liver, severe renal disease, and toxemia of pregnant women. 2. American diets may be low in magnesium compared to RDAs if diet is low in calories or contains mostly highly refined and processed foods. 3. Magnesium and calcium share a control system in the kidneys.

tine, with most excreted in the stool. When iron is absorbed in excess of body needs, it can be stored. Major storage areas are the liver, spleen, and bone marrow. The body has no mechanism for excretion of excess iron. Refer to Table 7-8.

Planning an iron-rich diet acceptable to most families is a challenge. If liver and other organ meats are not included in the diet, other foods must be selected to increase dietary iron. Some examples of such foods or food preparation methods include: raisin cookies and prune

TABLE 7-6
Chlorine (Cl)

Functions	Food Sources	Results of Deficiency or Excess	Conditions Requiring Increase	Specific Characteristics
Aids in maintaining fluid electrolyte balance and acid base balance. Aids in digestion and absorption of nutrients as a constituent of gastric secretions.	*Estimated minimum requirement:* 750 mg for a 24-year-old. table salt (60% chloride) protein foods: seafood, meats, eggs, milk	Intake is not usually a problem unless a condition as in next column exists.	Excessive vomiting Aging (decreased gastric secretions	1. Chloride is the chief *anion* of the fluid outside the cells. 2. The gastric (stomach) contents are primarily hydrochloric acid (HCl). 3. Chloride is a buffer in a reaction in the body known as the chloride shift. This has the effect of maintaining the delicate pH balance of the blood.

TABLE 7-7
Sulfur (S)

Functions	Food Sources	Results of Deficiency or Excess	Conditions Requiring Increase	Specific Characteristics
Participates in detoxifying harmful compounds. Component of amino acids.	RDA: not established protein foods that contain the amino acids methionine, cysteine, and cystine (cheeses, eggs, poultry, and fish)	No specific descriptions of a deficiency or excess	No specific conditions requiring an increase	1. Much information remains to be learned about the role of sulfur in human physiology. 2. Greatest concentration is in hair and nails.

TABLE 7-8
Iron (Fe)

Functions	Food Sources	Results of Deficiency or Excess	Conditions Requiring Increase	Specific Characteristics

Plays essential role in formation of hemoglobin. Is found in *myoglobin*, the iron-protein molecule in muscles.	RDA for a 24-year-old:
	10 mg (male)
	15 mg (female)
	liver, kidneys, lean meats, whole grains, parsley, enriched breads, cereals, legumes, almonds dried fruit: prunes (and juice), raisins, apricots approximately 2–10% of iron in vegetables and grains can be absorbed, compared to 10–30% absorption of iron from animal protein
		Deficiency iron-deficiency anemia
		
		Excess hemosiderosis: a condition where iron is deposited in the liver and body tissues. The cell becomes distorted and dies. The liver is damaged.
			Girls and women of childbearing age due to menstrual losses (about 30 mg per month lost) Pregnancy (supplementation with iron and folacin needed) Acute or chronic blood loss Inadequate protein intake	1. Approximately ¾ of functioning iron in the body is in hemoglobin.
				2. Hemoglobin is the principal part of the red blood cell, and carries oxygen from the lungs to the tissues. It assists in returning CO_2 (carbon dioxide) to the lungs.
				3. Iron is only absorbed in an acid medium. Absorption is enhanced by ascorbic acid.
				4. Milk is a very *poor* source of iron, containing only a trace.
				5. Iron is not well absorbed in the body, even under good conditions. Generally about 10% in a mixed diet is absorbed.
				6. Iron is the most difficult nutrient to meet through diet for women.
				7. The following nutrients are essential for the manufacture of red blood cells:
				  a. iron, vitamin B_6, and copper for hemoglobin formation
				  b. protein for globin formation
				  c. vitamin C to aid the absorption of iron
				8. The populations at risk for iron-deficiency anemia are:
				    infants (6–12 months)
				    adolescent girls
				    menstruating women
				    pregnant women

TABLE 7-9
Iodine (I)

Functions	Food Sources	Results of Deficiency or Excess	Conditions Requiring Increase	Specific Characteristics
Basic component of *thyroxin*, a hormone in the thyroid gland that regulates the basal metabolic rate (BMR). Contributes to normal growth and development of the body.	*RDA:* 150 *mcg* adults iodized salt (major source) seafood: salt water fish food additives: dough oxidizers, dairy disinfectants, coloring agents foods containing seaweed	*Deficiency* cretinism (stunted growth, dwarfism) goiter (enlargement of thyroid gland) *Excess* hyperthyroidism (toxic goiter)	Wherever soil is low in iodine In areas where goiter is endemic In pregnant women with deficient diets	1. Certain foods contain substances that block absorption of iodine: cabbage, turnips, rutabagas. 2. Iodine-containing food additives may cause excess intake of iodine in some areas of the U.S.

bread (especially with whole wheat flour); casseroles with dried beans and peas; substituting molasses for sugar; and adding parsley to dishes. Slow cooking in an iron pot increases available iron by 50 to 75 percent.

Implications for Health Personnel _____

Of all the essential minerals, iron probably poses the most clinical problems. All health care professionals should pay special attention to the following information and guidelines.

TABLE 7-10
Zinc (Zn)

Functions	Food Sources	Results of Deficiency or Excess	Conditions Requiring Increase	Specific Characteristics
Contributes to formation of enzymes needed in metabolism. Affects normal sensitivity to taste and smell. Aids protein synthesis. Aids normal growth and sexual maturation. Promotes wound healing. May help in the treatment of acne.*	RDA for adults: 15 mg (male) 12 mg (female) oysters, liver, meats, poultry, legumes, nuts	*Deficiency* associated with extreme malnutrition impairs wound healing decreases taste and smell dwarfism and impaired sexual development in children *Excess* toxicity associated with ingestion of acid foods stored in zinc-lined containers	Following surgery, especially when diet has been inadequate prior to surgery Those with alterations in taste and smell Certain diseases of dark-skinned races, such as sickle cell anemia	Availability of zinc is greater from animal sources; vegetable sources contain phytates, which bind it, causing its excretion.

*Latest studies indicate that zinc supplements can be effective in treating acne in some subjects.

TABLE 7-11
Fluorine (F)

Functions	Food Sources	Results of Deficiency or Excess	Conditions Requiring Increase	Specific Characteristics
Protects against dental caries.	*Estimated safe and adequate daily intake:* 1.5–4.0 mg for all adults seafood fluoridated drinking water (1 PPM* added to water)	*Deficiency* 50–70% cases of tooth decay from fluorine deficiency *Excess* mottled stains on teeth	Areas where no fluoride available	Fluoride is being used to assist in regenerating bone loss due to osteoporosis in selected studies.

*PPM = parts per million

1. Since iron is a nutrient likely to be deficient in the human body, the following tips will be helpful when instructing a client:
    a. Cooking foods in larger pieces and in smaller amounts of water reduces the amount of iron lost in preparation.
    b. The use of meat drippings and fruit pulp conserves iron.
    c. A diet high in bulk reduces iron absorption; clients at risk of iron deficiency should use only moderate fiber content.
    d. High intake of antacids makes the gastric juices alkaline and reduces iron absorption.
    e. An adequate calcium intake increases iron absorption because the calcium will bind with the phosphates, phytates, oxalates, and cellulose and leave the iron free for absorption.

TABLE 7-12
Copper (Cu)

Functions	Food Sources	Results of Deficiency or Excess	Conditions Requiring Increase	Specific Characteristics
Considered "twin" to iron; aids in formation of hemoglobin and energy production. Promotes absorption of iron from gastrointestinal tract. Aids bone formation. Aids brain tissue formation. Contributes to myelin sheath of the nervous system.	RDA (safe and adequate estimates): 1.5–3.0 mg adults liver, kidney, shellfish, lobster, oysters, nuts, raisins, legumes, corn oil	*Deficiency* occurs in association with disease states such as: PEM (Protein Energy Malnutrition) kwashiorkor (extreme protein deficiency) sprue (disease marked by diarrhea) cystic fibrosis kidney disease iron deficiency anemia *Excess* ingestion of large amounts is toxic to humans	Disease states noted under deficiencies	1. Copper is concentrated in the liver, brain, heart, and kidneys. 2. Absorption takes place in small intestine. 3. Other minerals can interfere with copper absorption. 4. Zinc is an antagonist to copper because it reduces absorption.

TABLE 7-13
Cobalt (Co)

Functions	Food Sources	Results of Deficiency or Excess	Conditions Requiring Increase	Specific Characteristics
Acts as a component of vitamin B$_{12}$.	*RDA:* not established (see Specific Characteristics) organ meats, muscle meat, vitamin B$_{12}$	No specific deficiency in humans; deficient production of B$_{12}$ noted in animals	No specific conditions requiring an increase	1. RDAs for cobalt not established, but 15 mcg/day is suggested.

TABLE 7-14
Manganese (Mn)

Functions	Food Sources	Results of Deficiency or Excess	Conditions Requiring Increase	Specific Characteristics
Appears necessary for bone growth and reproduction. Acts as an enzyme activator.	*Estimated safe and adequate daily intake:* 2.0–5.0 mg nuts, legumes, tea, coffee, grains	No deficiencies noted in humans	No specific conditions requiring an increase	1. Manganese has not been demonstrated to be an essential nutrient in man.

TABLE 7-15
Selenium (Se)

Functions	Food Sources	Results of Deficiency or Excess	Conditions Requiring Increase	Specific Characteristics
Part of an enzyme that functions as an antioxidant. With vitamin E repairs damage caused by oxygen.	*RDA for 24-year-old:* 70 µg (male) 55 µg (female) *Main sources* meats, eggs, seafoods *Other* vegetables grown in selenium rich soil	*Deficiency* increased risk of cancer causes one type of heart disease *Excess* Selenosis*	Pregnancy and lactation Children living in countries where no selenium exists in soil or water, e.g., parts of China	1. Found in all body cells as part of an enzyme system. 2. Adequate RDA intakes believed to have a role in cancer prevention. 3. Excess selenium toxic. 4. The line between health and overdose is very thin. 5. Daily dose should not exceed 70 µg.

*Selenium toxicity

f. Spinach is not a good source of iron. It contains a large amount of the oxalates that hinder iron absorption.

g. Since ascorbic acid promotes iron absorption, eating foods containing iron and vitamin C together produces the best results.

2. Iron-poor foods are pale in color (lack pigment). Iron salts are colored and impart their color to the foods they are in. Examples are milk (iron-poor) and liver (iron-rich).

3. Since the body cannot excrete excess iron, and it can therefore pose health hazards if consumed in large amounts:

   a. keep iron medication out of the reach of children (iron poisoning among children is the fourth most common type of poisoning).

   b. read labels on over-the-counter preparations (some are high in iron and, when mixed with other iron compounds, may create excess).

4. Iron medications interfere with some antibiotic absorption. Patients taking both preparations need to take them at different times.

The health team should also pay attention to the following information to ensure clients are at their optimal mineral status.

1. Both the quality and quantity of food intake should be monitored.

2. The use of diuretics may lead to alteration in the fluid and electrolyte balance in the body, especially high losses of sodium (hyponatremia) and potassium (hypokalemia).

3. Hypokalemia (potassium deficiency) may become severe in the following disorders: vomiting, diarrhea, wound drainage, diabetic acidosis, and in those taking digitalis for heart conditions.

4. Person with poor food intake may suffer from multiple mineral deficiencies.

5. Alcoholics, psychiatric patients, drug abusers, the aged, the poverty stricken, and those with malabsorptive disorders are most likely to suffer mineral deficiencies.

6. Certain foods and conditions of the intestinal tract will greatly influence the absorption of minerals. Each mineral should merit separate consideration, since not all react to the same conditions and foods.

7. Calcium deficiency (hypocalcemia) results from insufficient intake, malabsorption, or lack of vitamin D. Acute hypocalcemia (which can cause death) causes tetany. Hypocalcemia from inadequate intake over long periods of time results in osteoporosis, which occurs in three out of five women over the age of 60 and is a severe disorder.

8. Recognize the factors that promote or inhibit iron absorption. Be able to plan an iron-rich diet that excludes least-liked foods high in iron.

9. Recognize major symptoms that may indicate deficiencies of minerals and follow up with treatment.

10. Be able to list the best food sources of the mineral(s) that the client is deficient in.

11. Find resources for those who have inadequate mineral intake due to lack of money for food or ignorance of nutrition needs.

ACTIVITY 2: Water and the Internal Environment

Next to oxygen, water is the most important nutrient for the body. Lack of water causes the cells to become dehydrated. A total lack of water can cause death in a few days. Fifty to seventy percent of body weight is water; and an individual's body water content does not vary significantly. The body does not tolerate much fluctuation, since it upsets the delicate balance and concentration of dissolved substances and causes a rapid loss of cell integrity. The major nutrient electrolytes (Na^+, K^+, Cl^-, Mg^{++}, Ca^{++}, HPO_4^- and $H_2PO_4^=$) have already been discussed in Activity 1. Small changes in diet can cause changes in water content and affect fluid balance. Low carbohydrate intake can increase water loss, as can low protein intake, although for different reasons. The water loss associated with low carbohydrate intake appears much faster than that associated with low protein intake. Omitting sodium from the diet may result in a small fluid loss. Individuals who reduce their sodium intake usually lose a little body weight. This is due, however, to fluid loss, not actual fat

loss. The output of water is normally balanced by input. If extra water is ingested, urinary output increases. The body maintains a steady water content state.

Functions and Distribution of Body Water

Water serves many important functions. In the human body, water acts as

1. a solvent

2. a component of all body cells, giving structure and form to the body

3. a body temperature regulator

4. a lubricant

5. a medium for the digestion of food

6. a transport medium for nutrients and waste products

7. a participant in biological reactions

8. a regulator of acid-base balance

In the body, water is distributed in the following manner:

1. ECF, or extracellular fluid (surrounding the cells): 20 to 25 percent of the body water is outside the cells. ECF includes the vascular system.
2. ICF, or intracellular fluid (inside the cells): 40 to 45 percent of the body water is inside the cells. The ICF contains twice as much water as the ECF.

Body Water Balance

Water requirements are dependent upon many factors, including the amount of solids in the diet, air humidity, environmental temperature, type of clothing worn, type of exercise performed (amount and energy output), respiratory (breathing) rate, and the state of health. The human body obtains water from

1. Beverages.
2. Foods, including dry ones like meat and crackers.
3. Metabolic breakdown of food for use by the body (oxidation of energy nutrients). This amount of metabolic water is not large, but it is significant, especially in certain disease conditions.

Water is lost from the body in many ways:

1. Most water is lost from the kidneys as urine.
2. Water is lost from skin as perspiration. Some insensible (unnoticed) perspiration occurs because it evaporates rapidly. Sweating, the key means of cooling the body, causes large water loss.
3. Water is lost from the lungs in breathing (water vapor).
4. Water is lost in the feces.
5. Certain disease conditions and injury can result in great water losses, creating crisis situations if not replaced at once. Some examples are acute diarrhea, burns, and blood losses.

A deficiency or excess of water can produce harmful effects to the body. The major outcome of water deficiency is dehydration. Prolonged dehydration leads to cell death, and multiple cell losses kill the organism. The very young, whose bodies contain a higher percentage of water, and the very old, whose bodies contain less water than younger persons, are the most susceptible to dehydration. In these individuals, it occurs more rapidly and is more severe.

Excessive consumption of liquids is usually not a problem for a healthy body, because the kidney controls the excretion of fluids, balancing intake with output. During kidney or other disorders where the body suffers a fluid imbalance, edema, ascites, and congestive heart failure may result. In these patients, water intake is restricted. Drinking excess liquids with a low mineral content (such as distilled water) may cause a condition known as water

intoxication. Mineral replacement will normalize fluid and electrolyte balance.

Maintenance of fluid and electrolyte balance within and between the cells is important for normal health. Control of these shifts is accomplished by complex mechanisms in the body. An extended analysis is not appropriate here, but the following points will help explain the mechanism of body water distribution.

1. Pressure balance: this kind of pressure controls fluid balance and hydrostatic-capillary blood pressure, osmotic pressure, and serum proteins (albumin) movement.
2. Hormonal influence: antidiuretic hormone (ADH), a hormone from the pituitary gland, and aldosterone from the adrenal gland regulate the excretion of fluid from the kidneys.
3. Thirst or lack of thirst: this response controls how much liquid is ingested.
4. Shifts of electrolytes (Ca, P, Mg, Na): for example, when the shifts move from bone to serum, the concentration of electrolytes in the body fluid is changed.

Water Requirements for Athletes

Since water is the nutrient most often depleted, its replacement should be of prime concern. Fortunately, it is the most easily restored nutrient of all. Anyone engaged in prolonged activity or enclosed in a hot environment can become dehydrated and should ingest fluids. Athletes are especially prone to dehydration. A fluid loss of up to 2 percent body weight is harmless, but a 4 to 5 percent loss is harmful.

Most athletes need to drink fluid during exercise. Long distance runners may lose 8 to 15 pounds of fluid during a race. This is equivalent to 16 to 30 cups of water. They should drink liquids before, during, and after a race. Since sweetened liquids or those with a high mineral content tend to hasten dehydration and cause diarrhea, plain water, unsweetened fruit juices, tomato or V-8 juice, and diluted colas and gingerale are preferred. The so-called "electrolyte" replacements that contain sugar, sodium, and potassium have no special value.

Extra fluids and minerals should be consumed cautiously in long distance events. Small amounts of sugar, for example, consumed every 1/2 to 1 hour during the long event is the preferred consumption method. Short-term events do not require special replacement other than water. Water can be taken at any time during an event.

Minerals affected by heavy exercise are sodium and potassium. Iron deficiency is common in female athletes. For athletes, mineral supplements are a temporary measure. They should consume foods with a high content of sodium, potassium, and iron.

Responsibilities of Health Personnel _____

1. Recognize the factors that promote or inhibit adequate fluid intake.
2. Recognize symptoms of dehydration and water intoxication.
3. Be aware that diet can cause changes in the fluid balance of the body, and make adjustments as necessary.
4. Recognize the importance of sodium-potassium and water in the body's fluid and electrolyte balance.
5. Understand the significance of equal input and output of fluid in maintaining homeostasis by knowing the ways the body gains fluid, loses fluid, and how water is distributed in the body.
6. Question scheduling of tests that require withholding fluids to such an extent that it might lead to dehydration.
7. Be aware that rising blood pressure may indicate retention of fluids.
8. Advise persons engaged in prolonged activity about appropriate replacement of water and body fluids.
9. Watch for symptoms of dehydration and replace lost electrolytes as well as fluids if needed.
10. Provide information to consumers regarding appropriate food and fluid intake.

Summary _____

The concentration of each electrolyte in the body fluid must be maintained within a narrow range so that the delicate balance will not be disturbed. Changes in electrolyte concentration, acidity, and alkalinity can adversely affect the whole body. The system of body fluid and electrolyte balance is so important that the body provides various mechanisms for regulation. A deficit in water or minerals can rapidly become life threatening.

PROGRESS CHECK ON MODULE 7

Multiple Choice

Circle the letter of the correct answer.

1. The vitamin most closely related to calcium utilization is
   a. vitamin A.
   b. vitamin D.
   c. vitamin K.
   d. phosphorus.

2. Three nutrients needed for bone growth are
   a. ascorbic acid, vitamin D, and magnesium.
   b. calcium, potassium, and vitamin D.
   c. phosphorus, calcium, and vitamin D.
   d. magnesium, manganese, and calcium.

3. Functions of sodium in the human body include
   a. maintenance of water balance.
   b. maintenance of acid–base balance.
   c. aiding glucose absorption.
   d. all of the above.

4. A mineral which is important in normal functioning of the heart is
   a. chlorine.
   b. potassium.
   c. phosphate.
   d. bicarbonate.

5. Calcium is
   a. used in muscle building.
   b. part of the blood clotting mechanism.
   c. used in blood clotting.
   d. found in abundance in soft tissues.

6. Phosphorus
   a. absorbs best when calcium is present.
   b. is found in many of the same foods as calcium.
   c. is needed in greater amounts during pregnancy.
   d. all of the above.

7. The only known function of iodine in human nutrition is synthesis of the thyroid hormone. Which of the following functions does this hormone perform?
   a. protects the cells from oxidation
   b. controls the basal metabolic rate
   c. lowers the oxygen intake
   d. controls nerve impulses

8. The mineral needed to strengthen the teeth to resist decay is
   a. calcium.
   b. phosphorus.
   c. iron.
   d. fluorine.

9. Which two foods are both rich sources of potassium?
   a. cooked rice and fortified margarine
   b. mashed potatoes and apple juice
   c. bananas and orange juice
   d. cranberry juice and grape juice

10. The two minerals whose major function is regulating the fluid balance of the body inside the cell (ICF) and outside the cell (ECF) are
    a. calcium and phosphorus.
    b. sodium and potassium.
    c. magnesium and iodine.
    d. chlorine and iron.

11. Sodium intake may need to be increased
    a. when vomiting, exudating burns, or diarrhea occur.
    b. to regulate acid-base balance and to prevent headaches.

c. when nausea, anorexia, muscle spasms, or mental confusion occur.

d. when hypertension and edema occur.

12. Which of the following would be considered the best source of iodine?

a. baked potato with iodized salt

b. tossed green salad with iodized salt

c. baked salmon with iodized salt

d. broccoli with iodized salt

13. Chloride

a. is directly necessary for protein synthesis in cells.

b. protects bone structures against degeneration.

c. is the body's principal intracellular electrolyte.

d. helps maintain gastric acidity.

14. Magnesium functions

a. in production of thyroid hormone.

b. as a catalyst in energy metabolism.

c. to transport oxygen.

d. in prevention of anemia.

15. Potassium

a. is directly necessary for protein synthesis in cells.

b. protects bone structures against degeneration.

c. is necessary for wound healing.

d. helps maintain gastric acidity.

16. Sulfur is present in all

a. carbohydrates.

b. fatty acids.

c. proteins.

d. vitamins.

17. A high need for calcium, such as during pregnancy,

a. increases calcium absorption.

b. decreases calcium absorption.

c. does not affect calcium absorption.

d. is related to other nutrient intake.

18. Heart failure related to potassium loss may occur except

a. during fasting.

b. with severe diarrhea.

c. in children with iron-deficiency anemia.

d. in hypokalemia.

19. The food source from which calcium is obtained in the highest concentration and most absorbable form is

a. dark green vegetables.

b. bone meal.

c. milk.

d. meats.

20. The most reliable food source of chloride is

a. meats and whole grain cereals.

b. salt.

c. dark green vegetables.

d. public water.

21. Potassium supplements

a. should always be taken with diuretics.

b. should be taken only under a physician's direction.

c. are necessary because food sources are limited.

d. increase muscle strength.

22. Which of the following contains the least sodium?

a. lemon juice

b. soy sauce

c. canned tomato juice

d. boiled ham

23. Which of the following substances is an electrolyte?

a. water

b. sodium

c. fatty acid

d. amino acid

24. The force that moves water into a space where a solute is more concentrated is

a. caloric energy.

b. osmotic pressure.

c. buffer action.

d. electrolyte imbalance.

25. A mineral found in higher concentrations in hard water than in soft water is

a. sodium.

b. potassium.

c. calcium.

d. fluoride.

26. A mineral found in higher concentrations in soft water than in hard water is

a. calcium.

b. magnesium.

c. sodium.

d. potassium.

27. Which of the following minerals is a cofactor in hemoglobin formation?

a. iodine

b. copper

c. sodium

d. calcium

28. Fluoride seems helpful in preventing

a. osteoporosis.

b. cancer.

c. diabetes.

d. heart disease.

29. Which nutrient enhances iron absorption from the intestinal tract?

a. biotin

b. vitamin C

c. vitamin D

d. calcium

30. Women have a higher RDA than men for
    a. copper.
    b. zinc.
    c. iron.
    d. ergosterol.

31. An iodine deficiency can cause
    a. anemia.
    b. hypertension.
    c. goiter.
    d. gout.

32. Fluoride is added to fluoridate water at a level of
    a. 1 part per million (PPM).
    b. 2 ppm.
    c. 3 ppm.
    d. 4 ppm.

33. Vitamin B$_{12}$ contains
    a. iron.
    b. cobalt.
    c. molybdenum.
    d. zinc.

34. A high salt diet may cause
    a. mottling of the teeth.
    b. a high cholesterol level.
    c. elevated blood pressure.
    d. reduced blood pressure.

35. Iodine is stored in the body in the
    a. stomach.
    b. thyroid gland.
    c. liver.
    d. muscles.

36. An excellent source of phosphorus is
    a. vitamin capsules.
    b. meat.
    c. celery.
    d. watermelon.

37. The best sources of zinc are
    a. shellfish, meats, and liver.
    b. breads, cereals, and grains.
    c. fruits and vegetables.
    d. milk products.

38. Contraction of the heart muscle is regulated by the level of
    a. iron.
    b. copper.
    c. calcium.
    d. manganese.

39. The best source of iron in the following list is
    a. egg yolks.
    b. polished rice.
    c. oranges.
    d. coconut.

40. Iron ordinarily is
    a. reused in the body.
    b. excreted efficiently in the urine.
    c. exhaled through the lungs.
    d. destroyed after it is released from hemoglobin.

41. Copper is needed
    a. to catalyze the formation of hemoglobin.
    b. to form elastin.
    c. for energy release in metabolic reactions.
    d. to regulate nerve impulses.

42. A valuable source of copper is
    a. olives.
    b. oranges.
    c. shellfish.
    d. meats.

43. A rich source of magnesium is
    a. cod liver oil.
    b. milk.
    c. breads and cereals.
    d. liver.

44. Good food sources of potassium include all except
    a. dried fruits.
    b. instant coffee.
    c. meats.
    d. olives.

True/False

Circle T for True and F for False.

45. **T** F Adequate calcium, ascorbic acid, and hydrochloric acid from the stomach are necessary for good absorption of iron.
46. T **F** Iron balance is controlled by urinary excretion.
47. **T** F The liver is the body's main storage site for iron.
48. **T** F Most iron is lost from the body whenever old blood cells wear out.
49. T **F** Hemorrhagic anemia is caused by a dietary deficiency of iron.
50. **T** F Pregnancy and lactation require supplementary iron.
51. T **F** Iron is widespread in foods, so a deficiency is rare.
52. **T** F Hemoglobin formation is the major function of iron.
53. **T** F The lack of calcium in the diet may cause muscle spasms, particularly in the extremities.
54. **T** F Growth, including wound healing, could be retarded by a zinc-deficient diet.
55. **T** F Food sources of zinc include meat, nuts, legumes, and shellfish.
56. **T** F Using large quantities of table salt may increase the risk of hypertension.

57. (T) F Foods that are high in protein are usually good sources of sodium.
58. (T) F Phosphorus is usually adequate in a diet that contains sufficient calcium and protein.
59. (T) F Most minerals that are essential in trace amounts are toxic in larger amounts.

Matching

Match the statements in Column A to their corresponding statements in Column B to complete the sentence.

	Column A		Column B
e	60. A function of water is	a.	outside the cells and inside the cells
a	61. Water is found in the body	b.	breathing, perspiring, urinating, defecating
c	62. Water is gained in the body by	c.	drinking, eating, cell metabolism
b	63. Water is lost from the body by	d.	dehydration, cell death
d	64. Output of water exceeding intake causes	e.	maintenance of a stable body temperature

References

Allen, L. H. 1986. Calcium and age-related bone loss. *Clinical Nutrition* 5(4):147.

Allen, L. H. 1986. Calcium and osteoporosis. *Nutrition Today* 21(3):6.

Cunningham, J. J. 1983. *Introduction to nutritional physiology.* Philadelphia: G. F. Stickley.

Fairbanks, V. F., and E. Beutler. 1988. Iron. In *Modern nutrition in health and disease,* 7th ed. M. E. Shils and V. R. Young (eds.). Philadelphia: Lea & Febiger.

Fregly, M. J. 1984. Sodium and potassium. In *Present knowledge in nutrition,* 5th ed. New York: Nutrition Foundation.

Goldberger, E. 1986. *A primer of water, electrolyte and acid-base syndromes,* 7th ed. Philadelphia: Lea & Febiger.

Hearney, R. P., and M. J. Barger-Lux. 1988. *Calcium and common sense.* New York: Doubleday.

Kee, J. L. 1986. *Fluids and electrolytes with clinical applications: A programmed approach.* New York: John Wiley & Sons, Inc.

Levander, O. A. 1988. Manganese. In *Modern nutrition in health and disease,* 7th ed. M. E. Shils and V. R. Young (eds.). Philadelphia: Lea & Febiger.

Levander, O. A. 1988. Selenium. In *Modern nutrition in health and disease,* 7th ed. M. E. Shils and V. R. Young (eds.). Philadelphia: Lea & Febiger.

Lindsay, R. 1987. Managing osteoporosis: Current trends, future possibilities. *Geriatrics* 42:35.

Lit, A. K. C. et al. 1980. *Fluid, electrolytes, acid-base and nutrition.* New York: Academic Press.

Markel, H. 1987. "When it rains it pours": Endemic goiter, iodized salt, and David Murray Cowie, MD. *American Journal of Public Health* 77:219.

Randall, H. T. 1988. Water, electrolytes, and acid-base balance. In *Modern nutrition in health and disease,* 7th ed. M. E. Shils and V. R. Young (eds.). Philadelphia: Lea & Febiger.

Schwartz, M. W. 1987. Potassium imbalances. *American Journal of Nursing* 87:1292.

Smith, K. T. (ed.). 1988. *Trace minerals in foods.* New York: Marcel Dekker.

Solomons, N. W. 1988. Zinc and copper. In *Modern nutrition in health and disease,* 7th ed. M. E. Shils and V. R. Young (eds.). Philadelphia: Lea & Febiger.

Stanbur, J. B. 1988. Iodine. In *Modern nutrition in health and disease,* 7th ed. M. E. Shils and V. R. Young (eds.). Philadelphia: Lea & Febiger.

West, J. 1985. *Best and Taylor's physiological basis of medical practice,* 11th ed. Baltimore: Williams & Wilkins.

Part II

PUBLIC HEALTH NUTRITION

Nutritional Assessment and Health Care Model

Time for completion
Activities: _____1½_____ hours
Optional examination: _½_ hour

Academic credit
Semester units: _⁴⁄₁₀_
Quarter units: _⁵⁄₁₀_

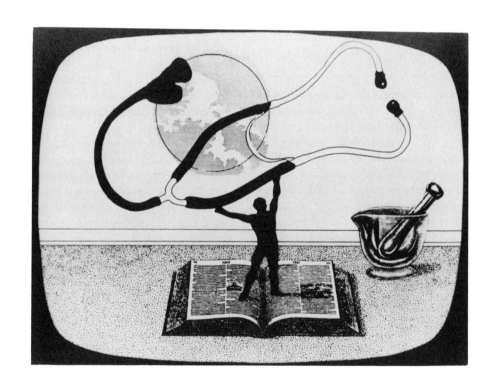

Outline

Objectives

Upon completion of this module the student should be able to:

1. Identify some physical signs of malnutrition.
2. Describe tools used in the assessment of nutritional status, such as
    a. diagnostic tests (radiologic/laboratory data)
    b. anthropometric measurements
    c. dietary history and recalls
    d. physical findings and sociological data
3. Recognize some common nutrition problems and propose corrective measures.
4. Be familiar with the responsibilities of health personnel in educating clients about nutritional needs.
5. Use the problem-solving process or model to promote health maintenance.

Glossary

Anthropometrics: measurement of the physical body, such as height and weight, chest and head circumferences.

Assessment: gathering of data about a person in order to logically identify his or her physical, psychological, social, and economic assets and liabilities.

Malnutrition: general term indicating an excess, deficit, or imbalance of one or more of the essential nutrients. May be used to describe an excess or deficit of calories. Psychosocial, economic, geographic, and physical factors can contribute to the development of malnutrition.

Nutrient: chemical substance in food that is needed by the body.

Nutritional status: the condition of the body as it relates to the consumption and utilization of food. (1) "Good nutritional status" refers to the intake of a balanced diet containing all the essential nutrients to meet the body's requirements for energy, maintenance, and growth. (2) "Poor nutritional status" refers to an inadequate intake (or utilization) of nutrients to meet the body's requirements for energy, maintenance, and growth.

Objective and subjective data: objective data are based on facts; subjective data are influenced by feelings, perceptions, and judgment rather than fact.

Serum: the watery portion of the blood that remains after the cells and clot-forming material (fibrinogen) have been removed; plasma is unclotted blood. In most cases serum and plasma concentrations are similar to one another. The serum sample often is preferred because plasma samples occasionally clog the mechanical blood analyzers.

Background Information

Health professionals, health care workers, and the client or patient comprise the health team in institutions and public health facilities. However, there are many types and kinds of noninstitutionalized health services, accompanied by an increasing number of private health practitioners.

The role of health care professionals is defined by law and based on educational preparation. They are required to receive certification, registration, licensing, or a combination of these.

An independent health practitioner may or may not be credentialed. However, as increasing numbers of people want to be responsible for their own health, these independent practitioners often serve as health resources. Through their counseling, health practitioners can influence the attitudes and health of many people. But, the practice of self-care must be preceded by the acquisition of information about health; that is, both the health care worker and the client need a solid background in the assessment of nutritional status, the techniques of health promotion, and accurate nutrition information.

This module is designed to assist the student to understand how to assess the nutritional status of clients or patients. The student will also learn the tools necessary to assist a health care professional to restore and promote health. Finally, the module teaches a student the problem-solving process in a health care system.

ACTIVITY 1: Assessment of Nutritional Status

In this activity we will explore four major techniques to assess nutritional status: (1) physical findings; (2) anthropometric measurements; (3) laboratory data; and (4) health and diet history.

Physical Findings

There are many clinical signs of good and poor nutrition. Although some of these signs are not related to a person's nutritional status, they serve as a general indicator of health. Data from a physical assessment are considered objective data and helpful to the health practitioner. Table 8-1 summarizes these findings.

Anthropometric Measurements

These measurements are relatively objective and are usually an important part of nutrition assessment. They are valuable in evaluating protein energy malnutrition (PEM). Figure 8-1 illustrates such measurements.

TABLE 8-1
Physical Indicators of Nutritional Status

Body Area	Signs of Good Nutrition	Signs of Malnutrition
1. Head to neck		
a. Hair	a. Shiny, lustrous; smooth healthy scalp	a. Dull, dry, thin, wirelike, sparse, brittle; scalp rough, flaky
b. Face	b. Skin smooth, moist, with uniform color	b. Pale or mottled, dark under eyes, swollen, scaling or flakiness, lumpiness
c. Eyes	c. Bright, clear, moist	c. Dry membranes, redness, fissures at corners, red rimmed, fine blood vessels or scars at cornea
d. Lips	d. Smooth, pink	d. Red, swollen, lesions or fissures
e. Tongue	e. Deep red, slightly rough surface	e. Scarlet or purplish color; raw, swollen, smooth
f. Teeth	f. Straight; none missing, no overlap, without cavities	f. Cavities, black or gray spots, erupting abnormally, missing
g. Gums	g. Firm, pink, smooth, no bleeding	g. Spongy, bleed easily, inflammation, receded, atrophied
2. Skin	2. Smooth, moist, uniform color	2. Dry, flaky, scaling, "gooseflesh," swollen, grayish, bruises due to capillary bleeding under skin, no fat layer under skin
3. Glands	3. No thyroid enlargement: No lumps at parotid juncture	3. Front of neck and cheeks become swollen, lumps visible at parotid; goiter visible if advanced hypothyroidism
4. Nails	4. Pink nail beds, smooth, firm, flexible, uniform shape	4. Brittle, ridged, pale nail beds, clubbed, spoon shaped
5. Muscle and skeletal system	5. Good posture, firm, well-developed muscles, good mobility; no malformations of skeleton	5. Flaccid, wasted muscles, weakness, tenderness, decreased reflexes, difficulty in walking Children: beading ribs, swelling at end of bones, abnormal protrusion of frontal or parietal areas
6. Internal systems		
a. Gastrointestinal	a. Flat abdomen, liver not tender to palpate, normal size	a. Distended, enlarged abdomen, ascites, hepatomegaly (enlarged liver) Children: "potbelly"
b. Cardiovascular	b. Normal pulse rate Normal blood pressure	b. Pulse rate exceeds 100 beats/min., abnormal rhythm, blood pressure elevated, mental confusion, edema

While physical appearances give us clues to internal problems, they can be misleading. They may not be nutrition-related. Physical findings must be coupled with other indications (lab test, anthropometrics, etc.) in order to validate them.

Approximately half the fat in our bodies is located directly below the skin (subcutaneous). In some parts of the body, this fat is more loosely attached, and can be pulled up between the thumb and forefinger. Such sites can be used for measuring fatfold thickness. Since fat stores decrease slowly even with an inadequate energy intake, a depletion of subcutaneous fat can reflect either long-term undernutrition or successful weight loss through dieting and exercise. Actual diagnostic tests used to determine nutritional status are usually made in the laboratory from blood and urine samples.

Laboratory Data _____

Laboratory tests are generally used to determine internal body chemistry. Though determined with great care and accuracy, these tests are influenced by many factors and subject to different interpretations.

The most common and useful biochemical techniques in evaluating malnutrition employ measurements of hemoglobin, blood cell counts (hematocrit), nitrogen balance, and creatinine excretion. The measurements are obtained from serum and plasma samples.

Laboratory tests valuable in assessing vitamin, mineral, and trace element status are listed in Table 8-2.

Health and Diet History _____

The type of data needed for health and diet history is subjective. Its accuracy depends on the skill of the interviewer and the client's memory, perception, and cooperation. From an interview, information can be obtained on the client's food intake history, presence of disorder, and drug usage. It is important that the interviewer learn something about the client's life and the factors that

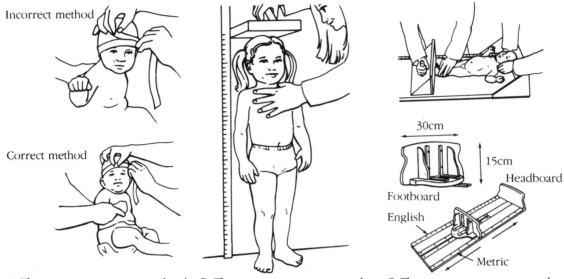

Incorrect method

Correct method

30cm

15cm
Headboard

Footboard

English

Metric

A. The proper way to measure head circumference.

B. The proper way to measure the height of a child older than 3 years.

C. The proper way to measure the length of a child under 3-years old.

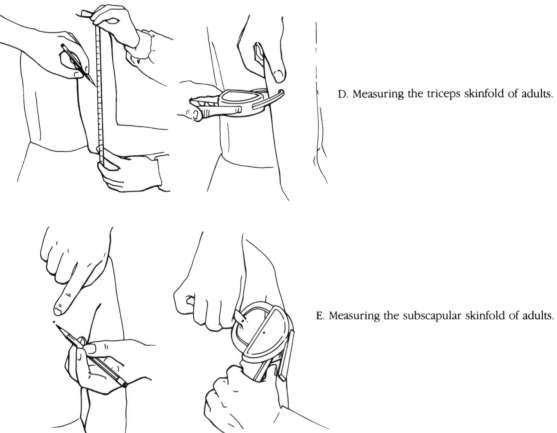

D. Measuring the triceps skinfold of adults.

E. Measuring the subscapular skinfold of adults.

Figure 8-1
Anthropometric Measurements

Assessment of growth and development by studying anthropometric measurements (physical measurements of the human body) provides important information about the nutritional status of infants, children, adolescents, and pregnant women. Standard measurements include weight, height, head circumference, midarm circumference, chest circumference, and skinfold thickness. These data provide developmentally significant ratios, including weight:height, midarm circumference:head circumference, chest circumference:head circumference, and midarm circumference:height. Data obtained over a period of time are especially helpful.

TABLE 8-2
Selected Blood Tests Useful for Determining Nutritional Status

	Nutrient	Laboratory Test	Acceptable Limits
1.	Carbohydrate	Plasma glucose	70–120 mg[1]/100ml[2]
2.	Fat	a. Serum cholesterol	140–220 mg/100ml
		b. Serum triglycerides	60–150 mg/100ml
3.	Protein	a. Visceral serum protein	above 6.5 gm[3]/100 ml
		b. Immune function:	
		(total lymphocyte count)	above 1200
4.	Fat-Soluble Vitamins		
	Vitamin A	a. Serum vitamin A	20-45 μg[4]/100 ml
		b. Serum carotene	40–300 μg/100 ml
	Vitamin D	a. Serum alkaline phosphatase	35–145 IU[5]/L[6]
		b. Plasma 25 hydroxy cholecalciferol	10–40 IU/L
	Vitamin E	Plasma vitamin E	above 0.6 mg/100 ml
	Vitamin K	Prothrombin time	12 seconds
5.	Water-Soluble Vitamins		
	a. Vitamin C	Serum ascorbic acid	above 0.3/100 ml
	b. B complex:		
	1. Thiamin	Red blood cell transketolase	0–15%
	2. Riboflavin	Red blood cell glutathione	below 1.2
	3. Niacin	Urinary nitrogen*	above 0.6 mg/gm creatinine
	4. Vitamin B_6	Tryptophan load*	below 50 μg/24 hrs.
	5. Vitamin B_{12}	Serum B_{12}	above 200 pg[7]/100 ml
	6. Folacin	Serum folacin	above 6.0 ng[8]/100 ml
6.	Minerals		
	Iodine	Serum protein bound iodine (PBI)	4.8–8.0 μg/100 ml
	Iron	a. Hemoglobin	male 14 mg/100 ml
			female 12 mg/100 ml
		b. Hematocrit	male 44%
			female 33%
	Calcium	Serum calcium	9.0–11.0 mg/100 ml
	Phosphorus	Serum phosphorus	2.5–4.5 mg/100 ml
	Magnesium	Serum magnesium	1.3–2.0 mEq[7]/L[8]
	Sodium	Serum sodium	130–150 mEq/L
	Potassium	Serum potassium	3.5–5.0 mEq/L
	Chloride	Serum chloride	99–110 mEq/L
	Zinc	Plasma zinc	80–100 μg/100 ml

*Urine analysis rather than blood sampling
Measurement terminology:
1. mg (milligram) 1,000 mg = 1 gm (gram)
2. ml (millileter) 1 ml = 1 cc (cubic centimeter)
3. gm (gram) 1,000 mg or 0.0001 kg (kilogram)

4. μg (microgram) 1,000 = 1 mg or 0.001 gm
5. IU (International Unit) not a metric measure
6. L (liter) 1,000 ml or 1,000 cc
7. pg (picogram) 10^{-12} gm
8. ng (nanogram) 10^{-9} gm

influence his or her eating habits (such as money, storage facilities, transportation, ethnicity).

Computerized diet analysis has become very popular in the last few years and is a valid tool to be used when specific types of information are being sought. One such diet analysis is used in Activity 2 to test the students' skills in assessment and client education.

More details on the assessment of nutritional status are presented later in this module.

Responsibilities of Health Personnel _____

The general responsibilities of health practitioners include recognizing a problem when it exists; correcting the problem if experience permits; and, most importantly, referring the client to another health professional if special expertise is needed. This responsibility can only be appropriately met if the health practitioner is familiar with and advises clients with accurate information on

1. the kinds of nutrients the body needs
2. the estimation of nutrients a person needs

3. the body's method of obtaining and maintaining adequate supplies of nutrients
4. the functions of various nutrients in the body
5. the relationship between nutrition and health
6. the relationship between food, exercise, and health
7. resources needed to facilitate nutritional education of the public
8. skill in applying the problem-solving process
9. use of anthropometric, physical, biochemical, and historical data to
   a. assess growth, weight changes, fat stores, muscle mass, and skeletal development
   b. plan nutrition program suitable to individual needs
   c. cooperate fully with other health professionals

Summary

Many parameters are useful in assessing nutrition status, including anthropometric, laboratory, physical, and historical data. These data form the basis for interpreting nutrient needs and determining how they will be met. Each client's individual needs in all the areas must be considered. Needs can change as people change—aging, recovering from diseases, or adopting different lifestyles are some of the important changes that require different nutritional patterns. Health practitioners should employ any or all of the tools described to assist them in determining the nutritional status of a person.

PROGRESS CHECK ON ACTIVITY 1

Fill-in

1. List and define the four factors generally used for assessment data: _____

   _____

   _____

2. This progress check contains exercises that will help the student apply the information just covered. List the areas identified in the Practices below that will require health education (use a separate sheet of paper to answer Practices A through D).

   Practice A
   Using the Nutritional Assessment and Diet History (Table 8-3), interview a family member or friend and try to determine his or her nutrient intake.

   Practice B
   Using Table 8-1, Physical Indicators of Nutritional Status, observe the person you are interviewing closely. Try to determine if he or she meets any of the physical criteria for malnutrition.

   Practice C
   Using a scale and tape measure, weigh and measure your subject.

   Practice D
   Compile the data and determine what kind of health education this person may need to improve his or her nutritional status.

3. List one indicator of good nutritional status for each of the following areas:

   a. hair _____

   b. skin _____

   c. eyes _____

   d. lips and tongue _____

   e. teeth and gums _____

   f. nails _____

   g. muscles _____

4. List five laboratory tests that are useful in assessing deficiencies and one finding associated with each:

   a. _____

   b. _____

   c. _____

   d. _____

   e. _____

Matching

Match the data listed on the left to the data-type listed on the right.

5. 5'6", 154 lb.
6. 30 percent above ideal body weight.
7. "I don't eat very much."
8. "I receive Social Security benefits."
9. "I think food is for enjoying."
10. "My stomach hurts when I eat spinach."

   a. objective data
   b. subjective data

TABLE 8-3
Nutritional Assessment and Diet History

Identification and Activity

1. Personal Data:
   Identifying number or name _____
   Age _____   Sex _____   Martial status _____
   Race _____   Religious preference _____   Ethnic origin _____
   Education _____ (Highest completed grade/degree)
   Employment: type _____   hours _____   approximate income _____
   Unemployed _____   Public assistance _____   Other _____
   Family composition (all living at one residence, ages and relationships) _____
   Person(s) most responsible for purchase, preparation of food _____
   Housing: type _____   facilities for storage, preparation of food _____

2. Health Data:
   A. Anthropometric: Height _____
      Present weight _____ (lbs) _____ (kg)
      Usual weight _____ (lbs) _____ (kg)
      Recent changes in weight _____
      Planned change? _____
      Triceps skinfold _____ (mm) Standard _____
      Midarm circumference _____ (cm) Standard _____
   B. Physical: Appearance of:
      1. Skin _____   7. Mouth, tongue, lips _____
      2. Hair _____   8. Teeth: Dentures _____
      3. Eyes _____   Edentulous _____
      4. Ears _____   Chews well _____
      5. Nails _____   Chews with difficulty _____
      6. Posture _____   9. Swallowing good _____ poor _____
      10. Any other pertinent physical data _____
   C. Laboratory: CBC _____   Hbg _____   Hct _____
      Serum levels of albumin/transferrin _____
      Urinary values _____
      Creatinine clearance _____
      Other _____
   D. Habits:
      1. Meals: number per day _____   Snacks: number per day _____
      2. Alcohol: amount daily _____   type _____
      3. Smoking: amount daily _____   type _____ (include cigars, pipes, and marijuana)
      4. Drugs: amount daily _____   specific kinds _____
      5. Exercise: kind _____   frequency _____   amount of time _____
   E. Other
      1. Gastrointestinal function:
         Appetite: good _____   fair _____   poor _____   recent changes _____
         Taste/smell: good _____   fair _____   poor _____   recent changes _____
         Indigestion: often _____   seldom _____ never _____
            If yes, list foods that cause _____
         List any foods that cause nausea/vomiting _____
         List any foods that cause diarrhea _____
         Bowel elimination: frequency _____   consistency _____
      2. Emotional state:
         calm _____   agitated _____   anxious _____   depressed _____
         Other: (Explain) _____

(continues)

TABLE 8-3 (Continued)

24 Hour Intake Record

3. Dietary History:

A. Food Preferences	Foods Acceptable	Food Dislikes	Food Allergies	Other

B. Meals: Usual	Serving Size	Time	Where	Special occasions weekends/holidays
Breakfast				
Lunch/dinner				
Dinner/supper				
Snacks				

C. Vitamin, mineral supplements taken: kind _____ amount _____
   Reason for taking _____

D. Usual preparation method (bake, boil, broil, fry, etc.)
   1. Meats _____
   2. Vegetables _____

Analysis

Nutritional Diagnosis/Planning (for nurse's use)

1. Review the assessment and diet history and list the potential needs for nutrition education.
2. Questions to guide the beginning practitioner:
   a. Was daily intake adequate in Kcal, nutrients, kinds and amounts of food?

      If *no*, indicate:
      1. Which food groups have been omitted or are in inadequate amounts?

      2. Which of the RDAs for major nutrients have not been met?

(continues)

TABLE 8-3 (Continued)

24 Hour Intake Record

3. Does the caloric intake provide for maintenance of normal weight?

Too low? _____ Too high? _____ For recovery from illness/injury? _____

b. What foods will need to be added/subtracted/substituted to meet the assessed needs of this person and maintain individuality?

c. Identify areas of patient teaching that need to be included as you plan your nursing care and interventions.

Explanatory Notes

The nutritional assessment should be a part of every health practitioner's relationship to the client. It is one of the tools that provide information to identify and meet client needs.

The purpose of nutritional assessment is to provide an essential part of the overall nursing assessment. Some people, because of their nutritional status at the time of disease or injury, may be at high risk for nutritional problems that affect the outcome of the disease process. This assessment may become critical in the overall recovery.

Some forms of food survey/intake should be obtained for every client at admission. If the client is unable to respond, information should be obtained from family or others who know the client's eating patterns in order to individualize the diet. Some of the data may be collected from other recorded observations and tests.

The nutritional assessment and diet history can be used as a basis for planning a diet with a patient that will speed recovery, as well as for teaching sound nutrition principles and promoting health maintenance.

ACTIVITY 2: Health Care Model: The Problem-Solving Process

Members of a health team work together to provide care for clients in an institution, a community, or a home setting. The health team consists of health professionals, health care workers, and the client. Some functions are delegated and many of them overlap. Cooperative effort of the team members assists clients in meeting their nutritional needs and achieving better overall care. A health team member should know the functions of other health professionals in order to support their efforts on behalf of the clients.

Studies suggest that the health of individuals in any setting can be improved through education. The rising cost of health care makes it necessary to maintain good health status to reduce risk of diseases. Proper nutritional care is one way to achieve the goal. This activity helps a care provider to learn a health care model that will identify and meet a client's needs.

Although such a health care model has many names, such as clinical care process, nursing process, or scientific method, for general purposes, we will call it the problem-solving process.

The problem-solving process consists of a series of logical steps to approaching and solving problems. It is a flexible model. Some practitioners choose a five-step plan,

some four, and some three. This exercise will use the four-step plan. It consists of these four components: assessment, planning, implementation, and evaluation.

Assessment

Assessment of a client identifies areas requiring assistance and provides a baseline for later evaluation of a client's nutritional status. It is made up of two parts:

1. Gathering careful and systematic data about the client's lifestyle, economic status, nutritional knowledge, the meaning of food and health to the client, and other pertinent information (some of this information is subjective and some is objective, as defined in Activity 1).

2. Identifying the problem(s) based on data obtained. (Nutritional Diagnosis)

Planning

After specific health problems have been identified, the practitioner plans the steps to solve them. Planning also helps each team member implement his or her respective responsibility in the overall care program. At this stage, decisions on implementing the plan and evaluating the results are made. Planning includes

1. Establishing client-oriented goals.
2. Establishing a care plan, including specific measures and objectives to be carried out.

Implementation

Implementation of health care involves carrying out the activities that were planned and outlined in the care plan. The following steps should be taken:

1. Coordinate the care. Cooperation and consistency among health care members are essential.
2. Provide for teaching and counseling. Be specific about who provides for each component; who initiates the plan; and who reinforces the plan and follows up.
3. Help the client to make necessary changes in eating and/or activities.

Evaluation

Identify the extent to which objectives have been met. Each objective should be evaluated separately. Plans for revisions are made whenever the desired effectiveness is not obtained. The process is made up of the following steps:

1. Measure the client's progress.
2. Evaluate the teaching.
3. Revise the plan and reteach the objectives not met.

Case Study

The following case study shows the use of the problem-solving process:

1. Assessment

A. Information collected about the client.
    1. Female, 43-years old, three children ages 13, 10, and 7. Marital status: divorced.
    2. Employed as an elementary teacher.
    3. History of hypertension.
    4. Five feet three inches tall, weight 165 lb., daily intake is 3,000 calories.
    5. Uses salt in cooking and frequently snacks.
    6. Uses fast foods, convenience foods, and eats rapidly.
    7. Older children have poor eating habits.
B. Identified problems based on data collected:
    1. Excess calorie intake for occupation, age, and so on, resulting in excessive fat storage.
    2. Excessive salt intake (fast foods, snacks).
    3. Elevated blood pressure (hypertension).

4. Lack of nutrition information and/or desirable eating behaviors.

Based on these problems, a diet low in calories and sodium is indicated. Basic nutrition information and techniques to modify eating behaviors will be needed to improve compliance with the diet.

2. Planning

Because this client's solutions involve major changes in lifestyle for the family, the health team decides to segment the educational process. The level of education is such that the criteria for evaluation can be very specific. Goals are set up with the client:

A. The client will reduce her salt and calorie intake to attain and maintain a normal body weight and blood pressure.
B. The client will modify the eating behaviors of the whole family to provide a healthier lifestyle.

3. Implementation

A. Coordinating care
    1. A registered dietitian will be the primary teacher.
    2. Reinforcement, follow up, and observations will be made by other health team members.
    3. A physician's approval with a physical examination and a 1,200 calorie, 2 gram sodium diet order is obtained prior to beginning.
    4. Resources and referrals are obtained as needed.
    5. A support system that includes a social worker and other personnel is instituted.
    6. All family members are included in the care process.
B. The care program is done in three segments as planned. The care plan objectives are as follows:

    Plan 1: The client will be able to plan, purchase, prepare, and serve a balanced diet. The client will also be able to achieve the following subobjectives:
    1. Identify the Basic Four food groups and state four foods from each group.
    2. Plan a day's menu, using the daily food guide.
    3. Make a purchase order for one week, using only foods allowed in food plan.
    4. State three acceptable methods of food preparation.
    5. Identify ways to attractively serve food.

    Plan 2: The client will be able to select foods that are acceptable on a 1,200 calorie, 2 gram sodium diet. The client will also be able to achieve the following subobjectives:
    1. List eight foods not allowed because of reduced calorie content of diet.

2. List eight foods not allowed because of 2 gram sodium restriction.
3. Differentiate between a diet that follows the Basic Four food pattern and one reduced in calories.
4. Make a list of acceptable seasonings to be used in place of salt.
5. Discuss the food preparation methods required for this diet and how they differ from those in Plan 1.

Plan 3: The client will be able to identify behavior modifications useful in complying with diet changes. The client will be able to achieve the following subobjectives:

1. List behavior techniques for:
   (1) eating slowly
   (2) eating small portions
   (3) stopping other activities while eating
2. Include other modifications identified from client profile.

4. Evaluation

A. Measuring progress
   Every objective in each plan needs to be evaluated separately. For example:
   1. The client stated the four food groups and four foods from each group verbally.
   2. The client planned an adequate menu based on the foods in the daily food groups.

B. Evaluating teaching
   Teaching evaluation is done by the health team conference, peer evaluation, and so on.

C. Revising objectives
   Any objectives not met during the first teaching process will be revised.

Responsibilities of Health Personnel

The responsibilities of the health personnel are as follows:

1. Provide or assist in the provision of nutrition education.
2. Provide referrals, resource personnel, and supportive nutritional services as needed.
3. Work cooperatively with other members of the health team.
4. Stay within the parameters of the health care practitioner's own role and recognize limitations.
5. Seek assistance as necessary.
6. Document appropriate information.

Summary

The health care practitioner has an important role in providing or assisting in the provision of quality nutritional care. The roles of a facilitator, advocate, and liaison cannot be negated. It is important that the skills of observation, interviewing, and problem solving be incorporated at every level in the health care systems. The clients will be the ultimate beneficiaries of these skills, and the clients themselves may well be the health care providers.

PROGRESS CHECK ON ACTIVITY 2

Fill-in

Review the Idaho diet analysis shown in Table 8-4 and answer all questions listed below based on the information given about the client in the analysis and the information given below.

1. A balanced diet should contain no less than 12 to 14% protein and no more than 35% fat. The remainder should be carbohydrate. In your client's diet, 12% of her calories came from proteins, 47% came from fats, and 41% came from carbohydrates. List at least three ways for each nutrient that your client's diet could be altered to fit the balanced diet guidelines given above.

   a. _____

   b. _____

   c. _____

2. The RDA range for potassium for a healthy individual of your client's age group is 1,875–5,625 mg per day. Her potassium intake was 1,349.5 mg. List at least three good sources of potassium.

   a. _____

   b. _____

   c. _____

3. The RDA range for sodium for a healthy individual of your client's age group is 1,100–3,300 mg per day. Her sodium intake is 2,018 mg. Does this sodium intake need to be lowered? Explain your answer. _____

   _____

   _____

4. Your client's food intake shows that she is low in some nutrients. Check the total diet analysis for the day and list all the nutrients that are below the RDAs in the 24-hour intake. _____

   _____

   _____

TABLE 8-4
Idaho Diet Analysis

			Activity Level	Hours
Today's Date	Age: 25 years		Sleeping or reclining:	7
Your Name	Female		Very light:	14
Your Address	Height (in): 66		Moderately active:	3
Your City, Your State	Current weight: 160 lbs		Very active:	
Your Zip Code	Desired weight: 140 lbs		Exceptionally active:	

Foods Eaten		# Servings
Breakfast:		
(Code)		
123	Unsweetened frozen reconstituted orange juice (½ cup)	0.5
200	Cooked cream of wheat (½ cup)	2
5	Natural American/cheddar cheese (1 oz.)	1
176	Commercial whole wheat bread (1 slice)	1
290	Butter (1 tsp.)	2
Lunch:		
244	Instant noodle soup (1 cup)	1
268	Lemon meringue pie (⅛ of 9" diameter)	1
218	Saltine cracker (1 square)	2
Dinner:		
45	Breaded fried cod filet (1 oz.)	4
181	Raised yeast doughnut (1 doughnut)	1
274	White sugar (1 tsp.)	1
290	Butter (1 tsp.)	1
301	Thousand island salad dressing (1 tbsp.)	1
Snacks:		
195	All bran (1 cup)	0.5
18	2% milk (1 cup)	0.5

A food or meal is a good source of a nutrient when the length of the nutrient line (%RDA line for that nutrient) is as long as or longer than the calorie line. The food or meal is not a good source of a nutrient when the length of the nutrient line is shorter than the calorie line.

Analysis for Breakfast

Nutrient	Amount	%RDA
Calories	385.0	16.7
Protein (g's)	13.5	23.2
Vitamin A (IU's)	727.0	18.2
Vitamin C (mg's)	28.0	46.7
Thiamin (mg's)	0.2	23.5
Riboflavin (mg's)	0.2	18.7
Niacin (mg's)	2.0	15.3
Calcium (mg's)	253.5	31.7
Iron (mg's)	1.6	9.1
Vitamin B_6 (mg's)	0.1	5.5
Magnesium (mg's)	44.0	14.6

Analysis for Lunch

Nutrient	Amount	%RDA
Calories	421.0	18.2
Protein (g's)	8.9	15.3
Vitamin A (IU's)	706.0	17.7
Vitamin C (mg's)	4.0	6.6
Thiamin (mg's)	0.1	17.0
Riboflavin (mg's)	0.1	15.0
Niacin (mg's)	1.5	11.5
Calcium (mg's)	24.0	3.0

(continues)

TABLE 8-4 (Continued)

Analysis for Breakfast (Cont'd)

%RDA

Nutrient	Amount	%RDA	0	10	20	30	40	50	60	70	80	90	100	110	120	130	140	150	160+
Iron (mg's)	1.6	8.8																	
Vitamin B$_6$ (mg's)	0.0	2.5																	
Magnesium (mg's)	25.0	8.3																	

Analysis for Dinner

Calories	549.0	23.7
Protein (g's)	23.9	41.0
Vitamin A (IU's)	285.0	7.0
Vitamin C (mg's)	4.0	6.6
Thiamin (mg's)	0.1	14.0
Riboflavin (mg's)	0.1	14.1
Niacin (mg's)	2.4	18.5
Calcium (mg's)	31.0	3.9
Iron (mg's)	1.1	6.0
Vitamin B$_6$ (mg's)	0.1	9.0
Magnesium (mg's)	44.0	14.6

Analysis for Snacks

Calories	132.5	5.6
Protein (g's)	7.3	12.6
Vitamin A (IU's)	1573.0	39.2
Vitamin C (mg's)	17.0	28.2
Thiamin (mg's)	0.7	77.5
Riboflavin (mg's)	1.0	87.9
Niacin (mg's)	8.0	61.5
Calcium (mg's)	173.0	21.6
Iron (mg's)	3.7	20.7
Vitamin B$_6$ (mg's)	0.5	29.5
Magnesium (mg's)	122.5	40.7

Total Diet Analysis

Calories	1487.5	64.5
Protein (g's)	53.7	92.3
Vitamin A (IU's)	3291.0	82.3
Vitamin C (mg's)	53.0	88.3
Thiamin (mg's)	1.3	132.0
Riboflavin (mg's)	1.6	135.8
Niacin (mg's)	13.9	106.9
Calcium (mg's)	481.5	60.2
Iron (mg's)	8.1	45.0
Vitamin B$_6$ (mg's)	0.9	46.5
Magnesium (mg's)	235.5	78.5

A balanced diet should contain no less than 12–14% protein and no more than 30% fat; the remainder should be carbohydrate. In your diet, 10% of your calories came from protein, 44% came from fats, and 46% came from carbohydrates. The RDA range for potassium for a healthy individual of your age group is 1875–5625 mg per day. Your potassium intake was 1462 mg.
The RDA range for sodium for a healthy individual of your age group is 1100-3300 mg per day. Your sodium intake was 2195.

Your Food Intake Shows that You Are Low in the Following Nutrients:

Nutrient	Foods that are Good Sources for the Nutrient
Vitamin A (IU's)	Apricot, broccoli, cantaloupe, carrots, liver, mixed vegetables, nectarine, peach, spinach, sweet potatoes, tomato products, tossed salad, vegetable/vegetable beef soup, winter squash

(continues)

TABLE 8-4 (Continued)

Vitamin C (mg's)	Asparagus, broccoli, cabbage, cantaloupe, cauliflower, grapefruit (juice), honeydew melon, orange (juice), potato, spinach, strawberries, summer squash or zucchini, sweet green pepper, tomato products
Calcium (mg's)	Cheese, cottage cheese, cream soup, enchilada, ice cream, macaroni and cheese, milk, milkshake, pizza, cheese, pudding, salmon, spinach, whole grain and enriched breads and cereals, yogurt
Iron (mg's)	Beans (dried), beef, dried fruit, egg yolks, fortified ready-to-eat cereals, kidney, lamb, liver, liverwurst, oysters, peas, pork, spinach, turkey
Vitamin B$_6$ (mg's)	Banana, beef, cabbage, chicken, corn, fortified ready-to-eat cereals, halibut, ham, liver, milk, potato, salmon, tuna, turkey
Magnesium (mg's)	Asparagus, beef, broccoli, cauliflower, chocolate, dried beans, hulled sunflower seeds, lima beans, peanuts and other nuts, spinach, sweet green pepper, tomato products, tossed salad, whole wheat breads and cereals
Potassium	Avocado, banana, cantaloupe, dates, figs, flounder, grapefruit (juice), halibut, honeydew melon, nectarine, orange (juice), potato, prunes (juice), soybeans

Based on your current weight of 160 lbs., height, sex, age, and activity level, you need 2,226 calories of energy per day.

Based on your desired or ideal weight of 140 lbs., you need 2,044 calories of energy per day.

Your food intake shows that you ate fewer calories than your calculated needs.

To lose one pound of body fat, you need to eat 3,500 calories less than your body needs. If you decrease your calorie intake by 500 calories per day, you will lose 1 pound per week. If you decrease your calorie intake by 1,000 calories per day, you will lose 2 pounds per week.

Your planned daily calorie intake in order to reach your ideal weight is 1,200 calories.

At your intended level of daily calorie intake (1,200 calories), you should reach your desired or ideal weight in about 10 weeks.

Source: University of Idaho, Cooperative Extension Service.

5. List at least five foods that are good sources of each nutrient that the client is deficient in, as identified in Question 4 above. _____

_____

_____

6. Based on your client's current weight of 160 lb., height, sex, age, and activity level, she needs 2,226 calories of energy per day. In general terms, describe how this figure was obtained. _____

_____

_____

7. Based on your client's desired or ideal weight of 140 lb., she needs 2,044 calories of energy per day. Her food intake shows that she ate fewer calories than your calculated needs. How many fewer calories did your client consume than needed? _____

_____

_____

8. Your client's planned daily calorie intake to reach her ideal weight is 1,200 calories.

a. Will her present diet meet the criteria for a safe reducing diet? Explain. _____

_____

_____

b. How long will it take her to reach her ideal weight if she stays on the 1,200 calorie diet?

_____

_____

9. Using the assessment data you have gathered from the 24-hour recall and the meal planning with exchange lists (see Appendix), plan an adequate 1,200 calorie diet for your client. Show your calculations. _____

_____

_____

10. State three behavioral objectives to be used in a teaching plan for this client. _____

_____

_____

References

Allman, R. et al. 1986. Pressure sores among hospitalized patients. *Ann. Int. Med.* 105:337.

Aronson, V., and B. Fitzgerald. 1990. *Guidebook for nutrition counselors.* Englewood Cliffs, NJ: Prentice Hall.

Banister, E. W. et al. 1988. *Contemporary health issues.* Boston: Jones and Bartlett.

Bingham, S. A. 1987. The dietary assessment of individuals: Methods, accuracy, new techniques, and recommendations. *Nutritional Abstract Review* 57(10):705.

Blackburn, G. L. et al. (eds.). 1989. *Nutritional medicine: A case management approach.* Philadelphia: Saunders.

Burton, P. W. 1986. Using the computer as a referral source to find the patient at nutritional risk. *Journal of the American Dietetic Association* 86:1232.

Christensen, K. S. et al. 1985. Hospital-wide screening improves basis for nutrition intervention. *Journal of the American Dietetic Association* 85(6):704.

Clay, B. et al. 1988. A comprehensive nutrition case management system. *Journal of the American Dietetic Association* 88(2):196.

Dikoviks, A. 1986. *Nutritional assessment: Case study methods.* Philadelphia: George F. Stickley Co.

Doak, C. C. et al. 1985. *Teaching patients with low literacy skills.* Philadelphia: Lippincott.

Dwyer, J. T. 1988. Assessment of dietary intake. In *Modern nutrition in health and disease,* 7th ed. M. E. Shils and V. R. Young (eds.). Philadelphia: Lea & Febiger.

Escott-Stump, S. 1988. *Nutrition and diagnosis-related care,* 2nd ed. Philadelphia: Lea and Febiger.

Estabrook, S. G. 1988. *The 1988 annual journal of dietetic software.* Norman, OK: Journal of Dietetic Software.

Ford, M. G. 1987. The computer as an aid in clinical management. *Journal of the American Dietetic Association* 87:497.

Frisancho, A. R. 1988. *Anthropometric standards for the assessment of growth and nutritional status.* Ann Arbor: Health Products.

Frisancho, A. R. 1988. Commentary: Nutritional anthropometry. *Journal of the American Dietetic Association* 88(5):553.

Gersovitz, M. et al. 1987. Validity of the 24-hour dietary recall and the seven-day record for group comparisons. *Journal of the American Dietetic Association* 73:48.

Gibson, R. S. 1990. *Principles of nutritional assessment.* New York: Oxford University Press.

Hallgren, B. et al. (eds.). 1986. *Diet and prevention of coronary heart disease and cancer.* New York: Raven Press.

Heymsfield, S. B., and P. J. Williams. 1988. Nutritional assessment by clinical and biochemical methods. In *Modern nutrition in health and disease,* 7th ed. M. E. Shils and V. R. Young (eds.). Philadelphia: Lea & Febiger.

Hodges, P. A. M., and C. E. Vickery. 1989. *Effective counseling: Strategies for dietary management.* Rockville, MD: Aspen.

Huyck, N. I. et al. 1987. Provision of clinical nutrition services by diagnosis-related groups (DRGs) and major diagnostic categories (MDCs). *Journal of the American Dietetic Association* 87(1):69.

Kamath, S. K. et al. 1986. Hospital malnutrition: A 33-hospital screening study. *Journal of the American Dietetic Association* 86(2):203.

Kane, J. K. 1987. *Exploring careers in dietetics and nutrition.* New York: Rosen Publishing Group.

Lang, C. E. (ed.). 1987. *Nutritional support in critical care.* Rockville, MD: Aspen.

McCool, A. C., and M. M. Garand. 1986. Computer technology in institutional foodservice. *Journal of the American Dietetic Association* 86:48.

National Institute of Health. 1988. *Eating for life.* Washington, DC: U.S. Department of Health and Human Services, Public Health Service, National Institute of Health.

National Institute of Health. 1989. *National Cholesterol Education Program: Expert panel on detection, evaluation, and treatment of high blood cholesterol in adults.* Washington, DC: U.S. Department of Health and Human Services, Public Health Service, National Institute of Health.

Orta, J. 1988. *Computer applications in the food and nutrition professions: An annotated bibliography.* New York: Garland Publishing.

Paige, D. M. et al. 1988. Nutritional assessment: An index to the quality of life. *Clinical Nutrition* 7(2):77.

Rubin, M. 1988. The physiology of bed rest. *American Journal of Nursing* 88(1):50.

Smith, F. B. 1985. Patient power. *American Journal of Nursing* 85(11):1260.

Snetselaar, L. G. *Nutrition counseling skills: Assessment, treatment, and evaluation,* 2nd ed. Rockville, MD: Aspen.

Sundberg, M. C. 1989. *Fundamentals of nursing with clinical procedures.* Boston: Jones and Bartlett.

Underwood, B. A. 1986. Evaluating the nutritional status of individuals: A critique of approaches. *Nutrition Review* 44(Suppl):213.

Wahlqvist, M. L., and J. S. Vobecky (eds.). 1987. *Patient problems in clinical nutrition: A manual.* London: John Libbey & Co.

Watson, R. R. (ed.). 1987. *Nutrition and heart disease.* Volumes I and II. Boca Raton, FL: CRC Press.

Module 9

Nutrition and the Life Cycle

Time for completion
Activities: _____1½_____ hours
Optional examination: _½_ hour

Academic credit
Semester units: _3/10_
Quarter units: _4/10_

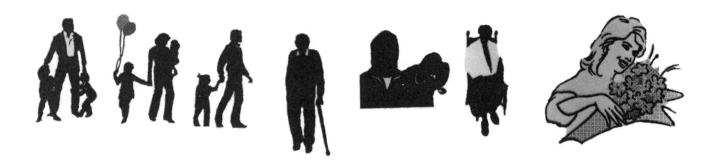

Outline

Objectives

Activity 1: Maternal and Infant Nutrition

Upon completion of the activity, the student should be able to:

1. Identify factors that influence the course and outcome of pregnancy with special reference to the client's health history, nutritional status, and food habits.
2. Describe the nutritional needs of women during pregnancy and lactation.
3. Explain the recommended weight gain pattern for a pregnant woman.
4. List health concerns during pregnancy and lactation.
5. Summarize the nutritional needs of the neonate/infant.
6. Compare the advantages and disadvantages of breast-feeding.
7. Discuss the introduction of solid foods to an infant's diet in relation to the sequence, process, and need for supplements.
8. Analyze the health concerns of the infant.

Activity 2: Childhood and Adolescent Nutrition

Upon completion of the activity, the student should be able to:

1. Describe the body changes that occur in the stages of:
   a. early childhood: toddler, preschooler
   b. middle childhood: school age to adolescence
   c. adolescence
2. Identify the nutritional needs of children and adolescents.
3. Discuss the health problems that often occur during childhood and adolescence.
4. Analyze areas of concern regarding eating behaviors of children and adolescents.
5. List ways to promote sound nutritional practices among children and adolescents.

Activity 3: Adulthood and Nutrition

Upon completion of the activity, the student should be able to:

1. Describe the body changes that occur during the span of the adult years.
2. Identify the nutritional needs during early, middle, and late adulthood.
3. Explain the health concerns of early, middle, and late adulthood.
4. Analyze the psychosocial, physiological, and economic influences on eating behaviors.
5. Evaluate the importance of maintaining a regular exercise program throughout the adult years.

6. List the effects of drugs, including alcohol, on nutrients and health.
7. Propose measures to promote healthful eating habits during adulthood, especially the later years.

Activity 4: Exercises, Fitness, and Stress Reduction Principles

Upon completion of the activity, the student should be able to:

1. Describe the major health concerns of adulthood.
2. Identify the nutritional components of keeping fit.
3. Describe the key elements of an exercise program.
4. Discuss the effects of nutrition and controlled exercise.
5. Describe an effective dietary regime for a person interested in staying healthy into old age.
6. Recognize the biological, psychological, and sociological factors that promote stress.
7. Counsel patients on techniques of stress reduction, relaxation, exercise, and optimal nutrition at any stage of the life cycle.
8. Follow the principles of a healthy lifestyle.

Glossary

Angina pectoris: intense chest pain resulting from myocardial anoxia.

Congenital anomalies: birth defects; abnormally formed organs or body parts.

Course and outcome of pregnancy: the absence or presence of complications.

Fetus: the developing baby during the third trimester.

Hypertension: Blood pressure elevated above normal limits.

Intrauterine device (IUD):   birth control device consisting of plastic or copper coils placed in the uterus for long periods of time to prevent conception.

Lactation: secretion of milk.

Low birth weight (LBW):   weight of baby lower than normal for calculated age.

Miscarriage: interrupted pregnancy prior to seventh month.

Mortality: death.

Myocardial infarction: technical term for a heart attack.

Neonate: a newborn child, from birth to twenty-eight days old.

Oral contraceptive agent (OCA):   oral medication (hormones) that can prevent conception.

Pica: the practice of eating nonfood items, such as laundry starch and clay.

Placenta: the structure that develops on the wall of the uterus during pregnancy and through which the fetus is attached by the umbilical cord to receive nourishment and excrete waste.

Premature: birth of a baby prior to 38-week gestational age.

Psychomotor: mind-directed muscle movements.

RBCs: red blood cells.

Small for gestational age (SGA): same as low birth weight (LBW).

Toxemia: a life-threatening condition associated with the presence of toxic substances in the blood.

Triglyceride: a form of fat found in food and blood.

Trimester: a three-month period during pregnancy; the nine-month pregnancy is divided into three trimesters.

Women, Infants, and Children (WIC): special supplemental food program for women, infants, and children (up to age five).

Background Information

The life cycle is the course of life from birth to death. Each stage in this cycle has effects upon the succeeding stages. In turn, each childbearing couple leaves its mark upon succeeding generations. The kind of nutrition a woman receives before and during pregnancy affects the growth and development of her child, as well as her own health. The nourishment that infants and children receive affects them as adults, and affects any offspring they may have.

Health practitioners must recognize that there are many different approaches to planning a diet for a pregnant woman, depending on factors such as culture, ethnicity, folklore, and others. The changing American lifestyle, with its distinct eating patterns and sedentary habits, is evaluated by health practitioners in terms of its health implications.

Every effort should be made to help people meet their nutritional needs at each stage of life. The health practitioner should develop approaches and knowledge appropriate to the various stages of life in order to promote sound nutritional practices for clients of all ages.

Every health practitioner should have a working knowledge of the interrelated effects of exercise, nutrition, and stress on the human body and practical applications to assist clients in healthy lifestyle changes.

ACTIVITY 1: Maternal and Infant Nutrition

Pregnancy: Determining Factors

A healthy, well-nourished woman whose nutritional status was good prior to becoming pregnant has a very good chance of delivering a health full-term baby of normal birth weight.

Food intake during pregnancy is important, but entering pregnancy with nutrient reserves has many advantages. It provides a margin of safety if food intake is interfered with during the early stages of pregnancy—for example, morning sickness (nausea and vomiting). The amount of each nutrient that can be stored in the body varies from small to large. However, a well-nourished body usually has a small surplus of all nutrients. This surplus can be crucial in the first trimester of pregnancy, when the ability to eat is impaired by the hormonal shifts and the tissues and organs of the embryo are being differentiated. This is the time when adequate nutrition is believed to help protect against some birth defects.

Good prepregnancy nutritional status also is an indicator of reasonably good eating practices. A woman who depends on a reliable food guide for regular meal planning will find it easy to adapt her diet to the higher requirements imposed during pregnancy. Because diet affects the course and outcome of pregnancy so greatly, the woman contemplating becoming pregnant in the near or distant future should learn to follow the principles of good nutrition. The adolescent female whose diet is considered to be unsatisfactory should be strongly encouraged to alter her nutritional habits before a planned pregnancy.

Teenage pregnancies are associated with many social and medical problems. The pregnant teenager under seventeen years of age is at particularly high risk. Nearly one-third of all teenage mothers are under the age of sixteen. The teenage mother faces two major concerns: her own development and that of the child, both of whom are likely to suffer. The course and outcome of teenage pregnancy are at risk and include the following complications: a higher incidence of maternal and infant mortality; premature or SGA (small for gestational age) infants; congenital anomalies; stillborns; and toxemia. While these complications are potential hazards for any pregnant and malnourished mother, their severity increases with the decreasing age of the mother. The teenager often fails to eat an adequate diet because she does not want to gain weight. Since a normal recommended pattern of weight gain is a major criterion in evaluating a healthy pregnancy, it is not surprising that diet counseling for a pregnant teenager is very important.

Pregnancy: Nutritional Needs and Weight Gain

The recommended pattern of weight gain is illustrated in Figure 9-1. This pattern is recommended even if the woman is overweight or obese at the beginning of pregnancy. While the pattern of weight gain is important, if a woman gains more during a trimester than was planned, she should not be advised to reduce caloric intake in the remaining weeks.

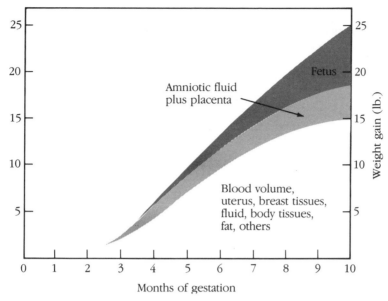

Figure 9-1
Weight Gain during Pregnancy

The recommended total weight gain during pregnancy is 24 to 30 pounds. The underweight woman will need to gain more weight. Usually a first-time pregnancy will sustain a higher net gain, especially in younger women. Of this weight, approximately 7 to 10 pounds is fetus, 1-1/2 to 2 pounds placenta, 2 pounds uterus, 8-1/2 pounds increase in blood volume and fluids, and 3 to 4 pounds increase in breast tissue and fat reserves. The increase in breast tissue and fat reserve is in preparation for breast-feeding.

The RDA specifies an increase of 300 kcal daily above the normal caloric requirement to meet the energy demands during pregnancy. This added intake should result in the recommended weight increase. Since 300 kcal is not a big increase, the calories should be obtained from nutrient-dense foods. The nutrients needed by pregnant women are the same as for nonpregnant women, but the amounts are sharply increased.

The pattern of weight gain is more important than the total amount gained. The desirable weight gain pattern is approximately 3 pounds during the first trimester of pregnancy and 1.0 pound per week for the remainder of the pregnancy. A sharp increase in weight gain after the twentieth week may signal excess fluid retention, a sign of the potential development of toxemia. Rapid weight gain from water is an effect, not a cause, of toxemia. Women who gain too much weight (fat) usually find it difficult to return to normal weight after pregnancy. Their babies may be fat, with an excess weight problem later in life.

All nutrients for the developing fetus must be supplied by the mother's diet or her body reserves. In addition, nutrients and energy must be available for increases in the mother's tissues and blood. Table 9-1 depicts the increased need for nutrients during pregnancy and lactation according to the 1989 RDAs.

The 30-gram increase in protein intake is important for a satisfactory pregnancy. Studies confirm that infants born to mothers with adequate protein intake are taller, have better brain development, and can resist diseases better. In addition, toxemia is more common in women with a low protein intake. Since protein will be used for energy if dietary energy is low, any diet below 1,800 calories may also negatively influence the outcome of pregnancy.

Even with a diet adequate in other respects, an iron supplement is recommended for pregnant women. Usually this is prescribed by the woman's physician, along with vitamins and minerals as a margin of safety. Some women misinterpret this to mean that if they take the supplements, they do not have to plan a careful diet. This is a dangerous interpretation, since the supplements contain no protein and usually only 25 to 30 percent of the recommended calcium. The prescription of a supplement by a doctor does not mean that megadoses of vitamins and minerals during pregnancy will guarantee better health. The opposite is true. The excess is stored in fetal tissues and can be toxic. High doses of vitamins A and D have been known to cause birth defects. Tables 9-2 and 9-3 summarize information related to vitamin intake during pregnancy. Although folic acid is not listed in these tables, it is a recommended supplement (see Table 9-1) during pregnancy to protect against megaloblastic anemia. Folic acid and vitamin C are usually given along with the iron supplement to improve absorption.

A sample meal plan and menu suitable for an adequate diet for a pregnant woman are given in Tables 9-4 and 9-5.

TABLE 9-1
1989 RDAs for a 25-Year-Old Woman at Three Physiological Stages

Nutrient	Daily Amount Needed	Additional Daily Amount Needed		
		Pregnancy	Lactation	
			1st 6 Months	2nd 6 Months
Energy (kcal)	2200	300[a]	500	500
Protein (g)	50	10	15	12
Vitamin A (μg RE)	800	0	500	400
Vitamin D (μg)	5	5	5	5
Vitamin E (mg α-TE)	8	2	4	3
Vitamin K (μg)	65	0	0	0
Vitamin C (mg)	60	10	35	30
Vitamin B_1 (mg)	1.1	0.4	0.5	0.5
Vitamin B_2 (mg)	1.3	0.3	0.5	0.4
Niacin (mg NE)	15	2	5	5
Vitamin B_6 (mg)	1.6	0.6	0.5	0.5
Folate (μg)	180	220	100	80
Vitamin B_{12} (μg)	2.0	0.2	0.6	0.6
Calcium (mg)	800	400	400	400
Phosphorus (mg)	800	400	400	400
Magnesium (mg)	280	40	40	40
Iron (mg)	15	15[b]	0	0
Zinc (mg)	12	3	7	4
Iodine (mg)	150	25	50	50
Selenium	55	10	20	20

Source: Recommended Daily Allowances, Revised 1989. National Academy of Sciences. Reprinted with permission.
[a]No additions for the first trimester.
[b]Since the increased pregnancy requirement cannot be met by the iron content of habitual U.S. diets or by the iron stores of at least some women, daily iron supplements are usually recommended.

Pregnancy: Health Concerns

Most of the health problems that occur during pregnancy can be reduced or prevented by nutritional adjustments. Among these problems are nausea, constipation, anemia, pica, heartburn, urinary urgency, muscle cramps, bloating, toxemia, and excessive alcohol consumption. While it is not possible in this module to discuss the probable causes, a brief summary of the nutritional adjustments designed to correct these conditions is given below:

1. Nausea: eat dry toast or crackers before arising; drink fluids between meals only; eat no fats and oils, use skim milk.
2. Constipation: eat high fiber foods such as fresh fruits, vegetables, prunes, and whole grain breads and cereals.
3. Anemias: increase intake of iron and the vitamins associated with red blood cell formation (folacin, B_6, B_{12}, and C).
4. Pica (the practice of eating nonfood items such as laundry starch and clay): educate the patient about the need to discontinue the practice.
5. Heartburn: eat bland foods; take antacids if prescribed; plan small and frequent meals.
6. Urinary urgency: generally avoid consuming tea, coffee, spices, and alcoholic beverages.
7. Muscle cramps: increase calcium and decrease phosphorus intake.
8. Bloating/cramping: plan frequent and small meals; eat no greasy foods; reduce roughage and cold beverages.
9. Excessive alcohol intake: consume few or no alcoholic beverages in view of documented birth defects from alcohol consumption.

Lactation and Early Infancy: An Overview

Breast-feeding is a preferred method of feeding infants and has advantages over other methods of feeding, but the mother, after consulting her physician, makes the decision on how to feed her infant. Many infants have been successfully fed by other methods. In some cases, it is detrimental to the infant to be breast-fed. These cases will be discussed later.

Lactation requires more energy and produces more stress on the body than does pregnancy. The mother must consume an adequate diet to replenish her reserves and produce enough milk for the baby.

TABLE 9-2
Water-Soluble Vitamins and Pregnancy

Vitamin	Remarks
C	Requirement increases during pregnancy; can cross placenta freely. Deficiency during pregnancy may lead to easy rupture of fetal membrane and increased newborn mortality rate. Excessive intake during pregnancy is suspected to lead to a higher requirement in the newborn.
B_1	Requirement increases during pregnancy because of a higher consumption of calories; a woman can retain more B_1 in the tissues. There is a claim that a large dose of this vitamin can alleviate the symptoms of morning sickness.
B_2	Requirement increases during pregnancy. Deficiency in a pregnant animal can cause birth defects in the offspring.
B_6	Requirement increases during pregnancy. Blood level decreases when some brands of oral contraceptive pills are used. Pregnant women who used these pills may have a low storage of the vitamin. Supplementation during pregnancy has been recommended, although the practice is not common. There is a claim that a large dose of this vitamin can alleviate the symptoms of morning sickness.
B_{12}	Although absorption increases during pregnancy, the fetus uses up a large amount. An inadequate intake reduces the blood level of this vitamin, which returns to normal after pregnancy. A woman who smokes has a smaller body storage than nonsmokers. The fetus can draw from its mother's minimal storage even if she is deficient in this vitamin, and a newborn baby has a fair storage of this vitamin. There is a suggestion that the baby may be premature if the mother's body storage is very low.

TABLE 9-3
Fat-Soluble Vitamins and Pregnancy

Vitamin	Remarks
A	In animals, deficiency or excess of this vitamin during pregnancy can produce adverse effects in newborns, including birth defects. In humans, a pregnant woman deficient in this vitamin may give birth to a child with arrested bone growth. It is claimed that excess intake during pregnancy may produce birth defects.
D	The intake of vitamin D during pregnancy must be carefully evaluated, since most foods are relatively low in this vitamin unless they are fortified. Deficiency or excess of this vitamin during pregnancy can be harmful to the newborn and may cause birth defects.
E	Although much is known about this vitamin concerning animal reproduction, little information is available concerning human pregnancy. By eating a well-balanced diet, the pregnant woman receives an adequate intake. Because very little vitamin E can cross the placenta, the infant has very little storage.
K	Hemorrhage in some mothers and newborns is caused by a lack of vitamin K. Vitamin K in the appropriate form and dosage can alleviate the bleeding problems. The wrong form and dosage of the vitamin can harm an infant.

The nutrient increases for lactation are described in Table 9-1. A nursing mother's diet is nearly the same as that of a pregnant woman, although her nutritional needs increase as the child's demand for milk increases. The nursing mother needs more protein, vitamins, minerals, and calories than she did during pregnancy.

Lactation is more stressful and requires more energy than pregnancy. The fat reserves in a woman's body will provide 200 to 300 calories and the remaining calories must be derived from the diet. Two to three months after childbirth, the mother should be back to her prepregnancy weight, although she will still be eating 500 to 1,000 calories more per day. If the food supply is adequate, the woman will usually eat well, lose weight, and maintain her figure while adequately nourishing her infant. Tables 9-6 and 9-7 describe an acceptable menu plan and sample menu for lactation.

Hormones that stimulate milk production are suppressed by anxiety and fatigue. These psychological conditions rather than any physical problem usually deter women from successful breast-feeding. When counseling new mothers, the health practitioner should discuss these factors as well as dietary considerations.

TABLE 9-4
Sample Meal Plan for a Pregnant Woman

Breakfast	Lunch	Dinner
Milk or milk products, 1 serving	Milk or milk products, 1 serving	Milk or milk products, 1 serving
Fruits or vegtables rich in vitamin C, 1 serving	Other fruits and vegetables, 1 serving	Green leafy vegetables, 2 servings
Grain products, 1 serving	Protein products, 1 serving	Protein products, 2 servings
	Grain products, 2 servings	
Snack*	**Snack***	
Milk or milk products, ½ serving	Milk or milk products, ½ serving	
Protein products, 1 serving		

*The snacks may be consumed at any time of the day.

The first year of life for an infant is marked by rapid growth. Birth weight triples and length increases by approximately 50 percent. Nutrition plays a major role in the rate of growth, although overall height will be genetically determined.

The period of the neonate, from birth to twenty-eight days, is one of rapid adjustment. Stomach capacity triples and kidneys become more efficient. In the first forty-eight hours, an infant must coordinate its breathing, sucking, and swallowing. It must also adjust its temperature control and regulation. The premature infant has very limited abilities to do these things and is likely to have immature liver and respiratory functions as well.

During the first two years of life, an infant will grow approximately twenty deciduous teeth and calcify its permanent teeth buds. The brain undergoes its most rapid growth period, increasing in cell size and number. The brain will have reached 80 percent of its growth by age two. Muscles and skeletal structures will strengthen and increase in size. Adequate nutrition is critical during the stage of infancy.

Breast-Feeding

The advantages of breast-feeding are as follows:

Nutritional Benefits

Breast milk offers some nutritional benefits not available in a formula. A higher level of lactose in breast milk creates

TABLE 9-5
Sample Menu for a Pregnant Woman, Including Protective (Basic) and Supplemental Foods

Breakfast	Lunch	Dinner
Orange juice, 4 oz.	Sandwich	Roast beef, 6 oz.
Oatmeal, ½ c.	whole wheat bread, 2 slices	Egg noodles, ½ c. with sauteed
Brown sugar, 1–2 tsp.	tuna fish, ½ c.	poppy seeds
Milk, 8 oz.	diced celery with onion	Cut asparagus, ¾ c.
Coffee or tea	mayonnaise	Salad
	lettuce	torn spinach, 1 c.
	Banana, 1 small	sliced mushrooms
	Milk, 8 oz.	radishes
	Coffee or tea	oil
		vinegar
		Milk, 8 oz.
		Coffee or tea
Snack	**Snack**	
Salted peanuts, ½ c.	Oatmeal raisin cookies, 2	
Milk, 4 oz.	Milk, 4 oz.	

TABLE 9-6
Sample Meal Plan for a Lactating Woman

Breakfast	Lunch	Dinner
Milk or milk products, 1 serving Fruits or vegtables rich in vitamin C, 1 serving Grain products, 1 serving	Milk or milk products, 1 serving Other fruits and vegetables, 1 serving Protein products, 1 serving Grain products, 2 servings	Milk or milk products, 1 serving Green leafy vegetables, 2 servings Protein products, 2 servings
Snack* Milk or milk products, 1 serving Protein products, 1 serving	**Snack*** Milk or milk products, 1 serving	

*The snacks may be consumed at any time of the day.

a better intestinal environment in the infant, permitting better bowel movements as well as better absorption of calcium, protein, and magnesium. Some formulas contain added lactose.

The fat in breast milk is high in linoleic acid, an essential fatty acid. The milk is also relatively high in cholesterol, which is essential for cell membranes, nerve tissue, and other compounds.

If the mother's diet is adequate, vitamin stores, even though small, are well utilized. If the diet is inadequate, the water-soluble vitamins may be low in her milk. Vitamin D and fluoride are not provided in adequate amounts in breast milk.

In the first few days after childbirth, the woman secretes a yellowish fluid called colostrum. It cannot be duplicated by any modern formula. It has an anti-infection property and provides immunity against several undesirable factors. The infant has less diarrhea and constipation, since some factors in colostrum inhibit the growth of bacteria. Colostrum contains antibodies which protect the infant from intestinal infections. Some reports indicate that colostrum can also protect against nonintestinal infections. Breast-fed babies have fewer respiratory infections and fewer allergies than non-breast-fed babies.

Psychological Benefits

Breast-feeding is believed to assist in establishing the bond between the woman and her child, but this claim receives mixed responses. The father may experience better bond-

TABLE 9-7
Sample Menu for a Lactating Woman, Including Protective (Basic) and Supplemental Foods

Breakfast	Lunch	Dinner

Orange juice, 4 oz.
Oatmeal, ½ c.
Brown sugar, 1–2 tsp.
Milk, 8 oz.
Coffee or tea
	Sandwich
	  whole wheat bread, 2 slices
	  tuna fish ½ c.
	  diced celery
	  mayonnaise
	  lettuce
	Banana, 1 small
	Milk, 8 oz.
		Roast beef, 6 oz.
		Egg noodles, ½ c. with sauteed poppy seeds
		Cut asparagus, ¾ c.
		Salad
		  torn spinach, 1 c.
		  sliced mushrooms
		  radishes
		  oil
		  vinegar
		Milk, 8 oz.
		Coffee or tea

Snack Salted peanuts, ½ c. Milk, 8 oz.	**Snack** Oatmeal raisin cookies, 2 Milk, 8 oz.	

ing if the infant is bottle-fed. A relaxed feeding atmosphere appears to be more important than the feeding method.

Other Considerations

Some research indicates that bottle-fed babies are more likely to become obese than breast-fed ones. The caloric content of both types of milk is the same (20 calories per ounce), but a breast-feeding mother is not as likely to overfeed the infant as the one who is bottle-feeding. Bottle-fed infants are also more likely to be given solid foods at an earlier age.

At present, the cost of breast-feeding cannot be differentiated from that of bottle-feeding. The cost of feeding the mother varies with food prices.

One of the hormones released when a woman is breast-feeding causes the uterus to contract and return to normal size. This helps the mother to regain her prepregnancy figure. Breast-feeding also helps delay ovulation, and while it has been used as a birth control method, it is not a sure method.

Bottle-Feeding _____

Some advantages of bottle-feeding are listed below:

1.   For those women who have an aversion to breast-feeding or whose spouses object, bottle-feeding may be a wise choice.

2.   Bottle-feeding is not as restrictive as breast-feeding. For mothers who work outside the home, this can be a major reason for bottle-feeding.

3.   When the mother suffers chronic conditions such as heart disease, tuberculosis, or kidney disorder, bottle-feeding is the preferred method.

4.   Whenever a mother is on prescribed or illegal drugs or has been sick during the pregnancy, bottle-feeding is preferred. Drugs pass from the mother into the milk and enter the infant. The infant is unable to detoxify and eliminate drugs. Even a small amount of drugs can result in overdose for the infant.

5.   A bottle-fed child grows equally as well as a breast-fed one. If a woman wishes to bottle-feed, she should do so. The cost, types, and techniques of formula-feeding should be taught by health personnel and emphasis should be placed on cleanliness. The problem of poor sanitation is especially common among families of low socioeconomic status.

Health Concerns of Infancy _____

Some health concerns of infancy are listed below:

1.   For infants allergic to milk, soybean preparations are used. They should be supplemented with the essential amino acid methionine to make them complete protein. Milk allergies are not the same as abnormal body protein metabolism from genetic predisposition. Infants with the latter type of trouble require special formulas.

2.   Overfeeding infants is common in the United States and obesity becomes a major concern. Overfeeding during this period can result in an excess formation of fat cells. The child will develop an overeating pattern, resulting in lifelong obesity problems. The use of skim or low-fat milk for infants, to prevent obesity, however, is to be avoided. These products are not appropriate for infants since they do not contain essential linoleic acid or the cholesterol necessary for building body compounds. Some infants develop diarrhea from a low fat intake. Preferred methods of preventing obesity include not introducing solid foods too early, not adding sugar to foods, and not offering formula to a fully fed child.

3.   Inadequacy of dietary iron and the onset of anemia are more common in infants after their fourth month when iron stores are depleted and birth weight has increased. If the prenatal diet of the mother was poor, and iron stores are lacking in the infant, anemia can begin earlier.

Introduction of Solid Foods _____

The decision on when to add solid foods to the infant's diet should be based on three factors: appropriate physical and physiological development, nutritional requirements, and the need to begin teaching lifelong dietary habits.

The ability to eat solid foods is a developmental task. Between three to six months of age, an infant can recognize a spoon and swallow nonliquid foods.

The enzyme system in the intestine must be ready to digest starches and nonmilk proteins before these foods are added. Usually starches can be digested after two to three months of age, but four to six months are required before infants acquire enzymes to digest nonmilk proteins.

When foods are added to a baby's diet, they should be introduced one at a time to detect allergic reactions. Only small amounts should be given. Mixtures of foods should be avoided. The use of sugar, salt, and other seasonings should generally be avoided. A wide variety of foods should be given to teach good eating habits, and the child should not be forced to eat more than he or she wants.

Baby food can be made at home, but the caretaker should be instructed about the type of foods to puree, and to omit foods high in spices, salt, and sugar. When the infant begins to eat table foods, the health practitioner should determine what the family diet is like. The child could begin receiving nutritionally inadequate foods if the family's diet is inadequate. Table 9-8 illustrates suitable supplemental foods that can be added to an infant's diet, and the usual age for introduction.

Responsibilities of Health Personnel

The pregnant woman should be counseled by the health professional to:

1. Select her diet with the help of a reliable food guide.
2. Include good food sources of folic acid.
3. Avoid skipping breakfast.
4. Eat to gain weight at the recommended pattern even if she is overweight.
5. Not reduce food intake or avoid gaining the recommended weight.
6. Use a moderate amount of iodized salt and extra liquids.
7. Call her physician immediately if weight increases suddenly.
8. Limit or quit smoking.
9. Avoid alcoholic beverages.
10. Avoid all drugs unless prescribed by a physician familiar with her pregnancy status.
11. Take nutrient supplements prescribed by a physician or nurse practitioner.
12. Adjust foods to minimize common problems, but without interfering with recommended intake.
13. Avoid fasting to reduce weight before a prenatal appointment. Fasting can lead to acidosis, which can cause fetal damage.

The lactating woman should be counseled by the health professional to:

1. Consume more food than during pregnancy and continue to do so as the infant eats more.
2. Continue to follow a reliable food guide.
3. Consume 400 I.U. of vitamin D daily from food or supplements.
4. Continue to take prenatal iron supplements for two to three months.
5. Drink at least three liters of fluid daily.
6. Rest and relax so that breast-feeding can be successful.
7. Consult the physician about the use of coffee, alcohol, and drugs, since they are excreted in the breast milk.

If bottle-feeding, the caregiver should be counseled by the health professional to:

1. Follow the directions exactly.
2. Not force the baby to drink every drop.
3. Practice aseptic technique when making formula.
4. Recognize developmental stages indicating when an infant should be started on solid foods.
5. Follow a reliable guide for addition of solid foods.
6. Offer single foods and note any allergies.
7. Introduce a variety of foods.
8. Reintroduce once-rejected food items at another time.
9. Avoid allowing the child to drink more than one quart of milk a day, to prevent refusal of other foods.

TABLE 9-8
Suitable Supplemental Food for Infants during the First Year

Food	Usual Age When Supplemented
Orange juice, tomato juice (source of vitamin C)*	10 days
Well-cooked cereals (iron fortified)	2–4 months
Strained, pureed vegetables and fruits	3–5 months
Carrots, squash, beans, peas	5–6 months
Pureed, strained meats	4–7 months
Dark green vegetables	6–7 months
Mashed home-cooked vegetables, potatoes, carrots	6–9 months
Mashed egg yolk	6–7 months
Crackers, zwieback, dried bread	7–9 months
Regular cooked cereals, meats, eggs, finger foods	10–12 months
Egg white	12 months or later

*If vitamin C supplementation is necessary and the child cannot tolerate juices, administer liquid ascorbic acid supplement.

10. Make mealtimes for the infant a pleasurable, special time.

The health practitioner should also offer the following advice to the caretaker:

1. Continue close physical contact with infant after breast- or bottle-feedings have been discontinued.
2. Note the following when using commercial baby foods:
   a. Items such as baby soups and mixed or prepared dinners have high water content and little meat. When meats and vegetables are selected separately, they provide better nutrition.
   b. Commercial baby foods are safe and most contain little sugar or salt.
   c. Items such as desserts contain extra sugar and should not be used frequently. Some may choose to avoid them completely.
3. Note the following when feeding toddlers:
   a. Allow toddlers their rituals during mealtime.
   b. Do not permit arguments at mealtime.
   c. Do not use rewards and reprimands to increase food consumption.

In general, a health practitioner should be aware of special problems of nutrition and provide information and service when needed.

PROGRESS CHECK ON ACTIVITY 1

Multiple Choice

Circle the letter of the correct answer.

1. A recommended pattern of weight gain during pregnancy is
   a. 8 pounds (first trimester), 8 pounds (second trimester), 8 pounds (last trimester) = 24 pounds
   b. 5 pounds (first trimester), 5 pounds (second trimester), 14 pounds (last trimester) = 24 pounds
   c. 3 pounds (first trimester), 10 pounds (second trimester), 11 pounds (last trimester) = 24 pounds
   d. 0 pounds (first trimester), 12 pounds (second trimester), 12 pounds (last trimester) = 24 pounds

2. When are caloric needs during pregnancy the highest?
   a. first trimester
   b. second trimester
   c. third trimester
   d. same each trimester

3. What is the RDA energy allowance for the pregnant woman?
   a. 100 kcal above nonpregnant energy needs
   b. 300 kcal above nonpregnant energy needs
   c. 500 kcal above nonpregnant energy needs
   d. 800 kcal above nonpregnant energy needs

4. What is the additional RDA allowance for the lactating woman above nonpregnant, nonlactating needs?
   a. 100 kcal
   b. 300 kcal
   c. 500 kcal
   d. 800 kcal

5. In addition to dietary sources, what mineral is recommended to be supplemented during pregnancy?
   a. potassium
   b. iron
   c. iodine
   d. zinc

6. What vitamin may need to be supplemented during pregnancy to prevent a type of megaloblastic anemia?
   a. folacin
   b. ascorbic acid
   c. riboflavin
   d. niacin

7. The factor(s) thought to assist the pregnant woman in meeting her calcium requirement include(s) all except
   a. absorption of calcium is increased during pregnancy.
   b. extra servings from the meat group are recommended.
   c. supplemental vitamins are prescribed.
   d. ascorbic acid is provided to increase absorption.

8. What mineral intake is no longer thought generally beneficial to restrict during pregnancy?
   a. iron
   b. sodium
   c. calcium
   d. potassium

9. Increased risks for the pregnant teenager include
   a. prematurity.
   b. toxemia.
   c. anemia.
   d. all of the above.

10. The most common dietary complaints during pregnancy include all except
    a. diarrhea.
    b. nausea and vomiting.
    c. constipation.
    d. indigestion.

11. Colostrum is needed by the infant to provide
    a. extra protein.
    b. antibodies.
    c. extra lactose.
    d. antigens.

12. Two nutrients for which supplementation is recommended to meet the increased requirements for pregnancy are
    a. iron and folacin.
    b. iron and phosphorus.
    c. zinc and folacin.
    d. iodine and calcium.

13. The mineral that is most related to the expansion of blood volume in pregnancy is
    a. magnesium.
    b. iron.
    c. sodium.
    d. calcium.

14. All but which of the following increases a pregnant woman's chances of having a low birth-weight infant?
    a. consuming a high protein diet during pregnancy
    b. having the first baby before age seventeen
    c. smoking cigarettes
    d. failing to gain the recommended amount of weight while pregnant

15. Which of the following statements about breast milk is true?
    a. It is lower in protein than cow's milk.
    b. It is generally less nourishing for infants than baby formula.
    c. It is more likely to cause allergy than formula.
    d. all of the above

16. If a mother finds she cannot breast-feed, the baby should be weaned onto
    a. whole milk.
    b. low-fat milk.
    c. formula.
    d. cereal gruel.

17. When the baby is eating solid foods, which food should be introduced first?
    a. fruits
    b. vegetables
    c. cereals
    d. eggs

18. To meet the food groups, a pregnant woman needs
    a. 4 glasses of milk a day.
    b. 6 servings of vitamin C-rich foods a day.
    c. 2 servings of breads and cereals a day.
    d. 1 fruit or vegetable serving.

19. Behavior by the mother that may be harmful to an unborn child is
    a. smoking.
    b. protein deprivation.
    c. drinking alcohol.
    d. all of the above.

20. Toxemia during pregnancy may be due to
    a. excessive sodium intake.
    b. excessive water intake.
    c. a low-protein diet.
    d. a high-protein diet.

21. An unnatural taste ("craving") for clay, ice, cornstarch, and other nonnutritious substances is

    a. a need for support, understanding, and love.
    b. called pica.
    c. a psychological abnormality.
    d. the body's signal for needed nutrients.

22. If a baby is thirsty, you should give it a bottle of
    a. fruit juice.
    b. sweetened water.
    c. formula.
    d. water.

23. Close physical contact after breast- or bottle-feeding
    a. will create an overly dependent child.
    b. will cause the infant to dislike others.
    c. is needed for the infant to thrive.
    d. is nice but not necessary.

True/False

Circle T for True and F for False.

24. T F The pattern of weight gain is more important than the total weight gain during pregnancy.
25. T F If a pregnant woman gains 25 pounds in her first trimester, she should avoid any further weight gain during the second and third trimesters.
26. T F The highest growth rate for an individual occurs during infancy.
27. T F An overweight or obese woman should try to gain little or no weight during pregnancy.
28. T F It is not possible to become pregnant while breast-feeding.
29. T F Breast milk is high in vitamin D.
30. T F Introducing solids to an infant will help it sleep through the night.

ACTIVITY 2: Childhood and Adolescent Nutrition

The basic social unit to which a child belongs, the family, is the primary source from which the child learns culturally acceptable food behaviors. In turn, these food habits are passed on to the next generation. Families can establish good nutrition by

1. Practicing good eating habits.
2. Providing wholesome, acceptable foods that promote good health.
3. Establishing eating patterns that are socially enjoyable and satisfying.

Childhood and adolescence are the growth periods from infancy to the beginning of adulthood and are marked by many body changes. Childhood spans the period from birth to prepuberty, with the period of the toddler (ages one to three years) as a transition. Adolescence ends when sexual organ development and physical maturity are complete.

This activity examines the nutritional needs of the toddler, early and late childhood, and adolescence.

Toddler: Ages One to Three _____

Children, ages one to three, should be introduced to good foods and healthy eating habits. Growth and development of children progress in an orderly manner. After the first year of life, the rate of growth slows. Early and middle childhood is marked by slow but steady growth increases. A toddler gains from 5 to 10 pounds per year and grows about 3 inches in height. The toddler has a reduced appetite and requires less food. He or she has cut twenty deciduous teeth generally by the age of two and a half to three. Foods that require more chewing can be added at this time. The toddler's psychomotor skills have improved, making use of utensils for eating possible. However, the toddler spills his or her food frequently and may appear clumsy. Time and practice will improve eating skills.

Because of their short attention spans, toddlers usually cannot stay seated to finish a meal. The developmental task of the toddler is to strive for autonomy and is reflected in the eating behavior. Children between the ages of two to three want to feed themselves; their favorite words are "want" and "no." They may say no even to foods they like to establish their own authority. This period is known as the "terrible twos" and it can be a frustrating experience for parents, especially new ones. Parents should recognize that offering a toddler choices between equally appropriate foods is acceptable and may increase desired eating habits.

Preschooler: Ages Three to Five

Children continue to develop new food behavior patterns while their growth continues at a slow rate. The preschool-aged child gains three to five pounds and grows two to three inches a year. Children between the ages of three and five are usually lean, raising concerns in their parents. An awareness of body changes will alleviate this concern.

The preschooler is energetic, active, and restless and has a high caloric need. Nutritious snacks that supply extra calories and essential nutrients should be offered. As muscle control improves, the child is better able to handle eating utensils. By age four or five, the child may be able to cut some of his or her own food.

Because preschoolers are inquisitive and learn by imitation, they will learn readily from the people with whom they are in contact. The food habits of the parents, such as food likes and dislikes, will be noted. Media and television capture preschoolers' attention. From the information so acquired they will form concepts about food. This is an ideal time to start teaching simple nutrition concepts such as equating foods that taste the best with those that are nutritious. However, children in this age group will request those foods preferred by their peers. Check the foods and snacks that are served preschoolers when they are away from home. Children cannot distinguish between good and bad foods at this stage. Tables 9-9 and 9-10 evaluate nutritious meals and snacks for toddlers and preschoolers.

Early Childhood: Health Concerns

The feeding of young children poses a number of concerns, including low food intake, manipulative behavior, food jags, and pica. With the exception of pica, all such concerns are easily remedied. Pica is the practice of eating nonfood items such as clay and laundry starch. Studies have shown that some children with pica are also anemic and most of them are from poor families in unclean environments. The greater concern, however, is lead poi-

soning that sometimes accompanies pica. Many children eat peeling paint from wall plaster because it has a slightly sweet taste. Lead poisoning adversely affects the nervous system, kidney, and bone marrow and may lead to death. Health care workers need to assist caretakers to prevent young children from playing near potential lead sources.

The four common health problems of young children in the United States are anemia, dental caries, obesity, and allergies.

Iron-Deficiency Anemia. Iron-deficiency anemia is a problem for all ages, but especially so for children. Many iron-deficient children come from low-income families with poor diets. However, some studies indicate that cultural traditions and ignorance of nutrition requirements are also factors contributing to iron deficiencies. Low blood-iron levels affect the child's resistance to disease, attention span, behavior, and intellectual performance. Iron-rich foods that children usually like include enriched breads, cereals and tortillas, eggs, dried fruit, molasses, lentils, and baked beans.

Obesity. Between the ages from birth to four years and seven to eleven years, the incidence of obesity is high.

TABLE 9-9
Daily Food Needs for Toddlers

Breads and Cereals
4 servings
Whole grain, enriched, or restored: cornmeal, crackers, breads, flour, macaroni and spaghetti, rice, rolled oats...

Vegetables and Fruits
4 servings
Include vitamin A- and C-rich foods
Vitamin A-rich foods:
(dark yellow or leafy green foods) apricots, broccoli, cantaloupe, carrots, pumpkin, spinach, sweet potatoes...
Vitamin C-rich foods:
oranges, grapefruit, cantaloupe, raw strawberries, broccoli, brussel sprouts, green peppers, lemon, asparagus tips, raw cabbage, potatoes and sweet potatoes (boiled in skins), tomatoes...

Milk & Dairy Products
3 servings
milk, cheese, ice cream, yogurt...

Meat, Fish, and Nuts
2 servings
beef, lamb, pork, liver, poultry, eggs, fish, shellfish...
dry beans, dry peas, lentils, nuts, peanut butter...

Source: Idaho Department of Health and Welfare.

TABLE 9-10
A Guide to Snacks for Toddlers

Planning Snacks

Choose snacks that are appropriate for the age of the child. Some foods are too hard for young children (3 years and under) to chew, and may even be dangerous.

In general, small, round foods (peanuts, cherry tomatoes, peas, raisins), or chunky and crunchy foods (carrots, celery, and other raw vegetables) should not be given to the young child.

Select Basic Foods

Almost everyone snacks. Snacks give us a lift when we need it and can help meet daily energy and growth needs. A good guideline for snack selection is to avoid high-sugar foods and choose from the basic food groups:

vegetables and fruits
breads and cereals
milk and dairy products
meat, fish, and nuts

Why Not Sugar Snacks?

Foods high in sugar content contribute to tooth decay and gum disease. Examples include:

jams and jellies	dried fruits	cake	pastries
honey	canned fruit	cookies	pie
syrups	gum	candy	carbonated drinks
sugar-coated cereals	breath mints	doughnuts	jello

Try to limit high-sugar foods to mealtimes.

Beware of Hidden Sugars

Many foods that we do not think of as sugar-foods do, in fact, contain sugar. For example:

peanut butter	chili sauce	salad dressings	lunch meats
soup	canned vegetables	white bread	flavored yogurt
catsup	crackers	snack bars	ice cream

When shopping, *read food labels* and select foods with little or no sugar. Ingredients are listed on labels in descending order according to their percentage of the total product. Sugar may be listed as sugar, sucrose, corn syrup, honey, dextrose, maltose, etc. (look for the "ose" ending). In general, avoid foods that contain sugar as a main ingredient.

Good Foods for Children

Juicy

apples	pears
blackberries	pineapple
cantaloupe	plums
cherries	raspberries
dill pickle	strawberries
grapefruit	tangerines
grapes	tomatoes
oranges	watermelon
peaches	

Hungry

cottage cheese	Vienna sausages
meat cubes:	sardines
chicken	shrimp
beef	cheese cubes
ham	eggs—hard cooked or deviled
lamb	peanuts and other nuts
lunch meat	plain yogurt with fruit added
pork	
turkey	

Crunchy

cabbage wedges	lettuce wedges
carrots	popcorn
cauliflower flowerets	radishes
celery	peppers, raw slices
cucumber strips	sunflower seeds
green onions	

Thirsty

white milk	juices—no sugar added:
buttermilk	orange juice
tomato juice	grapefruit juice
	pineapple juice
	apple juice
	other fruit juices

Source: Idaho Department of Health and Welfare

Most studies confirm that a fat child ingests the same number of calories as a lean child, but the fat child is less active. Some fat children have emotional problems. Some imitate family eating habits and each member in the family is usually overweight. A controlled caloric intake that permits growth and a regular exercise program are recommended. Behavior modification and a strong support system are useful in retraining the child's eating pattern. The whole family should participate in this effort.

Dental Caries.   Dental caries is a widespread problem for all age groups. It is easily prevented by a balanced diet and assisted by self-care oral hygiene. A daily intake of fluoride, either through water, tablets, or supplements, also reduces the incidence of cavities by 50 to 60 percent. Fluoridated toothpaste is not recommended for children under the age of three because they may ingest excess fluoride from swallowing the toothpaste.

Allergies.   Many childhood allergies are caused by food. In youngsters, milk allergy is common, followed by egg white, citrus, chocolate, seafood, wheat, and nut allergies. Symptoms can be respiratory difficulties or some forms of skin rash. The preferred and usually easiest treatment is to remove the offending food or foods. Frequently, an allergic reaction to one food will trigger a reaction to others. Some allergies run in families, and the parent should note any reaction as new food is introduced to a child. The health worker should counsel parents on how to substitute an offending food with a nonoffending one of equal nutritional value. Module 25 contains detailed information about food allergies.

Early Childhood: Nutritional Requirements

The following are recommended allowances and should be individualized by carefully recording a child's growth rate.

Calories

The requirements for calories are

1 to 3 years: 102 kcal per kg of body weight

4 to 6 years: 90 kcal per kg of body weight

7 to 10 years: 70 kcal per kg of body weight

Protein

The requirements for protein are

1 to 3 years: 16 g for a 13 kg child

4 to 6 years: 24 g for a 20 kg child

7 to 10 years: 28 g for a 28 kg child

The quality of protein ingested influences the growth rate and other nutritional requirements of the child. If inadequate amounts of carbohydrate and fat are ingested, the protein will be used for energy needs and growth will be arrested.

Fat

All children need fat in their diet. Thirty to forty percent of daily calories should come from fat.

Vitamins and Minerals

The requirements for these two nutrients are high for children. If a varied diet is consumed, supplements are unnecessary. If anemia is present, iron may be prescribed, along with other supplements. A diet deficient in one nutrient is likely to be deficient in others. Frequently, children's diets are low in calcium and vitamins A and C. Vitamin C is important for iron absorption. The RDAs for children appear in the appendix.

Middle Childhood: General Considerations

The physical changes that occur in the middle childhood years are not dramatic. Deciduous teeth are shed and permanent teeth are cut. The slow and steady increase in height and weight continues. Children in this age group spend more time away from home, as friends become important to them. Weekday school lunch meals are nutritionally adequate. However, many children complain of the appearance, taste, and texture of foods to which they are not accustomed. Although some lunches are not appetizing, generally it is peer-group pressure that fosters children's attitudes toward school lunches.

The nutritional concerns of middle childhood are characterized by obesity from overeating "empty" calories and insufficient exercise, skipping meals, and adopting negative eating behaviors. Stress from schoolwork and activities influences appetite and the overall eating habits of this group.

Tables 9-11, 9-12, and 9-13 describe various meal plans and sample menus for children ages one through twelve.

Adolescence: Nutrition and Diet

It is difficult to determine exactly the age at which adolescence begins. The boundaries marking the change vary among individuals. For example, there are marked differences in the rate and amount of physical changes, as well as psychological and social development, among individuals. Some researchers divide adolescence into early and late stages. The preteen or pubescence stage covers ages ten to twelve and puberty ages twelve to eighteen.

Adolescence is a transition period in the life cycle of individuals and carries many labels or names. There is a

TABLE 9-11
Suggested Meal Plan and Sample Menu for 1- and 2-Year-Olds*

Meal Plan	Sample Menu
Breakfast	*Breakfast*
Juice or fruit	Orange juice
Cereal (hot or dry) with milk	Hot oatmeal with milk
	Whole wheat toast
Toast or egg (soft-boiled)	Butter
Butter or margarine	Milk
Milk	
Snack	*Snack*
Milk or juice	Apple juice
Lunch	*Lunch*
Meat, cheese, egg, or alternate	Grilled cheese sandwich
Potato, bread, crackers, or alternate	Peas
Vegetable	Milk
Butter or margarine	Ice cream
Milk	
Dessert	
Snack	*Snack*
Milk, juice, pudding, or crackers with cheese or alternate	Rice pudding
Dinner	*Dinner*
Meat, cheese, poultry, or alternate	Meat loaf
Vegetable or salad	Spinach or carrots
Potato, bread, roll, or alternate	Roll
Butter or margarine	Butter
Dessert	Applesauce
Milk	Milk

*Serving size varies with the child. Other nutritious items not shown may be used, e.g., jams, oatmeal, cookies, peanut butter. Their inclusion must be integrated into the child's overall daily intake of calories and nutrients.

TABLE 9-12
Suggested Meal Plan and Sample Menu for 3- through 6-Year-Olds*

Meal Plan	Sample Menu
Breakfast	*Breakfast*
Juice or fruit	Apple
Cereal (hot or dry)	Bran flakes with milk
Egg, meat, or toast	Egg (soft-boiled) with whole wheat toast
Milk	Milk
Snack	*Snack*
Dry fruits or nutritious cookies	Dates
Lunch	*Lunch*
Meat, egg, or alternate	Peanut butter and jelly sandwich
Potato, bread, or alternate	Vegetable soup with rice
Vegetable	Margarine
Butter or margarine	Milk
Milk	Custard pudding
Dessert	
Snack	*Snack*
Milk or juice	Orange juice
Crackers, pudding, or dried fruits	Apple wedges with peanut butter
Dinner	*Dinner*
Meat, cheese, poultry, or alternate	Fish sticks
Vegetable or salad	Sweet corn
Potato, bread, roll, or alternate	Baked potato
Butter or margarine	Butter
Dessert	Fruit pudding
Milk	Milk

*Serving size varies with the child. Other nutritious items not shown may be used, e.g., jams, oatmeal, cookies, peanut butter. Their inclusion must be integrated into the child's overall daily intake of calories and nutrients.

dearth of scientific data regarding adolescents' growth, development, and nutritional needs. It is the second greatest growth spurt in the life cycle. Girls begin sooner than boys, usually between the ages of ten to twelve, while boys begin this growth between the ages of twelve to fourteen.

During the period of adolescence (ten to eighteen years), the average male doubles in weight, gaining approximately 70 pounds and thirteen to fourteen inches in height. Girls gain approximately 50 pounds and nine inches in height. Adequately nourished girls develop permanent layers of adipose or fat tissue. This is normal and

desirable, but the fat creates panic in the young girl wishing to be thin and fashionable.

The nutrient needs and energy requirements are very high during adolescence. The basal metabolic rate (BMR) is the highest in any life stage except during pregnancy. More food is needed and girls need to increase their intake earlier than boys.

Eating habits of the adolescent are generally poor, especially the eating habits of girls. The developmental aspect of adolescence urges them to separate from the family and establish their own identity. One way they assert themselves is to deviate from a normal food habit.

TABLE 9-13
Suggested Meal Plan and Sample Menu
for 7- through 12-Year-Olds*

Meal Plan	Sample Menu
Breakfast	*Breakfast*
Juice or fruit	Pear(s)
Cereal (hot or dry) with milk	Farina with milk
	Toast
Toast	Egg or sausages
Egg, meat, or alternate	Margarine
Butter or margarine	Milk
Milk	
Lunch	*Lunch*
Meat, cheese, or alternate	Macaroni and cheese
	Coleslaw
Potato, bread, or alternate	Milk
	Fresh peaches
Vegetable	
Butter or margarine	
Milk	
Dessert	
Snack	*Snack*
Dried fruits or nutritious cookies	Molasses cookies
	Apple juice
Milk or juice	
Dinner	*Dinner*
Meat, cheese, or alternate	Hamburger
	Carrots or peas
Vegetable	Shredded raw cabbage salad
Salad	
Potato or alternate	Baked potato
Bread or alternate	Bread
Butter or margarine	Butter
Dessert	Ice cream
Milk	Milk

*Serving size varies with the child. Other nutritious items not shown may be used, e.g., jams, oatmeal, cookies, peanut butter. Their inclusion must be integrated into the child's overall daily intake of calories and nutrients.

Social acceptance by the peer group is more important than family approval, and only peer approval is valued.

The adolescent's diet tends to be low in calcium, iron, and vitamins A and C. Meals are skipped, particularly breakfast, since more time is spent on appearance than eating. Body weight, skin, and hair problems, either real or imagined, take precedence over nutritional concerns. Health does not play a role in the adolescent's food choices. Among teenagers in parts of the country, the incidence of tuberculosis and other respiratory illness is high, probably due to severe nutrient deficiencies which lower resistance in these individuals. Adolescents, preoccupied as they are with self, do not seem to relate nutrition to body function. They do not think that what they eat today will reflect their health status in the future.

Adolescence: Health Concerns

The major health concerns of adolescence are as follows:

Smoking, Alcohol, and Drugs

Experiments with these substances often begin in the early teens. They affect the nutritional status in different ways: they can lessen the sense of taste and smell, decrease appetite, and reduce vitamin C level in the body. Some adolescents overdose on vitamin or mineral supplements in an effort to "get more energy" or "look better." Poisoning from excess vitamins A and D has been documented.

Physical Development

With the exception of young athletes who maintain a good physique, the majority of preteens and teens are physically poorly developed. Their muscle mass is less dense, with poor tone and endurance. Good physical fitness programs and appropriate nutrition classes in the curriculum should be mandated from kindergarten to grade 12.

Obesity

Teenagers who are obese usually have been overweight or obese since childhood. Since adjusting sexual roles, planning careers, and beginning adult lifestyles create great stress at this time, food is sometimes overused as a comfort and security measure and the teen can become obese. Their favorite food is usually high-fat, high-calorie food with little nutritional value. Obese adolescents tend to eat less food than their lean counterparts, but they also exercise less. Girls particularly often adopt bizarre eating behaviors because of fad dieting.

If the adolescent needs to diet, it must not be so restricted as to delay growth and maturation. Teenage boys require 45–55 kcal per kg of body weight per day, while girls require 40–47 kcal per kg of body weight a day. The RDA for other nutrients for this group is higher than for others except pregnant and nursing mothers. A diet should be only mildly limited in calories and the adolescent's activity should increase. Realistic goals to lose weight should be established. Teenagers should be taught that a body cannot lose more than one or two pounds a week without starving. Emotional and peer support is essential, but careful monitoring is also important. If a teenager is not given guidance or follows an unsound fad diet practiced by adults, there may be severe weight loss with associated health problems.

Studies have indicated that teenagers do not consume adequate amounts of iron, calcium, and vitamins A and C.

Anemia

A number of surveys indicate that iron-deficiency anemia is a widespread problem beginning in childhood and continuing through adolescence, particularly among girls. Iron requirements are high because blood volume increases with the rapid growth increases in both sexes. The onset of the menses in the female adds to the need. Poor dietary habits are responsible for this problem and improved habits can eliminate iron deficiencies.

Dental Caries

Cavities occur mainly from the consumption of too much fermentable carbohydrates (sugars and sweets, especially the sticky type) and from poor hygiene (inadequate brushing and flossing). However, an adequate total diet which includes a source of fluoride is also necessary for good teeth and oral tissues.

Acne

Acne may or may not be related to certain foods, such as fats and chocolate. Some scientists suggest that a low zinc intake and increased consumption of alcoholic beverages may be responsible for acne.

Cardiovascular Concerns

Because of the excess fat and salt in the preferred foods of teenagers, the blood cholesterol and triglycerides levels and blood pressure in these individuals may be adversely affected. They may have a higher risk of coronary heart disease later in life. The National Cholesterol Education Program has addressed this concern.

In April 1991, the expert panel on blood cholesterol levels in children and adolescents (the National Heart, Lung, and Blood Institute and the National Institutes of Health) drafted a report to include screening and dietary therapy for these populations, and the final report became available in the summer of 1991. A brief summary of this report follows.

1. Compelling evidence exists that early coronary atherosclerosis or its precursors often begin in childhood and adolescence.
2. Children and adolescents with elevated serum cholesterol, especially LDL-Cholesterol, frequently come from families in which there is a high frequency of CHD among adult members.
3. Children and adolescents with high cholesterol levels are more likely than the general population to have high cholesterol levels as adults.
4. The panel recommends selectively screening, in the context of regular health care, those children who are at greatest risk of having high cholesterol levels as adults, thus increasing their risk of CHD.

The following recommendations are intended for all healthy children of more than two years of age and for healthy adolescents. The aim of the recommendations is to lower the average levels of blood cholesterol among all American children and adolescents:

1. Nutritional adequacy should be achieved by eating a wide variety of foods.
2. Energy (calories) should be adequate to support growth and development and to reach or maintain desirable body weight.
3. The following nutrient intake is recommended:
   a. Saturated fats: less than 10 percent of total calories
   b. Total fat: no more than 30 percent of total calories
   c. Dietary cholesterol: less than 300 mg/day

These recommendations refer to an average intake over a period of several days. The recommendations are *not* intended for infants from birth to two years, whose fast growth requires a large percentage of calories from fat. Toddlers between two and three years of age may safely make the transition to the recommended eating patterns.

Acceptable LDL-Cholesterol ranges are <110 mg/dL. Borderline LDL-Cholesterol range is 110–129 mg/dL. High LDL-Cholesterol range is ≥ 130 mg/dL. Selective diet therapy is used to lower the borderline and high LDL-Cholesterol to acceptable levels (<110 mg/dL). This is the step 1 and step 2 diet for lowering cholesterol discussed in Module 13. For a more detailed analysis, students and instructors may wish to refer to *Nutrition Today* May/June 1991.

Teenage Pregnancy

A major health problem for teenage girls is pregnancy. In this country there are one million teenage pregnancies every year. One hundred thousand pregnancies are in women under the age of eighteen and 30,000 pregnancies are in females under fifteen years of age. Nearly one-third of the pregnant teenagers in the United States are under the age of sixteen. Many become pregnant again within a year.

Pregnant teenagers are at great risk of developing toxemia and delivering stillborn, premature, or low birth weight (LBW) babies. Fetal-maternal mortality rates of this group are higher than those for the adult woman. A young mother's nutritional status has a profound effect on the course and outcome of her pregnancy. A pregnant teenager has the unusually high nutrient demands of pregnancy superimposed over a rapid growth spurt. Without careful planning and support, the results can be hazardous.

Nutrition Education

Adolescents desperately need nutrition education. While health concerns are not effective in motivating good eating habits, some guidelines that relate to their concerns can be used to help adolescents.

1. Stress immediate effects, such as improved vitality, increased endurance, and better hair, nails, complexion, and general appearance.
2. Give basic facts so they can make informed choices.
3. Encourage them to eat breakfast and more meals with the family, try new foods, select nutrient-dense snacks, and recognize self-responsibility.
4. Stock only foods that are nutrient-dense and preferred.
5. Set a good example. The use of fad diets and the practice of skipping breakfast are noted by the teenager as acceptable eating patterns.

Effective nutrition education is possible only if teenagers realize and accept responsibility for their health. Examples include

1. Emphasizing that teens are responsible for their own health.

2. Acquiring a knowledge of body changes and nutrient requirements.

3. Recognizing teen health problems and understanding that the immediate consequences (appearance, vitality) are more pertinent to the teenager than long-term consequences.

4. Understanding that pregnancy is a time for special support and requires counseling, assistance, and resources.

5. Realizing that peers, coaches, heroes, media idols, and other similar individuals are more influential in a teen's life than parents or caretakers. Examples, suggestions, and encouragement from these individuals through personal contacts or public messages can result in better eating habits.

6. Knowing that nutrient requirements for the teen years are higher because of rapid development.

7. Accepting snacking as a part of teen life. It can contribute to good nutrition if good food choices are made.

8. Recognizing that the use of alcohol and other drugs has negative effects on eating habits.

Responsibilities of Health Personnel

A health practitioner has the following responsibilities:

1. Provide adequate knowledge of the adolescent phase of the life cycle to the caretakers.
2. Practice good eating habits as a role model for children.

3. Relate the use of food to developmental tasks.
4. Relate nutritional requirements to adolescents' stage of the life cycle.
5. Describe body changes to caretakers and children.
6. Be aware of nutritional health problems that can develop during the life cycle and attempt to prevent them.
7. Identify changing food behaviors at each stage and take measures to accommodate them.
8. Emphasize safety in handling and eating food, such as washing hands, avoiding touching food, not eating and drinking from others' plates or utensils, returning food to the refrigerator, and the like.
9. Promote healthy eating behaviors by beginning a child's nutrition education early and continuing throughout the formative years.
10. Share guidelines for promoting sound nutrition habits at every opportunity.

PROGRESS CHECK ON ACTIVITY 2

Multiple Choice

Circle the letter of the correct answer.

1. Which of these characteristics is not typical of the toddler?
   a. slow but steady growth rate
   b. very big appetite
   c. food jags
   d. has 20 teeth

2. Which of these characteristics is not typical of the preschooler?
   a. develops self-control
   b. is energetic, restless
   c. imitation and inquiry are learning methods
   d. food habits learned now last throughout life

3. The most common health problem(s) of young children in the United States is/are
   a. anemia.
   b. dental caries.
   c. obesity.
   d. all of the above.

4. Lead poisoning often affects young children with pica. This occurs because they eat
   a. laundry starch.
   b. peeling paint from wall plaster.
   c. clay.
   d. mud.

5. Iron-deficiency anemia may be caused by all except
   a. poor dietary intake.
   b. cultural traditions.
   c. ignorance of requirements.
   d. hemorrhage.

6. The iron-rich foods that children usually like include
   a. spinach, prunes, and liver.
   b. green beans, chicken, and milk.
   c. baked beans, eggs, and dried apricots.
   d. all of the above.

7. From the following list, choose the one factor most likely to cause obesity in childhood.
   a. too much food
   b. not enough supervision
   c. not enough exercise
   d. too much pressure/stress

8. Dental caries can be prevented by
   a. regular brushing and flossing.
   b. regular checkups with a dentist.
   c. a balanced diet.
   d. all of the above.

9. The nutrients most likely to be low in children's diets are
   a. iron, calcium, and vitamins A and C.
   b. iron, thiamin, riboflavin, and niacin.
   c. calcium, phosphorus, and vitamin D.
   d. iron, fluoride, and vitamins B_1 and B_2.

10. If a mother is trying to follow the basic food group pattern in feeding her three-year-old child, what would be an appropriate amount for a serving of meat, fruits, and vegetables?
    a. two tablespoons
    b. three tablespoons
    c. one-half cup
    d. three-fourths cup

11. The school lunch is intended to provide what part of the child's daily nutrient needs?
    a. one-fourth
    b. one-third
    c. one-half
    d. 15 percent

12. Which of the following are health concerns of the school-age child?
    a. skipping meals
    b. stress/exhaustion
    c. anorexia
    d. all of the above

13. Just before adolescence, the growth patterns of girls and boys are
    a. the same.
    b. different, in that girls have a larger percentage of fat.
    c. different, in that boys have a smaller lean body mass.
    d. different, in that boys start out taller.

14. During the period of adolescence, the average boy
    a. gains approximately 50 pounds and 10 inches in height.
    b. gains approximately 10 pounds and 1 foot in height.
    c. gains approximately 70 pounds and 13–14 inches in height.
    d. gains approximately 1 pound for every 1 inch of height.

15. To educate teenagers about nutrition
    a. encourage them to eat breakfast.
    b. stress health effects when they grow old.
    c. stock both nutrient-dense and nutrient-light foods at home.
    d. advise supplementation of diet.

16. Teenagers should not
    a. be responsible for their own health.
    b. snack indiscriminately.
    c. be concerned about physiological changes in the body.
    d. be influenced by others.

17. Which of the following are common health problems of teenagers?
    a. tuberculosis
    b. anemia
    c. dental caries
    d. all of the above

18. Pregnant teenagers are at high risk for all except
    a. delivering stillborns.
    b. delivering premature infants.
    c. developing toxemia.
    d. developing heart disease.

True/False

Circle T for True and F for False.

19. T F A toddler can be expected to gain 10 pounds a year and grow 2 inches in height.
20. T F Preschoolers gain approximately 3–5 pounds and about 2–3 inches per year.
21. T F Young children do not practice manipulative behavior.
22. T F Young children who are overweight should be put on skim milk.
23. T F A diet that is deficient in one nutrient is likely to be deficient in others as well.
24. T F Adolescence is the second greatest growth spurt in life.
25. T F Pregnant teenagers are less likely to have problem pregnancies than women in their twenties.
26. T F Smoking decreases the sense of taste and smell.
27. T F Obesity affects a significant number of teenagers.
28. T F Teenage girls' eating habits are better when compared to boys the same age.
29. T F Teenage girls require 2,200–2,400 calories daily, but boys need twice that amount.

Fill-in

30. Name four of the most common food allergies in young children:

a. _____

b. _____

c. _____

d. _____

ACTIVITY 3: Adulthood and Nutrition

Early and Middle Adulthood _____

The chronological ages of early and middle adulthood differ among expert opinions. For this discussion, the early adult stage covers eighteen to forty and the middle adulthood period covers ages forty to sixty-five.

During all stages of adulthood, body changes occur. In early adulthood, physical growth ceases. During the adult years, nutrients are mainly used for body repair and maintenance. Body composition changes include a decrease in lean mass, an increase in fat, and a reduction in bone density. Osteomalacia and arthritis may occur. With a reduction in basal metabolic rate (BMR), body functions and the capacity to perform physical work decline with advancing years. The fall in BMR and activity necessitates a decrease in caloric intake. Also, the lifestyles adopted by a person influence food habits and nutrient needs.

Nutrient needs during adulthood may be analyzed as follows:

1. The diet should be optimal in all essential nutrients except for calories. Energy needs decline because of a decrease in activity and BMR.
2. Calcium needs remain high during adulthood as calcium in bones is removed and replenished constantly.
3. Iron needs remain high in women until menopause.
4. Social development continues through adulthood and nutritional status affects the quality of life.
5. Many factors that adversely affect the health of the adult require a modification of the adult's dietary habits.
6. A regular exercise program benefits nutritional status.

The RDAs for the early and middle years are found in the appendix. The following health concerns and problems of early and middle years should be noted:

1. Psychological stress and sedentary lifestyles are social factors that can create health problems.
2. Alcohol, drug, and tobacco use negatively affect health and nutritional status.
3. Chronic exposure to environmental pollutants is a health hazard, especially in large cities.
4. Obesity, arthritis, and osteomalacia are common disorders of middle age. Osteoporosis is especially common in women.

5. Cardiovascular diseases and cancer are leading causes of death in the adult population.

Some concerns that specifically affect women in the adult years should be noted:

1. Pregnancy, lactation, and menopause change a woman's nutrient requirements.
2. Certain contraceptives can create health problems. The use of the intrauterine device (IUD) as a birth control measure causes a heavy menstrual flow and a greater need for iron. Oral contraceptive agents (OCAs), because they are hormones, affect the body's metabolism of nutrients. The changes mimic the nutritional status of pregnancy; that is, a higher nutritional intake is required. Protein metabolism is altered and serum cholesterol and glucose levels rise when OCAs are used. Requirements for vitamin C, vitamin B_6, and folacin are increased in these women.
3. Abortions affect iron status of women, as heavy blood loss usually accompanies the process.
4. Menopause decreases the need for iron, but calcium needs are increased in women of child-bearing age to retard or prevent osteoporosis.

The Elderly: Factors Affecting Nutrition and Diet _____

Aging individuals often face major adjustments in social and economic status as well as physical changes. The physical body changes due to old age greatly affect dietary habits.

Gastrointestinal Tract

Many changes occur in the gastrointestinal tract, including loss of teeth, reduced production of saliva, diminished taste and smell, and decreased ability to digest foods. When these changes occur, chewing may become painful and a diet with soft foods is preferred. Eating pleasure declines when taste and smell are impaired. Some adults prefer strongly flavored foods, while others avoid food because it does not taste good any more. The decrease of gastric secretions may interfere with the absorption of iron and vitamin B_{12}. Fat digestion may be impaired if the liver produces less bile or the gallbladder is nonfunctional.

Neuromuscular System

Neuromuscular coordination decreases with age and conditions such as arthritis may hamper food preparation and the use of eating utensils. Muscles in the lower gastrointestinal tract become weaker with advancing age and constipation is a common problem. Many of the elderly turn to laxatives, which can interfere with nutrient absorption. Kidney repair and maintenance deteriorates with age and renal function is impaired in some individuals. Fluid and electrolyte balance is difficult to maintain, especially during illness.

Eyes

Elderly persons may have difficulty in reading recipes or labels on foods.

Personal Factors

Apart from physical changes discussed above, personal factors affect an elderly person's dietary and nutritional status, including fixed income, loneliness, and susceptibility to health claims. Often the elderly are existing on a fixed income that prevents an adequate food supply. This income deficit also affects housing and facilities, limiting cooking frequency and food storage. Without transportation, the elderly often purchase food from a nearby store or one that will deliver groceries. Such stores usually charge more for foods.

Social isolation affects the eating behaviors of the aged to a great extent. Elderly persons living alone lose their desire to cook or eat. Lonely people become apathetic, depressed, and fail to eat. They are more susceptible to illnesses and other stresses.

Many of the elderly purchase foods and supplements from health food stores because of advertisements claiming that the foods have curative power and may in fact retard the aging process. Table 9-14 contains a week's sample menus for older people.

The Elderly: Health Problems _____

Many of the health problems of the elderly are nutrition-related. Some examples are discussed below.

1. *Nutrient deficiencies.* Recent studies have shown that the elderly are often deficient in protein, iron, calcium, and vitamins A and C. This increases the incidence of iron-deficiency anemia and osteoporosis, decreases resistance to infections, and lowers overall health status.

2. *Alcoholism.* This is a major problem among the elderly, especially for those living alone. Other drugs, either prescribed or illegally obtained, also interfere with the body's use of nutrients. Alcohol-drug interactions influ-

TABLE 9-14
A Week's Sample Menus for Older People

Snacks: Some suggested items are fresh fruit; soft, dried prunes; whole wheat crackers with cheese; cheese sticks; juices; peanut butter on toast; and yogurt. Snacks may be served in mid-morning, mid-afternoon, and/or before bedtime. Five to six oz. wine before meals may improve appetite.

Monday

Breakfast

½ c. orange juice
1 poached egg
Whole wheat toast/margarine
½ c. skim milk
Coffee or tea

Lunch

1 c. braised beef tips on noodles
Celery or carrot sticks
Rye bread/margarine
1 c. skim milk
1 orange, sliced

Dinner

Chicken breast, broiled
½ c. buttered spinach
½ c. wild rice
Hot roll/margarine
Fresh fruit: banana, melon, other
Decaffeinated coffee

Tuesday

Breakfast

½ c. grapefruit juice
½ c. cooked oatmeal, sugar, and skim milk
English muffin, 1 oz. cheese

Lunch

Vegetable soup/crackers
Cottage cheese with pineapple salad
Banana
Toasted raisin bread with butter
Tea or decaffeinated coffee

Dinner

3 oz. broiled fish/lemon
Boiled new potato/parsley
½ c. creamed peas
Green onions
Whole wheat bread/margarine
Gingerbread, 1 square
Decaffeinated coffee

Wednesday

Breakfast

Sliced banana and milk
2 bran muffins/margarine/jelly
Cottage cheese
Coffee or tea

(continues)

TABLE 9-14 (Continued)

Lunch

1 c. split pea soup/whole wheat crackers
Tomato and shredded lettuce salad/dressing
Skim milk
1 pear

Dinner

1 c. beef and vegetable stew/cornbread sticks, margarine
½ c. cabbage coleslaw
½ c. rice pudding with raisins
Decaffeinated coffee/ice tea

Thursday

Breakfast

2 stewed prunes
2 French toast slices with butter and syrup
8 oz. skim milk
Decaffeinated coffee/tea

Lunch

1 hamburger with onions/catsup/mustard/mayonnaise
Pickles, lettuce
French fries/catsup
Ice cream or sherbet
Skim milk

Dinner

Roast beef
½ c. mashed potatoes
½ c. buttered broccoli
1 sliced tomato with dressing
2 oatmeal cookies
Fruit cup

Friday

Breakfast

Sliced orange
1 c. puffed rice with skim milk and sugar
Scrambled egg/wheat toast/margarine
Hot tea/coffee

Lunch

Tomato and rice soup/crackers
⅔ c. potato salad with 2 oz. turkey/ham
Celery or green pepper sticks
½ c. strawberries/whip topping
Skim milk

Dinner

1 c. tuna noodle casserole
½ c. mixed lettuce salad

1 slice angel food cake with fruit cocktail
Decaffeinated coffee

Saturday

Breakfast

Melon or fresh fruit
2 hot cakes/margarine/syrup
1 sausage pattie
8 oz. skim milk
Coffee/tea

Lunch

Chicken nuggets
½ c. green peas with mushrooms
½ c. carrot and raisin salad
Whole wheat bread/margarine
Banana pudding
Skim milk

Dinner

1 c. spaghetti and meatballs in tomato sauce/garlic bread
½ c. string beans
½ c. fruit gelatin
Decaffeinated coffee

Sunday

Breakfast

3 stewed figs
½ c. hot cream of wheat/sugar
Skim milk
Cinnamon roll/margarine
2 slices crisp bacon
8 oz. hot chocolate made with skim milk
Coffee or tea if desired

Lunch

2-egg cheese omelet
½ c. steamed rice
½ c. asparagus
Celery or carrot sticks
Toast/margarine/jelly
Peach halves
8 oz. skim milk

Dinner

1 baked pork chop with applesauce
½ c. buttered carrots
Mashed potatoes
Lettuce wedge/dressing
½ c. custard
Decaffeinated coffee

Note: Each day's caloric contribution is about 1,800 kcal. The amount can be increased or decreased by adjusting the serving sizes. Thus, the serving sizes of some items are not provided. To provide adequate RDAs, use the snacks to complete the foundation diet as discussed elsewhere. If there is concern about the cholesterol in eggs, replace some egg servings with lean meat (e.g., turkey, fish and so on) or use cholesterol-free egg substitutes.

ence the entire life span, as does the abuse of prescription drugs. (See Module 10.)

3. *Obesity.* This results from reduced activity and caloric need and can complicate any existing problems as well as increase the development of others. Obesity also reduces mobility, increasing risk of falling accidents. As respiratory and cardiovascular functions deteriorate and arthritis conditions worsen, the quality of life is generally diminished. Lack of exercise is a factor in obesity throughout the

life span. Exercise is discussed later in this module.

4. *Osteoporosis*. This disorder (see also Module 7) remains a major health problem among the elderly, especially women past the age of sixty. While the symptoms appear after menopause, researchers agree that the disorder begins as early as age thirty. The 1989 RDAs reflect the young woman's increased needs. At present, no known preventive measure exits, but symptoms can be minimized with an adequate diet and regular exercise. Some believe that limited alcohol and caffeine consumption and a moderate fiber intake can also help. Extra calcium may be helpful and some studies indicate that fluoride may increase bone density and relieve some symptoms.

5. *Diabetes*. Noninsulin-dependent diabetes is a common problem among middle-age and elderly people. Approximately 75 percent of those with diabetes of this type are overweight or obese. In most patients, the disease can be controlled by diet alone, and the most effective treatment is to reduce to and maintain a normal body weight. (See Module 16.)

6. *Diverticulosis*. This widespread problem is characterized by a weakening of the intestinal walls, resulting in diverticulosis. Low-fiber diets, along with weakened muscle tissue, are believed to be a causative agent in this disease.

7. *Hypertension*. This is a common disorder in the United States and tends to increase with age in many adults. Two nutritional factors believed to play a role in hypertension are salt and body fat. Excessive weight or obesity appears to be a more important factor than a high intake of salt. Recent studies indicate that a calcium deficit may also contribute to the incidence of hypertension.

8. *Atherosclerosis*. This is a leading medical problem in the elderly and can result in heart attack or stroke. Coronary heart disease is the leading cause of death in the United States. Diet is one of the risk factors involved in the development of the plaque that narrows the lining of the arteries and blocks the blood flow. This subject is discussed in more detail in Module 14.

9. *Cancer*. The second leading cause of death in the United States is cancer. Cancer has been the subject of much research in recent years, especially in the areas of pollutants, food additives, smoking, and diet. While the debate continues, the American Cancer Society's committee on diet and nutrition has issued four guidelines as preventive measures:

1. Limiting fat intake to 30 percent of total (calories).
2. Assuring an adequate (but not excessive) fiber intake to include fresh fruits, vegetables, and whole grains. Fruits and vegetables high in vitamin A are especially encouraged.

3. Limiting intake of cured, smoked, and charcoal-broiled meats.
4. Limiting intake of alcohol.

Three other major issues related to food habits and nutritional status are nutrition quackery; drug and nutrient interactions, including alcohol; and an appropriate exercise program. Because these issues affect all stages of life, a brief summary of each follows.

Nutrition Quackery

Many people fall prey to claims made by medical quacks, especially people who are trying to cope with aging, clinical disorders, or psychological problems. Individuals who buy these products because of their claims for cures, longevity, youthful appearance, and painless weight loss are uselessly spending billions of dollars per year. They pay high prices for worthless and unnecessary products. Such products are sometimes actually harmful, and many people delay seeking competent medical advice until it is too late.

It is important to distinguish between valid nutritional or health claims and false advertisements designed to sell ineffective and potentially harmful products. Recognizing valid claims from false ones can be aided by noting the following characteristics of faddist publications and products:

1. Citing research from bogus health care facilities (such as Granada Institute for Scientific Research and Holistic Health), or renowned ones (such as Mt. Sinai).
2. Making undocumented claims of success through testimonial evidence.
3. Advertising unsubstantiated or unproven claims for products and services. Such advertising includes wrongful claims such as
   a. "Most people are poorly nourished."
   b. "Sugar is a deadly poison."
   c. "All people need megavitamin Brand X because modern processing has taken all the nutrients from food."
   d. "All food additives and preservatives are poisonous."
   e. "Natural vitamins are better than synthetic ones."
   f. "It's easy to lose weight; lose seven pounds overnight."
   g. "Most diseases are due to faulty diet."
4. Promising quick dramatic cures. Examples include
   a. "The medical community will not use these products because they would lose business."
   b. "Thousands cured of _____ (cancer, arthritis, balding) by using Pangamic Acid."
5. Selling certain substances as "vitamins," although scientifically they are not vitamins. Examples include
   a. *Vitamin P*. Claims include curing ulcers, inner

ear disorders, and asthma; preventing miscarriages, bleeding gums, acne, hemorrhage, rheumatic fever, hemorrhoids, and muscular dystrophy; and protecting the body from the danger of x-rays.

b. *Vitamin B₁₅.* Claims include curing high blood pressure, asthma, rheumatism, alcoholism, atherosclerosis, and cancer.

c. *PABA.* Claims include preventing hair from graying, delaying aging, restoring depigmented skin.

d. *Vitamin T.* Claims include curing hemophilia, memory loss, and anemia.

e. *Vitamin B₁₃.* Claims include curing multiple sclerosis, cancer, and hypertension.

f. *Vitamin F.* Claims include curing cancer, eczema, psoriasis, dermatitis, and preventing heart disease.

Scientists identify the substances listed in Item 5 as follows:

a. *Vitamin P.* A bioflavinoid of a group of substances from citrin, found in the white segment of citrus fruits. Gives characteristic taste, but is not a vitamin. Gives citrus fruit its flavor and holds the segments together.

b. *Vitamin B₁₅.* No known composition; no vitamin activity; unknown safety. Not legally recognized as food or drug in the United States and Canada.

c. *PABA.* A water-soluble substance found with folacin (a vitamin). Body makes its own PABA and it is not recognized as a vitamin.

d. *Vitamin T.* A product made from sesame seeds; not a vitamin.

e. *Vitamin B₁₃ (orotic acid).* Unknown activity and not a vitamin.

f. *Vitamin F.* An unsaturated fatty acid and not a vitamin.

PROGRESS CHECK ON ACTIVITY 3

Multiple Choice

Circle the letter of the correct answer.

1. The basic biological changes in old age center on
    a. an increased basal metabolic rate.
    b. a gradual loss of functioning cells and reduced cell metabolism.
    c. an increased drug–nutrient absorption rate.
    d. all of the above.

2. Fewer calories are needed in the later years because
    a. the aged tend to have less appetite.
    b. work will be reduced for the body processes.
    c. there is a gradual decrease in the rate of body metabolism.
    d. there is a decrease in the need for body repair.

3. Feelings (mental attitude) common in the aging process that may affect the nutritional status are
    a. a sense of rejection and loneliness.
    b. weakness and insecurity.
    c. disgust at the inability to chew foods thoroughly.
    d. discomfort from poor digestion.

4. The increased use of salt and sugar as an individual grows older is because
    a. of a special liking for very sweet or salty foods.
    b. of the development of poor food habits.
    c. such seasonings are familiar ones and are not expensive.
    d. of a decreased sense of taste and smell.

5. The nurse who works closely with elderly patients should recognize that the resistance to new foods, or to the familiar foods prepared in a different way, is one evidence of
    a. feelings of insecurity.
    b. selfishness.
    c. decreased judgment.
    d. their reluctance to eat.

6. Which of the following food lists should be emphasized in planning a diet for an older person?
    a. whole grain breads and cereals, meat, potatoes, and other vegetables
    b. bread, jelly, fruits, butter, milk, and eggs
    c. fresh fruits, vegetables, milk, eggs, lean meat, and whole grain breads/cereals
    d. bland soft-cooked foods

7. An aged patient may best be helped to keep up an interest in food by
    a. urging the patient to eat everything on the plate or tray.
    b. offering sweets between meals occasionally.
    c. including at least one food that the patient especially likes.
    d. explaining that the body needs that food to keep well.

8. Mrs. A. tells you that she has trouble with constipation and that when she was at home she took mineral oil several times a week. Your best response to her would be based on the awareness that mineral oil
    a. has 5 calories per gram which are "empty calories."
    b. is an ineffective laxative.
    c. increases the problem of constipation.
    d. interferes with the absorption of fat-soluble vitamins.

9. Mrs. A., because of her age and need for good nutrition with minimal caloric intake, should avoid "empty calories" found in
    a. carbonated drinks.
    b. black coffee.

c. tomato juice.

d. iced tea.

10. To help you, your family, or patients, which one of these statements offers the best guide to good nutrition?

a. Eating large amounts of food is one of the surest ways of being well nourished.

b. Reading and following the latest information on diets is a good plan to follow to attain good nutrition.

c. Eating a variety from the food groups is one of the surest ways to achieve good nutrition.

d. Taking vitamin and mineral supplements in recommended amounts is the surest way to a well-nourished body.

11. In selecting the protein food for Mr. O., who is on a fat-restricted diet, which of these groups is the best?

a. pork, cheese, and veal

b. chicken, legumes, and ham

c. eggs, cold cuts, and lean beef

d. chicken, fish, and lean beef

12. A person with a decline in neuromuscular coordination or severe arthritis may find difficulty in

a. food preparation.

b. use of eating utensils.

c. shopping for food.

d. all of the above.

13. The RDA for a 50-year-old for calcium is

a. 500 mg.

b. 700 mg.

c. 800 mg.

d. 1,000 mg.

14. To prevent the development of osteoporosis one needs to

a. have a lifelong adequate supply of calcium.

b. have a lifelong adequate intake of fluoride.

c. schedule physical workouts as part of a regular routine.

d. all of the above.

15. The group of foods most neglected by the elderly is the

a. milk group.

b. meat group.

c. fruit and vegetable group.

d. bread and cereal group.

16. Malnutrition among the elderly is most often due to

a. loneliness.

b. lack of education.

c. poor housing.

d. multiple disabilities.

17. Drugs commonly used that may interfere with nutrition include

a. laxatives.

b. diuretics.

c. vitamin/mineral megadoses.

d. all of the above.

18. Women who take OCAs may have low levels of

a. B vitamins and vitamin C.

b. vitamin C and iron.

c. calcium and magnesium.

d. vitamin A and calcium.

19. Women who use an IUD may be low in

a. B vitamins and vitamin C.

b. vitamin C and iron.

c. calcium and magnesium.

d. vitamin A and calcium.

True/False

Circle T for True and F for False.

20. T F There is about a 7.5 percent increase in the need for calories in each decade past the age of twenty-five years.

21. T F The simplest basis for judging adequacy of caloric intake is the maintenance of normal weight.

22. T F Most elderly persons require additional supplements of vitamins and minerals.

23. T F Older persons are frequent victims of food faddists' claims.

24. T F Obesity may be considered a form of malnutrition.

25. T F Chronologically, the aging process begins after age 65.

26. T F The elderly person is likely to experience reduced body functioning due to physiological changes, disease, and/or psychological factors.

27. T F Taste and smell acuity decreases with advancing age.

28. T F The need for essential amino acids lessens considerably during the aging process.

Fill-in

29. Why may an elderly person find it necessary to shop for food at markets that may be higher in cost but close to his or her home? _____

_____

30. What are two contributing factors in the reduced caloric needs of elderly persons? _____

_____

31. Nutrient needs for the elderly _____ compared to younger adults (remain the same/decrease).

32. Obesity is an increased risk for many elderly persons, especially women. What are three problems experi-

enced by obese elderly persons?

_____

_____

_____

33. What might be one factor contributing to iron-deficiency anemia in the elderly? _____

_____

34. What three nutrients besides iron are often found

deficient in the diets of elderly persons?

_____

_____

_____

35. What are two unique benefits of food supplementation through the Nutrition Program for the Elderly?

_____

_____

ACTIVITY 4: Exercise, Fitness, and Stress Reduction Principles

Adulthood covers a broad chronological span in which many physical and physiological changes occur. Clearly, genetic factors play a large part in longevity, but recent research indicates that regular exercise, fitness, especially cardiovascular fitness, and reduction of stress lead to extended life spans. The quality of life is also enhanced.

One major concern of adults of any age is physical appearance. Physical appearance is largely a matter of genetics, having inherited the general size and shape that we now possess. However, a determination of body fat may reveal that size and shape can be altered. Since there is a national disdain for fat and since poor body image contributes to social stigma as well as health problems, it is desirable to attain and maintain a healthy body weight.

The role of exercise in maintaining positive body image and physical fitness cannot be overlooked. It is especially beneficial when combined with a healthy eating pattern.

Physical Fitness _____

Although recent polls show that well over half of the adults in the United States participate in some form of exercise, most people are not educated to physical fitness requirements. The key elements to physical fitness include frequency of activity, duration of activity, intensity of activity, and type of activity. The first step in beginning a quest for physical fitness involves program selection. In order to become physically fit, a program must be selected to reach individual goals. This is important for continued good health.

Exercise testing can calculate the functional capacity of the cardiovascular system, a measurement important to exercise program selection. The goal in such testing is to determine predicted heart rate without causing chest pain.

Exercise and Nutritional Factors _____

The effects of controlled exercise are clearly beneficial. Experts believe that the recent decline in cardiovascular mortality is a result of increased health consciousness

throughout society and the practice of a regular exercise regimen combined with proper nutrition.

Most studies have shown that exercise decreases blood pressure in hypertensive patients, though such findings have not been conclusive. Similar studies have demonstrated that active men have blood pressure lower than inactive men. Exercise has been shown to decrease smoking. Numerous studies have confirmed that exercise lowers the levels of triglycerides in the blood. The blood levels of HDL cholesterol, thought to provide protection against heart disease, increase with exercise. In response to such findings, exercise has become a basic part of the rehabilitation program for patients who have undergone bypass surgery, as well as for those who have angina pectoris or who have suffered a myocardial infarction. Except for patients with certain diseases, such as congestive heart failure, acute myocarditis, or unstable angina pectoris, exercise programs can decrease morbidity and mortality.

An Ideal Program _____

The ideal physical fitness program must be suited to both health considerations and goals. For example, certain programs will yield increased strength; others will yield increased flexibility; yet others will increase cardiac and respiratory endurance. Although all these goals are worthwhile and can be achieved simultaneously if desired, the most important goal is stimulating the heart and circulatory system. A physical fitness training session is characterized by a warm-up period, an endurance phase, occasional competition, and finally a cooling-down period. Typically the session will last up to an hour in total. Patients undergoing rehabilitation will normally be limited to about half that time.

Frequency and intensity vary according to the individual's medical and exercise history, but three sessions weekly, performed at 70 percent or greater of a person's maximum heart rate, usually provides sufficient exercise to keep the body conditioned. Three days per week allows ample time for recovery, so the body in general, and critical organs in particular, do not become stressed. The duration of a physical fitness program depends on the body's condition when training is begun. For flexibility and strength programs, exercise must continue after the goal is attained to prevent loss of what has been achieved. An effective program includes good dietary habits that provide optimal nutrition and adequate calories, a diet low in fat but high in energy foods, such as complex carbohydrates.

Caloric Cost and Running

Exercise spends calories. For example, studies of running have determined that pace has little effect on calorie expenditure. Two men of equal body weight who run the same distance will expend about the same number of calories, regardless of whether one is in top physical condition and the other is a neophyte runner. Put another way, a 150-pound man will utilize approximately 1 kcal per pound in running 1½ miles in 10 minutes. The same man would utilize about 140 calories in covering the same distance in 16 minutes.

When caloric costs are known, exercise can be used to control weight. If 100 extra calories per day is expended, a weight loss of 10 pounds per year can be expected. Or, an individual who eats 3,000 calories per day and expends 200 calories per day through exercise can eat an additional 200 calories per day without gaining weight.

The key to physical fitness lies in tailoring a program to meet individual needs. If exercise uses more calories than are consumed, weight loss results. Attempts to gain or lose can affect both health and performance and should therefore be under supervision. Attempts to gain or lose weight should follow certain basic health guidelines, and nutritious foods from all four food groups should be included. Supplements should not be necessary, except for female athletes, who may require iron and folic acid. Sufficient time to achieve weight loss should be allowed.

Stress and Special Populations

The developmental tasks at each stage of the life span offer different stresses and challenges. Successfully completing these tasks is a form of growth. Failure to meet the tasks results in stress, which has multiple effects on the body systems.

Stressors can be biological, psychological, or sociological. Some of the effects of stress at different stages in the life cycle are included in the following examples.

Parents of newborns often find that their lifestyles have been disrupted in many ways they had not expected. Parents of toddlers are stressed by the inquisitiveness shown by children this age. As children grow, their parents' stress increases. Adolescence, the age at which children begin to assert their independence, is particularly painful. Adults who are responsible for the care of their aging parents also experience distress at this added responsibility.

Working adults experience overload and burnout and the symptoms become progressively more serious over time unless stress reduction can be achieved. Older adults moving from the work force to retirement encounter many stresses. They may feel a loss of productivity and thus a loss of usefulness. Loneliness and boredom may also be present in those who make no attempt to alleviate these feelings. Primary losses of the aging are losses of physical capacity to care for oneself, lapses of memory, diminished physique, and the death of old friends.

Adults who develop good coping mechanisms such as aerobic exercise, positive nutritional habits, and planned relaxation can stop the progression of symptoms and reverse extreme stages of stress. A word of caution: although stress management is a popular topic, some of the advertised products to fight stress, such as special "stress" vitamins, cassette recordings, and machines of various kinds, may, in fact, cost the consumer much more financially than the consumer will receive in benefits, and thus may increase stress. The prudent course is still to follow proven avenues for health maintenance. *Health maintenance* refers to measures that will enable an individual to stay young and healthy in body and mind for as many years as possible. These measures include becoming aware of the consequences of imprudent dieting, and often, changing a lifetime of poor eating habits. It also means educating oneself to refute invalid claims for quick fixes and to recognize valid basic factors. It includes paying attention to body signals and learning in what ways and how to relax, when and how to exercise, and, best of all, how to make healthy choices and enjoy the rest of life.

PROGRESS CHECK ON ACTIVITY 4

Fill-in

1. Name the key elements of establishing a physical fitness regime.

    a. _____

    b. _____

    c. _____

    d. _____

2. Exercise testing is done primarily to determine the

    _____

3. List three beneficial effects of regular exercise.

    a. _____

    b. _____

c. _____

4. Name the components of a physical fitness training session.

   a. _____

   b. _____

   c. _____

   d. _____

5. An effective fitness program includes good dietary habits. Describe the eating pattern that will meet this criterion.

   _____

   _____

   _____

   _____

6. Situation: If Mary drinks 6 oz. of regular soda pop per day, and it contains approximately 100 calories more than her caloric output of 2,000 calories, what will be the outcome if she does this each day for one year? Choose an answer from below and give your rationale.

   a. Nothing will happen; 100 calories extra per day shouldn't count.
   b. She'll probably lose weight, as her diet is unbalanced.
   c. She'll gain about 10 pounds over the year's time.
   d. It will increase her fluid intake, which is healthy.
   e. She will have higher energy levels.

7. Identify four health problems brought about by unrelieved stress.

   a. _____

   b. _____

   c. _____

   d. _____

8. Name three ways to help alleviate some of the stress encountered by adults of all ages.

   a. _____

   b. _____

   c. _____

9. "Stress Tabs" are a popular vitamin supplement on the market and a lot of people buy them. They contain primarily vitamin C and the B complex. Evaluate this product designed for stress management based on your previous knowledge.

   _____

_____

_____

10. Define health maintenance. _____

_____

_____

Summary

Nutrition plays an important role throughout all phases of the life span. The information below summarizes the key points discussed in Activities 1, 2, 3, and 4 of this module.

Optimal nutrition during pregnancy is critical. New tissue is formed at this time, including the developing baby, materials for nourishing the embryo and fetus, and the mother's own body. Pregnancy is divided into three trimesters with each trimester covering three months. Each trimester requires more nutrients than the last. When the fetus's cells are dividing rapidly, the mother's intake of unhealthy food or other substances can have dramatic and sometimes tragic consequences. The desirable weight gain for a healthy pregnant woman ranges between 24 and 30 pounds. The pattern of weight gain and the foods eaten to achieve the gain are most important. The diet should be chosen for nutrient density and balance and must be carefully planned. Certain supplements are usually recommended and should be prescribed.

The first year of life is the most rapid growth period of all and, consequently, the infant has the highest nutrient needs. A healthy full-term infant will have some reserve supplies of some nutrients, but will need replenishing after four to six months.

Both breast- and bottle-feeding can produce a healthy child, each having advantages and disadvantages. While breast milk is uniquely suited to infant needs, formulas can be satisfactory. Psychological, cultural, safety, and health factors need to be considered before choosing the feeding method. Infants need solids added to their diet at about four to six months of age. Developmental readiness is a consideration. Solid foods should be added one at a time and the child observed for reactions.

The food intake of young children is erratic. While their growth has slowed, muscle and skeletal tissue is developing. Their nutrient needs remain high, although caloric intake may decrease. During these years, the most important thing a caregiver can do for a child is to provide a basis for sound eating habits. This is sometimes difficult and always challenging, as advertising, peer pressure, and poor examples influence the child as well as his or her own developmental tasks. Understanding childhood behavior patterns is necessary in order to cope with the growing child. Obesity and iron-deficiency anemia are nutritional problems in this age group.

The second greatest growth spurt of life happens in the adolescent years. Again, nutrient demands are high. Many factors, except concern for the state of health, influence a teenager's eating habits. There is an intense obsession with physical appearance, especially as it relates to weight for girls and athletic performance for boys. The bizarre eating habits of the teenage girl not only make her the least well-nourished of any group in the United States but may also precipitate eating disorders, such as anorexia nervosa and bulimia.

Teenage pregnancies present many medical and nutritional problems, putting both mother and baby at great risk. Since one in five babies is born to a teenage mother, these young women should receive nutrition counseling, government support, and some form of health monitoring by health agencies. Common health problems among teenagers include anemia, calcium deficiency, vitamin C deficiency, alcohol and drug abuse, and obesity.

Having completed the growth cycle of adolescence, the adult settles into maturity, which requires consuming adequate nutrients to maintain and repair body tissue, maintaining a normal weight, getting regular exercise, and avoiding excess stress. These health maintenance measures are believed to prevent or delay the onset of chronic degenerative diseases and improve the quality of later life. The loss of tissue and organ functioning that accompanies the aging process takes place gradually. Generally, scientists believe that the aging process is genetically determined, but most agree that a lifelong commitment to good eating habits and adequate exercise can modify health and longevity. No studies have shown that any special foods or supplements can prolong life any longer than can a regular balanced diet. Nutrition status in the later years is affected not only by food intake and physiological factors but also by stress, poverty, loneliness, and low self-esteem. Middle-aged and older adults are especially susceptible to nutritional quackery.

Drugs and alcohol affect the nutrition of the adult and many drug-nutrient reactions are harmful. Cardiovascular, renal, hepatic, and neuromuscular disorders often develop in these years.

Adults of all ages can get the nutrients they need by following the guidelines for a balanced diet, such as the Dietary Guidelines for Americans, the basic food groups, and other guides as described in Module 1.

Nutrition plays a role in each stage of the life cycle. Good eating habits should be developed on a continuum throughout life, so that each stage meets the current needs and passes on good nutritional status to the next stage.

The quality of life is enhanced throughout the life cycle whenever principles of optimum nutrition, physical fitness, a healthy weight, and positive mechanisms for coping with stress are recognized, understood, and followed. All of these principles can be learned, thus changing behavior patterns and contributing to a long, healthy, and happy life.

Responsibilities of Health Personnel _____

A health worker should impart the following information to clients:

1. Young adults who use oral contraceptives should be informed that they need extra folacin, riboflavin, and vitamins C, B_6, and B_{12}.
2. Young women who use IUDs should be informed that they need to compensate for extra menstrual losses with extra iron and vitamin C.
3. A basic food guide should be followed by adults of all ages for optimum nutrition. The only nutritional decrease should be in the caloric intake as aging occurs. The RDA for energy for ages fifty to seventy-five is 90 percent of that for the young adult. The RDA for energy for ages over seventy-five is approximately 75 percent of that for the young adult.
4. The older adult may need to avoid foods that are difficult to chew.
5. Older adults should be discouraged from overusing laxatives.
6. Adults should be aware that both physiological and psychological factors affect their nutritional well-being.
7. Drugs (including alcohol) can adversely affect nutritional status and foods can interfere with some drug therapies.
8. Adults benefit from using foods that are good sources of fiber.
9. Consuming more high-calcium foods may help to alleviate osteoporosis, a leading disorder in later adulthood.
10. People should not delay adopting good dietary habits until middle age. The dietary guidelines are sensible eating guides and should be followed from adolescence to old age.
11. People on medication should ascertain from their health care professional if nutrient supplements are needed to counteract adverse effects of a drug.
12. People treated for a disease requiring a modified diet should seek assistance from a professional, preferably a registered dietitian.
13. Various programs are designed to help adults meet their nutritional requirements.
14. Elderly people cope better with changes brought on by aging if they are advised or assisted to
    a. Select nutrient-dense foods that are low in fat, permitting adequate nutrients without weight gain.
    b. Drink plenty of liquids, two to three quarts a day. Water is good for the body and has no calories.

c.   Accommodate chewing problems by cutting, chopping, or grinding food when necessary.

d.   Follow a modified diet, if one is prescribed.

e.   Avoid excess salt and try new spices to make food taste better.

f.   Find and use outside resources to improve social interactions and eating habits, such as senior centers, neighborhood groups, exercise groups, Meals on Wheels, extension services, voluntary community services for elders (e.g., free transportation, discounts, etc.).

g.   Interact with family and friends, stay in touch, and not become isolated.

h.   Keep physically fit.

15.   Many acceptable exercise and fitness programs are designed for people of all ages and various states of health and mobility. The health worker should encourage selecting and following a suitable plan.

16.   Stress reduction techniques and materials should be provided whenever the client indicates need.

References

Aloia, J. F. 1989. *Osteoporosis: A guide to prevention and treatment.* Champaign, IL: Leisure Press.

Armbrecht, J. et al. (eds.). 1984. *Nutritional intervention in the aging process.* New York: Springer-Verlag.

Behrman, R. E. et al. 1987. *Nelson textbook of pediatrics.* Philadelphia: Saunders.

Berger, H. (ed.). 1988. Vitamins and minerals in pregnancy and lactation. *Nestle Nutrition Workshop Series.* Vol. 16. New York: Raven Press.

Bidlock, W. R. et al. 1986. Nutritional requirements of the elderly. *Food Technology* 40:61.

Boston Children's Hospital. 1986. *Parents' guide to nutrition.* Reading, MA: Addison-Wesley.

Canada's National Guidelines on Prenatal Nutrition. 1987. *Nutrition Today* 22(4):34.

Chen, L. H. (ed.). 1986. *Nutritional aspects of aging.* Volumes I and II. Boca Raton, FL: CRC Press.

Chernoff, R. 1987. Aging and nutrition. *Nutrition Today* 22(2):4.

Chernoff, R., and D. A. Lipschitz. 1988. Nutrition and aging. In *Modern nutrition in health and disease,* 7th ed. M. E. Shils and V. R. Young (eds.). Philadelphia: Lea & Febiger.

Elliott, R. 1987. *The vegetarian mother and baby book: A complete guide to nutrition, health and diet during pregnancy and after.* Westminister, MD: Pantheon.

Epstein, L. H. et al. 1985. Childhood obesity. *Pediat. Clin. N. A.* 32:363.

Erick, M. (ed.). 1988. *D.I.E.T. during pregnancy (Developing Intelligent Eating Techniques).* Brookline, MA: Grinnen-Barrett.

Fomon, S. J., and W. C. Heird (eds.). 1986. Energy and protein needs during infancy. *Bristol-Myers Nutrition Symposia.* Vol. 4. Orlando, FL: Academic Press.

Gong, E. J., and F. P. Heald. 1988. Diet, nutrition, and adolescence. In *Modern nutrition in health and disease,* 7th ed. M. E. Shils and V. R. Young (eds.). Philadelphia: Lea & Febiger.

Hess, M. A., and A. E. Hunt. 1987. *Pickles & ice cream: The complete early pregnancy nutrition course.* Winnetka, IL: Hess and Hunt.

Hutchinson, M. L., and H. N. Munro (eds.). 1986. Nutrition and aging. *Bristol-Myers Nutrition Symposia* Vol. 5. Orlando, FL: Academic Press.

Kaplan, S. et al. 1986. Considerations for those providing nutritional care to the elderly. *J. Nutr. Elderly* 5:53.

Leonard, R. 1987. Focusing elderly nutritional programs. *Food Management* 22:34.

Leville, G. A. et al. 1986. Role of the food industry in meeting the nutritional needs of the elderly. *Food Technology* 40:82.

Munro, H. N. 1985. Nutrient needs and nutritional status in relation to aging. *Drug-Nutrient Interactions* 4(1/2):55.

Munro, H. N., and D. E. Danford (eds.). 1989. *Nutrition, aging, and the elderly.* New York: Plenum Press.

National Institute of Health. 1991. National Cholesterol Education Program Description. National Heart, Lung, and Blood Institute. Bethesda, MD.

National Cholesterol Education Program. Expert Panel on Blood Cholesterol Levels in Children and Adolescents. *Nutrition Today.* May-June 1991, pp. 36–41.

Natow, A., and J. Heslin. 1988. *No-nonsense nutrition for your baby's first year.* New York: Prentice Hall.

Natow, A. B. et al. 1986. *Nutritional care of the older adult.* New York: Macmillan.

Picciano, M. F. 1987. Nutrient needs of infants. *Nutrition Today* 22(1):8.

Posner, B. M. et al. 1987. Nutrition, aging, and the continuum of health care. ADA technical support paper. *Journal of the American Dietetic Association* 87(3):345.

Ranno, B. S. et al. 1988. What characterizes women who overuse vitamin and mineral supplements? *Journal of the American Dietetic Association* 88(3):347.

Rathbone-McCuan, E., and B. Havens. 1988. *North American elders: United States and Canadian perspective.* Westport, CT: Greenwood Press.

Ritchey, S. J., and L. J. Taper. 1983. *Maternal and child nutrition.* New York: Harper-Row.

Roe, D. A. 1987. *Geriatric Nutrition,* 2nd ed. Englewood Cliffs, NJ: Prentice-Hall.

Rowe, J. W. et al. 1987. Human aging: Usual and successful. *Science* 237(4811):143.

Rozin, P., and T. A. Zollemecke. 1986. Food likes and dislikes. *Annual Review of Nutrition* 6:433.

Satter, E. 1987. *How to get your kid to eat . . . but not too much*. Palo Alto, CA: Bull Publishing Co.

Schneider, E. L. et al. 1986. Recommended dietary allowances and the health of the elderly. *New England Journal of Medicine* 314:157.

Story, M. et al. 1988. Adolescent nutrition: Self-perceived deficiencies and needs of practitioners working with youth. *Journal of the American Dietetic Association* 88:591.

Tramposch, T. S. et al. 1987. A nutrition screening and assessment system for use with the elderly in extended care. *Journal of the American Dietetic Association* 87(9):1207.

Whitehead, R. G. 1988. Pregnancy and lactation. In *Modern nutrition in health and disease*, 7th ed. M. E. Shils and V. R. Young (eds.). Philadelphia: Lea & Febiger.

Worthington-Roberts, B. S. et al. 1989. *Nutrition in pregnancy and lactation*, 4th ed. St. Louis: Mosby.

Module 10

Drugs and Nutrition

Time for completion
Activities: _____ 1½ _____ hours
Optional examination: _½_ hour

Academic credit
Semester units: _²⁄₁₀_
Quarter units: _³⁄₁₀_

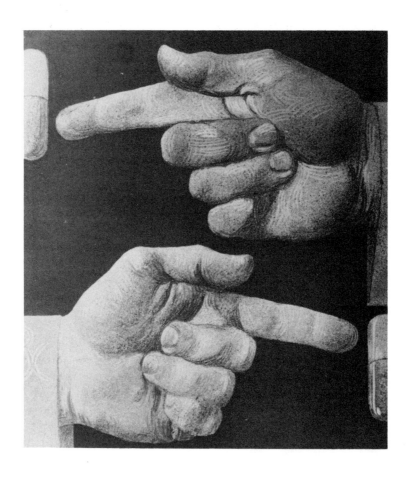

Outline

Objectives

Upon completion of this module the student should be able to:

1. Describe the effects of drugs on the utilization of nutrients.
2. Describe the effects of nutrients on the utilization of drugs.
3. Identify food and drug incompatibilities.
4. Accurately assess a client's response to food and drug interactions.
5. Provide specific instructions to clients regarding their diet and drug therapy.

Glossary

Actions: Drug actions are grouped according to the body system for which they are specific. The student should consult a Physicians' Desk Reference (PDR) or Pharmacopoeia for details. General actions of drugs are listed here.

1. *Additive:* effects of two drugs are equal to the sum of each.
2. *Cumulative:* concentration of a drug in the body increases with each successive dose.
3. *Synergistic:* combined effects of certain drugs are greater than that of the individual drugs.
4. *Tolerance:* drug must be increased to produce the same effect.
5. *Toxicity:* potentially harmful side effects from the use of a drug.

Anti: against. Many drugs work against diseases or disorders. Examples include antibiotics (against infections), antidepressants (against depression), etc.

Bioavailability: degree to which a drug or other substance becomes available for body use after administration.

Chelate (kee-late):   form a chemical compound (with another drug or food).

CNS: central nervous system.

MAO: monoamine oxidase, a drug used to treat psychiatric illness.

OCA: oral contraceptive agent.

OTC: over the counter.

pH: acidity or alkalinity of fluids and compounds.

Physicians' Desk Reference (PDR):   Physicians' desk reference.

Teratogen: agent capable of producing adverse effects.

Background Information

General Considerations

Only in the past decade has the multiple effect of the interactions of drugs and nutrients been recognized. Many drugs and nutrients that are prescribed produce a different effect than was originally intended. Drugs affect taste, appetite, intestinal motility, absorption, and metabolism of nutrients. Many of these interactions compromise nutritional status and health.

The effect of nutrients on drugs is equally important. Food may delay drug absorption, alter drug metabolism by enzyme induction or inhibition, or alter the rate of drug excretion and drug response.

Most people are tremendously concerned about the relationship between drug usage and nutrition. This concern involves not only illicit drugs such as cocaine or marijuana, but many prescription and over-the-counter drugs as well.

The effects of drugs on the body can vary widely. Numerous factors produce these varying results. Consider, for example, the usage difference that can occur. The drug can vary; the dosage can vary; time and frequency of consumption can vary. Reactions also vary according to the health status of the drug user. If body nutrition is good, the body can effectively deal with a larger drug dose than it could otherwise handle. Conversely, a malnourished person may require a higher dosage to produce a desired therapeutic effect. Finally, the ability to absorb drugs and nutrients varies; for example, because of age or differences in digestive juice production, drug response can vary.

Nutritional status can be affected by single or multiple drug therapy. Effects may be short-term or long-term. In the digestive system, effects such as diarrhea, constipation, nausea and vomiting, and altered taste and smell sensitivity may occur, changing intestinal absorption, utilization, storage, synthesis, and metabolism of nutrients. Of special concern is how drugs can affect the body's ability to manufacture and metabolize nutrients.

The effects of drugs on nutrients are profound. They may directly destroy or change the nutrient, damage intestinal walls, and/or lower absorption. Drugs can directly destroy, displace, or change the nutrients themselves.

Inside the human body, a drug can join with a nutrient, rendering the nutrient incapable of being utilized normally. When this occurs, the nutrient will simply be excreted by the kidney.

Drugs affect all nutrients—carbohydrates, fat, protein, vitamins, minerals—to varying extents. For example, drugs can cause fat to be deposited in the liver, can cause blood insulin levels to fluctuate, can reduce body vitamin storage, and can increase excretion of minerals in the urine.

Ingestion

Drugs affect nutrient ingestion by causing changes in appetite, taste, and smell. Common side effects of many medications administered orally or parenterally are nausea and vomiting, resulting in decreased food intake. Some drugs, such as antidepressants, antihistamines, and oral contraceptives increase appetite. A small amount of alcohol before meals will increase saliva and gastric secretions and stimulate the taste buds.

Drugs that decrease food intake include amphetamines, cholinergic agents, some expectorants, and narcotic analgesics. In the elderly patient, tranquilizers often cause a decrease in food intake because of slow metabolism and disinterest in food and surroundings.

Bulk-forming medications may reduce appetite by creating a feeling of fullness. Some may decrease appetite by inhibiting gastric emptying.

Drugs that affect taste or have offensive odors decrease intake. Examples include penicillamine, streptomycin, potassium chloride, vitamin B complex liquids, and some chemotherapies.

Nausea and vomiting may occur with many drugs, causing a decrease in food intake. Examples include oral hypoglycemic agents, cancer chemotherapeutic agents, and many antibiotics given orally.

Patients on diets with sugar or sodium restrictions should be monitored for intake of drugs containing glucose and sodium or other restrictive nutrients. Cough syrups, expectorants, and elixirs contain large amounts of glucose. Many antibiotics and parenteral solutions contain large amounts of sodium.

Absorption

The most frequently reported diet-drug interaction involves alteration of the bioavailability of the drug because of concurrent food ingestion. At the same time, the drug may alter the absorption of various nutrients.

Absorption of drugs and nutrients occurs by different means. Drug absorption is governed by its physical form, particle size, gastrointestinal pH, and solubility in fats. Nutrient absorption, on the other hand, depends upon an intact enzyme system, and gastrointestinal secretions. The small intestine is the major site for drug and nutrient interactions.

Drugs causing malabsorption induce diarrhea, steatorrhea, and weight loss. Abdominal pain, flatulence, and nutrient deficits may also occur.

Metabolism

Alterations in metabolism can be due to drug interference with the enzyme system or drug-induced vitamin antagonists.

Nutritional imbalances are known to affect the metabolism of drugs. To handle a drug properly, the body requires many nutrients: niacin, riboflavin, pantothenic acid, ascorbic acid, folic acid, vitamin B_{12}, protein (amino acids), fat, glucose, iron, copper, calcium, zinc, and magnesium. If any nutrient is lacking, normal drug metabolism can be diminished. The toxicity of the drug may be increased or decreased by the metabolic alteration. In effect, the altered metabolism yields a change in the dosage's planned therapeutic effect, rendering the dosage either too high or too low under the circumstances.

In humans, an extreme nutrient deficiency or an extreme nutrient excess can be expected to unbalance drug metabolism. When protein is lacking, manufacture of important enzymes involved in drug metabolism is reduced. For example, many protein-deficient children are infested with hookworms. The drug used to combat hookworms, tetrachloroethylene, is known to be toxic in high doses, yet undernourished children do not exhibit toxic effects when given large doses of the drug. It is thought that because of the depressed quality of the enzymes involved, the drug forms fewer of the usual toxic byproducts.

Excretion

Drugs affect nutrient excretion by altering reabsorption or transport. It may also alter the kidneys' ability to concentrate. Some drugs affect specific nutrients more than others. Examples include the effect that diuretics have on calcium and potassium excretion, and the increased excretion of ascorbic acid due to aspirin therapy. Aspirin in large doses also depletes potassium.

Foods affect drug excretion by changing urine pH and causing the precipitation of certain drugs. Retention of salt and fluids is another undesirable effect associated with drug-nutrient interactions. Examples include steroids, antihypertensives, and estrogens.

PROGRESS CHECK ON BACKGROUND INFORMATION

Fill-in

Define:

1. Cumulative _____

   _____

2. Synergistic _____

   _____

3. Toxicity _____

   _____

4. Antibiotic _____

   _____

5. Chelate _____

   _____

6. OCA _____

   _____

7. OTC _____

   _____

8. Teratogen _____

_____

9. Drugs profoundly affect nutrient utilization. List five ways in which this effect is accomplished.

a. _____

b. _____

c. _____

d. _____

e. _____

10. Describe the most common symptoms exhibited by the digestive tract in response to drug therapy.

a. _____

b. _____

c. _____

11. Drug effects on the body depend on five major variances. Name them.

a. _____

b. _____

c. _____

d. _____

e. _____

12. Metabolism alterations may be due to what two major factors?

a. _____

b. _____

13. The body requires fourteen nutrients in adequate amounts in order to properly metabolize a drug. Name five of them.

a. _____

b. _____

c. _____

d. _____

e. _____

14. Drugs affect nutrient excretion by altering _____ and _____.

15. Foods affect drug excretion by causing _____ or _____.

ACTIVITY 1: *Food and Drug Interactions*

Effects of Food on Drugs _____

Food can make a drug more or less effective. Just as drugs can interfere with our food utilization, so too can foods and nutrients affect the action of drugs (Lamy, 1980). Foods can change drug absorption, neutralize drug effects, interact with drugs, and influence their excretion rate.

Doctors prescribe drugs for maximum therapeutic effect. Yet, it has long been assumed that the presence of food in the intestinal tract, the primary absorption site, affects the absorption of most drugs. The extent of this effect remains unclear. Food can increase or decrease acidity, digestive secretions, and intestinal motility. Such effects directly determine whether a drug will be easily destroyed, how long it will stay in the intestine, whether a drug will become crystals, whether a drug will be absorbed at all, and other technical changes.

Dietary minerals such as iron, magnesium, calcium, and aluminum salts demonstrate how food chemicals or nutrients can affect drug absorption. These minerals can chemically join with tetracycline, a commonly used antibiotic, to form tiny solid particles (insoluble precipitate). Simultaneous ingestion of these minerals and tetracycline causes the drug to lose its therapeutic value, requiring a large dose to offset the loss. This example shows that the common practice of taking such drugs with food or liquids to mask

the drug taste may be questionable. Patients should be given specific directions about combining drugs with meals or snacks, including the rationale for them.

Vitamins are considered drugs if they are used for pharmacological effects. For example, if a person has a bladder infection and a megadose of vitamin C is prescribed, the vitamin C is not being used for its characteristics as a vitamin but rather is being prescribed to acidify the urine. Such use is pharmacological rather than nutritional. Niacin, a B vitamin, is similarly used to lower blood cholesterol.

Administering medications with meals is common practice to reduce gastrointestinal side effects, but this practice can also result in reduced, delayed, or altered drug action. Using food as a vehicle to administer crushed tablets or to disguise taste can also affect the drug's action if the food alters the pH or chelate of the drug. Oral medications are affected by food in the gastrointestinal tract, the pH of the stomach and small intestine, and the motility of the gastrointestinal tract.

Fatty foods and high-fat, low-fiber meals slow the emptying of the stomach by as much as two hours. The action of a drug administered with or after such a meal would be similarly slowed. High-protein meals increase gastric blood flow and increase the absorption of some drugs. Meals high in glucose cause a slight, transient decrease in blood flow to the gastrointestinal tract, which tends to decrease drug absorption.

Effect of Drugs on Food _____

There is increasing evidence that drug and food interactions can compromise a patient's nutritional status—and ultimately a patient's health.

Impaired absorption is a common mechanism by which drugs interfere with vitamin homeostasis. Mineral oil, the first agent found to cause malabsorption, forms an insoluble complex in which the fat soluble vitamins (A, E, D, and K) pass through the gut before absorption takes place. Elderly patients who are chronic users of mineral oil may be at risk for developing rickets due to malabsorption of vitamin D.

Certain drugs induce enzyme systems that require vitamin cofactors. This may increase vitamin needs. Some drugs compete with vitamins for the sites of action. Additionally, some drugs decrease endogenous nutrient synthesis. For example, the broad spectrum antibiotics interfere with vitamin K synthesis by microorganisms normally present in the colon.

It is now firmly established that oral contraceptives definitely result in a deficiency of vitamin B_6 in about 10 to 30 percent of pill users. The high incidence of headache and depression among these patients is now traced to a lack of this vitamin. Apparently, reduction of vitamin B_6 participation in body metabolism of brain chemicals indirectly causes the depression and headache.

Various efforts have been made to remedy the adverse effects of the pill on the patient's nutritional status. Including vitamins and minerals in the pill has been suggested. Regular blood and urine checking for the levels of vitamins and minerals is another alternative. However, medical politics, clinical philosophies, technical uncertainties, and other factors have prevented any major health policy from being adopted.

Even common aspirin can cause nutritional problems. Chronic salicylate therapy has been shown both to decrease uptake of vitamin C in leukocytes and impair the protein-binding ability of folate.

The more common drug-induced deficiencies that are known have been presented here. Very likely many drug-nutrient interactions that have not yet been recognized take place in acute or chronic therapy, and more data are needed about the interactions that are known.

Both preventive and corrective measures are needed to ensure that therapeutic drug use will not harm a patient's nutritional status. More clinical studies are needed, as are long-range programs, since the complexities regarding the relationship between drugs and nutrition require careful study. Further study is especially needed among populations who take drugs for long periods; for example, women taking oral contraceptives and older Americans.

Food and Drug Incompatibilities _____

Certain foods and beverages are known to be incompatible with therapeutic drugs. These incompatible reactions occur as the result of pharmacologically active ingredients in the food, notably ethyl alcohol and various amines. These food ingredients react especially with drugs for treating psychiatric illness (monoamine oxidase inhibitors) and alcohol abuse (disulfiram).

Cheese and other foods contain the chemical tyramine (and its related amines). Drugs such as these are often prescribed for treating depression. Tyramine can react with procarbazine to create a "hypertensive crisis" in a patient. Reaction can occur within one-half to one hour after consuming the incompatible substance.

Alcohol, hot beverages, and antacids should not be given with sustained-release tablets or capsules because these substances can cause premature erosion of the pH-sensitive coating on the drug. Enteric-coated tablets should not be given with alkaline meals or antacids.

Many drugs, particularly central nervous system depressants, should not be taken in conjunction with alcohol because of a cumulative depressant effect. Other drugs combined with alcohol intake produce an effect similar to disulfiram (Antabuse), with an acute onset of facial flushing, dyspnea, nausea and vomiting, palpitation, headache, and hypotension. Alcohol consumed with some drugs increases the potential for gastric irritation and bleeding.

The severity of reaction depends on the drug dosage, amount of food ingested, patient susceptibility, and the interval between drug and food consumption. The severity of reaction can also be affected by the condition of the food.

Practicing physicians and all health professionals are encouraged to be familiar with drug-nutrition relationships. They are also encouraged to be at the forefront of efforts to reduce drug-induced malnutrition.

PROGRESS CHECK ON ACTIVITY 1

Fill-in

1. Name four changes food and nutrients can cause on a drug.

   a. _____

   b. _____

   c. _____

   d. _____

2. Incompatibility of food and drugs results from what two major active ingredients in food?

   a. _____

   b. _____

3. Use of MAOs in treating depression has declined due to what major reaction? _____

_____

4. The severity of drug reactions with food is due to five factors. Name them.

   a. _____

   b. _____

   c. _____

   d. _____

   e. _____

5. Cocaine ingestion affects nutritional status by what method?

_____

_____

6. Anticholinergics, useful for treating peptic ulcers, will affect nutritional status by causing _____

_____

Multiple Choice

7. Vitamins are considered drugs if/when
   a. they are prescribed.
   b. they are recommended.
   c. they are used for pharmacological effects.
   d. vitamins are not drugs; they are nutrients.

8. Administering drugs with meals is a common practice used to

   a. reduce GI side effects.
   b. disguise taste.
   c. chelate the drug.
   d. a and b.
   e. all of these.

9. Oral medications are affected by food in the GI tract in which of the following ways?
   a. pH of the stomach
   b. motility of the gut
   c. chelate of the medication
   d. all of the above

10. A fatty meal affects passage of a drug by
    a. absorbing it so that it is unable to pass.
    b. delaying it by as much as two hours.
    c. speeding it by as much as two hours.
    d. all but c.

11. A meal high in protein affects drug therapy by
    a. increasing absorption of the drug.
    b. decreasing absorption of the drug.
    c. delaying passage of the drug.
    d. neutralizing the effects of the drug.

True/False

12. T F Manufacturers now include vitamins and minerals in oral contraceptives.

13. T F Drugs often require extra vitamins because they use vitamins as cofactors.

14. T F Broad spectrum antibiotics interfere with vitamin K synthesis.

15. T F Headache and depression among OCA users have been traced to a deficiency of vitamin B_6.

ACTIVITY 2: Drugs and the Life Cycle

Effects on Pregnancy and Lactation _____

A number of drugs, some of which are also classified as food components, have shown harmful effects on the course and outcome of pregnancy. These include alcohol, caffeine, some food additives, and food contaminants.

Alcohol

Alcohol consumption has many adverse effects on fetal development. Infants born to alcoholics exhibit anomalies of the eyes, nose, heart, and central nervous system, as well as mental retardation (the fetal alcohol syndrome: FAS). More moderate consumption of alcohol leads to what is termed fetal alcohol effect. These effects include less severe but similar symptoms to FAS. The women also demonstrate higher rates of spontaneous abortion, abruptio placenta, and low birth weight delivery. Deficiencies of folic acid, magnesium, and zinc also may occur in the pregnant female and may play an important role in FAS.

Caffeine

Data is very limited in relation to human pregnancy and ingestion of caffeine, although it has been shown to be teratogenic in rats. A general warning is issued to pregnant women regarding limitation of caffeine intake.

Additives

Food additives, such as saccharin and aspartame, show no ill effects on the developing fetus, although moderation in the use of these substances during pregnancy (as well as non-pregnancy) is encouraged. Women who carry the PKU heterozygous gene should limit (or avoid) their intake of aspartame during pregnancy, as aspartame contains phenylalanine.

Contaminants

Mercury poisoning poses severe risks to the fetus including neurological problems and permanent brain damage. Other heavy metals, such as nickel, cadium, and selenium, also pose heavy risks to the fetus and infant. Fetal growth retardation is seen in offspring of cigarette smokers due to effects from carbon monoxide, nicotine, and the decreased supply of oxygen transport to the fetus.

Other Food Components

Often overlooked for being potentially threatening, or most often believed to be beneficial rather than harmful, is the use of excessive amounts of vitamins and minerals. Congenital renal anomalies, multiple CNS malformations, cleft palate, and other severe defects have been reported in infants whose mothers took large doses of vitamin A during pregnancy. Other fat-soluble vitamins exhibit toxicity symptoms to the developing fetus and newborn when taken in large doses, though not as severe as that with hypervitaminosis A. Zinc in excess given to pregnant women appears to cause premature delivery and possible incidence of stillbirth.

Recreational and Medicinal Drugs

Recreational and medicinal drugs exert negative and damaging effects to the fetus. The effects are especially severe in the first trimester. Barbituates, hydantoin, anticonvulsants, and anticoagulants are chemicals known to be associated with fetal abnormalities, as well as over-the-counter drugs. All "street" drugs are extremely dangerous. A great spurt in brain growth occurs in the third trimester. Damage to the CNS at this critical stage of development potentially alters later brain functions.

Drugs and Breast-Feeding

For centuries, breast milk has been considered the perfect food for infants. But long-standing jokes about infants rejecting breast milk because the mother gorged on garlic, onion, or other strong foods are now gaining credence through clinical findings. Chemical ingredients in onion, garlic, and chocolate apparently produce an unpleasant reaction in nursing babies. A greater concern is that drugs can also appear in breast milk and affect nursing infants. Doctors are justifiably concerned about the possibility that therapeutic drugs and nondrug chemicals can make their way from mother to infant.

Several factors have contributed to the heightened concern in the medical community. First, breast-feeding has regained popularity and is steadily on the increase.

Second, drug use is also on the increase. Numerous new drugs are available, and the number of over-the-counter (OTC) drugs has substantially increased. In addition, more women are taking oral contraceptives while nursing, and industrial and household chemicals have contaminated the environment. For example, pesticides have been found in breast milk.

Drug Passage to Breast Milk

The amount of a drug appearing in the milk primarily depends on the type of drug consumed, the concentration of the drug, and the time elapsed between drug ingestion and breast-feeding. Contrary to popular belief, the quantity of milk secreted has little to do with the amount of the drug passing to breast milk. Method of drug administration does affect passage, since injected drugs appear faster than oral doses. The amount appearing in the milk may range from high to insignificant. For various reasons, the drug's presence may be harmless. For example, it may be nontoxic or ineffective, may be destroyed by the infant's system, or may not be absorbed by the infant. Certain drugs may be harmless unless they reach the infant in large quantities, whereas others may be harmful in small quantities.

Physicians must be especially careful when prescribing drugs for a nursing mother and must also determine whether the patient is using OTC drugs and whether environmental chemicals are inadvertently present. If the mother has a recognizable disease such as high blood pressure, edema, diabetes, and arthritis, she must be informed of the potential risk to the child. Of course, physicians can recommend interruption of breast-feeding if a drug that passes to breast milk must be used. Other professionals such as nurses, dietitians, and nutritionists should be equally familiar with the drugs that can pass to breast milk.

Effects on Adults

As consumers of many types of over-the-counter and prescription drugs, as well as recreation drugs, the young adult is at great risk for overmedicating. They are also prone to use several kinds of drugs at the same time. Prescription medications are not necessarily safer just because they are physician supervised. A person is at high risk whenever OTCs are taken along with prescription medication. Add to this the frequent use of alcohol and the combination is life-threatening. The many reactions and contraindications from these habits are beyond the scope of this module, but the health professional must be aware of all such practices because they are commonplace in our society.

Probably the most common of the chronically used drugs that can profoundly affect nutrition are the estrogen-containing oral contraceptives. Women using these drugs are at risk of a clinical folate deficiency if they have marginal stores of this vitamin. Moreover, certain oral contraceptives reduce pyridoxine levels, a fact that may be associated with the common complaints of depression heard from some women on the pill. In some cases, impaired glucose tolerance related to OCA use has responded to pyridoxine supplementation. And, although no clinical significance has been attached, many users of oral contraceptives are found to have low vitamin C levels.

Oral contraceptives are known to affect the metabolism of virtually all nutrients. Such effects are subject to variables such as dosage, length of time used, prior nutritional status, nutrient intake, and individual susceptibility.

Effects on the Elderly

The use of multiple drugs by the elderly poses many problems, yet more drugs are prescribed for them than for any other segment of the population. Ninety-nine percent of nursing home patients are multiple drug users, averaging four to six different drugs per day, depending on which surveys are reported. This author has observed as many as 20 different drugs on the chart of one nursing home patient. Elderly people living outside a facility also take many prescription drugs, although in lesser quantities as a usual rule.

The aged commonly have adverse reactions to many drugs, possibly because of deficiency of vitamin C, an important nutrient necessary for the normal process of drug metabolism. The elderly cannot metabolize and excrete drugs as well as younger adults. Therefore, the action of the drug may last longer. In addition, drugs can interact, resulting in toxic and other undesired effects.

Nutrient absorption and metabolism are particularly affected by drug therapies in the elderly. The ability to digest, absorb, and metabolize nutrients decreases with aging without the additional burden of drug usage, yet many of the drugs may be necessary.

Further study is especially needed among populations who take drugs for long periods; for example, women taking oral contraceptives and older Americans need further study.

Practicing physicians are encouraged to be familiar with drug-nutrition relationships. They are also encouraged to be at the forefront of efforts to reduce drug-induced malnutrition. Such efforts include legislation to bring certain nonprescription drugs under tighter control, constraints on excessive use of prescription drugs, and educational efforts. Although nurses, nutritionists, dietitians, and other allied health professionals do not prescribe drugs, their concerned participation in these efforts is obviously important.

PROGRESS CHECK ON ACTIVITY 2

Fill-in

1. Describe the most severe effects of hypervitaminosis A on an infant. _____

   _____

   _____

2. The amount of drugs appearing in breast milk depends upon three primary factors. Name them.

   a. _____

   b. _____

   c. _____

3. Describe the FAS infant. _____

   _____

   _____

4. Describe the effects of alcohol on the pregnant woman.

   _____

   _____

   _____

5. The effects of OCAs depend upon four characteristics of the user. What are the four characteristics?

   a. _____

   b. _____

   c. _____

   d. _____

6. List the three most important reasons that the elderly have adverse reactions to drugs.

   a. _____

   b. _____

   c. _____

7. Give three examples of the most common drug-nutrient interactions among the elderly.

   a. _____

   b. _____

   c. _____

Multiple Choice

8. Zinc taken during a pregnancy can cause
   a. premature deliveries.
   b. liver damage.

c. stillbirths.
d. a and b.
e. a and c.

9. Pregnant women who are carriers, or who have phenylketonuria, should avoid aspartame ingestion because it
   a. makes the infant hyperactive.
   b. causes birth defects.
   c. contain phenylalanine.
   d. contains caffeine.

10. The effects of recreational and/or medicinal drugs are most severe in the
    a. third trimester of pregnancy.
    b. first trimester of pregnancy.
    c. second trimester of pregnancy.
    d. entire pregnancy.

True/False

11. T F Prescription medications are safer than OTC medications.
12. T F Overmedicating means taking a larger dose than prescribed.
13. T F Drug-induced malnutrition is not a problem since so many supplements are available.
14. T F Education is the best method of preventing drug-induced malnutrition.
15. T F Some drugs are harmless to infants.
16. T F The physician is the person who must provide patient education regarding drug use.

Nursing Responsibilities

Nurses should be aware that generalities cannot assure proper administration, but knowledge of general principles may assist them in determining the many interactions.

1. Dietary nutrients affect drug actions, altering the pH, chelating, or changing the motility of the GI tract.
2. Drugs profoundly affect the action of the nutrients, interfering with absorption time and depleting body stores of essential nutrients.
3. Some diet and drug interactions create severe adverse side effects.
4. Some drug-nutrient interactions are synergistic.
5. Nutrients affect the distribution process by which drugs are delivered from the site of absorption to areas throughout the body. This process is also true for the effect of drugs on nutrients.
6. Drug-nutrient interactions profoundly affect digestion, absorption, metabolism, and elimination.
7. Many foods and drugs given together are totally incompatible, especially psychotropic drugs.
8. Since these processes are complicated, be prepared to repeat instructions to patients many times.
9. Effects of specific diet-drug reactions should be observed and documented. The patient should be informed.
10. Diet-drug interactions must be assessed on an individual basis for each drug and each individual.

References

Basu, T. K. 1988. *Drug-nutrient interactions*. New York: Croom, Helm and Methuen.

Bodinski, Lois. 1987. *The nurses' guide to diet therapy* (2nd ed.). New York: J. Wiley and Sons Medical Division.

Carruba, M. O., and J. E. Blundell (eds.). 1986. *Pharmacology of eating disorders: Theoretical and clinical developments*. New York: Raven Press.

Gilman, A. et al. 1985. *Goodman and Gilman's pharmacological basis of therapeutics* (7th ed.). New York: Macmillan.

Green and Harry. 1987. *Nutrition in contemporary nursing practice* (2nd ed.). New York: J. Wiley and Sons Medical Division.

Groisser, D. S., P. Rosso, and M. Winict. 1982. Coffee consumption during pregnancy, *Journal of Nutrition* 112:829.

Hui, Y. H. 1986. *Principles and issues in nutrition*. Monterey: Wadsworth Health Sciences.

Lamy, P. P. 1980. How our patients' diet can affect drug response. *Drug Therapy* 10.

Lillian, L. J. et al. 1982. Diet and ethanol intake during pregnancy. *Journal of the American Dietetic Association* 81:252.

Loebl, S., and G. R. Spratto. 1986. *The nurse's drug handbook* (4th ed.). New York: Wiley.

Malseed, R. T. 1985. *Pharmacology: Drug therapy and nursing considerations* (2nd ed.). Philadelphia: Lippincott.

McCabe, B. J. 1986. Dietary tyramine and other pressor amines in MAOI regimens: A review. *Journal of the American Dietetic Association* 86(8):1059.

Pagliaro. 1986. *Pharmacologic aspects of nursing*. St. Louis: Mosby.

Potter, P., and A. G. Perry. 1988. *Fundamentals of nursing*. St. Louis: Mosby.

Spiller, G. A. (ed.). 1981. Nutritional pharmacology. In *Current topics in nutrition and disease*, Vol. 4. New York: Alan R. Liss.

Roe, D. A. 1987. *Drug-induced nutritional deficiencies*. Westport, CT: AVI Publishing Co.

Roe, D. A. 1988. *Diet and drug interactions*. New York: Van Nostrand Reinhold.

Roe, D. A. 1988. Diet, nutrition, and drug reactions. In *Modern nutrition in health and disease* (7th ed.). M. E.

Shils and V. R. Young (eds.). Philadelphia: Lea & Febiger.

Rosett, H. L. et al. 1983. Patterns of alcohol consumption and fetal development. *Obstetrics and Gynecology* 61:539.

Sandler, M., and T. Silverstone (eds.). 1986. *British Association for Psychopharmacology Monograph No. 7. Psychopharmacology and food*. New York: Oxford University Press.

Smith, C. H., and W. R. Bidlack. 1984. Dietary concerns associated with the use of medications. *J. Amer. Diet. Assoc.* 84:901.

Spiller, G. A. (ed.). 1981. Nutritional pharmacology. In *Current topics in nutrition and disease*, Vol. 4. New York: Alan R. Liss.

Worthington-Roberts, et al. 1988. *Nutrition in pregnancy and lactation*. Times/Mirror College Publishing. St. Louis: Mosby.

Module 11

Food Ecology

Time for completion
Activities: _____1_____ hour
Optional examination: _½_ hour

Academic credit
Semester units: _²⁄₁₀_
Quarter units: _³⁄₁₀_

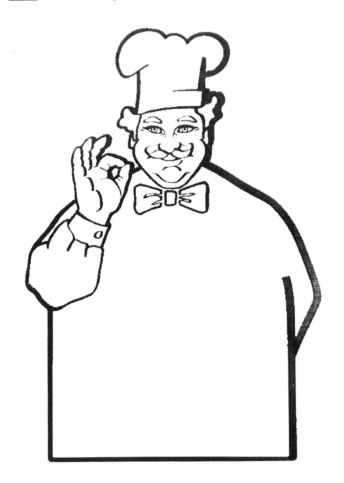

Outline

Objectives

Upon completion of this module, the student should be able to:

1. Describe the appropriate methods for the safe handling, storage, and preparation of food to prevent illness by:
   a. recognizing agents that cause food-borne illness;
   b. knowing ways to minimize contamination;
   c. becoming familiar with regulations regarding the protection of food.
2. Describe the appropriate methods for handling, storing, and preparing food to conserve nutrients by becoming knowledgeable about:
   a. nutrition labeling;
   b. pasteurization, enrichment, and fortification of foods.

Glossary

Bacteria: small unicellular microorganisms. They are spherical (cocci), rod shaped (bacilli), comma shaped (vibrios), or spiral (spirochetes). The symptoms produced by the bacteria depend on the type of bacteria ingested.

Enrichment: the addition of thiamin, niacin, riboflavin, and iron to bread and cereal products. The amount added to foods is set by the federal government.

Fortification: the addition of one or more nutrients not originally present in the food.

GRAS: generally recognized as safe. These are additives that have been used for a long time without known ill effects. Substances and additives sanctioned by the Food and Drug Administration prior to 1958.

Pasteurization: the practice of heating milk to 140 degrees Fahrenheit for 30 seconds to kill disease-producing bacteria, or to 161 degrees for 15 seconds.

Restoration: replacing food nutrients that were present before processing but were destroyed by the processing.

URI: upper respiratory infection.

Virus: a minute microorganism much smaller than a bacterium. It has no independent cell activity. Viruses reproduce inside a host cell. More than 200 disease-producing viruses have been identified.

Background Information

No matter how thorough an individual's knowledge is regarding the nutritional value of foods, unless the food is safe, there can be no optimal diets. No matter how carefully selected, food can only provide nourishment and health if it has been handled in such a way that it is neither contaminated nor a source of food-borne illness. Certain organisms that are transmitted to humans through food cause illness and sometimes death.

Modern food technology and sanitation practices have greatly reduced the threat of commercial food contamination. Food labelings have enabled consumers to be aware of the contents of food purchased. However, unsafe food handling practices and nutrient losses from food preparation persist and continue to create problems even in modern societies. This is especially true in any group-eating environments, including health care facilities, shelter and retirement centers, schools, and restaurants.

ACTIVITY 1: Food Safety

Causes of Food-Borne Illness

The three most common biological agents of illness, which are transmitted to people from the food supply, are bacteria, parasites, and viruses. The two most common factors causing transmission are human carelessness and lack of knowledge of food handling. Examples of causative factors include

1. Contamination of the water supply.
2. Sewage seeping into livestock food.
3. Poor personal hygiene—for example, from the oral-fecal route, not washing hands after using the toilet.
4. Improper storage of raw foods, especially eggs, meats, fish, poultry, and dairy products.
5. Improper storage of cooked foods—for example, using deep pans for storage of hot food which slows the cooling of food.
6. Improper preparation of foods—for example,

undercooking food, especially pork and pork products.

7. Improper holding temperatures—that is, above 40 degrees and below 140 degrees Fahrenheit. Improper thawing of frozen food, such as at room temperature.
8. Poor health practices, especially in group settings. Examples include sneezing and coughing into food, blowing nose over food, not washing hands before handling food, and handling food with hands that have open sores or boils.
9. Contamination by organisms transmitted from food handler to food or equipment and cross contamination between foods.
10. Lack of knowledge by food handlers of the potential hazards of the organisms they carry.

For reference purposes, Table 11-1 describes the characteristics of some common food-borne diseases.

TABLE 11-1
Characteristics of Different Food-Borne Diseases

Disease and Organism That Causes It	Source of Illness	Symptoms	Prevention Methods
Salmonellosis *Salmonella* (bacteria; more than 1,700 kinds)	May be found in raw meats, poultry, eggs, fish, milk, and products made with them. Multiplies rapidly at room temperature.	Onset: 12–48 hours after eating. Nausea, fever, headache, abdominal cramps, diarrhea, and sometimes vomiting. Can be fatal in infants, the elderly, and the infirm.	Handling food in a sanitary manner. Thorough cooking of foods. Prompt and proper refrigeration of foods.
Staphylococcal food poisoning Staphylococcal enterotoxin (produced by *Staphylococcus aureus* bacteria)	The toxin is produced when food contaminated with the bacteria is left too long at room temperature. Meats, poultry, egg products, tuna, potato and macaroni salads, and cream-filled pastries are good environments for these bacteria to produce toxin.	Onset: 1–8 hours after eating. Diarrhea, vomiting, nausea, abdominal cramps, and prostration. Mimics flu. Lasts 24–48 hours. Rarely fatal.	Sanitary food handling practices. Prompt and proper refrigeration of foods.
Botulism Botulinum toxin (produced by *Clostridium botulinum* bacteria)	Bacteria are widespread in the environment. However, bacteria produce toxin only in an anaerobic (oxygenless) environment of little acidity. Types A, B, and F may result from inadequate processing of low-acid canned foods, such as green beans, mushrooms, spinach, olives, and beef. Type E normally occurs in fish.	Onset: 8–36 hours after eating. Neurotoxic symptoms, including double vision, inability to swallow, speech difficulty, and progressive paralysis of the respiratory system. **Obtain medical help immediately. Botulism can be fatal.**	Using proper methods for canning low-acid foods. Avoidance of commercially canned low-acid foods with leaky seals or with bent, bulging, or broken cans. Toxin can be destroyed after a can is opened by boiling contents hard for 10 minutes—**not recommended.**
Perfringens food poisoning *Clostridium perfringens* (rod-shaped bacteria)	Bacteria are widespread in environment. Generally found in meat and poultry and dishes made with them. Multiply rapidly when foods are left at room temperature too long. Destroyed by cooking.	Onset: 8–22 hours after eating (usually 12). Abdominal pain and diarrhea. Sometimes nausea and vomiting. Symptoms last a day or less and are usually mild. Can be more serious in older or debilitated people.	Sanitary handling of foods, especially meat and meat dishes and gravies. Thorough cooking of foods. Prompt and proper refrigeration.

(continues)

Bacteria and Food Temperature

In order to minimize the risk of food-borne illnesses, all individuals should take care to keep food clean to prevent bacteria from multiplying and to adequately cook fresh and frozen meat, fish, poultry, and eggs.

The majority of cases of food poisoning are from bacteria or toxin from the bacteria. If we know what causes bacteria to multiply, we can take preventive measures.

Given a few pathogens and favorable conditions, a harmless food can quickly become a source of illness.

Bacteria thrive in foods that are moist, warm, good sources of protein, and low in acid. A few thrive in the absence of oxygen supply (anaerobic). These bacteria are usually in home-canned low acid foods where they produce the deadly "botulism" toxin.

The time-temperature factor is critical in preventing bacteria from multiplying. After purchasing food, it is

TABLE 11-1 (Continued)

Disease and Organism That Causes It	Source of Illness	Symptoms	Prevention Methods
Shigellosis (bacillary dysentery) *Shigella* (bacteria)	Food becomes contaminated when a human carrier with poor sanitary habits handles liquid or moist food that is then not cooked thoroughly. Organisms multiply in food stored above room temperature. Found in milk and dairy products, poultry, and potato salad.	Onset: 1–7 days after eating. Abdominal pain, cramps, diarrhea, fever, sometimes vomiting, and blood, pus, or mucus in stools. Can be serious in infants, the elderly, or debilitated people.	Handling food in a sanitary manner. Proper sewage disposal. Proper refrigeration of foods.
Campylobacterosis *Campylobacter jejuni* (rod-shaped bacteria)	Bacteria found on poultry, cattle, and sheep and can contaminate the meat and milk of these animals. Chief food sources: raw poultry and meat and unpasteurized milk.	Onset: 2–5 days after eating. Diarrhea, abdominal cramping, fever, and sometimes bloody stools. Lasts 2–7 days.	Thorough cooking of foods. Handling food in a sanitary manner. Avoiding unpasteurized milk.
Gastroenteritis *Yersinia enterocolitica* (nonspore-forming bacteria)	Ubiquitous in nature, carried in food and water. Bacteria multiply rapidly at room temperature, as well as at refrigerator temperatures (4° to 9° C). Generally found in raw vegetables, meats, water, and unpasteurized milk.	Onset: 2–5 days after eating. Fever, headache, nausea, diarrhea, and general malaise. Mimics flu. An important cause of gastroenteritis in children. Can also infect other age groups and, if not treated, can lead to other more serious diseases (such as lymphadenitis, arthritis, and Reiter's syndrome).	Thorough cooking of foods. Sanitizing cutting instruments and cutting boards before preparing foods that are eaten raw. Avoidance of unpasteurized milk and unchlorinated water.
Cereus food poisoning *Bacillus cereus* (bacteria and possibly their toxin)	Illness may be caused by the bacteria, which are widespread in the environment, or by an enterotoxin created by the bacteria. Found in raw foods. Bacteria multiply rapidly in foods stored at room temperature.	Onset: 1–18 hours after eating. Two types of illness: (1) abdominal pain and diarrhea, and (2) nausea and vomiting. Lasts less than a day.	Sanitary handling of foods. Thorough cooking of foods. Prompt and adequate refrigeration.
Cholera *Vibrio cholera* (bacteria)	Found in fish and shellfish harvested from waters contaminated by human sewage. (Bacteria may also occur naturally in Gulf Coast waters.) Chief food sources: seafood, especially types eaten raw (such as oysters).	Onset: 1–3 days. Can range from "subclinical" (a mild uncomplicated bout with diarrhea) to fatal (intense diarrhea with dehydration). Severe cases require hospitalization.	Sanitary handling of foods. Thorough cooking of seafood.
Parahaemolyticus food poisoning *Vibrio parahaemolyticus* (bacteria)	Organism lives in salt water and can contaminate fish and shellfish. Thrives in warm weather.	Onset: 15–24 hours after eating. Abdominal pain, nausea, vomiting, and diarrhea. Sometimes fever, headache, chills, and mucus and blood in the stools. Lasts 1–2 days. Rarely fatal.	Sanitary handling of foods. Thorough cooking of seafood.

(continues)

TABLE 11-1 (Continued)

Disease and Organism That Causes It	Source of Illness	Symptoms	Prevention Methods
Gastrointestinal disease Enteroviruses rotaviruses parvoviruses	Viruses exist in the intestinal tract of humans and are expelled in feces. Contamination of foods can occur in three ways: (1) when sewage is used to enrich garden/farm soil; (2) by direct hand-to-food contact during the preparation of meals; and (3) when shellfish-growing waters are contaminated by sewage.	Onset: After 24 hours. Severe diarrhea, nausea, and vomiting. Respiratory symptoms. Usually last 4–5 days but may last for weeks.	Sanitary handling of foods. Use of pure drinking water. Adequate sewage disposal. Adequate cooking of foods.
Hepatitis Hepatitis A virus	Chief food sources: shellfish harvested from contaminated areas, and foods that are handled a lot during preparation and then eaten raw (such as vegetables).	Jaundice, fatigue. May cause liver damage and death.	Sanitary handling of foods. Use of pure drinking water. Adequate sewage disposal. Adequate cooking of foods.
Mycotoxicosis Mycotoxins (from molds)	Produced in foods that are relatively high in moisture. Chief food sources: beans and grains that have been stored in a moist place.	May cause liver and/or kidney disease.	Checking foods for visible mold and discarding those that are contaminated. Proper storage of susceptible foods.
Giardiasis *Giardia lamblia* (flagellated protozoa)	Protozoa exist in the intestinal tract of humans and are expelled in feces. Contamination of foods can occur in two ways: (1) when sewage is used to enrich garden/farm soil; and (2) by direct hand-to-food contact during the preparation of meals. Chief food sources: foods that are handled a lot during preparation.	Diarrhea, abdominal pain, flatulence, abdominal distention, nutritional disturbances, "nervous" symptoms, anorexia, nausea, and vomiting.	Sanitary handling of foods. Avoidance of raw fruits and vegetables in areas where the protozoa is endemic. Proper sewage disposal.
Amebiasis *Entamoeba histolytica* (amoebic protozoa)		Tenderness over the colon or liver, loose morning stools, recurrent diarrhea, change in bowel habits, "nervous" symptoms, loss of weight, and fatigue. Anemia may be present.	Sanitary handling of foods. Avoidance of raw fruits and vegetables in areas where the protozoa is endemic. Proper sewage disposal.

Source: C. L. Ballentine and M. L. Herndon, *FDA Consumer*, July-August 1982, pp. 25–28.

essential to minimize the opportunity for bacteria incubation by properly storing, preparing, and handling food. Figure 11-1 depicts the effects of temperature on potential disease-producing organisms.

Observation of safe food preparation practices is an effective way to prevent food-borne illness. These practices, which all family members should observe, are listed below.

Safe Food Preparation Practices _____

Observe personal hygiene:

1. Hands should always be clean whenever food is handled. Hot water and soap should be used to wash hands after going to the bathroom, before handling cooked foods, and after handling raw food.
2. A person who is ill should not prepare food.
3. During food preparation, contact between hands and the mouth, nose, or hair should be avoided, as should coughing and sneezing over foods. Tissues or handkerchiefs should be used to prevent contamination.
4. Tasting food with fingers and utensils used during preparation is not advised, even if the cooking temperature is very hot.

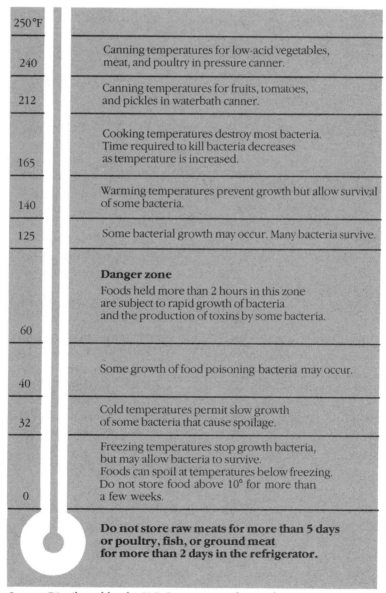

Source: Distributed by the U.S. Department of Agriculture.

Figure 11-1
Temperature Guide to Food Safety

The following guidelines apply to the food environment:

1. All kitchen equipment and utensils should be thoroughly cleaned before being used with any foods.

2. Cooked foods should not be allowed to stand at room temperature for more than two to three hours whenever feasible. Exposure of food to temperatures between 5 degrees and 60 degrees Celsius (40 degrees and 140 degrees Fahrenheit) should be kept to a minimum. The practice of preparing foods a day or several hours before eating should be done with care and avoided if possible.

3. Hot foods should never be allowed to cool slowly to room temperature before refrigerating. The slow cooling period provides an ideal growth temperature for bacteria. Foods should be refrigerated immediately after removing from a steam table or warming oven. A shallow pan, cold running water, or ice bath can be used to cool foods rapidly for storage. A large amount of food in a big container requires additional cooling time before all the contents are below 7 degrees Celsius (45 degrees Fahrenheit), potentially creating an environment for bacteria to grow.

4. When leftovers are served, the food should be heated until all parts reach a temperature of 74 degrees Celsius (165 degrees Fahrenheit). This destroys all vegetative cells of bacteria. Whenever applicable, food should be chopped into small pieces and boiled to destroy any susceptible vegetative cells of the bacteria. No cooling should be permitted after preparation—the food should be served hot.

5. Certain popular foods—stuffed turkey, gravies, cream pies and puddings, sandwiches, and salads—are frequent culprits in food poisoning. When preparing roast turkey, do not stuff the bird but cook the stuffing separately. If turkey is stuffed with raw fillers, avoid stuffing it the night before. If stuffing is cooked separately, it should be cooked immediately after mixing, especially if in a large quantity. Stuffing is an excellent place for bacteria to grow, and if a large amount of lukewarm stuffing is permitted to stand at room temperature, the organisms will surely multiply.

6. Gravies and broths are quite susceptible to bacterial contamination, especially as leftovers. These foods should be placed in the refrigerator as soon as possible. Gravy or broth should not be held in the refrigerator more than one or two days, and it should be reheated or boiled for several minutes before serving. A reheated dressing should not be permitted to stay at room temperature.

7. Cream pies and puddings are also often involved in food poisoning. People dislike keeping these items in the refrigerator, because they can become soggy. However, leaving them at room temperature can allow bacteria to multiply rapidly. Ideally, such pastries should be prepared as close to serving time as possible.

8. Items such as ham sandwiches, turkey and chicken salads, and deviled eggs require special attention. One good practice is to freeze the sandwiches immediately after preparation and thaw them whenever they are needed. Chicken salads may be prepared by using frozen chicken cubes, which will thaw as the salad stands. The entire salad dish should be kept cool.

Responsibilities of Health Personnel

A health practitioner should emphasize the following when educating a client, an institution, or the general public:

1. Observe sanitary practices that minimize the likelihood of food-borne illness.
2. Teach all family members the principles of cleanliness.
3. Check closely for sanitary, safe practices being followed among all personnel working in a health care setting.
4. Make your clients aware that bacteria are a major cause of food-borne illness, and that they thrive in a warm, moist environment.
5. Foods kept at a temperature between 60 degrees and 125 degrees Fahrenheit for more than two hours may not be safe to eat.
6. Observe good hand washing technique.
7. Advise individuals not to work with or around food when they are ill or have any skin lesions.
8. If insecticides are used, counsel extreme caution in cooking and eating areas to prevent contamination of food.
9. Regularly inspect all areas where food is stored and prepared.
10. Perform laboratory cultures on a regular basis in health care facilities.
11. Encourage mandatory regular teaching of food personnel and demonstrations of appropriate techniques of safe food handling.
12. Check the source of supply of food items (supplier).
13. Purchase only those food items that meet government regulations for safety, such as pasteurized milk and dairy products, USDA inspected meats, and fish.

PROGRESS CHECK ON ACTIVITY 1

Fill-in

1. Describe five ways in which a food may be contaminated by a food handler.

   a. _____

   b. _____

   c. _____

d. _____

e. _____

2. The storage temperature of perishable foods must be *below* _____ degrees F or *above* _____ degrees F in order to retard the growth of bacteria.
   a. 32 degrees F, 200 degrees F
   b. 40 degrees F, 140 degrees F
   c. 60 degrees F, 170 degrees F
   d. 80 degrees F, 190 degrees F

3. What is the major causative agent in food-borne illness? _____

   _____

4. Describe how temperature and moisture affect the growth of organisms. _____

   _____

5. List five prevention methods for contamination of foods.
   a. _____
   b. _____
   c. _____
   d. _____
   e. _____

6. List the most common gastrointestinal symptoms of food-borne illness. _____

   _____

True/False

Circle T for True and F for False.

7. T F Leftover food should be cooled completely before it is refrigerated.
8. T F Cooking reduces the number of pathogenic bacteria, but does not destroy all of them.
9. T F Cooking may not provide protection against food contaminated with staphylococcus.

10. T F Cooking destroys most parasites and viruses.

Case Study

You are invited to the residence of a friend who runs a day care center for the elderly. She has six residents plus her own family, and has hired a person to cook who has had no previous training. While you are visiting, you observe the following procedures (comment on the food handling practices in each instance given):

11. A pot of homemade beef vegetable soup was made the night before and left on the counter overnight because there was not room to refrigerate it. The cook is not concerned because she has plans to reheat it before serving. _____

    _____

    _____

12. The cook takes several cans of green beans from a cupboard to heat and two of them are rusty at the seams. One has a little leakage, but none of the cans are bulged. Should you warn her not to use them? Explain. _____

    _____

    _____

13. The cook assembles the ingredients for potato salad before she begins preparation. She then takes a break and runs a few errands before she prepares the potato salad. _____

    _____

    _____

14. The cook takes the cutting board from under the sink near the water pipes and cuts and finely chops all the vegetables, fruits, and meats she plans to use for the next two meals. She then puts them in a deep, open pan and refrigerates them. _____

    _____

    _____

ACTIVITY 2: Nutrient Conservation

Nutrients can be lost during storage, preparation, and cooking of foods, as demonstrated in Activity 1. Nutrients may also be lost during processing or preservation of foods.

Using good food preparation methods to maximize nutrient retention is especially important when the diet is limited or low in certain nutrients. The following measures are recommended to minimize loss during storage, preparation, and cooking.

Storage

1. Avoid bruising soft fresh produce such as berries and peaches.
2. Store perishable items at the recommended temperature, usually in the refrigerator or freezer.
3. Store foods, except fresh meats, in containers that allow little room for air to circulate, or wrap the foods in moisture/vapor-proof material.

4. Package green vegetables in such a way that they stay crisp. Keep them slightly moist, not wet. (Washed lettuce keeps well if wrapped loosely in a clean towel and enclosed in a plastic bag.)

5. Store less perishable items (such as canned foods, dry cereals, cooking oils) in a cool dry place.

6. If foods are not stored in opaque or colored glass containers, store away from the light.

7. Use fresh foods as quickly after harvesting as possible.

8. Store food in glass jars in a dark place.

9. Plan for fast turnover of food on the shelf or in the refrigerator to avoid long storage times. Use leftovers as soon as possible.

Preparation

1. Prepare fresh produce as close to time of use as is practical.

2. Use very sharp knife for cutting fresh produce.

3. Avoid soaking cut fruits and vegetables, especially if they are your major source of any water-soluble nutrients.

4. When appropriate, scrub vegetables instead of paring them and leave them whole instead of cutting them.

5. If paring is desired, pare as thinly as possible. If practical (as for beets and potatoes), peel after cooking.

6. Use clean fresh vegetable parings for making stock for soup.

7. Use the liquid from canned fruit as an ingredient in homemade fruit punch.

8. Save time, fuel, and nutrients by eating raw fruits and vegetables often.

9. Avoid reheating leftover cooked vegetables by using them in cold salads.

10. Discard bruised or dried outside leaves of vegetables.

Cooking

1. Cook vegetables for the shortest time possible, just until tender.

2. If cooking any type of vegetable in water, make sure it is boiling rapidly before vegetable is added.

3. Cook vegetables in the smallest amount of water practical for the type of pan, but take care not to scorch them. A small volume of water is especially helpful to reduce nutrient loss when cooking vegetables that are cut into small pieces. Cover the pan tightly to minimize the amount of water needed.

4. Steam, microwave, or pressure cook clean, whole, unpeeled vegetables.

5. Stir-fry vegetables the Chinese way.

6. Plan meals so that vegetables can be served as soon as they are cooked.

7. Heat canned vegetables in the liquid in which they are packed.

8. Use cooking liquid from vegetables and drippings from meat for gravy, sauces, soup stock, or for cooking grains such as rice. Small amounts of cooking liquid can be saved and stored in the freezer.

9. Do not add baking soda when cooking vegetables, even though it makes green vegetables stay brightly colored.

Food Additives as Nutrients

In order to process food and preserve nutrients, chemical substances are added to foods. While these procedures are necessary, they have confused the consumer and changed the nutrient content of many foods. In addition, new foods are being introduced to the consumer daily for which the nutrient content is unknown. Some measures to protect and enlighten the consumer have been established by the government.

The Food and Drug Administration (FDA) enforces laws and regulations to ensure that food is safe, wholesome, and properly labeled. Outside substances are present, intentionally and accidentally, in food as a result of processing, storage, or packaging. Some additives are intentionally added to food to enhance its nutritional value. This takes three forms:

1. *Enrichment.* The addition of thiamin, niacin, riboflavin, and iron to bread, flour, and cereal products in amounts set by the government.

2. *Restoration.* The addition of nutrients to a food to restore it to its original quality. These are nutrients that have been lost through manufacturing or processing.

3. *Fortification.* Addition to food of one or more nutrients not originally present or occurring only in minute amounts. Some examples are: adding vitamin D to milk; adding vitamins A and D to skim milk and nonfat dry milk; adding iodine to salt; and adding fluoride to water.

Nonnutritive additives do not improve quality. They preserve food and prevent unwanted changes (for example, antioxidants).

All additives to food must be approved by the FDA. There is a category of additives generally recognized as safe (known as GRAS). These substances are sanctioned by the FDA and have been in widespread use over a long period of time without known ill effects. All others must undergo rigid testing before being added to foods.

In order to protect consumers and educate them about their nutrient intakes, the FDA has established regulations for food labeling.

Nutritional labeling is mandatory on FDA-regulated products as of January 1993 (see Module 1). There is a standardized format for presenting the information.

Summary

The government's role and the individual's role in conserving nutrients are important considerations for health personnel.

Safeguarding the food supply, appropriate selection and purchase of foods, label reading, and knowledge of nutrition principles can prevent illness and improve health.

Responsibilities of Health Personnel

When counseling a client, an institution, or the general public, a health practitioner should

1. Teach clients that many foods lose nutrients, especially vitamins, during storage.
2. Teach clients that food storage at warm temperatures increases nutrient loss as well as bacterial and insect growth.
3. Make clients aware that nutrients are lost by unnecessary trimming, dissolving, soaking, or cooking foods in water.
4. Teach clients that nutrients are lost by overcooking.
5. Teach clients and families that proper food storage, preparation, and cooking techniques can improve their nutritional status.
6. Educate consumers about the advantages and proper reading of nutrition labels.
7. Encourage clients to learn the general principles of nutrition.
8. Encourage food producers to maintain high quality products.

PROGRESS CHECK ON ACTIVITY 2

Fill-in

1. Nutrition labeling is not mandatory in what two circumstances?

   a. _____

   b. _____

2. List three advantages to nutrition labeling.

   a. _____

   b. _____

   c. _____

3. Identify three practices to preserve nutrient content of foods during storage.

   a. _____

   b. _____

   c. _____

4. Identify at least six food preparation and cooking practices that keep nutrient loss at a minimum.

   a. _____

   b. _____

   c. _____

   d. _____

   e. _____

   f. _____

Define the following terms:

5. Enrichment _____

6. Fortification _____

7. Restoration _____

8. Name two types of food additives and give one example of each.

   a. _____

   b. _____

References

Ballentine, C. L., and M. L. Herndon. *FDA Consumer.* July-Aug. 1982. pp. 25–28.

Branen, A. L. et al. 1990. *Food additives.* New York: Marcel Dekker.

Cheeke, P. R. 1989. *Toxicants of plant origin.* Boca Raton, FL: CRC Press.

Chia, J. K. et al. 1986. Botulism in an adult associated with foodborne intestinal infection with *Clostridium botulinum. New England Journal of Medicine* 315:239.

Cohen, S. M. 1986. Saccharin: Past, present, and future. *Journal of the American Dietetic Association* 86:929.

Concon, J. M. 1987. *Food toxicology, contaminants, and additives,* vols. 1, 2. New York: Marcel Dekker.

Lawler, P. F. 1986. *Sweet talk: Media coverage of artificial sweeteners.* Washington, DC: The Media Institute.

Lewis, R. J. Sr. 1989. *Food additives handbook.* New York: Van Nostrand Reinhold.

Monahan, J. P. 1984. *Food poisoning.* Lackawazen, PA: Medical-Info Books.

Newberne, P. M. 1988. Naturally occurring food-borne toxicants. In *Modern nutrition in health and disease* (7th ed.). M. E. Shils and V. R. Young (eds.). Philadelphia: Lea & Febiger.

Nightingale, S. L. 1987. Foodborne disease: An increasing problem. *Am. Family Physic.* 35:353.

Noah, N. D. 1985. Food poisoning. *British Medical Journal* 291:879.

Rechcigl, M., Jr. (ed.). 1983. *Foodborne diseases of biological origin*. Boca Raton, FL: CRC Press.

Rogan, A., and G. Glaros. 1988. Food irradiation: The process and implications for dietitians. *Journal of the American Dietetic Association* 88:833.

Ryser, E. T., and E. H. Marth. 1989. New foodborne pathogens of public health significance. *Journal of the American Dietetic Association* 89:949.

Senti, F. R. 1988. Food additives and contaminants. In *Modern nutrition in health and disease* (7th ed.). M. E. Shils and V. R. Young (eds.). Philadelphia: Lea & Febiger.

Walker, R., and E. Quattrucci (eds.). 1988. *Nutritional and toxicological aspects of food processing*. Philadelphia: Taylor and Francis.

Part III

NUTRITION AND DIET THERAPY FOR ADULTS

Nutri-Calc
Nutrition Software for the 90's

Since 1985 CAMDE has offered the Nutri-Calc series of nutrient analysis software programs. These programs can be used to analyze recipes, diets, or meals for their nutrient content. Each offers fast and easy selection of foods, graphical analysis displays, expandable food databases, adjustable food quantity measures, and many other advanced features.

As a special offer made to purchasers of this book, CAMDE's programs can be purchased at a substantial discount. These are the full regular programs, not limited student versions.

Nutri-Calc   **Regularly $95   Only $57!**
It has 1600+ foods, with 30 nutrients. Compare diets to the RDA's, Canadian RNI's, or enter other dietary goals. Enter exercise and other activities to estimate caloric expenditure. Nutri-Calc requires an IBM PC or compatible with 512K RAM.

Nutri-Calc HD   **Regularly $225   Only $135!**
This is a more comprehensive program for use on IBM PC compatibles. It has 3400+ foods, with 30 nutrients. In addition to the features in Nutri-Calc, Nutri-Calc HD can save and plot history data, has extensive printing options, ability to save and include notes, and several other features. The program requires a Hard Disk and 512K RAM.

Nutri-Calc Plus   **Regularly $225   Only $135!**
For use on the Apple Macintosh, this top-rated nutrition program allows diets and recipes to be analyzed for 32 nutrients. The program has extensive graphical displays. History data is maintained, so nutrient intake can be plotted over time. The program includes 3800+ foods.

To order, please call CAMDE at (602)821-2310, or complete this form and mail it to:

CAMDE Corporation
P.O. Box 2006
Chandler, Arizona 85244-2006

If ordering by phone, please be sure to mention this book when ordering.

* *

[   ] Please send one copy of _____

Name: _____

Address:_____

City, State, Zip: _____

Phone: _____ Disk Size: [ ] 5.25"   [ ] 3.5"

Payment: Check [   ]   Mastercard [   ]   Visa [   ]

Name On Card:_____

Card #: _____ Exp. Date: _____

Signature: _____

Orders subject to approval of CAMDE. Prices subject to change without notice.

Overview of Therapeutic Nutrition

Time for completion
Activities: _____1_____ hour
Optional examination: _½_ hour

Academic credit
Semester units: _²⁄₁₀_
Quarter units: _³⁄₁₀_

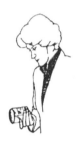
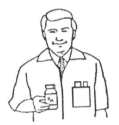
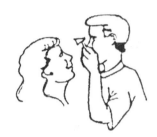
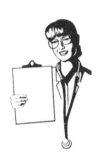
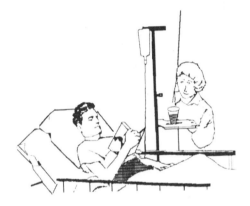

Outline

Objectives

Upon completion of this module, the student should be able to:

1. Define the principles of diet therapy.
2. Explain the objectives of diet therapy.
3. Describe the methods used to adapt a normal diet to treat a specific clinical disorder.
4. Identify the most common therapeutic diets used in clinical care.

Glossary

Acculturation: traditions, values, or religious beliefs that comprise a way of life (see Module 2, Part 1).

Ascites: an abnormal accumulation of fluid in the peritoneal cavity resulting in distention of the abdomen.

Diet therapy: The use of any diet for restoring or maintaining optimal nutritional status and body homeostasis.

Distention: stretching, enlarging.

Edema: abnormal accumulation of fluid in body tissues (intercellular space).

Gastritis: inflammation of the stomach.

Liquid diet: a modified diet consisting of foods that pour or become liquid at body temperature (see Activity 2).

Milieu: surroundings, environment.

Modified diet: a regular diet that has been altered to meet specific requirements of individuals with a disease or disorder.

Peritoneal: pertaining to the serous membrane lining the walls of the abdominal and pelvic cavities.

Satiety: feeling of fullness, satisfaction.

Soft diet: a regular diet that has been modified in texture and/or seasoning, depending on the medical needs of the patient (see Activity 2).

Background Information

Basic Principles

Therapeutic nutrition is based on the modification of the nutrients or other aspects of a normal diet to meet a person's nutritional needs during an illness. An understanding of the basics of normal nutrition is a prerequisite to the study of the principles of diet therapy. A nurse's background in anatomy, physiology, and pathophysiology will facilitate the clinical application of these principles.

The purpose of diet therapy is to restore or maintain an acceptable nutritional status of a patient. This is accomplished by modifying one or more of the following aspects of the diet:

1. basic nutrient(s)
2. caloric contribution
3. texture or consistency
4. seasonings

In adapting a normal diet to treat a disease, one or more of the above modifications may be needed to restore or maintain the good nutritional status of a given patient. In general, all therapeutic diets must consider physical factors, clinical disorders, and the patient's total acculturation.

In many cases the patient may require an alteration of feeding methods in order to accomplish the stated purpose of diet therapy. It may also become necessary to alter the feeding intervals. These changes will be discussed in Activity 2.

The nurse's role is critical in helping a patient adjust to a modified diet by acting as the coordinator, interpreter, and teacher of diet therapy. Meeting the patient's nutritional needs involves the coordination of the medical, dietary, and nursing staff. In larger hospitals, the nurse maintains liaisons among the patient, the physician, and the dietitian; assists the patient at meals; observes the patient's response to foods and beverages; charts pertinent information; and supports and supplements the primary instruction given by the dietitian. In small hospitals, nursing homes, and community nursing services, the nurse may be responsible for planning, supervising, and teaching the modified diet. In many cases, the nurse may need to interpret the diet and make food selections both for the patient and the kitchen personnel.

Kinds and Uses of Exchange Lists

Exchange lists for calculating various modified diets are employed by nutritionists, dietitians, and other health professionals to accurately calculate the amounts and kinds of foods required. These include exchange lists for diabetes, weight reduction or gain, renal disorders, and phenylketonuria. The bases for all these lists are the food groups for selecting a balanced diet. Food lists are classified primarily on their key nutrients, all the foods in a particular group having approximately the same set of nutrients. When diets are calculated, for whatever reason, the recommended servings are intended to provide at least 80 percent of the RDAs for all nutrients. When the health professional instructs a client, he or she does not use the figures from nutrients when instructing. Instead, figures are given in terms of foods that will meet the nutrient requirement. The basic food groups, therefore, are very practical. The patient can use them to plan menus, order meals in restaurants, and make grocery lists. Checking the foods selected from each group can give the patient and counselor an estimate of how adequate the diet is. The food groups do not account for ethnic and mixed dishes, and will need to be interpreted according to variations acceptable to the client. Supplements to the food groups can be added whenever the diet is not adequate for a particular individual.

The Food Exchange System of Dietary Control. This system is widely used in planning all kinds of diets. It is based on six exchange lists, which group foods according to their carbohydrate, protein, and fat content. Caloric content of the diet can be calculated when these are known. Diets can therefore be designed to modify basic nutrients, energy value, texture, and/or seasonings (primarily sodium content). (See Activity 3.) The percentage of each of the energy nutrients (carbohydrate, protein, and fat) in the diet can be figured to meet the dietary guidelines for Americans. The exchange system is presented in Appendix E.

Renal Diet Exchange System. For patients with renal disease, the exchange lists become even more detailed. These individuals must be able to pick foods from each of the lists in a renal exchange diet that do not exceed their prescribed levels of sodium, potassium, calcium, and protein, as well as managing total calories and any fluid restrictions. Renal patients are usually counseled several times by the health team and closely followed to assess compliance and needed nutrient changes. Since these diets are very individualized, an exchange list for renal patients is not included in this book. See Module 19 for details on the treatment of renal disorders.

Exchange Lists for Phenylketonuria (PKU). By nature of the metabolic error that creates an infant with PKU, the exchanges are created for two main purposes: to furnish adequate nutrition for rapid growth and a healthy child while keeping the phenylalanine level low enough to prevent the mental retardation and other unacceptable changes that take place when rigid diet control is not imposed.

The exchange lists for PKU infants and children are not within the scope of this book, but the health professional should be aware that these lists are available and be proficient in providing caregivers of these children with instructions concerning them. See Module 26 for more details on PKU, the disease and treatment.

The use of the new labeling laws as discussed in Module 1 will add to the ability of the professional to provide additional information to consumers when they are interpreting these lists. Consumers who learn to read the labels will find that they are more confident and better able to follow diet instructions when using any of the lists.

PROGRESS CHECK ON BACKGROUND INFORMATION

Fill-in

1. What is the major principle of therapeutic nutrition?

   _____

   _____

2. State the purpose of diet therapy. _____

   _____

3. Describe the methods used to adapt a normal diet to a disease condition. _____

   _____

   _____

4. What are the four most common therapeutic diet modifications?

   a. _____

   b. _____

   c. _____

   d. _____

5. Identify four illness factors that affect food consumption.

   a. _____

   b. _____

   c. _____

   d. _____

6. Explain the nurse's role in helping a patient adjust to a therapeutic diet modification.

   a. _____

   b. _____

   c. _____

   d. _____

ACTIVITY 1: *Principles and Objectives of Diet Therapy*

Health professionals in care of the hospitalized patient must consider the physiological, psychological, cultural, social, and economic factors of the patient. Illness may alter any of these factors.

The stress of illness brings about many fears in the hospitalized patient and often causes personality changes.

Immobilization can disrupt nutritional balance and interfere with patient care. In addition, drug therapy often reduces food intake and interferes with nutrient utilization. The disease process itself modifies food acceptance. Food preferences may revert to those of childhood favorites. Symbolic security foods may be desired. Some patients express their fear, frustration, and hostility by rejecting food and showing resentment toward everyone connected with it.

Another major stress is the frequent necessity to modify the diet. When confronted with this necessity, patients frequently respond irrationally and refuse to accept the change. The health team can help a hospitalized patient accept a therapeutic diet by recognizing the many factors that affect the patient and then helping with the adjustment. In this milieu, the nurse becomes the key to the success or failure of a modified diet.

The patient's nutritional needs are evaluated according to past nutrition practices and the clinical disorder. If nutritional status was poor before admission, the patient's needs will be greater than those of a well-nourished patient. Each analysis must be individualized.

The focus of diet therapy is on the patient's identified needs and problems. The diet plan should be relevant to the nature of the illness and its effects on the body. It should be based on sound, scientific rationale in line with current nutrition concepts. The nurse should question a prescribed diet that shows no apparent relationship to the disease. It is helpful to educate the patient by providing a rationale and expected effects of the modified diet.

PROGRESS CHECK ON ACTIVITY 1

Fill-in

1. List five factors that affect the nutritional care of the hospitalized patient.

    a. _____

    b. _____

    c. _____

    d. _____

    e. _____

2. List four ways that the stress of illness affects food acceptance.

    a. _____

    b. _____

    c. _____

    d. _____

3. What is the focus of diet therapy? _____

    _____

    _____

4. Upon what principle is therapeutic nutrition based?

    _____

    _____

5. What is the purpose of diet therapy? _____

    _____

    _____

    _____

ACTIVITY 2: Routine Hospital Diets

Regular Diets

The "normal," "regular," or "house" diet is the most frequently used of all diets in hospitals. A normal diet, like a modified diet, is of great importance in a therapeutic sense. When a patient eats well, the body's damaged tissues (from the illness) are continuously repaired and maintained.

The normal diet in a hospital must meet the Recommended Dietary Allowances (RDAs). During illnesses, the additional stress is often accommodated by increasing these allowances. The daily food groups are often the basis for dietary planning. The normal hospital diet has no restrictions of food choice.

Soft Diets

The soft diet is the second most common hospital diet. It differs from a normal diet in texture and seasonings. Usually ordered as "mechanical soft" or fiber-restricted, depending on the needs of the patient, the soft diet is a

nutritionally adequate diet. The following differentiates these two types of soft diet.

Mechanical Soft Diet

The mechanical soft diet is limited to soft foods for those who have difficulty chewing food because of missing teeth or poorly fitting dentures. The seasonings and preparation of this diet are the same as those for a normal diet.

Table 12-1 describes foods permitted in a mechanical soft diet.

Soft Diet (Fiber-Restricted)

The soft fiber-restricted diet differs from the normal diet in being reduced in fiber content and soft in consistency. It serves as a transition between a full-liquid diet and a normal diet following surgery, in acute infections and fevers, and in gastrointestinal disturbances. Table 12-2

TABLE 12-1
Foods Permitted in a Mechanical Soft Diet

Food Types	Foods Permitted
Milk	All forms
Cheeses	All forms
Eggs	Any cooked form
Breads	White, rye without seeds, refined whole wheat; corn bread; any cracker not made with whole grains; French toast made from permitted breads; spoon bread; pancakes; plain soft rolls
Cereals	All cooked, soft varieties; puffed flakes and noncoarse ready-to-eat varieties
Flour	All forms
Meats, fish, poultry	Small cubed and finely ground or minced forms; as ingredients in creamed dishes, soups, casseroles, and stews
Seafoods	Any variety of fish without bone (canned, fresh, or frozen; packaged prepared forms in cream sauces); minced, shredded, ground, and finely chopped shellfish
Legumes, nuts	Fine, smooth, creamy peanut butter; legumes (if tolerated) cooked tender, finely chopped, mashed, or minced
Potatoes	White potatoes: mashed, boiled, baked, creamed, scalloped, cakes, au gratin; sweet potatoes: boiled, baked, mashed
Soups	All varieties, preferably without hard solids such as nuts and seeds
Fruits	Raw: avocado, banana; cooked and canned: fruit cocktail, cherries, apples, apricots, peaches, pears, sections of mandarin oranges, grapefruits, or oranges without membranes; all juices and nectars
Vegetables	All juices; all vegetables cooked tender, chopped, mashed, canned, or pureed; canned, pureed, or paste forms of tomato
Sweets	Marshmallow and chocolate sauces; preserves, marmalade, jelly, jam; candy: hard, chocolate, caramels, jellybeans, marshmallows, candy corn, butterscotch, gumdrops, plain fudge, lollipops, fondant mints; syrup: sorghum, maple, corn; sugar: granulated, brown, maple, confectioner's; honey, molasses
Desserts	All plain or certain flavored varieties (permitted flavorings include liquids, such as juice; finely chopped or pureed fruits without solid pieces of fruit, seeds, nuts, etc.); gelatins, puddings; ice cream, ice milk, sherbet; water ices; cakes, cookies, cake icing; cobblers
Fats	Butter, margarine, cream (or substitutes), oils and vegetable shortenings, and bacon fat; salad dressings, tartar sauce, sour cream
Seasonings	Salt, pepper, soy sauce, vinegar, catsup; all other herbs, especially finely chopped or ground, that can be tolerated

describes foods permitted and prohibited in a soft diet. Table 12–3 provides a sample menu for the diet.

Liquid Diets

A liquid diet consists of foods that will pour or are liquid at body temperature. The nutritive value of liquid diets is low and, consequently, such diets are used only for very limited periods of time. Liquid diets may be clear-liquid or full-liquid. They are standard hospital diets. The liquid diet is used for various reasons. One objective is to keep fecal matter in the colon at a minimum. The clear-liquid diet may be used after surgery. The diet can replace fluids lost from vomiting or diarrhea. The clear-liquid diet is composed mainly of water and carbohydrates. It is only a temporary diet, since it is nutritionally inadequate. Its use is typically limited to 24 to 36 hours. The meals, which are small and frequent, are usually served every two, three, or four hours. Such a diet regimen is usually followed by the full-liquid diet. Each of these two diets is described below.

Clear-Liquid Diet

This diet permits tea, coffee or coffee substitute, and fat-free broth. Gingerale, fruit juices, flavored gelatin, fruit ices, and water gruels (strained and liquefied cooked cere-

TABLE 12-2
Foods Permitted and Prohibited in a Soft Diet (Fiber-Restricted)

Food Types	Foods Permitted	Foods Prohibited
Milk	All milk and milk products without added ingredients; condensed and evaporated milk, chocolate milk and drink; cocoa and hot chocolate; yogurt and whey	Any milk product with prohibited ingredients
Cheese	Cottage cheese, cream cheese, mild cheese, and any cheese not prohibited	Any sharp, strongly flavored cheese; any cheese with prohibited ingredients
Eggs	Poached, scrambled, soft- and hard-cooked eggs; salmonella-free egg powder (pasteurized)	Raw or fried eggs
Breads and equivalents	Breads: white, Italian, Vienna, French, refined whole wheat, corn bread, spoon bread, French toast, seedless rye; muffins, English muffins, pancakes, rolls, waffles; melba toast, rusk, zwieback; biscuits, graham crackers, saltines, and other crackers not made with whole grains	Breads: any variety with seeds or nuts; Boston brown, pumpernickel, raisin, cracked wheat, buckwheat; crackers: all made with whole grain; rolls: any made with whole grain, nuts, coconut, raisins; tortillas
Cereals	Cooked and refined dry cereals	Dry, coarse cereals such as shredded wheat, all bran, and whole grain
Flours	All varieties except those prohibited	Any made with whole-grain wheat or bran
Beverages	All types	None
Meat, fish, poultry*	Meats: beef, liver, pork (lean and fresh), lamb, veal; poultry: turkey, chicken, duck, Cornish game hens, chicken livers; fish: all types of fresh varieties, canned tuna and salmon	Fried, cured, and highly seasoned products such as chitterlings, corned beef, cured and/or smoked products, most processed sausages, and cold cuts; meats with a lot of fat; geese and game birds; most shellfish; canned fish such as anchovies, herring, sardines, and any strongly flavored seafoods
Legumes, nuts	Fine, creamy, smooth peanut butter	Most legumes, nuts, and seeds
Fruits	Raw: avocado, banana; canned or cooked: apples, apricots, cherries, peaches, pears, plums, sections of oranges, grapefruits, mandarin oranges without membranes, stewed fruits (except raisins), fruit cocktail, seedless grapes; all juices and nectars	All raw fruits not specifically permitted; all dried fruits; fruits with seeds and skins
Vegetables	All juices; canned or cooked: asparagus, beets, carrots, celery, eggplant, green or wax beans, chopped kale, mushrooms, peas, spinach, squash, shredded lettuce, chopped parsley, green peas, pumpkin; tomato: stewed, pureed, juice, paste	All those not specifically permitted
Fats	Butter, margarine, cream (or substitute), oil, vegetable shortening, mayonnaise, French dressing, crisp bacon, plain gravies, sour cream	Other forms of fats and oils, salad dressings, highly seasoned gravy
Soups	Any made from permitted ingredients: bouillon (powder or cubes), consommé, cream soups; strained soups: gumbos, chowders, bisques	Soups made from prohibited ingredients; split pea and bean soups; highly seasoned soups such as onion
Potatoes	White potatoes: scalloped, boiled, baked, mashed, creamed, au gratin; sweet potatoes: mashed	White potatoes: fried, caked, browned, and in salad; yams

(continues)

TABLE 12-2 (Continued)

Food Types	Foods Permitted	Foods Prohibited
Rice and equivalents	Rice (white or brown), macaroni, spaghetti, noodles, Yorkshire pudding	Wild rice, bulgur, fritters, bread stuffing, barley
Sweets	Sugar: granulated, brown, maple, confectioner's; candy: hard, jellybeans, mints, marshmallows, butterscotch, candy corn, chocolate, caramels, fondant, plain fudge, gumdrops; syrups: maple, sorghum, corn; jelly, marmalade, preserves, jams; honey, molasses, apple butter; marshmallow and chocolate sauces	All candies containing nuts, coconut, and prohibited fruits
Desserts	Cake, cookies, custard, pudding, gelatin, ice cream, cobblers, ice milk, sherbet, water ice, cream pie with graham cracker crust; all plain or flavored without large pieces of fruits	Any products containing nuts, coconut, or prohibited fruits
Miscellaneous	Sauces: cream, white, brown, cheese, tomato; vinegar, soy sauce, catsup; all finely ground or chopped spices and herbs served in amounts tolerated by the patient	Spices and sauces that the patient is unable to tolerate, such as red pepper, garlic, curry, mustard; pickles; olives; popcorn, potato chips; Tabasco and Worcestershire sauces

*Cooked tender—may be broiled, baked, creamed, stewed, or roasted.

als are sometimes given. Small amounts of fluid are given to the patient every hour or two. For example, the diet is used for 24 to 48 hours following acute vomiting, diarrhea, or surgery.

The primary objective of the diet is to relieve thirst and to help maintain water balance. Broth provides some sodium, and fruit juices contribute potassium. The inclusion of carbonated beverages, sugar, and fruit juices furnishes a small amount of carbohydrate. This diet is deficient in nutrients and provides about 600 calories per day.

Severe malnutrition results from an extended use of this diet. A sample menu for a clear-liquid diet is shown in Table 12-4.

Full-Liquid Diet

This diet consists of liquids and foods that liquefy at body temperature. It is used for acute infections of short duration and for patients who are too ill to chew. It may be ordered after a short period on the clear-fluid diet follow-

TABLE 12-3
Sample Menu for a Soft Diet

Breakfast	Lunch	Dinner
Orange juice, ½ c.	Tomato soup, ½ c.	Soup, creamed, ½ c.
Farina, ½ c.	Cod, broiled, 2–3 oz.	Beef, stew meat, tender, 3–4 oz.
Egg, soft-boiled, 1	Potato, baked, medium, 1	White rice, ½ c.
Bacon, crisp, 2 strips	Toast, 1 slice	Asparagus, canned, ½ c.
Toast, 1 slice	Butter or margarine, 1 tsp.	Toast, 1 slice
Butter or margarine, 1 tsp.	Pudding, plain, ½ c.	Butter or margarine, 1 tsp.
Jam, 1–3 tsp.	Coffee or tea, 1–2 c.	Gelatin, flavored, ½ c.
Milk, 1 c.	Sugar, 1–3 tsp.	Coffee or tea, 1–2 c.
Coffee or tea, 1–2 c.	Cream, 1 tbsp.	Cream, 1 tbsp.
Sugar, 1–3 tsp.	Salt, pepper	Sugar, 1–3 tsp.
Cream, 1 tbsp.		Salt, pepper
Salt, pepper		

TABLE 12-4
Sample Menu for a Clear-Liquid Diet

Breakfast	Lunch	Dinner
Clear juice, ⅔ c. Coffee or tea Sugar **Snack** Juice, ⅔ c. or broth, clear, ½ c.	Clear juice, ⅔ c. Broth (chicken, beef, or vegetable), ⅔ c. Flavored gelatin, ½ c. Coffee or tea Sugar **Snack** Flavored ice, ½ c.	Clear juice, ⅔ c. Broth (chicken, beef, or vegetable), ⅔ c. Fruit ice or flavored gelatin, ½ c. Coffee or tea Sugar **Snack** Carbonated beverage

ing surgery or in the treatment of acute gastrointestinal disorders.

The diet is offered in six feedings or more. Table 12-5 describes foods permitted in a full-liquid diet and Table 12-6 provides a sample menu. Initially, amounts smaller than those indicated are given.

Standard hospital progressive diets usually include clear-liquid, full-liquid, soft, and regular diets. However, any one of the diets may be used exclusively throughout the patient's hospital stay. When the patient is on a clear-liquid diet for an extended period, the nurse must remind the health team regarding potential undernutrition.

TABLE 12-5
Foods Permitted in a Full-Liquid Diet

Milk and milk products	Whole milk, skim milk, chocolate, buttermilk, smooth or plain yogurt, whey, milk shakes, cocoa
Cheeses	Cheese soup
Eggs	Eggnog from pasteurized mix or other egg forms prepared in a beverage; scrambled or soft-cooked eggs if tolerated
Cereals	Cream of Rice; Cream of Wheat; cooked, refined cereals such as farina, grits, cornmeal, strained thin oatmeal, and granulated rice, gruels
Meats, fish, poultry, legumes, and nuts	Strained and pureed forms added to broth and cream soup
Potatoes	Pureed form added to soup
Soups	Any pureed or strained soup; cream soup, broth, bouillon
Fruits	All juices, including nectars
Vegetables	All juices and pureed forms used in preparing soups
Beverages	Coffee (regular, decaffeinated, or substitute), tea, carbonated types, lemonade, commercial instant types, other tolerated varieties
Desserts	Custards, plain or flavored (no fruits) gelatin, smooth ice cream, plain water ices, ice milk, puddings, sherbets, Popsicles
Sweets	Honey, molasses, sugar, syrup, hard candy, jellies
Fats	Margarine, butter, cream, oils
Miscellaneous	Nutritious protein supplements (homemade or commercial); salt; any finely ground herbs, spices, or flavorings tolerated by the patient

TABLE 12-6
Sample Menu for a Full-Liquid Diet

Breakfast	Lunch	Dinner
Orange juice, ½ c.	Pineapple juice, ½ c.	Grapefruit juice, ½ c.
Cream of Rice, ½ c.	Cream soup, strained, ⅔ c.	Vegetable soup, strained or pureed, ⅔ c.
Milk, ½ c.	Milk, ½ c.	Pudding, ½ c.
Coffee or tea, 1–2 c.	Gelatin, strawberry flavored, ½ c.	Coffee or tea, 1–2 c.
Cream	Coffee or tea, 1–2 c.	Cream
Sugar	Cream	Sugar
Salt	Sugar	Salt
	Salt	
Snack		**Snack**
Apple juice, 1 c.	**Snack**	Custard, ½ c.; or nutritional supplement
	Ice cream, 1 c.	

PROGRESS CHECK ON ACTIVITY 2

Multiple Choice

Circle the letter of the correct answer.

1. The clear-liquid diet
    a. replaces lost body fluids.
    b. provides a nutritionally adequate diet.
    c. includes any food that pours.
    d. is never used after surgery.

2. Which of the following groups of food would be allowed on a clear-liquid diet?
    a. strained cream of chicken soup, coffee, and tea
    b. tomato juice, sherbet, and strained cooked cereal
    c. raspberry ice, beef bouillon, and apple juice
    d. tea, coffee, and eggnog

3. The full-liquid diet
    a. is always nutritionally adequate.
    b. is followed by clear-liquid diet.
    c. does not include milk in any form.
    d. is sometimes given to patients with acute infections.

4. The full-liquid diet
    a. is given to all patients on the first day of their hospital stay.
    b. includes no protein foods.
    c. includes no highly fibrous foods.
    d. is commonly given immediately after surgery.

5. The protein content of the full-liquid diet
    a. can be increased by adding lactose to beverages.
    b. can be increased by adding dried milk to beverages.
    c. cannot be varied.
    d. is always adequate.

6. The clear-liquid diet
    a. is given to all patients with chewing difficulties.
    b. may be used after surgery.
    c. includes milk foods.
    d. is nutritionally adequate.

7. The soft diet
    a. is a standard diet in health facilities.
    b. is always served to children under 12 years old.
    c. is similar to a high-residue diet.
    d. does not nourish as well as a full-liquid diet.

8. A major difference between the regular and the soft diet is the
    a. nutrient content.
    b. texture of the foods.
    c. energy values.
    d. satiety value of the food.

9. It is not unusual for the soft diet to be
    a. ordered to precede the clear-liquid diet.
    b. ordered to precede the full-liquid diet.
    c. ordered to succeed the full-liquid diet.
    d. used in place of the clear-liquid diet.

10 Which of the following foods would not be included in a soft diet?
    a. ground beef
    b. leg of lamb
    c. roast chicken
    d. grilled pork chops

11. Cellulose is
    a. a complete protein.
    b. an indigestible carbohydrate.
    c. a saturated fat.
    d. an essential mineral.

12. Texture of food refers to its

a. color.
b. flavor.
c. consistency.
d. satiety value.

13. Which of the following groups of food would not be allowed on the soft diet?
    a. coffee, bananas, and sponge cake
    b. salt, sherbet, and scrambled eggs
    c. butter, angelfood cake, and fried chicken
    d. gingerale, chocolate ice cream, and cocoa with marshmallows

Fill-in

14. Adapt the following menu to meet the needs of a patient on a soft diet: fresh fruit cup, oatmeal with milk and sugar, bran muffin, and butter. _____

15. Indicate which of the following foods would be allowed on a soft diet by writing Y (yes) and N (no):
    _____ a. banana nut bread
    _____ b. roast chicken breast
    _____ c. baked halibut
    _____ d. french fries
    _____ e. angelfood cake
    _____ f. black coffee
    _____ g. celery sticks
    _____ h. tapioca pudding
    _____ i. coconut cookies
    _____ j. tossed salad

ACTIVITY 3: Diet Modifications for Therapeutic Care

The underlying concept in planning a therapeutic diet is that it is based on a normal balanced diet. The regular or house diets used during acute care can be modified to meet specific conditions, since they are already balanced diets. In addition to meeting specific needs, the changes that may be required must take into account many specific factors affecting the patient.

The modifications most generally used deal with four aspects of foods: basic nutrients; energy value; texture or consistency; and seasonings.

Modifying Basic Nutrients

The quantity and quality of the protein, fat, carbohydrate, vitamins, water, and minerals in a diet may be modified. An increase is used to correct deficiencies or provide extra nutrients for repair of body tissue. The increase may involve one or more nutrients, but combinations are frequent, since all nutrients have interrelated functions. Examples are a high-protein, high-carbohydrate, and high-vitamin diet for postoperation and an iron-rich diet for iron-deficiency anemia. The diet for a malnourished patient upon admission to the hospital may require increases in all the nutrients. A nutrient-rich diet is not necessarily accepted by the patient. The patient with a chronic, debilitating illness may be anorexic and present quite a challenge to the health team.

Nutrients may be reduced in a diet because the patient can metabolize only a certain amount. For example, a person with high blood sugar requires a diet low in simple carbohydrate. High serum lipids require a low-fat diet. When a diseased kidney cannot excrete excess minerals, a reduced intake of minerals is prescribed, as well as a monitored fluid intake.

Modifying Energy Value

The calculated diet is used to adjust caloric intake to regulate body weight. Calculations are based on the caloric value of foods—the number of calories per gram a food will furnish when metabolized by the body. Adjustments are made in the amounts of carbohydrate, protein, and fat contained in the diet. For example, an underweight patient may need a 3,000-calorie diet while an overweight patient may need only 1,500 calories. The diabetic diet is also a calculated diet. The nutrient values are calculated individually in order to ensure that daily requirements for each are met. A 1,000-calorie diet containing only fat and carbohydrate can be developed, if there is no concern for nutrient adequacy. Patients with certain malabsorptive disorders may require diets with increased energy value along with adjustments in the amount of a specific nutrient.

Modifying Texture or Consistency

Modification of foods' texture or consistency is used to: provide ease of chewing, swallowing, or digestion; rest the whole body or an affected organ; and bring a patient back to a regular diet. It is widely used in combination with other modifications—for example, low-residue, soft, and liquid diets. Patients with gastrointestinal diseases or trauma to the mouth and throat frequently are given diets altered in texture. Post-surgery patients may progress from liquid, to soft, to regular diets, as tolerated. Patients with heart disorders may be prescribed diets altered in texture to ease digestion to rest the damaged heart.

Modifying Seasonings

Seasonings are usually adjusted to individual tolerances, but a few are not advised in certain diseases. Salt restriction is prescribed for various conditions, including sodium retention in the body, edema, ascites, and others. Some physicians forbid certain spices for ulcers, acute gastritis, and other intestinal disorders.

Whatever the modification, the goal of diet therapy remains the same: to restore and maintain good nutritional status. Nutrient supplements of vitamins, minerals, and high protein formulas are needed for highly restricted diets, anorexia, and impaired absorption and metabolism.

A planned diet is successful only when it is eaten. The diet must be individualized to take into account the psychological and cultural factors that influence food acceptance. In addition, the food must be attractively presented, palatable, and safe. The patient's environment at mealtime is also an important factor, as is the attitude of the individuals serving the meals.

PROGRESS CHECK ON ACTIVITY 3

Fill-in

1. What are the four basic modifications made in a diet?

   _____

   _____

   _____

   _____

2. Give an example and the rationale for decreasing a nutrient in the diet. _____

   _____

   _____

   _____

3. Name three situations where diet supplementation

would be needed.

   a. _____

   b. _____

   c. _____

4. Explain how a diet can be individualized and still provide the correct modifications. _____

   _____

   _____

   _____

   _____

Nursing Implications

1. Recognize the unique position of the nurse in promoting dietary compliance to modified diets.
   a. Assess nutritional status.
   b. Observe and document nutritional intake.
   c. Evaluate response to diet therapy.
   d. Teach or support the diet teaching and diet therapy ordered for the client.
2. Be aware that diet therapy, alone or in conjunction with other treatment, may play an important role in the prevention and treatment of disease by
   a. Lessening severity of symptoms.
   b. Decreasing need for medication.
   c. Delaying onset of disease or delaying progression.
   d. Increasing resistance to diseases or speeding recovery.
3. Provide the client and caregivers with nutrition information, encouragement, education, and referrals as needed.
4. Recognize the social, cultural, and psychological aspects that influence nutritional status of hospitalized clients and intervene when needed.
5. Continue to update knowledge regarding diet therapy.

ACTIVITY 4: Alterations in Feeding Methods

It is estimated that protein energy malnutrition (PEM) is present in 25 to 50 percent of all medical surgical patients. The most common reason is exhausted nutrient reserves when entering a facility. In addition, hospitalized patients who were previously stable can experience malnutrition in as little as two weeks.

Of particular significance are those patients at high risk for whom oral feedings are inadequate, such as being on five days or more of clear liquids. Other high-risk patients who may require alternate feeding methods are those with eating disorders, malabsorption syndromes, cancer, or a hyper-metabolic condition such as burns. Whenever a patient cannot or will not eat, for any one of myriad reasons, an alternate method of feeding should be employed.

There are two parenteral or intravenous feeding methods. One method injects nutrients into the blood via a peripheral vein (for example, a vein in the arm, near the surface). The other method injects nutrients into the blood via a central vein (those deeper into the central portion of the system; for example, the subclavian located under the collarbone).

Special Enteral Feedings (Tube Feedings)

A tube feeding is a nutritionally adequate diet of liquified foods administered through a tube into the stomach or duodenum. These foods may be commercially available or prepared in-house. From the standpoint of accuracy in measuring, sanitation, and convenience, most hospitals prefer commercial mixtures. These mixtures can be blenderized table foods, milk-based formulas, lactose-free formulas, meat-based formulas, and residue-free formulas. Patients prescribed hospital-prepared formula after discharge can be taught to make their own, using common ingredients (see Table 12-7). Tube feedings, whether commercially or in-house prepared, usually furnish 1 calorie per milliliter. A 24-hour intake of 3 liters would furnish 3,000 calories.

Enteral feedings have several advantages, including the following:

1. It is more economical to feed enterally than intravenously, considering equipment, time, and foods used.
2. It is safer to feed enterally than intravenously. The risk of fluid and electrolyte imbalances and infection is less than for intravenous feedings.
3. It may be more pleasant for the patients, especially if they tolerate conventional foods; they eat what the family does.

Some disadvantages of enteral feedings include

1. Nutritional inadequacy for certain patients (not enough protein and calories).

TABLE 12-7
Some Common Foods Used in Tube Feedings

Milk-based formulas
   whole or skim milk
   eggs
   syrup, honey , molasses, or sugar
   cream or half-and-half
   cooked strained cereals
   vitamin supplements in liquid form

Blenderized formulas
   Strained meats, fruits, and vegetables are added to
      the ingredients in the milk-based formula.

Meat-based formulas
   Milk and cream are omitted and juices added for
      desired consistency.
   Calcium supplementation may be necessary.
Other foods that may be added to increase nutrient
   content and/or calories:
   Salad oil
   Juices, fruit and vegetable
   Bread without crusts

2. Overnutrition for certain patients (excess calories and formula).
3. Diarrhea or constipation.
4. Vomiting.

Depending on the patient and the circumstances, some or all of the above problems can be avoided or remedied.

There is an increasing movement back toward use of more enteral feedings. Recent studies indicate that the intestinal bacteria will translocate to other areas, become pathogenic, and create sepsis when they are not fed.

Parenteral Feedings via Peripheral Vein

Nutrient fluids entering a peripheral vein can be saline with 5 or 10 percent dextrose (clinically represented by D5W or D10W); amino acids; electrolytes; vitamins; and medications. Intravenous fluids may be either isotonic, hypotonic, or hypertonic. Both hypotonic and hypertonic solutions create a shift in body fluids. Hypotonic solutions draw fluid from the blood vessels into the interstitial spaces and cells. Hypertonic solutions create the opposite effect; they draw fluids out of interstitial spaces into the blood.

When enteral feedings are contraindicated, feeding by a peripheral vein is often used. This type of feeding is safer than feeding by a central vein, but it fails to provide adequate calories and other nutrients for repair and replacement of losses. The dangers of overloading with fluid in order to meet caloric needs are inherent in using solutions via the peripheral vein. Some examples of nutrient quantities in these solutions will illustrate the clinical problem. For example, 2,500 cc of D5W provides 425 calories and 0 gram protein; 200 cc of 3.5 percent amino acid solution provides 70 grams protein, 280 calories, but 0 gram carbohydrate to spare protein. A 10 percent fat emulsion (intralipids may be used via the peripheral vein) furnishes 1 calorie per cc emulsion, contains no amino acids, and is not compatible with any other added nutrients. It elevates serum cholesterol levels and is questionable in its ability to promote nitrogen balance by sparing protein.

Parenteral Feeding via Central Vein (Total Parenteral Nutrition [TPN])

When a patient is severely depleted nutritionally or if the GI tract cannot be used, parenteral feeding via a catheter inserted into a central vein (usually the subclavian to the superior vena cava) can provide adequate nutrition. The solution for TPN is a sterile mixture of glucose, amino acids, and micronutrients. The intralipids are not given in this solution and may be administered via a peripheral vein. The amounts of micronutrients added are based on the individual's blood chemistry. Multivitamin preparations can be added to the TPN solutions, except for B_{12}, K, or folic acid, which are given separately.

TPN has many advantages. It can be used for long periods of time to meet the individual body's total nutritional needs. The solutions can be adjusted according to individual needs by increasing or decreasing any or all of the nutrients.

TPN also has many disadvantages. The solutions are very expensive, and they support rapid growth of bacteria and fungi. The rate of infusion must be adhered to rigidly, around the clock. Dressing changes are done using sterile technique. Careful monitoring of the patient's response and corrective measures when needed are mandatory for safe administration of these solutions.

Nursing Implications

The responsibilities or implications for nutritional support by the nursing staff are varied and many. A brief summary of some of these implications follows.

1. Discard all unused, cloudy, or sedimented fluids.
2. Do not add drugs and other mixtures to a solution containing protein.
3. Refrigerate solutions until they are used.
4. Be aware that dates should be on tube feedings, and that they should not be given past 24 hours of date.
5. Be alert for signs of gas, regurgitation, cramping, and diarrhea, and be prepared to intervene.
6. Take necessary precautions when using nutrient solutions because they are excellent sources for bacterial growth.
7. Be especially alert for signs of hypo- or hyperglycemia when TPN is used and intervene if necessary.
8. Assist the patient in adjusting to an alternate feeding method. Many patients experience stress due to fear and concern of unfamiliar feeding methods.
9. Encourage and practice good oral hygiene measures with the patient, even though he or she is not eating by mouth.
10. Encourage early ambulation, which makes use of the muscles and increases the use of calcium and protein. Physical activity also raises morale.

PROGRESS CHECK ON ACTIVITY 4

Multiple Choice

1. Which of the following is an important concern for the nurse who is providing nutrition by peripheral vein?
   a. calorie overload
   b. contamination of the injection site
   c. fluid overload
   d. all of the above

2. The solution used for TPN consists of
   a. glucose, amino acids, and micronutrients.
   b. glucose, amino acids, and fatty acids.
   c. 10% dextrose in saline and vitamins.
   d. commercial hydrolyzed mixtures.

3. Which of the following vitamins would need to be given separately instead of added to a formula?
   a. thiamin, niacin, and riboflavin
   b. the fat-soluble vitamins
   c. B_{12}, K, and folic acid
   d. none of these

True/False

4. T F Nutrient fluids via peripheral vein are as adequate for long-term feedings as those via central vein.
5. T F Tube feedings are always commercial preparations.
6. T F Parenteral feedings will sustain the fluid and electrolyte balance of a postoperative patient.
7. T F TPN can be used for long periods of time and still maintain cell integrity.
8. T F Enteral feedings are more likely to become contaminated than parenteral ones.

Matching

Match the statement to the appropriate fluid.

9. Draws fluid from interstitial spaces into the blood.
10. Does not create a fluid shift.
11. Draws fluid from blood into interstitial spaces.

   a. isotonic fluid
   b. hypotonic fluid
   c. hypertonic fluid

Fill-in

12. Define tube feedings. _____

13. List two advantages and two disadvantages of enteral feeding. _____

14. List two conditions requiring TPN.
   a. _____
   b. _____

15. List three important nursing measures for a patient receiving TPN.
   a. _____
   b. _____
   c. _____

16. List three types of formulas used in tube feedings and describe the major difference of each from the other.

_____

_____

_____

References _____

American Dietetic Association. 1988. *Manual of clinical dietetics*. Chicago: American Dietetic Association.

Beaton, G. H. 1988. Criteria of an adequate diet. In *Modern nutrition in health and disease,* 7th ed. M. E. Shils, and V. R. Young (eds.). Philadelphia: Lea & Febiger.

Drummond, K. E. 1989. *Nutrition for the foodservice professional*. New York: Van Nostrand Reinhold.

Food and Nutrition Board, National Research Council, National Academy of Sciences. 1989. *Recommended dietary allowances*. 10th ed. Washington, DC: National Academy Press.

Halsted, C. H., and R. B. Rucker. 1989. *Nutrition and the origin of disease*. San Diego, CA: Academic Press.

Massachusetts General Hospital Department of Dietetics. 1984. *Diet reference manual,* 2nd ed. Boston: Little, Brown, and Co.

Mayo Clinic. 1988. *Mayo Clinic diet manual*. Philadelphia: B. C. Dekker.

Miller, S. A., and M. G. Stephenson. 1987. The 1990 national nutrition objectives: Lessons for the future. *Journal of the American Dietetic Association* 87:1665.

National Institute of Health. 1989. *Eating to lower your high blood cholesterol*. United States Department of Human Services/Public Health Service National Institute of Health Publication No. 89-2920. Baltimore, MD: National Institute of Health.

National Research Council. 1986. *Nutrient adequacy*. Washington, DC: National Academy Press.

Nieman, D. C. et al. 1990. *Nutrition*. Dubuque, IA: W. C. Brown.

Paige, D. (ed.). 1983. *Manual of clinical nutrition*. Pleasantville, NJ: Nutrition Publication.

Puckett, R. P., and B. B. Miller (eds.). 1988. *Food service manual for health care institutions*. Chicago: American Hospital Publishing.

Renner-McCaffrey, J., and A. H. Leyshon. 1989. *Quality assurance in hospital nutrition services*. Rockville, MD: Aspen Publishers.

Shils, M. E., and V. R. Young (eds.). 1988. *Modern nutrition in health and disease,* 7th ed. Philadelphia: Lea & Febiger.

Sullivan, C. 1990. *Management of medical foodservice*. New York: Van Nostrand Reinhold.

United States Department of Agriculture. 1985. *Thrifty meals for two. Home and Garden Bulletin No. 244*. Washington, DC: United States Department of Agriculture.

Wardlaw, G. M., and P. M. Insel. 1990. *Perspectives in nutrition*. St. Louis: Mosby.

Diet Therapy for Surgical Conditions

Time for completion

Activities: _____1_____ hour

Optional examination: ½ hour

Academic credit

Semester units: ²⁄₁₀

Quarter units: ³⁄₁₀

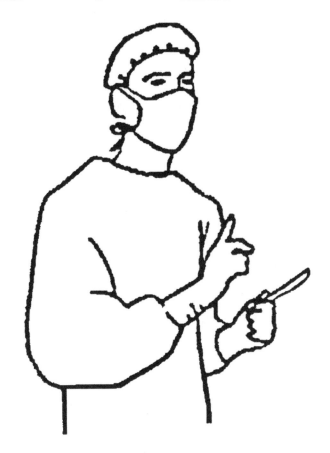

Outline

Objectives

Upon completion of this module, the student should be able to:

1. Identify the physiological and psychological effects of body trauma or stress.
2. Contrast the outcomes of surgery in a patient with poor nutritional status and in a patient with good nutritional status.
3. Explain the rationale for the importance of the nutrients most needed during the surgical experience.
4. List the major nutritional problems encountered in preoperative patients and possible solutions to these problems.
5. Describe the diet therapy regime for the postoperative patient and rationale for its use.
6. Identify common foods and fluids suitable for replacing losses and promoting healing in the surgical patient.
7. Relate nursing interventions to the nutritional care of the surgery patient.

Glossary

Acidosis: an accumulation of excess acid or depleted alkaline reserve (bicarbonate content) in the blood and body tissues. It almost always occurs as part of a disease process.

Ambulatory: able to walk; not confined to bed.

Calcification: process in which organic tissue becomes hardened by deposition of lime salts in the tissues.

Capillary walls: the sides of the minute blood vessels (capillaries). Capillaries connect the smallest arteries with the smallest veins.

Coenzymes: enzyme activators, such as vitamins, which enter into a variety of body processes.

Collagen: the protein in connective tissue and bone matrix.

Colloidal osmotic pressure: the pressure that develops on either side of a membrane. The colloid does not pass through the membrane, so therefore keeps the concentration of the solution approximately equal to that of circulating blood. The colloidal substance is a protein; therefore, when protein in the diet is depleted, edema develops because the solution can then pass from inside the membrane into the tissues.

Connective tissue: fibrous insoluble protein that holds cells together; collagen represents approximately 30 percent of body protein.

Decubitis ulcers: inflammation, sore, or ulcer over a bony prominence (exercise, movement, good skin care, and a high-protein, high-vitamin diet are needed for prevention).

Dehiscence: splitting open; separation of all the layers of a surgical wound.

Dehydration: the loss or deprivation of water from the body or tissues.

Diuresis: increased excretion of urine.

Duodenum: the first portion of the small intestine extending from the pylorus to the jejunum. It is about 10 inches long and both the common bile duct and pancreatic duct empty into it.

Edema: swelling; the body tissues contain an excess amount of tissue fluid.

Enteral nutrition: fed by way of the small intestine.

Evisceration: extrusion of the internal organs; disembowelment.

Exudate: fluid with a high content of protein and debris that has escaped from blood vessels and deposited on tissues.

Hyperalimentation: the intravenous infusion of a solution of amino acids, glucose, vitamins, and electrolytes to sustain life and maintain normal growth and development. The solution is infused into the superior vena cava via the subclavian vein.

Hyperglycemia: glucose in the blood elevated above the normal limit.

Hypoglycemia: blood sugar below the normal limit.

Interstitial: pertaining to or situated between parts or in the interspaces of a tissue.
a. *fluid:*   the extracellular fluid bathing most tissues, excluding fluid with the lymph and blood vessels.
b. *tissue:*   connective tissue between cells.

Intravenous: within the veins.

Parenteral nutrition: not fed through the alimentary canal but rather by subcutaneous, intramuscular, intrasternal, or intravenous injection.
a. *via central vein:*   in the central portion of the system.
b. *via peripheral vein:*   near the surface.

Peripheral veins: veins away from the central portion of the system; near the surface.

Peristalsis: the wormlike movement by which the alimentary canal propels its contents, consisting of a wave of contractions passing along the tube.

Plasma protein: the liquid part of the blood and lymph is the plasma. Plasma contains numerous chemicals and protein, glucose, and fats. Protein in plasma prevents undue leakage of fluids out of the capillaries.

Prothrombin: a chemical substance in the blood that interacts with calcium salts to produce thrombin, which clots blood.

Subclavian vein: a large vein located under the collarbone that unites with the interior jugular and forms the innominate vein.

Superior vena cava: the principal vein draining the upper portion of the body. Formed by the junction of right and left innominate veins, it empties into the right atrium of the heart.

Background Information _____

The nutritional status of the patient before, during, and after surgery is important to a rapid and successful recovery. Factors affecting pre- and postoperative conditions are introduced below.

Effects of Stress

All kinds of stress or trauma deplete body stores and interfere with ingestion, digestion, and metabolism. Injury, accidents, trauma, burns, cancer, illness, fever, infections, loss of blood and other fluids, loss of body tissues, and other conditions requiring surgery can significantly deplete body substances in a patient. Such injuries or stress require an increased amount of nutrients for repair. These problems are usually compounded by psychological stress such as anxiety, fear, and pain, which greatly interfere with the desire or ability to eat.

During stress periods there may be reduced function of the gastrointestinal (GI) tract. Muscular activity is lowered in the digestive tract. This may cause abdominal distention, gas pains, and constipation. In some cases, the nervous system may be stimulated by these conditions, resulting in nausea, vomiting, and diarrhea. Prolonged stress results in depleted liver glycogen and the wasting of muscle tissue.

Effects of Nutrition

Good nutrition prior to surgery leads to effective wound healing, increases resistance to infection, shortens convalescence, and lowers the mortality rate.

Poor nutrition prior to surgery leads to poor wound healing, dehydration, edema, excessive weight loss, decubitis ulcers, increased infections, potential liver damage, and a high mortality rate.

Most patients are not at optimum nutritional status when they are admitted to a health care facility. If surgery is to be performed, the patient's nutritional status must be improved by an appropriate dietary regimen prior to surgery. This minimizes surgical risk. Unfortunately, this is not always possible due to the acute need for surgery. Some also believe that such consideration is given low priority because of poor hospital practice, limited staffing, lack of communication, relatively low urgency, and so on.

Nutrients for the Surgical Experience

The nutrients that are considered important for persons undergoing surgery are

1. *Protein.* Needed to build and repair damaged tissue.
2. *Carbohydrate and fat.* Needed to spare protein and furnish energy.
3. *Glucose.* Needed to prevent acidosis and vomiting.

4. *Vitamins.*
   a. *Vitamin C:* needed to hasten wound healing and collagen formation.
   b. *Vitamin B complex:* needed to form the coenzymes for metabolism, especially of carbohydrates.
   c. *Vitamin K:* needed to promote blood clotting.
5. *Minerals.*
   a. *Zinc:* needed to aid wound healing.
   b. *Iron:* needed to permit hemoglobin synthesis to replace blood loss.

PROGRESS CHECK ON BACKGROUND INFORMATION

Multiple Choice

Circle the letter of the correct answer.

1. Effects of stress on the body include all except
   a. stimulation of the desire to eat.
   b. depletion of body tissues.
   c. depressed GI functioning.
   d. decreased liver glycogen.

2. Poor nutrition prior to surgery may result in all of the following except
   a. increased resistance to infection.
   b. dehydration.
   c. edema.
   d. liver damage.

Fill-in

List four effects of good nutritional status on the outcome of surgery.

3. Good wound healing
4. ↑ infection resistance
5. ↓ death rate
6. ↓ convelesent period c̄ ↓ complications

Matching

Some nutrients have been identified as being very important in the surgical experience. Match the nutrient at the left with the letter of its major function at the right.

E 7. Glucose   a. builds and repairs tissue
D 8. Vitamin C   b. blood clotting
A 9. Protein   c. synthesis of hemoglobin
F 10. B Complex   d. aids in wound healing and collagen formation
C 11. Iron   e. prevents acidosis and vomiting
       f. provides coenzymes for metabolism

Match the word with its definition.

D 12. Dehiscence   **a.** excessive urine

E 13. Evisceration   **b.** connective tissue

B 14. Collagen   **c.** between the cells

C 15. Interstitial   **d.** splitting open

A 16. Diuresis   **e.** disembowelment

True/False

Circle T for True and F for False

17. (T) F   Physical stress reduces function of all body organs.

18. (T) F   Psychological stress depletes body stores.

19. T (F)   If the patient is not fed orally he or she won't get edema and ascites.

20. T (F)   Most patients have adequate nutritional status prior to surgery.

ACTIVITY 1: Pre- and Postoperative Nutrition

Preoperative Nutrition

The major nutritional problems in the preoperative period are undernutrition and overnutrition. Both the undernourished and obese patients present special needs.

The undernourished patient, because of a lack of the major nutrients necessary for recovery, is at higher risk in surgery than a patient of normal weight. Protein deficiency is most common among these patients. Low body protein storage will predispose the patient to shock, less detoxification of the anesthetic agent by the liver, increased edema at the incision site, and decreased antibody formation. The last factor increases the risk of infection. Intravenous feeding of solutions that are more concentrated in nutrients (hyperalimentation) prior to surgery is one way to replenish body nutrient storage. This assumes that surgery can be postponed for a time. Aggressive oral nutrition, although more time consuming, can accomplish the same goals.

Obese patients are at higher health risk in surgery than those of normal weight. Excess fat complicates surgery, puts a strain on the heart, increases the risk of infection and respiratory problems, and delays healing. The risks of dehiscence and evisceration are greater in the obese patient. Preexisting conditions such as hypertension and diabetes which are prevalent in obese persons also increase risks. There is no quick way for an obese person to safely lose weight prior to surgery. If time permits, a low-calorie diet, high in the essential nutrients, should be attempted. Starvation or fad diets are obviously not recommended preoperatively. Conversely, a reduction diet after surgery is not in the patient's best interest when the need for all nutrients is high. If weight loss is needed, a low-calorie diet should not be instituted until healing is complete.

Dietary considerations presurgery for an adequately nourished patient are also important. The special nutritional needs of surgical interventions should be met. The preoperative diet for these persons should be rich in carbohydrate, protein, minerals, vitamins, and fluids. This diet will assist in a rapid recovery as it promotes wound healing and decreases the risk of infections and other complications.

If a patient has preexisting conditions—for example, diabetes—the blood sugar should be stabilized before surgery. Other problems such as anemia, dehydration, acidosis, or electrolyte imbalances should be corrected before the surgical procedure.

Postoperative Nutrition

The goal of postoperative diet therapy is to replace body losses as soon as possible. Energy, protein, and ascorbic acid are major factors in achieving rapid wound healing. Fluid replacement is another major concern. Minerals and other vitamins also play a vital role in recovery.

The postoperative diet may be liquid, soft, or of regular consistency, but it must be high in calories, protein, vitamins, minerals, and fluids.

Rationale for Diet Therapy

Protein

100–200 grams of high quality protein per day are needed.

1. Up to 1 pound of tissue protein per day may be lost through bleeding, high metabolic rate (using protein for energy), from exudate, and catabolism of muscle tissue as well as from surgery itself.

2. Plasma protein loss from hemorrhage or wound bleeding may occur. Loss of plasma protein and blood volume increases the risk of shock. Extra protein is required to replace these losses.

3. Fever and inflammation that may accompany surgery can be reduced by an increased supply of protein.

4. When antibody production decreases, infections increase. A high protein intake can reduce the risk of infection.

5. Edema may develop due to an imbalance of colloidal osmotic pressure. Serum protein levels must be increased to reduce edema. Edema at the incision site may also develop, slowing healing. This is another reason for protein intake.

6. Bone healing is delayed if the protein intake is not

high. The bone marrow is considered a special protein that anchors minerals and favors calcification.

7. Hormones and enzymes are protein substances. A lack of protein can lower production of these vital substances.

8. In the liver, protein combines with fat for removal. This prevents fatty infiltration. Thus, increased protein can protect the body against liver damage. When a protein combines with a fat, the product is a lipoprotein.

Fluids

There must be sufficient fluids to replace potential losses from vomiting, fever, diuresis, drainage, and exudates. Preventing dehydration is of great importance. Up to seven liters of fluid per day may be needed. Because the body tends to retain sodium and fluid postoperatively, total fluid intake and output must be measured and recorded to assure proper fluid balance.

Calories

If the caloric intake in the postoperative patient is inadequate, protein will be used for energy rather than for tissue rebuilding and wound healing. More than half of ingested proteins will be used to provide energy in the absence of sufficient carbohydrates and fats. A minimum of 2,800 calories per day from carbohydrates and fat must be available to spare protein for its primary purpose. The student should review the protein-sparing action of carbohydrates in Modules 4 and 5. An example of protein-sparing action is if a patient has had extensive surgery that requires 250 grams of protein for tissue building and repair, the total caloric content of the diet should range from 4,000–6,000 calories.

Vitamins

Vitamin C availability is imperative. The role of vitamin C, as the student will recall, is to supply the cementing material of connective tissue, capillary walls, and new tissue. Depending on the nature and extent of the surgery, the patient may need six to twenty times the RDAs.

Vitamin K is also of special concern because of its function in blood clotting. Intestinal bacteria synthesis of this vitamin is decreased because of the use of antibiotics. Any liver damage reduces prothrombin formation, which can be corrected by the presence of more vitamin K.

The need for B complex vitamins increases with rising caloric requirements. These vitamins function as coenzymes in carbohydrate and protein metabolism, the formation of hemoglobin, and the prevention of anemia.

Minerals

Minerals are of great importance in the replacement of electrolytes simultaneously lost with fluid from the body. The amount and kinds of minerals to be replaced are determined by the type of surgery and extent of loss in the patient. Certainly, sodium, chloride, phosphorus, potassium, and iron will need replacing and an increase in calcium supply is mandatory if bone surgery or loss is involved. Table 13-1 lists food sources of some of the most essential nutrients needed by surgical patients.

PROGRESS CHECK ON ACTIVITY 1

Multiple Choice

Circle the letter of the correct answer.

1. The major nutritional problems that the health team encounters among patients scheduled for surgery are ___B___ and ___D___.
   a. anxiety
   b. undernutrition
   c. pain
   d. overnutrition

2. Low body protein reserves can cause all except which of the following conditions?
   a. shock and edema
   b. muscle wasting
   c. anxiety
   d. liver damage

3. Sufficient fluids are supplied in the diet to replace losses from all except
   a. edema.
   b. diuresis.
   c. vomiting.
   d. drainage.

True/False

Circle T for True and F for False.

4. T F A minimum of 1,200 calories per day from carbohydrate and fat is required for protein-sparing of the postoperative patient.

5. T F The major problem in preoperative patients is under- or over-nutrition.

6. T F Decreased protein increases antibody formation.

7. T F It is more important to increase total calories than carbohydrate in the preoperative diet.

Fill-in

8. Using the following menu, indicate the major nutrients supplied by each food listed by placing an "X" in the appropriate column.

TABLE 13-1
Some Food Sources of the Nutrients Identified as Essential to a Successful Surgery

Protein		Vitamin C	Vitamin B Complex*		Vitamin K	Iron	Zinc
Complete:	Milk Eggs Meat Fish Poultry	Citrus fruits Sweet and hot peppers Greens Strawberries	1.	Thiamin: pork, oysters, organ meats, enriched bread and cereals	Green leafy vegetables† Fruits Cereals Meats	Liver Heart Eggs Raisins Prunes Whole wheat and enriched cereals and breads Apricots, dried Red meats Oysters Pork Almonds	Shellfish (especially oysters) Dairy products Eggs Whole grain cereals
Incomplete:	Vegetables Grains Nuts and seeds	Cantaloupe Cabbage	2.	Riboflavin: milk, milk products, organ meats, muscle meats, oysters, enriched bread and cereals			
			3.	Niacin: liver, tuna, peanuts and peanut butter, peas, pork, enriched bread and cereals			

*Others not listed of this group will be supplied if these 3 B vitamins in the diet are adequate.
†Best source

	Pro	CHo	Thia	Nia	Ribo	Fe	VitC
Oyster stew	X	X	X	_	X	X	_
Whole wheat garlic toast	X	X	X	X	X	X	_

	Pro	CHo	Thia	Nia	Ribo	Fe	VitC
Green pepper and cabbage slaw	X	X	_	_	_	_	X
Raisin rice pudding with orange sauce	X	X	_	_	_	X	X

ACTIVITY 2: The Postoperative Diet Regime

Goals of Dietary Management

The main goal of postoperative nutritional and dietary care is for the patient to regain a normal body weight. This is brought about by a positive nitrogen balance and the subsequent muscle formation and fat deposition. This goal can be achieved by first correcting all fluid and electrolyte imbalances and giving appropriate transfusions. The second step is to provide carefully planned dietary and nutritional support for the patient, with special emphasis on those nutrients discussed at the beginning of this module. The third step is to monitor food intake by maintaining a detailed record of what is consumed.

A postoperative dietary regimen also requires the aggressive nutritional support that is needed to maintain normal body functions and tissues. Tissue maintenance is especially important since additional losses may result from postoperative bed confinement and ensuing muscle atrophy. Nutritional supports should also attempt to replace tissue (such as muscle, bone, blood, exudate, and skin) that may have been lost during the trauma of surgery. Any malnourishment should be remedied if it has not already been treated. Plasma protein should be supplied to control or prevent edema and shock. Plasma protein also provides vital components for the synthesis of albumin, antibodies, enzymes, and other necessary substances, which may have been lost through bleeding or the escape of fluids. Finally, plasma protein also accelerates the healing of wounds.

Inadequate nutritional supports increase morbidity and mortality, delay the return of normal body functions, and retard the process of tissue rebuilding. Inadequate nutrition prevents wounds from healing at a normal pace and causes edema and muscular weakness. Most importantly, all of these consequences prolong convalescence and discomfort for the patient.

Feeding the Patient Immediately after the Operation _____

Since a patient usually cannot tolerate solid food immediately after an operation, it is withheld anywhere from a few hours to two or three days. A feeding that is too early may nauseate the patient and cause vomiting and possible aspiration. This results in further fluid and electrolyte losses, discomfort, and potential pneumonia. The following outline lists the various types of dietary support that can be used during this short part of the postoperative period.

1. No food by mouth (NPO)
2. *Intravenous feeding:* blood transfusion, fluids and electrolytes, 5 percent dextrose, vitamin and mineral supplements, protein-sparing solutions (with or without Intralipid), combination of above
3. *Oral feeding:* routine hospital progressive liquid diets with or without supplements, liquid protein supplements with or without nonprotein calories, combinations of above
4. A combination of oral and intravenous feedings

Many clinicians feel that it is not worthwhile to provide aggressive nutritional support during such a short period of food deprivation. This decision is justified in a well-nourished individual who can afford temporary catabolic losses and would not be able to efficiently use the supplied protein or calories. As described in Activity 1, the majority of patients do not fit this category. The attending physician must decide if the patient is well nourished and if enteral or parenteral feedings can be tolerated. If the feedings can be tolerated, a subsequent decision must be made on benefits of these exogenous nutrients. The health professional may, after his or her assessment of the patient's status, request the physician to evaluate the patient and prescribe additional feedings.

Blood transfusions and fluid and electrolyte compensation are administered to those patients needing them. Some doctors prescribe 5 percent dextrose solution in saline or water, but the amount given is limited by the patient's tolerance. Another problem is that a concentrated dextrose solution may cause thrombosis in the peripheral veins. Because of the relatively low nutrient density of dextrose solution, it should not be used as a long-term means of feeding. It has been claimed generally that the infusion of dextrose spares some body protein from breakdown to provide needed calories. Recently various medical centers have experimented with the infusion of protein-sparing solutions made up mainly of essential amino acids. The preliminary trials have been very encouraging. However, if such means are used every day, it may not only be expensive, but further deteriorate fragile peripheral veins. Some hospitals use vitamin and mineral supplements as well as protein-sparing solutions.

Although solid foods are withheld from patients immediately after an operation, most hospitals provide patients with oral feedings after their intestinal functions return to normal (as early as 24 hours after the operation). The feedings consist of routine hospital progressive diets (see Module 12). This stepwise postoperative feeding may cover 1 to 3 days, depending on the patient's tolerance, strength, and type of operation or trauma.

Some patients may be able to start with a soft diet, while others must begin with a clear liquid diet. Occasionally progressive feedings may be supplemented with commercial formulas. Some patients are given liquid protein supplements with or without non-protein calories if they can tolerate the feedings. Again, depending on the patient and his or her condition, a combination of feeding methods, including total parenteral nutrition (see Module 12), may be used. For patients requiring tube feeding, consult the detailed procedures described in Module 12.

At this early stage of postoperative recovery, physicians, nurses, and dietitians should work closely to determine whether dextrose solution or oral liquid diets should be continued. This is important, since both types of feeding may not be nutritionally sound without concentrated supplements. Nutritional supports, including fluids, electrolytes, protein, calories, and other nutrients, should be carefully reviewed. Finally, a long-term aggressive postoperative dietary treatment should be planned and executed to combat the catabolic consequences of trauma and to bring about a speedy recovery.

Dietary Management for Recovery _____

When a patient can tolerate regular hospital foods, the health team should plan and prescribe an appropriate diet. Experts in clinical nutrition have tried for a number of years to develop a postoperative diet that will provide patients with an optimal amount of nutrients. In general, the following diet prescription should satisfy most clinical conditions that involve trauma: (1) 40 to 50 kcal/kg body weight/d, (2) 12 percent to 15 percent of total calories as protein, (3) well-balanced intakes of the established RDAs, and (4) carefully monitored intakes of vitamins A, K, C, B_{12}, and folic acid and the minerals, iron and zinc. To illustrate the protein and calorie composition of such a diet, Table 13-2 includes two examples (40 kcal and 50 kcal/d) for a man weighing 70 kg.

If the patient has a minimal amount of tissue and blood loss, a sound preoperative nutritional status, a moderate to good appetite, and no sign of surgical complications, a diet of 35 to 40 kcal/kg is probably sufficient. However, the diet for a postoperative patient should be individualized, especially the serving sizes and the frequency of feeding. Patients usually tolerate solids better if the feedings are small and frequent.

TABLE 13-2
Approximate Protein and Calorie Content of a Postoperative Diet for a Male Patient Weighing 70 kg

kcal/kg Body Weight	Total Daily Kilocalories	Approximate Dietary Protein (g)	Total Calories from Protein (%)
40	2,800	84	12
50	3,500	131	15

Both carbohydrates and fats are important sources of calories, and they should be provided in about equal quantities to constitute 85 percent to 88 percent of the total calories. (If this reduces the patient's appetite, less fat should be consumed.) The calories from carbohydrates and fats used to correct hypermetabolism supply energy for all processes of rebuilding and repairing and spare protein for anabolic purposes.

If the patient is given solid food, a good quantity of fruits and vegetables should be included in meals in addition to protein, fat, and carbohydrate. Refer to Module 12 for planning a high-protein, high-calorie, balanced diet. The need for vitamins A, K, C, B_{12}, and folic acid in a postoperative regimen requires special attention. Vitamins A and C have been proven experimentally and clinically to assist in wound healing as well as tissue repair. Vitamin A is well known for its role in maintaining epithelial structures, and vitamin C is important for collagen synthesis. In addition, vitamin A acid (retinoic acid) has recently been shown to assist in wound healing and is currently suspected to be a possible curative agent for certain types of human cancer.

The body's ability to clot blood postoperatively depends on an adequate supply of vitamin K. Folic acid and vitamin B_{12} are necessary for the synthesis and turnover of all body cells, especially red blood cells, and should be amply provided. The postoperative use of antibiotics may inhibit the formation of these three important vitamins by the intestinal flora, thus partially reducing the body's supply. Therefore, patients must be monitored for deficiencies of these nutrients and given adequate supplementation.

The importance of iron and zinc cannot be underestimated. Iron is vital for hemoglobin synthesis and is used to compensate for blood loss and possible anemia. Zinc has a definitive role in wound healing and clinical supplementation with zinc postoperatively is now common. Zinc sulphate is the preferred form, given in dosage amounts of 25 to 250 mg. See Table 13-1 for food sources of these essential nutrients.

Nursing Implications

Recognizing that inadequate nutritional support may increase morbidity and mortality during the early postoperational period, the nurse should

1. Recognize that malnutrition even in the short period of 1–3 days postoperatively may retard the healing process.
2. Monitor the patient closely and provide nourishment as soon as bowel sounds are present.
3. If oral feedings are contraindicated, check for other feeding methods that will furnish adequate nutrients.
4. Assess total fluid intake carefully and compare total fluid losses to avoid circulating overload.
5. Be aware that any weight gain during this period may be indicative of excess fluids.
6. Recognize the need for extra nutrients and fluids if the patient has elevated temperature.
7. Request specific written orders for change of diet and/or feeding method as the condition indicates.
8. Provide aggressive nutritional support during the early postoperative period as well as in subsequent convalescence.
9. Refer to the nutritional support team for assistance if your facility has one. Otherwise, work within the health team of which you are part.
10. Document all changes, requests, and rationales carefully.

PROGRESS CHECK ON ACTIVITY 2

Fill-in

1. State the main goal of dietary management in the postoperative period. _Regain Norm Body Wt._

2. List three ways this goal can be achieved.
   a. _Correct Fluid & Electrolyt imbalance_
   b. _Plan Nutritional & Dietary Support_
   c. _Moniter food intake_

3. Describe the three major functions of plasma protein.
   a. _Prevent Edema/Shock_
   b. _Provide Synthesis of Albumin, Antibodies_
   c. _accelerates wound healing_

4. Identify five intravenous feedings that may be used in the immediate postoperative period.
   a. _Blood_
   b. _Fluid/Electrolytes_

c. _D5W – .45 NaCl_

d. _Hypercal/_

e. _Vitamin Supplement._

5. Describe the normal progression of *routine* hospital diets and approximate time periods of use for each (consult Module 12 if in doubt about the time periods). _Cl liquid 24 hr after bowel sounds return_
Full liquid 1-2.
Soft Reg - Remainder of Stay.

Situation

Johnny B., 5' 6", 150 pounds, wrecked his motorcycle. He was wearing a helmet, but sustained a mild concussion. In addition, he received a compound fracture of the left femur and multiple lacerations of the arms, face, and upper body. He was in surgery for three hours. The diet prescription is for a soft diet in 6 feedings with the following specifications: 45 kcal/kg/bw/d, 15 percent of total calories as protein, 55 percent as carbohydrate, and the remainder as fat. Answer the following questions about this situation.

6. What is the total kcal content of Johnny's diet? Round to nearest whole number. _____

7. How many grams of protein per day will he receive?
_____

8. How many grams of fat are in his diet order? _____

9. How many grams of carbohydrate will Johnny get?
_____

10. Write a one-day menu, including the three snacks, that will satisfy the diet requirements.

Breakfast
_____
_____
_____

Mid-AM
_____
_____

Lunch
_____
_____
_____

Mid-PM
_____
_____

Dinner
_____
_____
_____

H.S. (Hour of Sleep)
_____
_____

References

Aaron, M. et al. 1989. *Enteral parenteral handbook: A screening tool for nutritional replacement in the hemodialysis patient.* Redwood City, CA: Satellite Dialysis Centers.

American Journal of Clinical Nutrition. 1980. Symposium on surgical treatment of morbid obesity. 33:353.

ASPEN. 1987. Guidelines for use of total parenteral nutrition. *J. Soc. Parenteral Enteral Nutr.* 10(5):441.

ASPEN. 1987. Guidelines for use of home total parenteral nutrition. *J. Soc. Parenteral Enteral Nutr.* 10(5):441.

Becker, H. D., and W. F. Caspary. 1980. *Postgastrectomy and postvagotomy syndromes.* New York: Springer.

Bellow, J. et al. 1987. Oral nutritional supplementation: A prospective evaluation of use, compliance, and cost. *Nutr. Support Serv.* 7(8):16.

Bingham, S. et al. 1982. Diet and health of people with an ileostomy. I. Dietary assessment. *British Journal of Nutrition* 47:399.

Bisballe, S. et al. 1986. Food intake and nutritional status after gastrectomy. *Hum Nutr. Clin. Nutr.* 40C:301.

Brennan, M. F. et al. 1986. Branched-chain amino acids in stress and injury. *Journal of Parenteral and Enteral Nutrition* 10(5):446.

Broadwell, D. C., and B. S. Jackson (eds.). 1982. *Principles of ostomy care.* St. Louis: Mosby.

Chen, M. et al. 1987. A decision tree for selecting an appropriate enteral formula. *Nutrition* 3(4):257.

Church, J. M. et al. 1987. Assessing the efficacy of intravenous nutrition in general surgical patients: Dynamic nutritional assessment with plasma proteins. *J. Parenteral Enteral Nutr.* 11(2):140.

Deitel, M. (ed). 1980. *Nutrition in clinical surgery.* Baltimore: Williams and Wilkins.

Deitel, M. (ed.). 1985. *Nutrition in clinical surgery.* 2nd ed. Baltimore: Williams and Wilkins.

Feitelson, M., et al. 1987. Tube feeding utilization/a quality of care review. *Journal of the American Dietetic Association* 87:73.

Groenwald, S. L. (ed.). 1987. *Cancer nursing: Principles and practices.* Boston: Jones and Bartlett.

Haynes-Johnson, V. 1986. Tube feeding complications: Causes, prevention, and therapy. *Nutri. Support Serv.* 6(3):17.

Hui, Y. H. 1987. *Handbook of enteral and parenteral feedings*. New York: Wiley.

Kohn, C. L. et al. 1987. Techniques for evaluating and managing diarrhea in the tube-fed patient. *Nutr. Clin. Pract.* 2(6):250.

Krey, S., and R. Murray (eds.). 1986. *Dynamics of nutrition support*. Norwalk, CT: Appleton-Century-Crofts.

Lang, C. (ed.). 1987. *Nutritional support in critical care*. Rockville, MD: Aspen.

McNeil, N. I., et al. 1982. Diet and health of people with an ileostomy. 2. Ileostomy function and nutritional state. *British Journal of Nutrition* 47:407.

Mughal, M. M., et al. 1987. The effect of nutritional status on the morbidity after elective surgery for benign gastrointestinal disease. *Journal of Parenteral and Enteral Nutrition* 11(2):140.

Mullen, B. D., and K. A. McGinn. 1980. *The ostomy book—living comfortably with colostomies, ileostomies, and urostomies*. Palo Alto, CA: Bull.

Mullen, J. L. et al. 1979. Implications of malnutrition in the surgical patient. *Archives of Surgery* 114:121.

Schrock, T. R., and L. W. Way. 1978. Total gastrectomy. *American Journal of Surgery* 135:348.

Shils, M. E. 1988. Enteral (tube) and parenteral nutrition support. In *Modern nutrition in health and disease*, 7th ed. M. E. Shils and V. R. Young (eds.). Philadelphia: Lea & Febiger.

Sitrin, M. D. et al. 1980. Nutritional and metabolic complications in a patient with Crohn's disease and ileal resection. *Gastroenterology* 78:1069.

Skipper, A. 1986. Specialized formulas for enteral nutrition support. *Journal of the American Dietetic Association* 86:654.

Souba, W. W., and D. W. Wilmore. 1988. Diet and nutrition in the care of the patient with surgery, trauma, and sepsis. In *Modern nutrition in health and disease*, 7th ed. M. E. Shils and V. R. Young (eds.). Philadelphia: Lea & Febiger.

Watt, R. 1985. The ostomy. Why is it created? *American Journal of Nursing* 85:1242.

Yarborough, M. F. (ed.). 1981. *Surgical nutrition*. New York: Churchill Livingstone.

Module 14

Diet Therapy for Cardiovascular Disorders

Time for completion
Activities: _____1½_____ hours
Optional examination: _½_ hour

Academic credit
Semester units: _⁴⁄₁₀_
Quarter units: _⁵⁄₁₀_

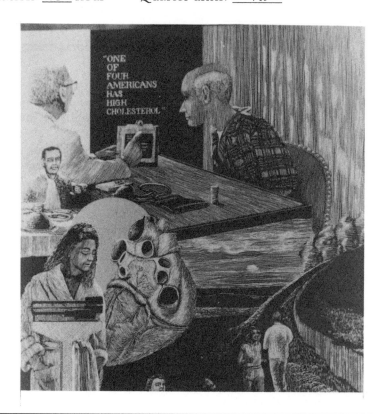

Outline

Objectives

Upon completion of this module, the student should be able to:

1. Discuss the controversies regarding the role of diet in preventing heart disease.
2. Describe and state the rationale of diet therapies used for the different heart disorders.
3. List the foods allowed, limited, and forbidden on selected therapeutic diets for heart disorders.
4. Identify resources available for patient education.
5. Identify nursing implications involved in the use of modified diets in cardiovascular disease.

Glossary

Atherosclerosis: thickening of the inside walls of arteries by deposits of fat or cholesterol substances (plaques).

Cardiovascular: of or relating to the heart and blood vessels.

Cerebrovascular accident (CVA):   when the blood vessels in the cerebrum (brain) are deprived of oxygen by an obstruction (occluded). This may be due to plaque formation, thrombus (blood clot), or aneurism (rupture of the blood vessel). Absence of oxygen to brain tissue for more than 5–6 minutes leads to irreversible cerebral changes and tissue death. Commonly called a "stroke."

Cholesterol: a fat-like substance manufactured in the liver from saturated fats, including body fat. It is widely distributed in the body tissues and serves many important functions.

Coronary: encircling (like a crown).

Coronary arteries: two large arteries that branch from the ascending aorta and supply the heart muscle with blood.

Coronary heart disease (CHD):   the coronary arteries supply all of the blood to the heart muscle. Occlusion, most often caused by narrowing of the vessels by plaque (atherosclerosis), deprives it of its nutrients and causes death to the part of the heart muscle that is occluded. When the occlusion is complete, myocardial infarction results (*see* Coronary occlusion).

Coronary occlusion: closing off of a coronary artery— most often caused by the plaques of atherosclerosis. When the occlusion is complete, myocardial infarction (MI) results.

Hyperlipoproteinemia: the presence of abnormally high levels of lipoproteins in the serum.

Hypertension: blood pressure elevated above the normal range for age and sex.

Lipoproteins: the form in which lipids are transported in the blood. There are four main classes of lipoproteins: chylomicrons, very-low-density lipoproteins, low-density lipoproteins, and high-density lipoproteins.

   a. low density lipoproteins (LDLs) transport 60–75% of the serum cholesterol. They carry *from* the liver *to* the body cells (including blood vessels). High serum levels of LDLs, therefore, increase the risk of CHD (see above).

   b. high density lipoproteins (HDLs) transport 20–25% of plasma cholesterol. They are believed to *collect* excess cholesterol from body cells and carry it *back* to the liver to be excreted or used for making bile.

Myocardial infarction (MI):   death of tissue of an area of the heart muscle as a result of oxygen deprivation, which in turn was caused by an obstruction of the blood supply (*see* Coronary heart disease). Commonly referred to as a "heart attack."

Triglycerides: the principal form of fat in foods and in the body, consisting of three fatty acids and glycerol.

Background Information

More than half the people who die in this country each year die of heart and blood vessel disease. About 75 percent of all adult hospitalized patients show symptoms of heart problems even though they are admitted for other causes. The high occurrence of these health problems means that the nurse should have accurate information about available dietary treatments for heart problems and the rationale for their use.

There is no known single cause of heart disease. However, the presence of a combination of certain factors predisposes a person to high risk of the disease. Some personal characteristics, such as a family history of heart disease, sex, and age cannot be changed, but dietary factors and stressful lifestyles can be modified. Therefore, the diets discussed in this module serve two goals: to reduce or prevent further damage to the cardiovascular system; and to prevent development of the disorder in yet unaffected individuals.

Current Consensus

National Cholesterol Education Program (NCEP).   The NCEP is one of three principal programs administered by the Office of Prevention, Education, and Control of the National Heart, Lung, and Blood Institute (NHLBI) of the National Institutes of Health (NIH). It came about after years of trials and scientific evidence that linked blood cholesterol levels to coronary heart disease. These trials showed that levels could be lowered safely by both diet and drugs. Hence, the National Cholesterol Education Program, today known as the NCEP, came into being.

Guidelines have been established for health professionals, patients, and the public. Among these important guidelines are two of particular interest to students of nutrition:

1.   To increase the knowledge of health professionals

regarding the major role that diet plays in reducing blood cholesterol.

2. To improve the knowledge, skills, and attitudes of students in the health professions regarding high blood cholesterol and its management.

Implementing dietary guidance with the use of nutrition labeling and standards of identity is one example of steps being taken to help Americans implement the guidelines. The major objective for this sweeping revision is to increase the availability of health-promoting foods.

In April 1991, the NCEP drafted an additional report that included children and adolescents. This report is included in other modules. Students should discuss these recommendations also while studying cardiovascular disease.

Nutritional Risk Factors in Heart Disease

The risk factors of heart disease include

1. Elevated serum cholesterol
2. Elevated serum triglycerides
3. Obesity
4. Hypertension
5. Generally poor eating habits and a sedentary lifestyle

All of these factors can be altered by diet and/or exercise.

ACTIVITY 1: The Lipid Disorders

Definitions

The term most frequently used in describing the lipid disorders is *hyperlipoproteinemia* (hyper = excess, lipoprotein = fat and protein, emia = in blood, which translates as excess level of fat/protein complex in blood). It refers to higher than normal levels of certain lipids in the blood. Because a lipid molecule is not water soluble, it must attach itself to a protein for transportation in the blood. Most dietary regimes aim at reducing serum levels of cholesterol and/or triglycerides.

Two other terms that are frequently used in discussions of lipid disorders are low-density lipoproteins (LDLs), "the bad guys" and high-density lipoproteins (HDLs), "the good guys." Although detailed discussion is not possible here, a brief explanation can clarify the matter.

The liver makes cholesterol from saturated fat. The amount of cholesterol synthesized is directly related to the quantity of saturated fat consumed. LDLs carry cholesterol to the artery plaques. Plaque formation is directly related to the amount of LDLs present. The connection is cholesterol, LDLs, plaques, and coronary heart disease. HDLs carry cholesterol away from the plaques, to the liver, to the gallbladder, and into the intestines, where it is excreted. HDLs, therefore, lower the risk of CHD. It appears that a person with a high HDL level is less likely to develop the disease than a person with a low HDL level. On the other hand, the reverse applies to blood LDL levels; that is, a high LDL level increases the risk of heart disease.

Cholesterol and Lipid Disorders

When we talk about blood cholesterol, we now refer to three forms: total, LDL, HDL. Some health-screening procedures measure the LDL cholesterol since it reflects the actual risk of atherosclerosis. To calculate LDL cholesterol, one may use the following formula:

$$\text{LDL cholesterol} = \text{Total cholesterol} - [(\text{Triglycerides} \times 5^{-1}) + \text{HDL}]$$

Normally, the plasma levels of different forms of lipid exist within certain limits. However, particular individuals may deviate from such norms and develop hyperlipidemia, or an elevated level of serum lipid. Three main types of lipid are involved in this condition: cholesterol (an excess of which is called hypercholesterolemia), triglyceride (hypertriglyceridemia), and certain forms of lipoprotein (hyperlipoproteinemia). Hyperlipoproteinemia is usually associated with hypercholesterolemia or hypertriglyceridemia, or both, although the reverse is not necessarily true. Any of the hyperlipidemias is undesirable because it may potentiate atherosclerosis or cause its associated clinical symptoms. The dietary management of these patients has two approaches: individual patients and the general public.

Dietary Management

To treat a patient with a lipid disorder, the attending physician uses laboratory data and clinical examination to type the patient. The typing uses many data: sex, age, symptoms, blood and laboratory tests, family history, and so forth. After the physician has typed the patient, the dietitian will use the appropriate dietary treatment according to the diagnosis. This chapter is not the proper forum to discuss details for treating individual patients with such diseases.

The second approach involves the public and is applicable to all individuals. It has one goal: to lower blood cholesterol. At present, the dietary management of a person with high blood (total or LDL) cholesterol is being promoted by three major groups: the American Heart Association (AHA); the National Cholesterol Education Program (NCEP); and other private health groups. All three groups target the amount and type of fats we eat.

The AHA and the NCEP have issued a two-step diet approach for the dietary management of blood cholesterol. This is presented in Table 14-1. The NCEP has also issued a guide to choose low-saturated fat, low-cholesterol foods (Table 14-2).

The NCEP has other recommendations that are of importance in patient care and public health programs. They are

1. The use of blood cholesterol as a means of classifying the risk of atherosclerosis for the population. The two classifications are based on plasma total cholesterol or LDL-cholesterol as shown in Table 14-3. These classifications can be applied if a person's blood cholesterol is known through screening or other means.

2. Using the LDL-cholesterol recommendations, one can make a careful study of a person's blood lipid and set goals as shown in Figure 14-1.

3. A combined flow chart that shows stage-by-stage the goals, monitoring, and follow-up recommendations of the NCEP. This is shown in Figure 14-2. This is extremely important in patient care as well as in public health programs.

Drug Management

As we have discussed, dietary management has two approaches: patient specific or the population as a whole. Obviously, when a person is under a physician's care, diet therapy is usually only part of the overall medical management. Under numerous circumstances, physicians have other tools that they can use to manage their patients. One such tool is medication. With advances in medicine, there are now many more choices when a physician has decided to lower the patient's blood cholesterol with the use of drugs. Table 14-4 provides a list of drugs with proven efficacy and those that are under active consideration.

Nursing Implications

Patients with lipid disorders have many diet modifications to make. In general, the nurse should

1. Follow the goals/objectives as shown in Figures 14-1 and 14-2.

2. Provide the patient with a list of foods to be used, limited, or omitted from the diet.

3. Provide an explanation of the reasons these foods are controlled.

4. Make arrangements for diet consultation with the dietitian or nutritionist to reinforce teaching.

5. If drug therapy is used, the patient should be provided with a list of possible side effects.

6. Be able to check the diet tray and recognize any errors in the food served.

7. Lend assistance to the patient in selecting an adequate menu within the limitations of the diet.

8. Remind the patient to check labels when shopping and describe what to look for. Meet with any others who are directly concerned in shopping and food preparation.

9. Discuss appropriate cooking methods.

10. Recommend reliable resources, either persons or materials, when necessary.

11. Use an approved diet manual or other sources of information when appropriate to answer questions and reinforce his or her own knowledge.

12. Stay abreast of new information regarding the use of these diets and incorporate any new findings into teaching.

TABLE 14-1
Dietary Therapy for High Blood Cholesterol Recommendations of the Adult Treatment Panel of the National Cholesterol Education Program

Nutrient	Recommended Intake	
	Step One Diet	*Step Two Diet*
Total fat	Less than 30% of total calories	
Saturated fatty acids	Less than 10% of total calories	Less than 7% of total calories
Polyunsaturated fatty acids	Up to 10% of total calories	
Monounsaturated fatty acids	10% to 15% of total calories	
Carbohydrates	50% to 60% of total calories	
Protein	10% to 20% of total calories	
Cholesterol	Less than 300 mg/day	Less than 200 mg/day
Total calories	To achieve and maintain desirable weight	

Source: Ernst, N. D. et al. 1988. National Cholesterol Education Program: Implications for dietetic practice. *Journal of the American Dietetic Association,* 88:1401.

TABLE 14-2
A Guide to Choosing Low-Saturated Fat, Low-Cholesterol Foods

Following a low-saturated fat, low-cholesterol diet is a balancing act: getting the variety of foods necessary to supply the nutrients you need without too much saturated fat and cholesterol or excess calories. One way to assure variety—and with it, a well-balanced diet—is to select foods each day from each of the following food groups. Select different foods from within groups, too, especially foods low is saturated fat (the left column). How many portions and the size of each portion should be adjusted to reach and maintain your desirable weight. As a guide, the recommended daily number of portions is listed for each food group.

	Choose	Go Easy On	Decrease

Meat, Poultry, Fish and Shellfish (up to 6 ounces a day)	Lean cuts of meat with fat trimmed, like:
	• beef
	   round, sirloin, chuck, loin
	• lamb
	   leg, arm, loin, rib
	• pork
	   tenderloin, leg (fresh),
	   shoulder (arm or picnic)
	• veal
	   all trimmed cuts except
	   ground
	poultry without skin,
	fish
	shellfish
			"Prime" grade
			Fatty cuts of meat, like:
			• beef
			   corned beef brisket, regular
			   ground, short ribs
			• pork
			   spareribs, blade roll, fresh
			goose, domestic
			duck
			organ meats
			sausage, bacon
			regular luncheon meats
			frankfurters
			caviar, roe

Dairy Products (2 servings a day, 3 servings for women who are pregnant or breastfeeding)	skim milk, 1% milk, low-fat buttermilk,
	   low-fat evaporated or nonfat milk
	low- fat yogurt
	low-fat soft cheeses, like cottage, farmer,
	   pot
	cheeses labeled no more than 2 to 6
	   grams of fat an ounce
		2% milk
		yogurt
		part-skim ricotta
		part-skim or
		imitation hard
		cheeses, like
		part-skim
		mozzarella
		"light" cream
		cheese
		"light" sour
		cream
			whole milk, like regular, evapo-
			   rated, condensed
			cream, half and half, most
			   nondairy creamers, imitation
			   milk products, whipped cream
			custard style yogurt
			whole-milk ricotta
			neufchatel
			brie
			hard cheeses, like swiss, American,
			   mozzarella, feta, cheddar,
			   muenster
			cream cheese
			sour cream

Eggs (no more than 3 egg yolks a week)	egg whites cholesterol-free egg substitutes		egg yolks

Fats and Oils (up to 6 to 8 teaspoons a day)	unsaturated vegetable oils: corn, olive,
	   peanut, rapeseed (canola oil)
	   safflower, sesame, soybean
	margarine, or shortening made from
	   unsaturated fats listed above: liquid,
	   tub, stick, diet
		nuts and seeds
		avocados and
		olives
			butter, coconut oil, palm oil, palm
			   kernel oil, bacon fat
			margarine or shortening made from
			   saturated fats listed above

(continues)

PROGRESS CHECK ON ACTIVITY 1

Fill-in

1. Complete the tables marked Exercise 14-1 and Exercise 14-2 (see page 208).
2. List four factors implicated in heart disease that are primarily of dietary origin.

a. _____

b. _____

c. _____

d. _____

TABLE 14-2 Continued

	Choose	Go Easy On	Decrease
Breads, Cereals, Pasta, Rice, Dried Peas and Beans (6 to 11 servings a day)	breads, like white, whole wheat, pumpernickel, and rye breads; pita; bagel; English muffin; sandwich buns; dinner rolls; rice cakes low-fat crackers, like matzo, bread sticks, rye krisp, saltines, zwieback hot cereals, most cold dry cereals pasta, like plain noodles, spaghetti, macaroni any grain rice dried peas and beans, like split peas, black-eyed peas, chick peas, kidney beans, navy beans, lentils, soybeans, soybean curd (tofu)	store-bought pancakes, waffles, biscuits, muffins, cornbread	croissant, butter rolls, sweet rolls, danish pastry, doughnuts most snack crackers, like cheese crackers, butter crackers, those made with saturated oils granola-type cereals made with saturated oils pasta and rice prepared with cream, butter, or cheese sauces; egg noodles
Fruits and Vegetables (2 to 4 servings of fruit and 3 to 5 servings of vegetables a day)	fresh, frozen, canned or dried fruits and vegetables		vegetables prepared in butter, cream, or sauce.
Sweets and Snacks (avoid too many sweets)	low-fat frozen desserts, like sherbet, sorbet, Italian ice, frozen yogurt, popsicles low-fat cookies, like fig bars, gingersnaps low-fat candy, like jellybeans, hard candy low-fat snacks like plain popcorn, pretzels nonfat beverages like carbonated drinks, juices, tea, coffee	frozen desserts, like ice milk homemade cakes, cookies, and pies using unsaturated oils sparingly fruit crisps and cobblers	high-fat frozen desserts, like ice cream, frozen tofu high-fat cakes, like most store-bought, pound, and frosted cakes store-bought pies most store-bought cookies most candy, like chocolate bars high-fat snacks, like chips, buttered popcorn high-fat beverages, like frappes, milkshakes, floats, and eggnogs

Label Ingredients

Go easy on products that list any fat or oil first or that list many fat and oil ingredients. The following lists clue you in to names of saturated fat ingredients (decrease) and unsaturated ingredients (go easy on).

		Go Easy On	Decrease
		carob, cocoa oils, like corn, cottonseed, olive, safflower, sesame, soybean, or sunflower oil nonfat dry milk, nonfat dry milk solids, skim milk	cocoa butter animal fat, like bacon, beef, chicken, ham, lamb, meat, pork or turkey fats, butter, lard coconut, coconut oil, palm or palm kernel oil cream egg and egg-yolk solids hardened fat or oil hydrogenated vegetable oil milk chocolate shortening or vegetable shortening vegetable oil (could be coconut, palm kernel, or palm oil)

Source: Eating to Lower Your High Blood Cholesterol. U.S.D.H.H.S./P.H.S./N.I.H., 1987.

TABLE 14-3
Summary Recommendations of the Adult Treatment Panel of the
National Cholesterol Education Program for Classification.

Classification Based on Total Cholesterol	Classification Based on LDL-Cholesterol
<200 mg/dL (<5.20 mmol/L) desirable blood cholesterol	<130 mg/dL (<3.35 mmol/L) desirable LDL-cholesterol
200–239 mg/dL (5.20–6.15 mmol/L) borderline-high blood cholesterol	130–159 mg/dL (3.35–4.10 mmol/L) borderline-high-risk LDL-cholesterol
≥ 240 mg/dL (≥ 6.20 mmol/L) high blood cholesterol	≥ 160 mg/dL (≥ 4.15 mmol/L) high-risk LDL-cholesterol

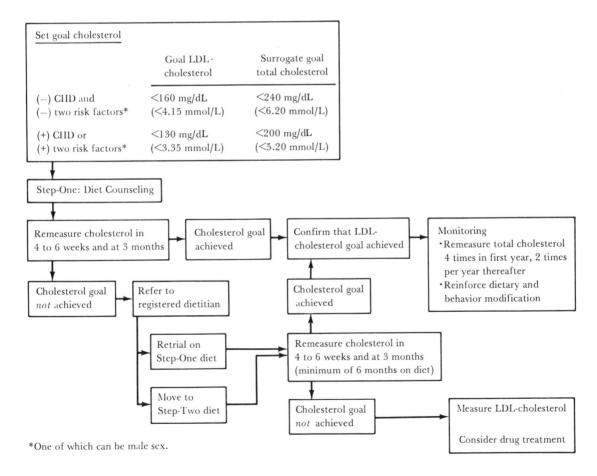

*One of which can be male sex.

Figure 14-1
Dietary Treatment Goals, Monitoring, and Follow-Up Recommendations of the Adult Treatment Panel of the National Cholesterol Education Program

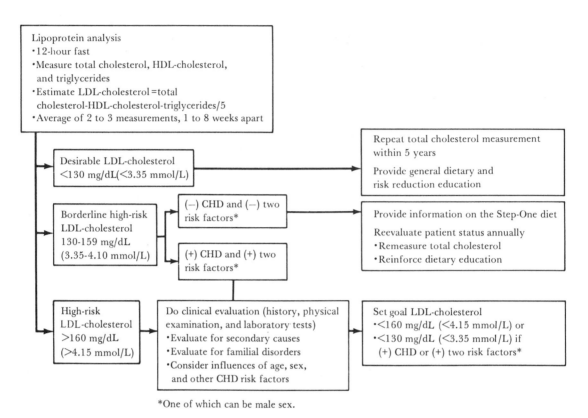

*One of which can be male sex.

Source: Ernst, N. D. et al. 1988. *Journal of the American Dietetic Association* 88:1401.

Figure 14-2
Classification of Patients Based on LDL-Cholesterol Recommendations of the Adult Treatment Panel of the National Cholesterol Education Program

Multiple Choice

Circle the letter of the correct answer.

3. Poor eating habits that can increase risk of heart disease include all except
   a. excessive amounts of alcohol.
   b. excess total daily calories.
   c. high consumption of ice cream and cake.
   d. eating a snack at bedtime.

4. The action of HDL in the blood is that of a carrier. Which of the following statements about HDL is true?
   a. HDL carries blood from the arteries to the liver.
   b. HDL carries cholesterol to the arteries and deposits it as plaque.
   c. HDL carries cholesterol from the arteries to the liver.
   d. none of the above

5. The most suitable of the following food groups for a patient on a Step 2 diet is
   a. lean pork, hamburger, lamb, and coconut.
   b. veal, chicken, trout, and peanut butter.
   c. duck, cheddar cheese, shrimp, and avocado.
   d. liver, bologna, ice milk, and olives.

6. The most suitable of the following food groups for a patient on a Step 1 diet is
   a. lean pork, hamburger, lamb, and coconut.
   b. veal, chicken, trout, and peanut butter.
   c. duck, cheddar cheese, shrimp, and avocado.
   d. liver, bologna, ice milk, and olives.

True/False

Circle T for True and F for False.

7. T F Cholesterol is manufactured in the heart and vessels.
8. T F Hyperlipoproteinemia refers to excess protein in the blood.
9. T F LDL is a term used to identify the process of lowering blood cholesterol.
10. T F Cholesterol gets into the blood only from ingested foods that contain it.
11. T F Exercise lowers cholesterol levels.
12. T F Exercise raises high-density lipoprotein levels.

TABLE 14-4
Drugs Recommended by the NCEP Adult Treatment Panel
for Consideration in Lowering Cholesterol

Drugs Highly Effective in Lowering LDL-Cholesterol*	Starting Dose	Maximum Dose	Usual Time and Frequency	Side Effects	Monitoring
cholestyramine colestipol	4 gm twice daily 5 gm twice daily	24 gm/day 30 gm/day	twice daily, within an hour of major meals	dose-dependent upper and lower gastrointestinal tract	during schedules of coadministered drugs
nicotinic acid	100–250 mg as single dose	3 gm/day, rarely doses up to 6 gm are used	three times a day with meals to minimize flushing	flushing, upper gastrointestinal and hepatic	uric acid, liver function, glucose
lovastatin	20 mg once daily with evening meal	80 mg/day	once (evening) or twice daily with meals	gastrointestinal tract and hepatic, miscellaneous, including muscle pains	liver function, creatine kinase, lens

Other Drugs for Consideration	Reduce CHD Risk	Long-Term Safety	Maintaining Adherence	LDL-Cholesterol Lowering %	Special Precautions
gemfibrozil†	not proven	preliminary evidence	relatively easy	5–15	may increase LDL-cholesterol in hypertriglyceridemic patients; should not be used in patients with gallbladder disease
probucol	not proven	not established	relatively easy	10–15	lowers HDL-cholesterol; significance of this has not been established; prolongs QT interval

*LDL is low-density lipoprotein, and HDL is high-density lipoprotein.
†Not approved by the Food and Drug Administration for routine use in lowering cholesterol. The results of the Helsinki Heart Study showed a decline in CHD risk.
Source: Ernst, N. D. et al. 1988. *Journal of the American Dietetic Association* 88:1401.

ACTIVITY 2: Heart Disease and Sodium Restriction

Dietary sodium restriction is an important part of the medical treatment for hypertension and congestive heart failure. Although hypertension is a symptom, not a disease, it is one leading contributor to heart attack and stroke and is also associated with diseases of the kidney. For these reasons, controlling hypertension is one way to prevent the development of these conditions. Congestive heart failure occurs when the heart fails to pump out the returning blood fast enough, allowing blood to accumulate in the right side of the heart. This raises venous pressure (pressure in the vein from the accumulation of blood),

causing fluid retention (edema) in the heart and its associated parts.

Diet and Hypertension

Secondary hypertension is caused by some known factor, such as a kidney disorder. The cause of essential or primary hypertension is unknown. Dietary factors that may cause high blood pressure include obesity and excessive use of salt. Some believe that caffeine in coffee and alcoholic beverages can potentiate the condition. New research

EXERCISE 14-1
Complete the Chart by Filling In the Information for Each Column

Diet	Disease or Condition	Foods Allowed	Foods Limited	Foods Forbidden	Nursing Implications
Step 1					

EXERCISE 14-2
Complete the Chart by Filling In the Information for Each Column

Diet	Disease or Condition	Foods Allowed	Foods Limited	Foods Forbidden	Nursing Implications
Step 2					

TABLE 14-5
Foods Excluded in a 3 to 5 Gram Sodium Diet

Meat Group

1. Cured, canned, or smoked meats and fish
2. Canned dried beans, meat stews, soups
3. Meat analogs: i.e., imitation bacon bits
4. Cheeses: regular, processed
5. Frozen TV dinners
6. Ready-prepared meats in gravy or sauces
7. Kosher meats

Grain Group

1. Salty crackers
2. Rolls with salted tops
3. Seasoned mixes: i.e., stuffing, pasta, rice

Milk Group

1. Cheese spreads
2. Processed cheese (cheese spreads)
3. Cheese: roquefort, blue, camembert
4. Salted buttermilk

Fruit and Vegetable Group

1. Any vegetable prepared in brine
2. Sauerkraut
3. Canned tomatoes; tomato juice
4. Tomato sauce or paste
5. V-8 juice

Other

1. Salted sauces and seasonings: barbecue sauce, chili sauce, meat sauce, Worcestershire sauce, etc.; any type of salt, including tenderizers and flavor enhancers
2. Salted snacks: chips, pretzels, popcorn, nuts, pickles, olives, seeds
3. Miscellaneous: mustard, relishes, bacon drippings, bouillon cubes, catsup, etc.

indicates calcium deficiency may be a factor in hypertension.

A low-sodium diet is usually supplemented with drug therapy (antihypertensives). Most antihypertensives contain diuretics. While most diuretics remove water and sodium from the body, some also remove potassium. Since the patient frequently is overweight, a low-calorie diet is also prescribed. Weight loss by itself will often reduce blood pressure, especially in males. The diet should be individually prescribed and tailored to the patient's need for sodium and calorie reduction. Since there are different levels of sodium restriction and many levels of calorie restriction, the diet order must be specific to be effective. A diet order that reads "salt poor, low cal" is unacceptable. Sodium is ordered in milligrams or grams, and calories by a specific number designed to help the patient lose weight. An adequate diet under 1,200 calories daily is difficult to plan; it results in low patient compliance, especially with long-term usage. A normal level of protein of high biological value is recommended. Fats in the diet are moderately low and the types of fat flexible. Unsaturated fats used within the caloric allowance are more acceptable than saturated fats. Carbohydrates provide up to 50 percent of the total caloric intake, but concentrated sweets are not recommended. High potassium foods should be encour-

aged if drug therapy causes loss of this mineral in the urine. Some physicians prescribe special potassium supplements.

Diet and Congestive Heart Failure

The treatment for congestive heart failure consists of rest to reduce the demands on the heart; drug therapy to strengthen the heartbeat and slow it down; and diet therapy to reduce edema and decrease the workload on the heart. The dietary regimen is as follows:

1. *Reduce edema.* A low-sodium diet is used, usually in the moderate to low range. It is difficult to severely reduce the sodium intake of a patient, because such a diet is most unpalatable.

2. *Decrease workload.* The diet may be of soft consistency and divided into five or six small meals per day. If the patient is overweight, the diet may also be restricted in calories. Fluids are not usually restricted, but excess fluid intake is not allowed. Although individual need varies, 2,000 to 3,000 ml of fluid per day is acceptable.

Some patients with hypertension and/or congestive heart failure may also require a modification of fat or cholesterol intake.

The Sodium Restricted Diet

The average intake of sodium in the American diet ranges from 3 to 8 grams per day. Although some sodium is essential for body functioning, the amount needed is approximately 1/2 to 1 gram daily. The main source of sodium in our diets is table salt (sodium chloride). Salt is about 40 percent sodium by weight. It is used extensively in food processing for items such as processed meats (lunch meat, ham, bacon, canned meats, and fish), dried foods, sauerkraut, olives, and pickles. It is used in baking and cooking, and then used again at the dining table. In addition, most foods contain some sodium before any processing or cooking takes place. Some unprocessed foods are higher in naturally occurring sodium than others. For example, meats, milk, and eggs are high in natural sodium, whereas most plant foods are low. There are exceptions. Beets, spinach, chard, and kale are fairly high in sodium. Fruits, oils, sugars, and cereal grains contain only a trace of sodium or none at all, if no sodium chloride is added in processing. If a diet is based on the basic food groups, unsalted bread/butter and unprocessed grains and meats are used, and no salt is used during cooking or at the table, then the diet contains approximately 500 mg sodium. It is not difficult to see how we can "overdose" our foods with sodium.

The four levels of sodium restriction recommended by the American Heart Association are commonly prescribed by physicians to control a patient's sodium intake. The levels vary from 250 mg up to 3 to 5 grams of sodium daily.

Mild Sodium Restriction (3 to 5 Grams Daily)

This is a regular diet which omits only salty foods and the use of salt at the table. Salt may be used lightly in cooking; for example, use half the amount stated in the recipe. This diet is frequently used after discharge from the hospital, when edema is under control. A wide variety of foods from the basic food groups is recommended. Table 14-5 illustrates the foods to avoid within each food group.

Moderate Sodium Restriction (1,000 Milligrams Daily)

This diet is used both in the hospital and at home. In addition to avoiding the foods indicated for the 3 to 5 gram sodium diet, the diet has the following restrictions:

1. No more than 2 cups milk per day.
2. No more than 5 oz. meat per day. One egg may be substituted for 1 oz. meat.
3. No salt in cooking.
4. Bread and butter beyond 3 servings daily should be unsalted.
5. No commercial mixes or regular canned vegetables.

Strict Sodium Restriction (500 Milligrams Daily)

This diet is used primarily for hospitalized patients, though it may be followed at home. The restrictions, however, result in low patient compliance except in a hospital setting. In addition to the restrictions indicated for 3 to 5 gram and 1,000 mg sodium diets, two other restrictions are required to lower the dietary sodium to 500 mg:

1. No bread and butter that has salt added.
2. No vegetables that are naturally high in sodium content.

Severe Sodium Restriction (250 Milligrams Daily)

The substitution of low-sodium milk for regular milk in the 500 mg sodium diet will lower the dietary sodium content to 250 mg.

The "Exchange Lists for Meal Planning," issued by the American Dietetic Association and the American Diabetic Association (see Appendix E), may be modified for the various levels of sodium restriction. This booklet is a helpful tool for diet planning, particularly when a caloric or fat modification is also necessary.

Some drinking water is high in sodium, especially if water softeners are used. Patients on low-sodium diets should ascertain their drinking water's sodium content, and, if necessary, use distilled water.

Many drugs, both prescription and over-the-counter, contain high levels of sodium. Patients need to be made aware of these.

Nursing Implications

The nurse should follow the guidelines below.

1. Be aware that sodium-restricted diets are unpalatable, especially at very restricted levels.
2. Be prepared to offer alternative seasonings to enhance flavor and encourage the patient to consume an adequate diet.
3. Caution patients to read the labels on foods and to avoid self-medication. Check medications received in the hospital, and, if they are too high in sodium, ask about alternates.
4. Check trays of all patients on sodium-restricted diets to make sure salt has not accidently been included.
5. Recognize that patients with congestive heart failure tend to have poor appetites. Accurate intake and output records are necessary. Meal sizes and intervals may need adjusting.
6. Check for inadequate potassium intake when antihypertensives are used.
7. Be aware that iodine intake may be low when salt is restricted.
8. Do not suggest salt substitutes without asking the physician first: there may be impaired renal function or, if a potassium supplement is being used, a patient could develop hyperkalemia. Salt substitutes are high in potassium.

PROGRESS CHECK ON ACTIVITY 2

Fill-in

1. Complete the table marked Exercise 14-3, on p. 211.
2. Write a day's menu for a person on a 500 mg sodium diet with no calorie restriction (use separate sheet).
3. List 10 appropriate seasonings that may be used in place of salt.

   a. _____
   b. _____
   c. _____
   d. _____
   e. _____
   f. _____
   g. _____
   h. _____
   i. _____
   j. _____

EXERCISE 14-3
Complete Each Column with the Appropriate Information

Diet	Disease or Condition	Foods Allowed	Foods Limited	Foods Forbidden	Nursing Implications
5,000 mg sodium					
1,000 mg sodium					
500 mg sodium					
250 mg sodium					

ACTIVITY 3: Dietary Care after Heart Attack and Stroke

Myocardial Infarction (MI), "Heart Attack" _____

Priority is given to life-saving measures immediately following a myocardial infarction (MI). An intravenous line (IV) is prepared and inserted. If needed, the IV can be used to administer drugs and regulate fluid and electrolyte balance.

The goals of diet therapy are to reduce the workload of the heart, restore and maintain electrolyte balance, and, after a brief period of undernutrition, to maintain an adequate nutritional intake. The diet therapy progresses as follows:

1. For the first 24 to 48 hours after oral feedings are ordered by the physician, the patient receives only clear liquids.
2. The liquid diet is followed by a low-residue diet, and then a soft diet. Foods are divided into five to six small meals. The diet also may be restricted in sodium, if necessary.
3. Beverages containing caffeine are omitted.
4. The physician may prescribe fluid restriction, if intake and output records warrant.
5. Constipation may accompany a restriction of fiber and/or fluids. Nursing measures to solve this complication are needed.

6. A gradual return to regular foods, with a restriction of sodium, fat, and/or cholesterol for certain patients.

Cerebrovascular Accident (CVA), "Stroke" _____

As with a myocardial infarction, the first measures taken by health professionals after a cerebrovascular accident are life-saving, not dietary. Ongoing therapy focuses on restoring and maintaining adequate nutrition. Diet therapy after a CVA progresses as follows:

1. An intravenous line is used for the first 24 to 48 hours. A careful monitoring is necessary. Fluids must be restricted if cerebral edema is present.
2. If the patient is comatose, tube feeding will be the diet of choice after IV therapy. Oral liquid feedings may begin when the patient is conscious. If the patient develops paralysis of one side of the throat, he or she will choke more easily on liquids than on semi-solids. In the event of such paralysis, very thick liquids or very soft solids may be necessary.
3. Eventually, with training, the patient may return to a regular diet.
4. Depending on the patient, the diet may be low in calories, sodium, fat, and/or cholesterol.

Nursing Implications

The responsibilities of the nurse include the following:

1. Assess food deficits as soon as oral feedings are resumed and take measures to restore sufficient intake.
2. Allow self-feeding for both MI and CVA patients as soon as possible.
3. Position the patient to allow maximum use of his or her remaining abilities and to give the patient some control.
4. Schedule nursing care and treatment far enough in advance of meals to let the patient rest before eating.
5. Relieve pain before meals are served.
6. Promote comfort, relieve anxiety, and be very patient.
7. Explain all restrictions in the patient's diet.
8. Teach diet restrictions when the patient is able to listen (when anxiety and fear have diminished).
9. Make arrangements for those involved in food purchasing and preparation to be involved in the teaching session with the dietitian.

PROGRESS CHECK ON NURSING IMPLICATIONS

Fill-in

1. List four objectives of diet therapy for a patient who has had a myocardial infarction.

   a. _____

   b. _____

   c. _____

   d. _____

2. List as many nursing measures as you can think of to assist a stroke victim to ingest an adequate diet.

   a. _____

   b. _____

   c. _____

   d. _____

   e. _____

   f. _____

   g. _____

   h. _____

   i. _____

   j. _____

PROGRESS CHECK ON ACTIVITY 3

Fill-in

1. List five hidden sources of sodium.

   a. _____

   b. _____

   c. _____

   d. _____

   e. _____

2. List ten seasonings that may be used freely on a low-sodium diet.

   a. _____

   b. _____

   c. _____

   d. _____

   e. _____

   f. _____

   g. _____

   h. _____

   i. _____

   j. _____

3. State five nursing measures applicable to the feeding of a CVA patient with right-sided hemiplegia who is not comatose.

   a. _____

   b. _____

   c. _____

   d. _____

   e. _____

4. Explain the rationale for a diet therapy that specifies "soft 2 gram sodium in 6 feedings" for a 5-day post-MI patient. _____

   _____

   _____

   _____

Multiple Choice

Circle the letter of the correct answer.

5. Which of the following menus would be the best choice for a person on a 1 gram sodium, low cholesterol diet?
    a. split pea soup, crackers, tuna salad, ice cream, and tea
    b. scrambled eggs, baked potato, fruit salad, baked apple, and skim milk
    c. broiled fresh trout with lemon, baked potato, sliced tomato salad, skim milk, and peach halves
    d. prime rib roast, broccoli, mashed potato, sliced pineapple, and tea

6. From the following list, which foods would be most suitable for a person on a 500 mg sodium diet?
    a. tuna fish salad with lettuce
    b. sliced turkey with cranberry sauce
    c. scalloped potatoes and ham
    d. honey and peanut butter sandwich

References

American Dietetic Association. 1988. *Manual of clinical dietetics*. Chicago: American Dietetic Association.

American Heart Association. 1986. *Recommendations for treatment of hyperlipidemia in adults*. Publication No. 72-204-A. Dallas, TX: American Heart Association.

Ballard-Barbash, R., and C. W. Callaway. 1987. Marine fish oils: Role in prevention of coronary artery disease. *Mayo Clin. Proc.* 62:113.

Beare-Rogers, J. (ed.). 1988. *Dietary fat requirements in health and development*. Champaign, IL: American Oil Chemists' Society.

Bernard, M. A. et al. (eds.). 1986. *Nutritional and metabolic support of hospitalized patients*. Philadelphia: Saunders.

Bierman, E. L., and A. Chait. 1988. Nutrition and diet in relation to hyperlipidemia and atherosclerosis. In *Modern nutrition in health and disease*, 7th ed. M. E. Shils and V. R. Young (eds.). Philadelphia: Lea & Febiger.

Brauer, P. M. 1985. Nutritional support of the critically ill. Part 1: Review. *Journal of the Canadian Dietetic Association* 46:292.

Brauer, P. M. et al. 1985. Nutritional support of the critically ill, Part II: Guidelines for the clinical dietitian. *Journal of the Canadian Dietetic Association* 46:304.

Bursztyn, P. (ed.). 1987. *Nutrition and blood pressure*. London: John Libbey.

Clark, L. T. 1984. Alcohol use and hypertension. *Postgraduate Medicine* 75:273.

Connor, S. L., and W. E. Connor. 1982. The dietary treatment of hyperlipidemia. *Med. Clin. N. A.* 66(2):485.

Connor, S. L., and W. E. Connor. 1986. *The new American diet*. New York: Simon and Schuster.

Dustan, H. P. 1985. Obesity and hypertension. *Ann. Intern. Med.* 103:1047.

Einhorn, D., and L. Landsberg. 1988. Nutrition and diet in hypertension. In *Modern nutrition in health and disease*, 7th ed. M. E. Shils and V. R. Young (eds.). Philadelphia: Lea & Febiger.

Ernst, N. D. et al. 1988. National Cholesterol Education Program: Implications for dietetic practice. *Journal of the American Dietetic Association* 88:1401.

Food and Nutrition Board, National Research Council, National Academy of Sciences. 1989. *Recommended dietary allowances*. 10th ed. Washington, DC: National Academy Press.

Grundy, S. M. 1987. Monounsaturated fatty acids, plasma cholesterol, and coronary heart disease. *American Journal of Clinical Nutrition* 45:1168.

Grundy, S. M. et al. 1987. Workshop on monounsaturated fatty acids. *Arteriosclerosis* 7:644.

Henry, H. J. et al. 1985. Increasing calcium intake lowers blood pressure: The literature reviewed. *Journal of the American Dietetic Association* 85:182.

Jones, R. J. 1977. Dietary management in the coronary care unit (questions and answers). *Journal of the American Medical Association* 237:2645.

Kaplan, N. M. 1985. Nondrug treatment of hypertension. *Ann. Intern. Med.* 102:359.

Mayo Clinic. 1988. *Mayo Clinic diet manual*. Philadelphia: B. C. Dekker.

National Institute of Health. 1984. The Joint National Committee on Detection, Evaluation, and Treatment of High Blood Pressure. USDHHS/PHS/National Institute of Health.

National Institute of Health. 1984. Treatment of hypertriglyceridemia. *Journal of the American Medical Association* 251:1196.

National Institute of Health. 1985. *Cholesterol counts: NIH Publication No. 85-2699*. USDHHS/PHS/National Institute of Health.

National Institute of Health. 1986. Nonpharmacologic approaches to the control of high blood pressure. *Final report of the subcommittee on nonpharmacologic therapy of the 1984 Joint National Committee on Detection, Evaluation, and Treatment of High Blood Pressure. Publication No. 1986-491-292-41147.* USDHHS/PHS/National Institute of Health.

National Institute of Health Consensus Conference. 1985. Lowering blood cholesterol to prevent heart disease. *Journal of the American Medical Association* 253:2080.

Parrot-Garcia, M., and D. A. McCarron. 1984. Calcium

and hypertension. *Nutrition Review* 42:205.

Poindexter, S. M. et al. 1986. Nutrition in congestive heart failure. *Nutr. Clin. Prac.* 1:83.

Schaefer, E. J., and R. I. Levy. 1985. Pathogenesis and management of lipoprotein disorders. *New England Journal of Medicine* 312:1300.

Schlichtig, R., and S. M. Ayres. 1988. *Nutritional support of the critically ill*. Chicago: Year Book Medical Publishers.

Sorkin, M. I. 1980. Hyperkalemia—causes, management, and prevention. *Consult* 20:25.

USDA. 1986. Dietary guidelines for Americans: Avoid too much fat, saturated fat and cholesterol. *Home and Garden Bulletin No. 232-3*. United States Department of Agriculture, Human Nutrition Information Service.

Watson, R. R. (ed.). 1987. *Nutrition and heart disease. Vols. I and II*. Boca Raton, FL: CRC Press.

Widhalm, K., and H. K. Naito (eds.). 1988. *Progress in clinical and biological research: Volume 255, Recent aspects of diagnosis and treatment of lipoprotein disorders: Impact on prevention of atherosclerotic diseases*. New York: Alan R. Liss.

Diet and Disorders of Ingestion, Digestion, and Absorption

Time for completion
Activities: _____1½_____ hours
Optional examination: _½_ hour

Academic credit
Semester units: $^3/_{10}$
Quarter units: ___$^4/_{10}$___

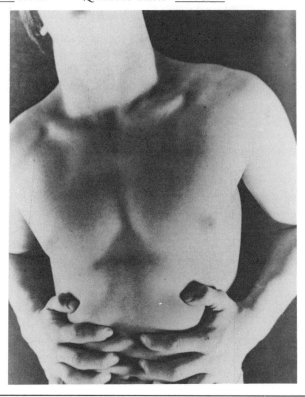

Outline

Objectives _____

Upon completion of this module, the student should be able to:

1. List the diet modifications used in certain gastrointestinal disorders.
2. Explain the rationale for the use of diet modifications.
3. Describe the diet modification sequence and progression.
4. List foods that meet the diet requirements.
5. State nursing implications for dietary care.

Glossary _____

Antiemetics: an agent (a drug) that relieves vomiting.

Aspiration: the act of inhaling. Pathological aspiration of vomitus or mucus into the respiratory tract (lungs) may occur when a patient is unconscious or under the effect of anesthesia.

Cachexia: general wasting of the body, especially during chronic disease.

Cholinergic: an agent (a drug) that stimulates the action of the sympathetic nerves.

Colostomy: creation of an opening between the colon and surface of the body. A surgical procedure.

Defecate: to eliminate waste and undigested food from the rectum.

Esophageal varices: varicose veins in the esophagus.

Flatulence: excessive formation of gas in intestinal tract.

Gall stones: precipitation of cholesterol crystals in the gallbladder to form stones.

Gastrectomy: removal of part of the stomach.

Hemorrhoidectomy: surgical removal of varicose veins in the mucosa either outside or just inside the rectum.

Ileostomy: creating an opening between the ileum and the surface of the body by establishing a stoma (see below) on the abdominal wall.

Ileum: distal portion of the small intestine extending from jejunum to cecum.

Immunotherapy: passive immunization of an individual with pre-formed antibodies. It activates the whole immune system to fight off disease. Most recently used in terminology relating to treatment of cancer.

Intraluminal: within the lumen (wall) of a tubular structure.

Jejunum: part of the small intestine extending from the duodenum to the ileum.

Mucosa (mucous membrane): the membrane that lines the tubular organs of the body.

Osteomate: one who has had an ostomy (colostomy or ileostomy). These are surgical procedures for creating an opening to the outside of the body for the elimination of waste.

Pectin: a carbohydrate that forms a gel when mixed with a sweetened liquid.

Pylorus: a distal part of the stomach opening into the duodenum. Contains many glands that secrete hydrochloric acid.

Stoma: a mouthlike opening. A surgical opening kept open for drainage and other purposes.

Varices: plural for varix; an enlarged, tortuous vein, artery, or lymph vessel.

Background Information _____

The gastrointestinal (GI) tract extends from the mouth to the anus. All disturbances related to food intake, digestion, absorption, and elimination affect the GI tract and usually require special diets. Such diets were among the very first ever used in the treatment of diseases. Unfortunately, many have not changed much since they were first used, even though recent research has shown that some of the diets used to treat diseases are ineffective and incompatible with the clinical conditions of patients. Two notable examples include the diets for diverticular diseases and peptic ulcer.

Psychological factors play a role when we consider many disorders of the GI tract. The digestive system is said to "mirror the human condition." If this is true, then specific foods do not cause the problem in all cases. Rather, the psychological state of the body that receives them can be responsible. Stress factors, such as anxiety, fear, work pressure, grief, emotional makeup, and coping patterns, have a great deal to do with how or if foods are tolerated. Obviously, if a person has specific food allergies or a physiological basis for food intolerance (such as an enzyme deficiency), then the offending foods should not be eaten. Otherwise, as in the case of an ulcer patient, there is no sound basis for the traditional diet therapy that permits only soft, white, or mildly flavored foods.

Frequently, patients with experience of traditional diet therapy will challenge a prescription of modern diet therapy. Nurses must understand and be prepared to explain the newer concepts of dietary management.

ACTIVITY 1: Disorders of the Mouth, Esophagus, and Stomach

Mouth

Cleft Lip and/or Palate

A congenital defect of newborns, cleft lip and/or palate is corrected by a series of surgeries after the infant reaches a weight safe enough to withstand a surgical procedure. These infants have a high nutritional requirement to prepare for surgery and rapid growth. The care provider must practice care in the positioning and feeding of these children to prevent aspiration. Certain types of nipples and/or tubing may be required for infant feeding. Families need counseling in the feeding and care of these infants. Nurses should receive additional training when caring for and teaching others to care for such patients.

Dental caries

Decayed teeth are epidemic in the United States. Nearly all children in the United States are afflicted and about 30 percent of Americans past the age of 25 wear full dentures. While poor dental hygiene (improper brushing, not flossing, and failing to get checkups) may account for part of the problem, much is dietary in nature. Lack of essential nutrients such as calcium, phosphorus, fluorine, and vitamins D, A, and C affect tooth and gum formation and development. Since both deciduous ("baby") and permanent teeth are formed in utero (before birth), the diet of the mother affects the offspring's teeth. Fetuses are not parasites and cannot necessarily derive adequate amounts of each nutrient needed for development from the mother. Some children are born without all of their permanent teeth buds, and, in this case, it is prudent to maintain deciduous teeth as long as possible.

A youngster's diet affects the strength and function of his or her teeth. Milk, juice, or sweetened drinks left in the bottle against an infant's gums during sleep can cause decay of newly erupted teeth. This is known as the "baby bottle syndrome." Children learn to like sweets if they receive them early in their diet. It is believed that the high use of concentrated sweets, especially the sticky type, is the main culprit in the formation of cavities (dental caries).

Health promotion measures that will benefit oral tissues throughout life include use of a well-balanced diet with adequate amounts of essential nutrients, limitation or omission of sweets, and proper oral hygiene and dental care.

Dentures

The wearing of dentures can be a mixed blessing. If properly fitted, they provide the ability to ingest a variety of foods not possible otherwise. Dentures are cosmetically attractive and improve self-esteem, but there are disadvantages associated with them. As bone recedes after teeth have been extracted, frequent realignments are mandatory for proper fit. Loose dentures may collect particles underneath them, causing pain. Rubbing between dentures and the gum tissue creates sore spots that can lead to inflammation or even tumors. The health of the gums on which dentures rest determines the success of wearing dentures. An adequate supply of vitamins A and C, along with other nutrients, is essential to gum tissue integrity.

Many older people have ill-fitting dentures or no dentures at all, even though they may have no teeth. This can cause great difficulty in chewing food, and therefore, in the digestion of food. This leads to a decreased intake of fiber and other essential nutrients, since unchewed and undigested foods are not absorbed. The effect of this condition on health is obvious.

Whenever dental problems exist or dentures are absent, the mechanical soft diet is preferred, since it provides adequate nutrition and ease of chewing. Module 12 provides additional information on the mechanical soft diet.

Fractured Jaw

The nutritional needs for a person following the trauma of a fractured jaw are high, as in other types of fractures. The treatment of choice is to wire the jaws together, which poses obvious problems with eating. A diet high in protein, calories, minerals, and vitamins is necessary for proper healing. Liquid food must pass through a straw without moving the jaw. Care must be taken to prevent choking, and a wire cutter must be close at hand to cut the wire if choking occurs. As the person is usually home for a considerable length of time before the wires are removed, the caretaker must be taught to use the wire cutter. Since the practice of oral hygiene is difficult, the oral tissues must be cleaned by a special and thorough procedure to prevent bacterial growth. Lack of adequate cleaning can cause cavities and produce odors that decrease the appetite. Table 15-1 lists examples of foods suitable for the person with a fractured jaw.

Esophagus: Hiatal Hernia

The esophagus is separated from the stomach by the diaphragm. When the stomach partially protrudes above the diaphragm because of the weakening of the diaphragm opening, hiatal hernia results. Hiatal hernia is usually treated with antacids and a low-fiber bland diet. Six small feedings per day are recommended and fluids are taken between meals. Foods that irritate esophageal mucosa are eliminated—for example, orange, tomato, or grapefruit

TABLE 15-1
Foods for a Patient with a Fractured Jaw

Composition of feedings	These are oral feedings composed of approximately
	    250 gms carbohydrate,
	    115 gms protein,
	    110 gms fat, and
	    2400 calories

General instructions	1. Follow the family menu as closely as possible, if the meal pattern is adequate. 2. Plan for the increase in protein by using meats of all kinds (beef, pork, poultry, lamb, veal, fish, organ meats) and meat substitutes such as eggs, cottage cheese, other soft cheeses, and yogurt. 3. All meats should be lean and, with the exception of beef, should be well cooked; beef may be used raw or rare if desired. Use sufficient broth when blending. 4. All meats, vegetables, breads should be cubed before being added to blender. Eggs should be added last when blending. 5. If butter or margarine is used, it should be very soft or melted before adding to mixture. 6. It may be necessary to strain the mixture after it has been blended to prevent clogging. 7. Variety can be obtained by using soups, vegetable juices, or broths for blending instead of milk, but be aware that this lowers total caloric intake. 8. The patient should participate in the selection of the various meats, vegetables, and pastas that go into the blender.

Meal plan for oral liquid feedings	*Breakfast* Strained juice Hot blended drink* Coffee/cream/sugar if desired or Beverage of choice	*Lunch* Fruit drink* Hot blended drink* Coffee/cream/sugar if desired or Beverage of choice	*Dinner* Fruit eggnog* Hot blended drink* Beverage of choice

	Supplemental Feedings To increase caloric intake over 2,400 add any of these: Choose from fruit drink,* fruit eggnog,* a thin milkshake, liquid gelatin, chocolate milk, malted milk, regular eggnog. Dry milk powder or vitamin supplements may be added to increase nutrients upon recommendation of the physician. Recipes follow for those items marked*.
Recipes for oral feedings	*Hot blended drink # 1* ½ c. cooked refined cereal such as farina, grits, cream of wheat, etc. 1 c. hot milk** 2 soft cooked eggs 1 tsp. melted butter or margarine ½ tsp. salt (optional) Mix all ingredients except fat. Blend to desired consistency and strain. Add the melted fat and salt. Reheat to desired temperature. *Hot blended drink # 2* ½ c. cubed poultry, veal, pork, lamb, or cheese ½ c. cooked rice or pasta ½ c. cooked vegetable of choice 1–2 slices whole wheat bread, cubed 1½ c. milk** 1 tsp. melted butter or margarine ½ tsp. salt (optional) Blend the meat or substitute separately with ½ c. of the milk for approximately 2 minutes. Add rice or pasta, vegetable, and bread. Add remaining milk and salt. Blend to desired consistency. Strain the mixture. Add the melted fat and reheat to desired temperature before serving. <div align="right">*(continues)*</div>

**All liquids used may be increased to thin the mixture to the consistency that will not clog a straw.

TABLE 15-1 (Continued)

Recipes for oral feedings (continued)	*Hot blended drink # 3*

Recipes for oral feedings
(continued)

Hot blended drink # 3
½ c. chopped raw or rare beef or ground beef patty
1 c. broth**
½ c. cooked or canned vegetable of choice
½ c. cooked potato (without skins)
1 c. milk, tomato juice, or cream soup**
1 tsp. melted butter or margarine
½ tsp. salt (optional)
Blend beef and broth together for approximately 2 minutes. Add other ingredients except fat. Blend together to desired consistency. Strain. Add fat and salt. Heat to desired temperature before serving.

Fruit drink
1 banana or ½ c. any canned or cooked fruit
⅔ c. fruit juice, preferable a vitamin C source (orange, grapefruit)**
Blend. Strain. Chill before serving.
Fruit eggnog
To the above recipe for fruit drink, add 2 teaspoons lemon juice, 1 tablespoon sugar, and 1 egg. Blend. Strain. Serve cold.

juices. Alcoholic beverages should be avoided. Patients should not eat within two hours of bedtime. Extra fluids and laxative foods help to prevent constipation which can put pressure on the esophagus. Patients should not lie down or bend over after eating. Extra height in the form of pillows or an elevated bed-head for sleeping is recommended. If the patient is obese, a weight loss will improve the clinical condition. Fats are usually avoided, since they tend to lower esophageal pressure and add calories.

The structural parts of brans, husks of whole grain products, hulls, skins, and seeds are important sources of fiber. Fiber and residue are not the same thing. Residue is the bulk that remains in the GI tract after digestion has taken place. The fiber content of a diet can be reduced with the following practices:

1. Use young, very tender cooked vegetables.
2. Omit foods with seeds, skin, and structural fiber, such as berries, celery, cabbage, corn, peas.
3. Peel fruits and vegetables and cook to soften fiber.
4. Puree or strain foods.
5. Use only refined white breads and cereals.
6. Omit fruits and vegetables and use only strained juices.

The very low-fiber diet, which uses only purees, is unpopular, but it is useful for tube-feeding patients or those with bleeding esophageal varices and post-GI surgeries such as a hemorrhoidectomy.

The more restricted a diet becomes, the less adequate it is in nutrients. The very low-residue diet should be prescribed for only short periods of time, as it is lacking in calcium, iron, and vitamins. This diet eliminates fiber and leaves a minimum of residue in the GI tract. See Table 15-2 for a low-to-moderate residue diet.

Stomach: Peptic Ulcer

Dietary Management

Peptic ulcer is the most common of the problems affecting the upper GI tract. An ulcer is an erosion of the stomach, pylorus, or duodenum. Ulcers occur only in areas affected by excess hydrochloric acid and pepsin (an enzyme). The most common location is the duodenal bulb, because the gastric contents emptying through the pyloric valve are most concentrated in acid at this point. Thus, the two main factors that can cause stomach ulcer are

1. Increased acidity and secretion of gastric juices.
2. Decreased secretion of the mucous lining and buffer.

However, we do not know what triggers these two conditions.

Treatment goals for the peptic ulcer are to relieve pain, heal erosion, and prevent recurrences. Therapy usually includes rest, antacids, and anticholinergics. Physicians recommend reduction of ulcer predisposing factors such as stress, hurried or skipped meals, and excess coffee, colas, smoking, and aspirin. Diet therapy has always played an important part in the treatment of ulcers, although its effectiveness has been questioned. Some experts believe that diet therapy can provide maximum healing and prevent further tissue damage. Others do not and prefer the use of drugs.

The general term "bland" has been used to describe various ulcer diets. It usually refers to a diet that is soothing, white, dull, strained, tasteless, unattractive, and uninteresting. This has been the traditional diet therapy for ulcer patients for many years. Recent research indicates that such diets are low in the nutrients necessary for wound healing (vitamin C, iron, protein), high in saturated fats

TABLE 15-2
Foods Permitted in Two Residue-Regulated Diets

	Foods and Daily Servings Permitted*	
Food Group	Low-to-moderate-residue diet (0–4 g fiber)	Minimum-residue diet (0–1 g fiber)
Meat, equivalents	Beef, veal, ham, liver, and poultry (broiled, baked, or stewed to tender); fish, fresh or salt (broiled, baked); canned tuna or salmon; shellfish, tender meat only	Beef, veal, ham, liver, and poultry (broiled, baked, or stewed to tender); fish, fresh or salt (broiled, baked); canned salmon or tuna
Milk, milk products	Whole, skim, chocolate; buttermilk, yogurt (2 c. daily including amount in food preparation)	None
Cheese	Cottage, cream, American, Muenster, and Swiss 1 c. milk = 1 oz. cheese	Cream, dry cottage, and American (in food preparation) Daily allowance: 1 oz. American or cream cheese or ¼ c. cottage cheese
Eggs	All varieties except fried	All varieties except creamed and fried
Grain, grain products	Bread (Italian, Vienna, or French); toast (French or melba); crackers (saltines or soda); rolls (plain, soft, or hard); others: biscuits, zwieback, rusk All above prepared with refined whole wheat or rye (without seeds), with no nuts or raisins Cereals (ready-to-eat, cooked, all prepared from refined grains); oatmeal Flours from refined grains other than graham or bran White rice Plain spaghetti, noodles, and macaroni	Same Same, except no oatmeal Same Same Same
Potatoes	Potatoes without skin (creamed, mashed, scalloped, boiled, baked); sweet potatoes without skin	None
Fruits	Daily allowance: 2 servings All juices and nectars; fruits, ripe and fresh (peeled, without seeds), frozen, or canned; grapes, bananas, apricots, plums, peaches, pears, cherries, avocados, citrus fruits (segments only); e.g., oranges, grapefruit, tangerine, honeydew, cantaloupe, pineapple, and nectarines	Citrus fruit juices (strained); other juices and nectars
Vegetables	Daily allowance: 1 serving for vegetables, with no limitation on juices Vegetables, well-cooked or canned: green and waxed beans, carrots, asparagus, beets, eggplant, mushrooms, onions, cauliflower, peas, winter squash, pumpkin, cabbage Vegetables, cooked, chopped: turnip greens, broccoli, spinach, kale, collards Vegetables, raw, chopped: lettuce	Daily allowance: 1 serving Vegetable juices (fresh, cocktail); tomato juice
Beverages	Coffee (regular, decaffeinated), tea; others: soft drinks, cereal beverages All drinks may be flavored with permitted fruits.	Same

(continues)

*When daily number of servings is not indicated, there is no restriction on the amount consumed by the patient. Also refer to the "soft diet" discussed in Module 12.

TABLE 15-2 (Continued)

| Food Group | Foods and Daily Servings Permitted* | |
	Low-to-moderate-residue diet (0–4 g fiber)	Minimum-residue diet (0–1 g fiber)
Soups	Broth and cream-based soups made from other permitted ingredients	Same
Candies, sweets	Plain candies, jelly, honey, syrup, sugar, jelly beans, mints	Plain hard candies, jelly, honey, syrup, sugar, jelly beans, mints
Fats	Cream: regular, dried substitutes, sour; dressings: mayonnaise and mayonnaise-type, all must be plain; regular smooth salad oil; butter, margarine, oils; others: crisp bacon, shortenings	Daily allowance: no limitation except heavy cream must be limited to ½ c. Cream: heavy, substitutes, nondairy, sour; dressings: mayonnaise and mayonnaise-type, all must be plain; regular smooth salad oil; butter, margarine, oils; others: crisp bacon, shortenings
Desserts	All must be plain and made from permitted ingredients: pie, cakes, cookies, pudding, gelatin, sherbet, ice cream	Cookies: plain sugar or vanilla wafers, arrowroot; cakes: sponge, angel food; puddings: tapioca or cornstarch made with fruit juices; others: meringues, plain gelatin desserts, plain water ices
Miscellaneous	Spices and herbs (ground or finely chopped); flavorings: soy sauce, vinegar, salt, monosodium glutamate, chocolate, catsup, and all commercial flavoring extracts; sauces and gravies: mild and made from permitted ingredients	Flavorings: salt, vinegar, commercial flavoring extracts; spices and herbs (ground or finely chopped, in small amounts, in food preparation only); gravies and sauces: made from permitted ingredients and used in minimal quantity

that can contribute to obesity and elevated blood lipid levels, low in fiber, able to increase acid production, and scientifically unsound.

For example, the protein in milk and cream is supposed to buffer stomach acid, but the high fat content of milk and cream frequently leads to elevated serum lipids and obesity, increasing the risks of coronary heart disease. The omission of spices from the diet has been another traditional therapy, but whether or not all spices irritate the gastric lining is debated. Foods containing fiber have also been omitted for fear of their potential abrasiveness to the tender stomach mucosa, as have many "gas-forming" foods. However, this restrictive and traditional "bland" ulcer diet is no longer prescribed by most health practitioners.

The present diet for ulcer therapy is called the "liberal bland" diet. This diet is an individualized modification of a regular diet and offers a wide range of foods. It is high in protein, moderate in fat (high in unsaturated type), and consumed in six moderate feedings per day. The patient is advised to avoid the following foods:

1. Coffee (all types), tea, and colas (their caffeine content increases gastric secretions).
2. Alcohol (this can damage stomach mucosa).
3. Meat extractives, such as broths (they stimulate gastric acid).

4. Any other food not well-tolerated by the patient. Such items include pickles, olives, fried foods, onions, and chili powder. Restriction must be individualized and not applied randomly.

Patients and physicians accustomed to the traditional diets have been slow to accept the liberal diet. Most hospitals generally offer the soft diet initially to ulcer patients (see Module 12). Individual changes are made toward a regular diet as the patients and their conditions indicate acceptance and improvement.

If a patient is in acute pain or is bleeding when admitted, stricter dietary measures may be necessary. The "graduated" or "progressive" ulcer regimes, which begin with Bland #1 and progress through Bland #4, may be found in most diet manuals in health care facilities. They are ordered by the physician if deemed necessary.

The principles of diet therapy for ulcer patients can be summarized in the following:

1. Optimum nutrition to promote healing and maintain health.
2. High protein for healing and buffering action.
3. Fat in moderate amounts to suppress stomach secretions (unsaturated fat is preferred).
4. Meal intervals and size adequate to maintain control of gastric secretions.

TABLE 15-3
Sample Menus for Regulated-Residue Diets

| Bland and Minimum-Fiber (Residue) Diet* | | |
Breakfast	Lunch	Dinner
Orange juice, strained, ½ c.	Chicken, tender, 3 oz.	Beef patty, well cooked, 3 oz.
Farina, ½ c.	Rice, ½ c.	Mashed potato, ½ c.
Milk, 1 c. (bland only)	Vegetable juice, 1 c.	White bread, 1 slice
Toast, white bread, 1 slice	White bread, 1 slice	Grapefruit juice, strained, ½ c.
Margarine	Ice cream, ½ c.	Custard, ½ c.
Sugar	Vanilla wafers, 2	Margarine
Jelly	Milk, 1 c. (bland only)	Coffee or tea (residue only)
Coffee or tea (residue only)	Coffee or tea (residue only)	

Snacks

Gelatin
Crackers

| Moderately Low-Fiber (Residue) Diet** | | |
Breakfast	Lunch	Dinner
Tomato juice, ½ c.	Melted cheese sandwich:	Roast beef, tender, 3 oz.
Egg, poached, 1	White bread, 2 slices	Potato, mashed, 1 c.
Toast, white bread, 1 slice	Cheese, mild, 2 oz.	Carrots, cooked, ½ c.
Bacon, 2 slices	Green beans, ½ c.	Orange juice, strained, ½ c.
Margarine	Apple juice, ½ c.	White bread, 1 slice
Jelly	Gelatin, 1 c.	Margarine
Coffee or tea	Vanilla wafers, 2	Ice cream, ½ c.
	Coffee or tea	Coffee or tea

Snacks

Milk, 1 c.
Cookies, plain, 2

* This menu contains about 1 g of fiber. Quantities of servings should be adjusted to meet the needs of the individual.
**This menu contains about 3 to 4 g of fiber. Quantities of servings should be adjusted to meet the needs of the individual.

5. A positive attitude and understanding of the factors related to both the causes and the possible healing of ulcers.

Nursing responsibilities in treating ulcer patients are listed below:

1. Explain the rationale for use of the newer diet therapy (some patients are very fearful and skeptical of the less restrictive diet).
2. Evaluate the diet for nutritional adequacy after individual changes have been made.
3. Encourage the consumption of laxative foods, especially if the patient is prescribed antacids, which cause constipation.
4. Explain the adoption of a less stressful lifestyle to help prevent a recurrence.

5. Intervene on the patient's behalf, if the prescribed diet is not tolerated.

Gastric Surgery

In some ulcer patients, stomach surgery is needed to manage the clinical condition—an uncontrollable bleeding ulcer. The necessity for optimum nutrition following gastric surgery is the same as in any other operation, but postgastrectomy diet therapy (which must be ordered by the physician) differs in some respects. In general the health practitioner should follow these basic principles:

1. Implement a progressive diet for a two-week course.
2. Keep meals small (1 to 2 oz. each) and frequent (hourly).

3. Increase the size of feedings by 1 oz. daily.
4. Use a six-meal ulcer diet by approximately day ten to day sixteen, if conditions permit.
5. Introduce simple, mild, low-fiber, and easily digested foods, such as cream soup, cream of wheat or rice, jello, custard, soft (poached) cooked eggs, mashed potatoes.
6. Resume a regular diet gradually.

The "dumping syndrome" is a complication of gastric surgery that may occur a short time after recovery from the operation, after eating is resumed. It may also be the delayed type, occurring from 1 to 5 years after a gastrectomy. It is more likely to occur in the patient who has had two-thirds or more of the stomach removed.

The process is as follows. Food reaches the jejunum ten to fifteen minutes after eating. With part of the stomach removed, the food is not digested properly and, instead of being delivered slowly, it is "dumped" quickly into the small intestine. The patient then experiences nausea, cramping, weakness, dizziness, cold sweating, a rapid pulse, and possibly vomiting. These symptoms of shock occur as the concentrated foodstuff draws water from the body tissues into the intestine. The symptoms are especially severe when the meal is high in simple carbohydrate, which can exert high osmotic pressure. Two to three hours after the meal, hypoglycemic symptoms may occur, because the absorbed monosaccharides, especially glucose, cause a rapid rise in blood glucose. This, in turn, stimulates the body to produce more insulin which quickly removes the excess glucose from the blood, resulting in hypoglycemia.

The aim of diet therapy is to provide the patient with optimum nutrition that will control these symptoms. The measures used and the rationale for each are listed below.

1. Small, frequent meals (which will not overload the jejunum), eaten slowly.
2. No liquid during meals and the following hour; the absence of liquid slows absorption.
3. High-protein foods for tissue repair and moderately-high-fat foods to add calories and delay the time food is emptied from the stomach.

4. Moderate to low amounts of complex carbohydrate foods (which are digested more slowly).
5. No milk, sugar, sweets, desserts, alcohol, or sweetened beverages. All of these pass rapidly into the jejunum and pull fluid there. Also, simple sugars stimulate insulin release and so should be avoided.
6. Raw foods as tolerated (low-fiber types are usually given).

Table 15-4 presents an antidumping diet and Table 15-5 provides a sample menu.

Nursing Implications

1. Encourage a supine position after meals to slow the flow of gravity.
2. Advise mouth rinsing before meals since cholinergic blocking agents can cause dryness of mouth.
3. Emphasize eating slowly in a relaxed, pleasant environment.
4. Explain the reasons for diet restrictions to the patient and family or care provider.
5. Be aware that vitamin B_{12} by injection may be necessary following total gastrectomy, because the intrinsic factor necessary for its absorption will be lost. Make sure that the patient understands the need for this treatment.
6. Check weight and caloric intake frequently.

PROGRESS CHECK ON ACTIVITY 1

Fill-in

1. Fill out the table in Exercise 15-1 (page 226) for the low-residue diet, listing all diseases/conditions for which this diet is applicable.
2. Fill out the table in Exercise 15-1 for the bland diet:
   a. traditional bland diet, listing all legitimate uses
   b. liberal bland diet, listing all disorders for which this diet is applicable
3. Locate a diet manual and write a one-day menu for Bland #2 diet in Exercise 15-1.

ACTIVITY 2: Disorders of the Intestines

Background Information

The most common of the intestinal disorders that occasionally affect people are constipation and diarrhea. Both disorders are usually managed with simple changes in diet and lifestyle. Other more severe intestinal conditions are diverticular disease, ulcerative colitis, and cancer.

Constipation

Since constipation is a symptom, many variables have been implicated in its treatment. One cause is related to the stress and strain of modern life. Poor personal habits may be responsible, including irregular routine and meals, inadequate rest and exercise, tension, and ignoring the

TABLE 15-4
Permitted and Prohibited Foods in an Antidumping Diet

Food Group	Foods Permitted	Foods Prohibited
Breads	All breads and crackers except those noted	Breads with nuts, jams, or dried fruits or made with bran
Fats	Margarine, butter, oil, bacon, cream, mayonnaise, French dressing	None
Cereals and equivalents	All grains, rice, spaghetti, noodles, and macaroni except those noted	Presweetened cereals
Eggs	All egg dishes	None
Meats	All tender meats, fish, poultry	Highly seasoned or smoked meats
Beverages	Tea, coffee, broth, liquid unsweetened gelatin, artificially sweetened soda (½–1 hour before and after meals)*	No milk or alcohol; carbonated beverages if not tolerated; beverages with meal unless symptoms begin to subside†
(The following are to be added as patient tolerance and condition progress.)		
Vegetables	Mashed potato, all tender vegetables (peas, carrots, spinach, etc.)	None creamed; gas-forming varieties if not tolerated (cabbage, broccoli, dried beans and peas, etc.)
Fruits	Fresh or canned (unsweetened or artificially sweetened); one serving citrus fruit or juice	None canned with sugar syrup; avoid sweetened dried fruits; e.g., prunes, figs, dates
Dairy products	Milk, cheese, cottage cheese, yogurt, all in small quantities	None
Miscellaneous	Salt, catsup, mild spices, smooth peanut butter	Pickles, peppers, chili powder, nuts, olives, candy, milk gravies

Note: Check for patient tolerance and acceptability of milk and milk products.

*Some practitioners prefer 1 to 2 hours before and after meals.
†Some practitioners permit 4 oz. of fluid with a meal.

body's need to defecate. Some medications that contain iron, aluminum, or calcium can cause constipation. Regular use of laxatives also is a contributing factor. Ideal treatment requires adopting good health habits to restore regularity and break the laxative cycle.

A regular balanced diet high in fiber and fluids is recommended to avoid constipation. Eight to ten glasses of fluids daily should be consumed. Foods high in fiber include whole grains and raw fruits and vegetables. If the patient cannot tolerate the latter, cooked ones may be used. Prune juice, apple juice, figs, and raisins are especially helpful. Bran with a high fiber content is an effective agent.

Nursing implications:

1. Explain the benefits of a high-fiber diet. In addition to increasing bulk, the foods that provide fiber are high in vitamins and minerals.
2. Discourage regular and excessive use of laxatives.
3. Reassure patients that a daily bowel movement is not an absolute necessity. It may not be normal for them.
4. Advise gradual inclusion of high-fiber foods in the diet. Excess dietary fiber at the beginning may cause cramping and gas. This can discourage patients from

continuing the diet.
5. Encourage a high fluid intake, especially of water.

Diarrhea

Diarrhea in infants, small children, and the elderly can be serious if prolonged, especially if an infection is present. Common mild diarrhea of short duration usually responds well to simple treatment. Diarrhea is functional when related to stress, irritation of the bowel, or a change in the regular routine, such as traveling. It is organic if it is caused by a GI lesion. Treatment includes eliminating the underlying cause, using antidiarrheal drugs as needed, and using appropriate diet therapy.

Diet therapy during severe diarrhea is characterized by the following:

1. No oral feeding for first 24 to 48 hours. Intravenous (IV) fluids to replace electrolytes and water. If the need for IV fluids continues beyond 72 hours, amino acids and vitamins may be added. If diarrhea is prolonged, total parenteral nutrition (TPN) will be necessary.
2. Resumption of oral feedings. First day: clear liquids

TABLE 15-5
Sample Menu Plans for Antidumping Diets

| | Soon after Surgery | | Later after Surgery | |
	Sample 1	Sample 2	Sample 1	Sample 2
Breakfast	Egg, poached, 1 Toast, 1 slice Butter, 1 tsp. Banana, ½	Egg, scrambled, 1 Toast, 1 slice Butter, 1 tsp. Peaches, ½ c.	Cream of Wheat, ½ c. Butter, 1 tsp. Egg, soft-cooked, 1 Cream, 1 oz.	Juice, tomato, 4 oz. Oatmeal, ½ c. Milk, 4 oz. Bacon, crisp, 2 slices Toast, 1 slice Butter, 1 tsp.
Snack	Gelatin, fruit-flavored, unsweetened, 1 c. Cream, 1 tbsp.	Cottage cheese, 2 oz. Crackers, 2	Custard, unsweetened, ½ c. Crackers, 4	Milk, 1 c. Crackers, 4
Lunch	Chicken breast, stewed, 3 oz. Potato, mashed, ½ c. Butter, 2 tsp.	Fish, 3 oz. Rice, ½ c. Spinach, ½ c. Butter, 2 tsp.	Roast beef, 3 oz. Rice, ½ c. Peas, buttered, ½ c.	Beef patty, 3 oz. Potato, ½ c. Asparagus, ½ c. Butter, 2 tsp.
Snack	Cottage cheese, 2 oz. Crackers, 4	Gelatin, fruit-flavored, unsweetened, 1 c.	Juice, orange, ½ c. Cheese, 1 oz. Crackers, 2	Cottage cheese, ½ c. Crackers, 4
Dinner	Meat, 3 oz. Rice with grated cheese, ½ c. Asparagus, tips, ½ c. Margarine, 1 tsp.	Turkey, sliced, 3 oz. Potato, baked, 1 Butter, 2 tsp. Tomato, 2 slices	Beef, 3 oz. Potatoes, mashed, 1 c. Carrots, ½ c. Tomato, sliced, ½ Butter, 2 tsp.	Chicken, 3 oz. Noodles, 3 oz. Spinach, ½ c. Margarine, 1 tsp.
Snack	Bread, 1 slice Meat, 2 oz. Margarine, 1 tsp.	Pudding, plain, unsweetened, with whipped cream, ½ c.	Pudding, unsweetened, ¼ c.	Sandwich: Bread, 2 slices Mayonnaise, 2 tsp. Meat, 2 oz.

with a minimum of sugar. Second day: progressively introduce a minimum-residue diet (see Tables 15-2 and 15-3), high in protein. Calcium supplements are provided. Applesauce and raw apples may be used for their pectin content, which can thicken the stools. Implement gradual progression of low-fiber, low-residue, soft, solid to regular diet as the situation improves.

Mild diarrhea usually responds to the following: reducing the total food intake, especially carbohydrate and fat; limiting residue; and replacing fluids. A bland low-residue diet may ease the discomfort.

Nursing implications for individuals or patients with diarrhea:

1. Note daily weight changes.
2. Keep accurate daily records of intake and output.
3. Do not permit carbonated beverages. Use flat coke or gingerale if carbonated beverages are desired.
4. Relieve any pain before serving meals.
5. Employ diversionary tactics during meals.
6. Offer replacements later, if patient does not finish food when it is first offered.

Diverticular Disease

Diverticuli are herniations (pockets or sacs) of intestinal mucosa through the muscles of the bowel wall. The process is referred to as diverticulosis. If accompanied by inflammation, the disorder is called diverticulitis. It is important to distinguish between the two, as the diet therapy used is different for each.

One cause of diverticulosis appears to be related to a lack of fecal bulk, which increases intraluminal pressure. The treatment of diverticulosis is aimed at preventing inflammation. A high-fiber diet is prescribed. Fiber sources include bran, whole grains, and fruits and vegetables. Pepper and chili powder, sometimes nuts and corn, may be eliminated.

Diverticulitis requires special attention. During acute

EXERCISE 15-1
Complete the Chart by Filling In the Information for Each Column

Diet	Disease or Condition	Foods Allowed	Foods Limited	Foods Forbidden	Nursing Implications
Low-Residue Diet					
Bland Diets a. Traditional bland					
b. Liberal bland					
Bland #2 Diet					

periods when the diverticuli are inflamed and there is pain, tenderness, nausea, vomiting, and distention, fecal residue may add to the discomfort. Diet therapy during this period may be limited to clear liquids progressing to full liquids, then to low-residue and to regular high-fiber diet as the inflammation subsides. Severe diverticulitis is usually treated by surgical methods (colostomy, bowel resection).

Nursing implications are as follows:

1. Patient education is most important here, as all diverticular disease was formerly treated with a low-residue diet.
2. The older patient should be especially reassured, as most diverticulosis occurs in the elderly and they become most anxious on a high-fiber diet.
3. A symptomatic patient should be encouraged to rest and to take medicines as prescribed.
4. Patients who are malnourished on admission should be replenished nutritionally to facilitate healing and recovery.

Inflammatory Bowel Disease _____

Inflammatory bowel disease is a term that is used for ulcerative colitis and Crohn's disease. Both may have the related condition of short bowel syndrome if there have been repeated surgeries that removed sections of the bowel as the disease progressed.

Both ulcerative colitis (U.C.) and Crohn's disease have increased in incidence in the United States. They have similar pathophysiology and clinical symptoms, but are prevalent in different groups. They both have severe nutritional consequences, but are separate diseases. Crohn's can occur anywhere in the GI tract, but U.C. is confined to the colon and rectum. The pattern of disease in Crohn's is that of a chronic disorder, often involving the entire intestinal wall. This may cause complications, such as partial or complete obstruction and the formation of fistulas. The inflammatory processes in U.C., on the other hand, are usually acute and are limited to the mucosa and submucosa of the intestine. The patient may have periods of remission.

Diet therapy for inflammatory bowel disease is based upon the common clinical symptoms of bloody diarrhea and the various associated nutritional problems.

Ulcerative Colitis (U.C.) _____

Primarily a disease of young adults, especially women, ulcerative colitis (U.C.) is a life-threatening disorder. While the cause is unknown, one major culprit is related to psychological factors. The disorder is characterized by widespread ulceration and inflammation of the colon, fever, chronic bloody diarrhea, edema, and anemia. The patient is severely malnourished, suffering from avitaminosis, negative nitrogen balance, dehydration, electrolyte imbalances, and skin lesions. Patients are nervous, anorexic, and in pain. The obvious need for maximum nutrition for a patient who cannot eat is a challenge to the health team.

The treatment of U.C. includes rest, sedation, antibiotics, antidiarrheal drugs, and rigorous diet therapy. Surgical removal of the diseased portion of the bowel is the treatment of choice, if other medical procedures fail. Diet therapy includes

1. Bland low-residue diet, supplemented with formula-feeding.
2. High protein: 125 to 150 grams.
3. High calorie: 3,000+ calories.
4. High vitamins/minerals, especially vitamins C, B complex, and K.
5. Moderate fat or as tolerated.
6. Dairy products usually eliminated to avoid secondary lactose intolerance, or lactose-free products used.
7. IV fluids used in addition to oral feedings to correct fluid and electrolyte losses due to diarrhea.
8. TPN is most effective when the bowel has been shortened or the disease is extensive.

Crohn's Disease

Crohn's disease is another manifestation of inflammatory bowel disease. It is particularly prevalent in industrial areas and among the 55 to 60 age group. It has an insidious onset and is characterized by tenderness, pain, diarrhea, and cramping in the right lower quadrant of the bowel. There is less blood in the stool than in ulcerative colitis, but increased secretion of mucus by the bowel. The patient runs a low-grade fever.

Widespread involvement of the small bowel results in malabsorption of fat, protein, carbohydrates, vitamins, and minerals and subsequent weight loss. Vitamin B_{12} deficiency may occur, leading to macrocytic anemia and neurologic damage. Bile salt losses lead to cholelithiasis, diarrhea, and steatorrhea. There may also be anemia due to loss of blood in the stool. Children with Crohn's disease show retarded growth patterns.

As with U.C., the effects of malabsorption are widespread. Malabsorption of vitamins C and K leads to capillary fragility, hemorrhagic tendencies, and petechiae. Malabsorption of calcium and vitamin D puts the patient at risk for osteomalacia and osteoporosis. The bone pain that is a frequent symptom of both U.C. and Crohn's is due to this impairment. Tetany and paresthesia are also related to calcium and magnesium malabsorption. The whole vitamin B complex is destroyed, giving rise to glossitis, cheilosis, skin changes, and peripheral neuritis.

The rational for diet therapy for both diseases is to restore nutrient deficits, prevent further losses, promote healing, and repair and maintain body tissue.

Nursing Implications

Nursing responsibilities for patients with ulcerative colitis or Crohn's disease include the following:

1. Be aware that the patient's need for high levels of food and fluids parallels that of a burn patient.
2. Interpret the diet to the patient and family member or care provider. A young person on a bland low-residue diet for long periods of time becomes discouraged.
3. Be aware that, if steroid-type medication is used, sodium restriction may also become necessary.
4. Do not confuse fluid retention with nutritional improvement (body weight gain).
5. Keep careful daily records: fluid intake and output, weight changes, nutrient intake, and calorie counts.
6. Seek outside resources for the patient (counselor, therapist) as needed. Work closely with dietitian and other health team members.
7. Provide the patient with the rationale for strict medical management and the side effects of same.
8. Provide education for continuing diet therapy for U.C. and Crohn's. It is based on
    a. restoring adequate nutrition intake.
    b. correcting deficits, usually with supplements.
    c. preventing further losses.
    d. controlling substances that do not absorb well, such as fats.
    e. promoting healing and repairing and maintaining tissue.
9. Any number of commercial preparations to add additional calories in easily digestible form may be obtained from the local pharmacy, i.e., MCT, Portagen, etc.
10. The diet for both U.C. and Crohn's remains
    a. high protein (125/150 gm/d) of HBV protein foods.
    b. high vitamin, especially those found to be most deficient.
    c. high minerals as needed by the individual (especially iron, which may be administered by transfusion, calcium, zinc, and potassium if diarrhea persists).
    d. low residue. See chart.
    e. high calorie to spare the protein for tissue healing and rebuilding.

Cancer

Although cancer may occur at any site along the GI tract and accessory organs, colon cancer is the second leading cause of cancer deaths in the United States among both males and females. Many individual foods and food additives have been implicated along with contaminated air, soil, and water. Much publicity has been given to the causative or preventive role of dietary fat, fiber, and other nutrients. Their excess or deficiency has been blamed for colon cancer, especially in the popular press and media. Most scientific data related to foods and cancer point to conclusive evidence that a change in diet to include several nutrients and fiber is beneficial. Unfortunately, many people have become unnecessarily fearful and have eliminated from their diets any item purported to cause cancer.

The fiber theory supports the direct relationship between a low-fiber diet and colon cancer. Low-fiber diets permit food residues to stay in the intestine. When they are fermented by intestinal bacteria, their byproducts stay against the intestinal wall for extended periods, exposing the mucosal lining to harmful substances. Residues from a high-fiber diet are rapidly eliminated and are subjected to less bacterial action. If we accept this explanation, what should we do about diet? A well-balanced diet using a variety of foods, moderately high in fiber and moderately low in fats, may not necessarily prevent cancer. However, it will improve nutrition in general and, perhaps, help reduce the risks of colon cancer development.

Weight loss, anorexia, weakness, vomiting, diarrhea, reduced absorption of nutrients, dehydration, and cachexia are all general symptoms in most cancer patients, and become more pronounced as the cancer progresses. The location of the cancer has specific effects on nutrition, metabolism, and modes of treatment, but many experts believe that more cancer patients die of malnutrition than of the disease.

Radiation, immunotherapy, and chemotherapy contribute to malnutrition because they result in changes in taste sensation, vomiting, diarrhea, anorexia, lack of saliva, and malabsorption of nutrients. At the same time, nutrient deficiencies reduce the effectiveness of medical treatment, thus prolonging recovery.

While the diet therapy for cancer is very individualized, some general factors apply to all cancer patients:

1. Improved nutritional status can enhance patient response to medical treatment.

2. Optimal nutritional care has increased survival rates of some patients.

3. Aggressive nutritional care improves a patient's quality of life.

4. Malnutrition in a cancer patient is no longer considered inevitable. Most patients can be adequately nourished, if properly planned and executed nutrition therapy is provided.

5. The psychological aspects of eating have a positive effect on the patient's emotional status. They denote caring, comfort, and concern. Emphasize eating to get well, i.e., health and wellness instead of illness.

6. Diets high in protein, calories, vitamins, and minerals are needed. Supplements, both oral and intravenous, may be needed. TPN is an excellent way to provide optimum nutrition, especially when the GI tract is impaired or malabsorption is present.

*There are no exact rules, but some general guidelines that fit many patients include these:

1. Liquid may be easier to consume than solids.
2. Choose foods high in nutrient density.
3. Liquid meals are better tolerated in the morning.
4. A flexible meal schedule may be followed (any time—frequent).
5. Highly seasoned or salty foods usually well tolerated.
6. Sweets and sour foods usually acceptable.
7. Foods with high fat content may be poorly tolerated.
8. Milk *may* or *may not* increase viscosity of mucous secretions—lactose-containing foods may be poorly tolerated (malabsorption).
9. Use cool, smooth liquids or semi-solids such as gelatin, applesauce, sherbets, pudding, popsicles.
10. Avoid citrus, tomato, pepper when mouth is sore.
11. Use smooth gravies, sauces, and broths (helps lubricate mouth).
12. Use cheese, beans, peanut butter if meat aversions arise.
13. Use food supplements like medication: small hourly doses may be better tolerated.
14. Avoid large volumes of hypertonic feedings.
15. Precede meals with antiemetics or pain-relief medications when needed.

See Module 20 for detailed explanation of cancer therapies.

Colostomy and Ileostomy

Many intestinal diseases not responsive to medical and dietary measures must be treated surgically. Depending on the location of the obstruction or disease, a colostomy or an ileostomy may be performed.

Colostomy

In a colostomy, the rectum and anus are removed. The remaining intestine is led to the outside through a hole in the abdomen. Because this surgical procedure diverts fecal material from the distal colon and rectum, where fluids are normally absorbed, patients with colostomies have stools with high water content.

Diet therapy is characterized by the following:

1. A well-balanced diet that is appropriate for the preoperative patient is indicated. See Module 13 for diet planning.

*Adapted from Beyer, Peter L. Update on supportive therapy in cancer patients. In *Cancer control for the professional.* 1980. July/August 7:4. Idaho Division of the American Cancer Society. Reprinted by permission.

2. The initial postoperative diet is clear-liquid, followed by a minimum residue regimen. Progress as rapidly as possible to a regular diet. Nutrient supplements are provided as needed.
3. General goals are to promote healing and prevent odor, constipation, and diarrhea.
4. Each patient must experiment with the diet. A patient can identify those foods to be limited or avoided.

The nursing implications in caring for this group of patients include the following:

1. Colostomy patients have real concerns about odors and flatulence. Help them with corrective measures. For example, spinach and parsley have deodorizing action and a commercial deodorant may be used in the bag.
2. A diet must be evaluated for adequacy, if certain food items are prohibited.
3. Eating slowly and thorough chewing can prevent swallowing air.
4. Patients with colostomy usually progress rapidly as they gain control over the elimination process and adapt well to changes in lifestyle.
5. Emotional support for the patient and family is mandatory.
6. Compile information regarding outside resources that will help patients.

Ileostomy

This surgery is indicated for intractable ulcerative colitis, Crohn's disease, and cancer of the colon. After removing the colon and rectum, the remaining intestine is led to the outside of the body through an opening in the abdomen. Since the surgery is performed higher in the intestine, the waste material is mainly in fluid form. There are great losses of fluid, sodium, vitamin K, and other essential nutrients. Fat absorption is poor and vitamin B_{12} absorption is reduced or absent. Body-weight loss is high.

Diet therapy after the operation is as follows:

1. The diet progresses from clear liquids to minimal-residue to low-residue. New foods are given one at a time to test the patient's tolerance.
2. Nutritional supplements and/or TPN may be needed in the early stages.
3. Vitamin B_{12} injections are given at scheduled times to prevent pernicious anemia.
4. Extra fluid is required. Orange juice and bananas are high in potassium, while extra salt with food increases sodium intake.
5. The progression to a regular diet is longer for the patient with an ileostomy than a patient with a colostomy.

Nursing implications for caring for this group of patients are to:

1. Provide emotional support and encouragement to eating adequately.
2. Work closely with the dietary department and plan for the family of the patient to participate.
3. Be aware that the same nursing measures are applicable to colostomy and ileostomy patients.

PROGRESS CHECK ON ACTIVITY 2

Matching

1. Indicate which of the following foods would be allowed on a minimum-residue diet by writing Y (yes) or N (no) in the blanks:
   - _N_ a. broccoli with hollandaise sauce
   - _Y_ b. bouillon
   - _N_ c. applesauce
   - _N_ d. fresh pears
   - _Y_ e. sherbet
   - _N_ f. fruitcake
   - _Y_ g. poached egg
   - _Y_ h. macaroni
   - _N_ i. pecan waffles
   - _Y_ j. broiled chicken

Multiple Choice

Circle the letter of the correct answer.

2. Residue is that part of food that
   a. remains longest in the GI tract.
   b. is indigestible.
   c. is left uneaten after the meal.
   d. is inedible.

3. Food residue
   a. is ultimately evacuated in the feces.
   b. never leaves the stomach.
   c. never leaves the intestines.
   d. results from incorrect cooking methods.

4. Large amounts of food residue cause
   a. a decrease in fecal matter.
   b. an increase in fecal matter.
   c. weight gain.
   d. diverticulosis.

5. Patients requiring low-residue diets usually have
   a. heart conditions.
   b. lung conditions.
   c. muscle conditions.
   d. gastrointestinal conditions.

6. The restricted-residue diet may be prescribed for patients with
   a. ulcerative colitis or Crohn's disease.
   b. measles or mumps.

c. atherosclerosis.
d. congestive heart failure.

7. The restricted-residue diet
   a. is always very high in calories.
   b. is very similar to the full-liquid diet.
   c. may be inadequate in vitamins and minerals.
   d. is nutritionally adequate.

8. The minimum-residue diet
   a. is always very high in calories.
   b. is very similar to the full-liquid diet.
   c. may be inadequate in vitamins and minerals.
   d. is nutritionally adequate.

9. Which of the following foods are allowed on a minimum-residue diet?
   a. milkshake, hamburger, and french fries
   b. tomato wedge, scrambled egg, and broiled bacon
   c. chicken sandwich on white bread with butter
   d. all of the above

10. Which of these foods would be included in a high-fiber diet?
    a. whole wheat bread, prunes, celery
    b. carrot sticks, bran cereal, apples
    c. coconut bars, pecan rolls, oatmeal
    d. all of the above

11. If the minimum-residue diet must be used for a period of time, the physician should
    a. alternate it weekly with the high-iron diet.
    b. substitute the full-liquid diet.
    c. add fresh fruit juices before each meal.
    d. prescribe a vitamin and mineral supplement.

Fill-in

12. Name 10 foods high in fiber content.
    a. *Any Whole Grain bread + cereals*
    b. *Any Fresh Fruits*
    c. *Any Fresh Veg.*
    d. *Nuts*
    e. *Prunes*
    f. *Figs*
    g. *Raisins*
    h. *broccoli*
    i. *Spinach*
    j. *Any cooked Fruit/Veg.*

13. List five goals for feeding a patient with an inflammatory bowel disease.
    a. *Correct Nutritional Deficet*

control substances not absorbed easily

b. *restore Adequate intake*
c. *prevent further loses*
d. *promote Repair + maintence of body tissue*
e. *promote healing*

14. List five nursing implications for nutritional care of the osteomate.
    a. *Concern of odor*
    b. *Eat slowly Chewing thuroughly*
    c. *Emotional support*
    d. *Referal information*
    e. *Diet eval Before food restriction ARE implyed*

References

American Journal of Clinical Nutrition. 1980. *Symposium on surgical treatment of morbid obesity.* 33:353.

Becker, H. D., and W. F. Caspary. 1980. *Postgastrectomy and postvagotomy syndromes.* New York: Springer.

Bingham, S. et al. 1982. Diet and health of people with an ileostomy. I. Dietary assessment. *Brit. J. Nutr.* 47:399.

Bisballe, S. et al. 1986. Food intake and nutritional status after gastrectomy. *Hum Nutr. Clin. Nutr.* 40C:301.

Brennan, M. F. et al. 1986. Branched-chain amino acids in stress and injury. *J. Parenteral Enteral Nutr.* 10(5):446.

Broadwell, D. C., and B. S. Jackson (eds.). 1982. *Principles of ostomy care.* St. Louis: Mosby.

Cashman, M. D. 1986. Principles of digestive physiology for clinical nutrition. *Nutr. Clin. Pract.* 1(5):241.

Center for Ulcer Research Education. Grossman, M. I. (ed.). *Peptic ulcer: A guide for the practicing physician.* Chicago: Yearbook Medical Publishers.

Church, J. M. et al. 1987. Assessing the efficacy of intravenous nutrition in general surgical patients: Dynamic nutritional assessment with plasma proteins. *J. Parenteral Enteral Nutr.* 11(2):140.

Cosnes, J. et al. 1985. Compensatory enteral hyperalimentation for management of patients with severe short bowel syndrome. *American Journal of Clinical Nutrition* 41(5):1002.

Deitel, M. (ed.). 1980. *Nutrition in clinical surgery.* Baltimore: Williams and Wilkins.

Desai, M. B. et al. 1988. Nutrition and diet in management of disease of the gastrointestinal tract. In *Modern nutrition in health and disease,* 7th ed. M. E. Shils and V. R. Young (eds.). Philadelphia: Lea & Febiger.

Durr, E. 1986. Nutritional intervention for patients with pressure sores. *Nutr. Supp. Serv.* 6(10):28.

Eastwood, G. L. 1984. *Core textbook of gastroenterology.* Philadelphia: Lippincott.

Freeman, H. J. (ed.). 1989. *Inflammatory bowel disease.*

Boca Raton, FL: CRC Press.

Fuchs, G. J. et al. 1985. Malnutrition and nutritional support in inflammatory bowel disease. *Nutr. Supp. Serv.* 5(6):28.

Gorman, M. A. et al. 1988. Position of the American Dietetic Association: Health implications of dietary fiber—technical support paper. *Journal of the American Dietetic Association* 88(2):217.

Greenwald, P. et al. 1987. Dietary fiber in the reduction of colon cancer risk. *Journal of the American Dietetic Association* 87(9):1178.

Heatley, R. V. et al. (eds.). 1986. *Clinical nutrition in gastroenterology.* London: Churchill.

Hermann-Zaidins, M. G. 1986. Malabsorption in adults: Etiology, evaluation, and management. *Journal of the American Dietetic Association* 86(9):1169.

Imes, S. et al. 1987. Diet counseling modifies nutrient intake of patients with Crohn's disease. *Journal of the American Dietetic Association* 87(4):457.

Kirsner, J. B., and R. G. Shorter. 1988. *Inflammatory bowel disease.* Philadelphia: Lea & Febiger.

Klurfeld, D. M. 1987. The role of dietary fiber in gastrointestinal disease. *Journal of the American Dietetic Association* 87(9):1172.

Kumar, N. et al. 1986. Effect of milk on patients with duodenal ulcers. *British Medical Journal* 293:666.

Lang, C. E. (ed.). 1987. *Nutritional support in critical care.* Rockville, MD: Aspen.

Lifshitz, F. et al. 1984. Food sensitivity and intolerance leading to diarrhea. *Clinical Nutrition* 3(1):5.

Linder, K. D. et al. 1985. Preoperative nutritional status and outcome in Crohn's disease. *Mayo Clin. Proc.* 60:393.

McNeil, N. I. et al. 1982. 1. Diet and health of people with an ileostomy. 2. Ileostomy function and nutritional state. *British Journal of Nutrition* 47:407.

Moore, F. D. 1986. Current thoughts on malabsorption: Parenteral, enteral, and oral feeding. *Journal of the American Dietetic Association* 86(9):1169.

Paige, D. M. et al. 1988. Nutritional assessment: An index to the quality of life. *Clinical Nutrition* 7(2):77.

Rathgeber, M. G. 1987. Nutrition and ostomies. A. D. A. practice group. *Dietitians in Nutrition Support Newsletter* 8(6):5.

Rubin, M. 1988. The physiology of bed rest. *American Journal of Nursing* 88(1):50.

Rydning, A. et al. 1986. Healing of benign gastric ulcer with low-dose antacids and fiber diet. *Gastroenterology* 91:56.

Schlichtig, R., and S. M. Ayres, 1988. *Nutritional support of the critically ill.* Chicago: Year Book Medical.

Simko, M. D. et al. 1984. *Nutrition assessment: A comprehensive guide for planning intervention.* Rockville, MD: Aspen.

Souba, W. W., and D. W. Wilmore. 1988. Diet and nutrition in the care of the patient with surgery, trauma, and sepsis. In *Modern nutrition in health and disease,* 7th ed. M. E. Shils and V. R. Young (eds.). Philadelphia: Lea & Febiger.

Szabo, S., and C. J. Pfeiffer (eds.). 1989. *Ulcer disease: New aspects of pathogenesis and pharmacology.* Boca Raton, FL: CRC Press.

Underwood, B. A. 1986. Evaluating the nutritional status of individuals: A critique of approaches. *Nutrition Review* 44(Suppl):213.

Wahlqvist, M. L., and J. S. Vobecky (eds.). 1987. *Patient problems in clinical nutrition: A manual.* London: John Libbey & Co.

Watt, R. 1985. The ostomy. Why is it created? *American Journal of Nursing* 85:1242.

Wilson, P. C., and H. L. Greene. 1988. The gastrointestinal tract: Portal to nutrient utilization. In *Modern nutrition in health and disease,* 7th ed. M. E. Shils and V. R. Young (eds.). Philadelphia: Lea & Febiger.

Woolf, G. M. et al. 1987. Nutritional absorption in short-bowel syndrome: Evaluation of fluid, calorie, and divalent cation requirements. *Digest Dis. Sci.* 32:8.

Module 16

Diet Therapy for Diabetes Mellitus

Time for completion
Activities: _____1½_____ hours
Optional examination: ½ hour

Academic credit
Semester units: ³⁄₁₀
Quarter units: ⁴⁄₁₀

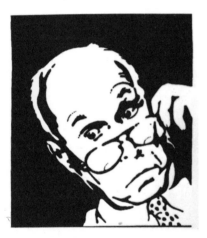
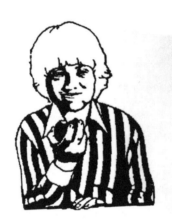
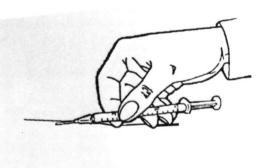
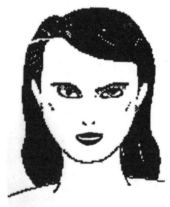
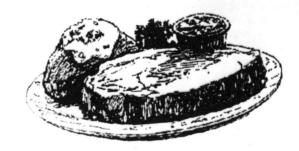
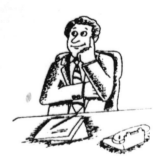

Outline

Objectives

Upon completion of this module, the student should be able to:

1. Explain the use of the Exchange System in dietary control.
2. Identify the six exchange lists.
3. List the carbohydrate, protein, fat, and energy values of each group of foods in the exchange lists.
4. Plan an appropriate menu for a person with a clinical condition that requires a calculated diet.
5. Describe the use of the calculated diet in controlling diabetes mellitus.
6. Describe the use of the calculated diet in controlling weight.
7. Describe the nursing implications appropriate to the disorders.

Glossary

High biological value: refers to complete proteins which supply abundant amounts of essential amino acids for synthesis of new tissues.

Hyperglycemia: condition that occurs when the glucose in the blood exceeds the normal range (the normal range for blood sugar levels is 70 to 120 mg per ml).

Hypoglycemic agent: a drug sometimes used by diabetics not receiving insulin to assist in lowering blood sugar levels. It is not a hormone.

Insulin: a hormone produced in the beta cells of the pancreas that controls blood glucose levels. It is the only hormone that lowers blood sugar.

Polyunsaturated: a fat that has two or more double bonds into which hydrogen can be added.

Triglycerides: the type of fat which is the body's main form of stored energy.

Background Information

The use of food exchange groups will not be new to the student who has studied the information on normal nutrition in Part 1. Only a brief review of the principles is provided here. The complete food exchange lists are located in Appendix E. These food groups are useful because they

1. Permit nutrients to be counted in foods.
2. Facilitate good meal planning by balancing the meal with choices from each group.
3. Enable a patient to comply with diet instructions with minimal effort because of their easy application.
4. Allow a certain flexibility and variety and reduce diet monotony.

5. Emphasize calorie-rich foods by completely omitting them from the lists.
6. Assure a reduced intake of saturated fats and cholesterol by a systematic procedure.
7. Enable a patient to raise or lower caloric content as needed.
8. Teach food selection in a practical way.
9. Regulate the intake of carbohydrate, protein, and fat and permit the calculation of a diet for the overweight, underweight, or diabetic patient.

The six exchange groups and their assigned values are listed in Table 16-1.

The student should remember the caloric values for the three major nutrients: carbohydrate: 1 gram = 4 calories; protein: 1 gram = 4 calories; fat: 1 gram = 9 calories. While alcohol is not a nutrient, it does furnish 7 calories per gram and is a factor to be considered in weight control. Because body fat contains some water, a pound of body fat equals 3,500 calories. Diet calculations are based on calories per kilogram (kg) of body weight. The conversion 1 kg = 2.2 lbs is important.

Foods may be exchanged within groups, but not between groups. This is because the caloric and nutrient contributions differ among groups. For example, if we substitute an apple for 1/4 cantaloupe, the contributions are similar. If we substitute an apple for one slice of bread, each contributes different amounts of calories, vitamins, minerals, and protein.

The caloric value of a diet can be regulated by the amount of fat permitted from all six lists. However, we can move the fat from group to group if we keep the total caloric level stable. For example, 1 cup skim milk = 80 calories and 1 cup whole milk = 150 calories. If whole milk is used in a diet, omit 2 fat exchanges elsewhere in the diet to account for the extra calories. Refer to the exchange groups in the appendix.

Certain raw vegetables for salads and other items containing negligible carbohydrate, protein, and fat are listed in "free" groups. A patient is instructed to consume them freely.

When the exchange method is used, the calculation of a diet requires that the patient refer to the nutritional values of the foods. Although patients prefer some foods to others, they should follow the daily food guide for the type of food and the amount to be included. The exchange list differs from the daily food guide in some aspects. The milk group in the daily food guide includes cheddar and cottage cheese, but these are listed with protein foods in the food exchange lists. Fruit and vegetables are grouped together in the daily food guide, but separately in the exchange list, primarily due to caloric considerations. The bread exchanges contain not only cereals, pastas, and breads but starchy vegetables as well.

TABLE 16-1
Outline of the 1986 American Diabetes Association Exchange Lists

Food Exchange List	Food Groups	Carbohydrate (g)	Protein (g)	Fat (g)	Kcal
1	Starch/bread	15	3	Trace	80
2	Meat				
	Lean	—	7	3	55
	Medium-fat	—	7	5	75
	High-fat	—	7	8	100
3	Vegetables	5	2	—	25
4	Fruit	15	—	—	60
5	Milk				
	Skimmed	12	8	Trace	90
	Low-fat	12	8	5	120
	Whole	12	8	8	150
6	Fat	—	—	5	45

ACTIVITY 1: Diet Therapy and Diabetes Mellitus

Background Information

Diabetes mellitus is characterized by an inability to metabolize carbohydrate due to a deficiency of insulin. The metabolism of protein and fat is also affected.

Glucose is the form of carbohydrate that is carried in the blood; all carbohydrate breaks down to glucose. Without glucose, the cells have no energy source and have to use muscle protein and tissue fat as an alternate. Without insulin, glucose cannot go from the blood into the cells. This glucose accumulates in the blood, producing hyperglycemia.

The sources of blood glucose are

1. Carbohydrate: 100 percent of digestible CHO converted to glucose
2. Protein: 58 percent converted to glucose
3. Fat: 10 percent converted to glucose
4. Glycogen (the liver's emergency supply of carbohydrate): converted to glucose when other sources are used up

Blood glucose is controlled by two hormones from the pancreas: insulin, which lowers blood sugar, and glucagon, which raises it.

Treatment and Diet Therapy

The cornerstone of treatment for diabetes mellitus is diet therapy. Many times it is the only treatment needed, especially in the 80 percent of the diabetic population who have the adult onset, noninsulin dependent type of diabe-

tes. The other 20 percent, which are usually juvenile onset, are insulin dependent and require both injections of insulin and diet therapy. Some diabetics can use the oral hypoglycemic agents. Exercise improves glucose tolerance and reduces insulin requirements.

The aim of diet therapy is to regulate carbohydrate intake while providing a nutritionally balanced diet designed for long-term use. Daily intake of calories and nutrients must be appropriately distributed among the various meals. In addition, the diet must be individualized according to the patient's growth, developmental stage, age, sex, cultural background, and ethnic factors.

Caloric Requirement

Daily caloric need includes basal metabolism, activity rate, and physiological stress (such as growth spurt, pregnancy). If the patient is overweight, the caloric range is usually 1,200 to 1,500 calories per day. If the patient is thin, young (growing), and male, it may be as high as 4,000 calories per day.

Nutrient Requirement

Past therapeutic diets for diabetics were low in carbohydrate and high in protein and fat. Newer diabetic diet plans, formulated from recent research, emphasize a definite increase in the complex carbohydrate: grains, potatoes, and other starchy vegetables such as legumes. Simple sugars (table sugar, sweets, jams, jellies, candy, soda pop) are still foods to avoid. There are exceptions. Prior to moderate or intense exercise and whenever a short-term illness disrupts a regular diet, simple carbohydrates may be added to or substituted in the diet. Daily carbohydrate intake provides 50–55 percent of the daily caloric requirement.

Protein of high biological value is stressed for diabetic diets, especially for children and adolescents. Protein provides 15 to 20 percent of the daily caloric intake.

Emphasis is placed on using polyunsaturated fats and limiting cholesterol in the remaining 30 percent of calories permitted for dietary fat.

An example will serve to illustrate the concept of nutrient balance:

Mr. X is placed on a 1,500 calorie per day diabetic diet. The nutrient balance is 50 percent carbohydrate, 20 percent protein, and 30 percent fat. What will be the number of grams of each nutrient used in the daily diet plan?

1. Carbohydrate
    1,500 calories × .50 = 750 calories
    750 calories ÷ 4 calories/gram = 187 grams carbohydrate, rounded to 190 grams
2. Protein
    1,500 calories × .20 = 300 calories
    300 calories ÷ 4 calories/gram = 75 grams protein
3. Fat
    1,500 calories × .30 = 450 calories
    450 calories ÷ 9 calories/gram = 50 grams fat

The diet prescription will be 190 g carbohydrate, 75 g protein, and 50 g fat. The amount of food from each of the six exchange lists will be chosen to satisfy these nutrient requirements.

Alcohol usage is determined by the attending physician. Since alcohol contains 7 calories per gram and no nutrients, it is usually substituted for fats in the diet. A chart showing the caloric content of individual servings of alcohol (1 glass of wine or 1 glass of beer, for example) helps those diabetics who drink.

Distribution Balance

When the daily amounts of protein, carbohydrate, and fat have been determined, they are converted into food servings and spread throughout the day into three meals and from one to three snacks, depending on the need for insulin injection, oral drugs, diet therapy, or a combination of these.

Large amounts of food, especially carbohydrates, should be avoided at any one time. A balance of meals throughout the day provides better control. The diabetic should eat at the same time each day.

There are many ways to calculate daily caloric need for a diabetic patient. One technique is as follows:

Patient's ideal weight   =   IW kg
    (IW)

Caloric need for sedentary patient	=	IW kg × 30 kcal/kg
Caloric need for patient with light activity	=	IW kg × 35 kcal/kg
Caloric need for patient with strenuous activity	=	IW kg × 40 kcal/kg
Total caloric need for obese or elderly	=	IW kg × 15–25 kcal/kg

After the patient's daily caloric need is determined, the physician (or dietitian) will prescribe the percentage of these calories from carbohydrate, protein, and fat, respectively. Then the permitted grams of these three nutrients can be calculated.

Food Exchange Lists

The Exchange System of dietary control is widely used to manage the diet of a diabetic patient. This system permits flexibility in planning and preparation and allows measuring instead of weighing. It also offers a variety of food choices.

However, the student will recognize, after studying the exchange lists, that it is not a suitable guide for planning meals for ethnic groups or in all clinical situations. People from many cultural backgrounds need dietetic counseling. Many times the illiterate or confused client will not understand the exchanges as written. At this time, students may wish to research the particular foods needed in order to individualize the diet or to simplify it. The dietitian in a nearby healthcare facility can be an excellent source for additional information and can assist in making appropriate diet instructions.

The Exchange System provides equivalent food value for each food within a list; for example:

Bread/cereal group: B vitamins, iron, protein, and carbohydrate.

Meat group: iron, zinc, B_{12}, protein, varying fat contents.

Milk group: carbohydrate, protein, varying fat contents, folacin, vitamins A and D, and B vitamins.

Vegetable group: vitamins A, E, C and K, B vitamins, fiber, protein, and carbohydrate.

Fruit group: vitamins, minerals, and carbohydrate.

Refer to Appendix E for these exchange lists.

Type I (Juvenile) Diabetes Mellitus

Caring for a diabetic child requires many special considerations, some of which are listed below:

A. Disease characteristics
    1. The patient may be normal or underweight.
    2. Disease onset is abrupt and increases in severity during growth periods.

3. Pancreatic cells cannot make insulin and a diabetic child is insulin dependent.
4. As the patient grows older, the requirement for insulin increases.

B. Dietary treatment goals
1. To permit normal growth and activity.
2. To control the disease.
3. To permit a normal school and social life with minimal restriction in freedom of movement and food choices.
4. To correspond with the action of insulin treatment.

To achieve the above goals, the diet must recognize the child's food preferences and differ little from that of the patient's peers. Also, the child must be provided adequate food to permit normal development and activities.

C. Diet prescription and meal planning
1. 75–90 kcal/kg of the child's ideal weight.
2. 3.3 to 2.2 g of protein per kg body weight, with decreasing amount for increasing age.
3. 50 percent of total calories from complex carbohydrate, 20 percent from protein, and 30 percent from fat.
4. Three meals and three snacks daily usually, with other meal patterns determined by patient's clinical condition, amount of insulin needed, daily activities, and other factors.
5. Meal plan coordinated with activities—sweets and extra fluids for strenuous and prolonged activities, eating a prescribed snack just before an exercise.

D. Patient compliance and education
1. A young diabetic will accept a diet if it is not too different from that of his or her peers and if it permits the child freedom in school and play.
2. The patient should learn how to use the exchange lists for fast foods. Such lists can be obtained from the American Diabetes Association. This permits the child to eat fast foods with his or her friends without deviating from the dietary prescription.

Illness and Diabetes Mellitus

A diabetic may become ill from causes such as infection, trauma, and so on. Patients with a short-term illness should follow the guidelines indicated in Exhibit 16-1.

Weight Control

Module 3 discussed obesity in great detail. It also described how the food exchange lists can be used to plan low-calorie diets. From Activity 1 in this module, the student has learned the application of the lists to calculate a diet with a specific caloric level. Module 3 also presented a table of diets (Table 3-4) of different caloric levels, with each diet divided into exchanges. Refer to it to familiarize yourself with the diets.

Nursing Implications

Responsibilities of the nurse include being familiar with the health concerns listed below.

A. Complications
1. Abnormal lipid metabolism is common among diabetic patients, especially Type IV and Type II hyperlipoproteinemias. The first one is treated by weight reduction. The second is managed by a diet with less than 30 percent of daily calories from fat, 20 percent of which is unsaturated.
2. Ketosis (acidosis) can be prevented if daily carbohydrate intake does not fall below 80 grams.

B. Diabetic foods
1. *Diabetic* foods are different from *dietetic* foods. The first group is either sugar-free or reduced in sugar content. The second refers to foods reduced in sugar, sodium, protein, or some other nutrients.
2. Diabetic foods are recommended for some but not all patients. Regular foods suitable for everyone are usually recommended, with only a few exceptions.

C. Drug usage
1. Obtain a detailed history of patient's use of drugs (prescription, over-the-counter, and illicit).
2. Experience has confirmed that prolonged excess vitamin C intake can lead to a false urinary glucose test.

D. Patient education
1. Dietary education forms the basis of successful diabetes control.
2. The nurse is an important coordinator in controlling diabetes.
3. Diet teaching begins from hospital admission and not after discharge.
4. A relative or caretaker who can assist with meal planning should be present during patient education.
5. The patient should be provided with as much information as possible. Some examples include
   a. food exchange lists
   b. diet plans
   c. scheduled meal times and frequency
   The patient's level of reading and comprehension must be considered.
6. Diabetic patients required to restrict sodium intake must be taught some basic knowledge of the sodium content of foods.

EXHIBIT 16-1
Sick Day Guidelines

1. Never omit the daily dosage of insulin, even if you feel too ill to eat your normal diet. You must consume some nourishment.
   a. If feasible, take fluids hourly. Keep a record. Use small amounts. Clear soups and broths will replace fluids lost in vomiting and in diarrhea.
   b. Liquids and carbohydrates are more easily tolerated during illness than proteins and fats. Determine the amount of carbohydrate you are allowed per meal and try to consume items listed below until you reach your carbohydrate allowance.

2. Check your diet plan. Food containing carbohydrates are fruits, milk, breads, and vegetables. Table 16-1 shows the amount of carbohydrate per exchange (serving) in each list. Multiply the carbohydrate amount by the number of exchanges allowed in each food group. An example for breakfast is

1 fruit	=	15 grams carbohydrate
1 milk	=	12 grams carbohydrate
2 bread	=	30 grams carbohydrate
1 meat	=	0 grams carbohydrate
1 fat	=	0 grams carbohydrate
TOTAL	=	57 grams carbohydrate

3. Fluids easily tolerated are listed below along with their carbohydrate equivalents:
   15 grams carbohydrate: 3/4 cup gingerale; ½ cup grape juice; ¾ cup orange juice; ⅓ cup apple, pineapple, or apricot juice.
   12 grams carbohydrate: 1 cup skim milk; 1 cup artificially sweetened eggnog; 1 cup cream soup made with equal parts of soup and water.
   15 grams carbohydrate: ¼ cup sherbet; ½ cup plain ice cream; ⅓ cup sweetened gelatin.

4. If you are still unable to eat after four or five liquid meals, call your physician for advice and take the following precautions:
   a. Stay warm in bed. If possible, have a relative or friend nearby in case of an insulin reaction.
   b. Test your urine for glucose (sugar) and acetone (ketone) every six hours or so. Have the results available when you call your physician. Even though you are now eating less (as a result of nausea and vomiting) than you usually do, your urine will show sugar and possible acetone. You will always need your normal insulin dose. Again, *do not omit* your daily insulin dose. Sometimes you may even need extra insulin. This may be in the form of regular insulin.

5. Call your physician if you are ill more than 48 to 72 hours or if vomiting or diarrhea persists for more than a few hours. It is better to call sooner than to put yourself in jeopardy.

6. Be prepared. Keep the following or similar items on hand: paregoric, Maalox, Tylenol, milk of magnesia, glucagon, usual insulin, and refrigerated regular insulin. Take prescribed item(s) with physician's consent.

Because of its importance, more information on patient education is provided below.

Patient Education

The diabetic patient must be considered a member of the health team. The success of the diet and of the treatment with insulin and oral drugs largely depends on patient cooperation. Therefore, a comprehensive and successful diabetic management program must always include patient education. The extent of patient education, of course, depends on the individual and the seriousness of his or her condition.

Educating a diabetic patient begins with the first visit to a clinic or upon admission to a hospital. The nurse, doctor, dietitian, and nutritionist work together to decide the best way to educate the patient. The advantages and disadvantages of treatments with diet, insulin, and oral

hypoglycemic agents should be stressed. When teaching a patient, some special points should be kept in mind.

Who to Teach and How

1. Teaching one patient instead of a group of patients is more useful to the patient, though more costly in time and money.

2. If group education is used, patients should be sorted by the type of diabetes; for example, young diabetics, insulin-dependent diabetics, obese patients using insulin, and thin patients using insulin. This sorting reduces confusion in the teaching process. If feasible, both individualized and group education is ideal..

3. The benefits and limitations of using paraprofessionals to teach the patient should be considered.

4. The patient's history should be studied, especially the type of diet instructions he or she has received. This

ensures that the patient will not receive contradictory information during an education session. Any information presented that seems to conflict with previous instructions can be explained to a patient's satisfaction.

5. At least one close relative or the patient's caretaker should be familiar with the information presented to the patient.

What to Teach

The characteristics of the disease should be explained as well as the role and interrelationship of insulin, diet, drugs, and exercise. The importance of instructions for coping with variations from the usual routine should be emphasized. Major differences between a lean and overweight diabetic also should be pointed out, and it should be emphasized that a lean diabetic has more flexibility in the amount of foods permitted.

Diet instructions must be written down. They should contain specific diet prescriptions and means of implementing them. Reasons for not eating certain foods should also be given. Instructions should include lists of the foods permitted, forbidden, and encouraged; recommended serving sizes; feeding schedules; guidelines about alcoholic beverages and the flexibility of meal planning; and so on. When food exchange lists are used, the patient should be able to make the calculations and to interchange food items. He or she should be familiar with the composition of food and the estimation of approximate contents of protein, carbohydrate, and fat. If the patient is functionally illiterate, this information must be given to others responsible, put in picture form, or recorded on tape.

Some teaching aids and counseling services for diabetes are listed below.

1. Local, city, and county diabetic programs.
2. Private and public diabetic (clinical) centers.
3. Professional sources of materials: drug companies, American Dietetic Association, American Diabetes Association, state health agencies.
4. Food models, films, and slides.
5. Ethnic teaching materials.
6. Demonstration kitchens and demonstration food portion sizes.
7. Recipes and cookbooks.

PROGRESS CHECK ON ACTIVITY 1

1. Fill out the table marked Exercise 16-1 for a calculated diet for diabetes mellitus.

Multiple Choice

Circle the letter of the correct answer.

2. Which of the following foods is not a member of the meat exchange group?
   a. eggs
   b. cheese
   c. peanut butter
   d. bacon

3. Which of the following statements correctly describes the action of insulin?
   a. Insulin controls the entry of glucose into the cell.
   b. Insulin regulates the conversion of glucose to glycogen.
   c. Insulin decreases the conversion of glucose to fat for storage as adipose fat tissue.
   d. Insulin allows fat to be converted to glucose as needed to return the blood glucose levels to normal.

4. The caloric value of a diabetic diet should be
   a. increased above normal requirements to meet the increased metabolic demand.
   b. decreased below normal requirements to prevent glucose formation.
   c. the individual's normal energy requirement to maintain ideal weight.
   d. contributed mainly by fat to spare carbohydrate.

5. In the Exchange System of diet control, an ounce of cheese may be exchanged for all except
   a. the same amount of meat.
   b. one cup of milk.
   c. two tablespoons peanut butter.
   d. one egg.

6. The Exchange System of diet control is based on principles of
   a. equivalent food values.
   b. flexible food choices.
   c. nutritional balance.
   d. all of the above.

7. How much orange juice would substitute for the CHO in an uneaten slice of bread?
   a. 1/2 cup
   b. 3/4 cup
   c. 1 cup
   d. 1 1/2 cups

8. The diabetic diet is designed for long-term use and contains a balance of
   a. energy.
   b. nutrients.
   c. distribution.
   d. all of the above.

9. Sources of blood glucose include
   a. carbohydrates.
   b. proteins.
   c. fats.

EXERCISE 16-1
Complete the Chart by Filling In the Information for Each Column

Diet	Disease or Condition	Foods Allowed	Foods Limited	Foods Forbidden	Nursing Implications
Calculated	Diabetes mellitus				

d.   all of the above.

10. If 50 percent of the total calories in a 1,500 calorie diabetic diet is from carbohydrates, how many grams of carbohydrate will the diet contain (round to nearest whole number)?
    a.   50
    b.   150
    c.   190
    d.   210

11. Emphasis is placed on using polyunsaturated fats and limiting foods high in cholesterol in the diet of the diabetic. The reason for this is
    a.   to aid in the prevention of cardiovascular diseases.
    b.   to aid in the digestive process.
    c.   to prevent skin breakdown.
    d.   to control blood sugar.

12. The daily intake of foods for the diabetic is spaced at regular intervals throughout the day. The reason for this is
    a.   to prevent hunger pangs.
    b.   to avoid symptoms of hypoglycemia or hyperglycemia.
    c.   to modify eating habits.
    d.   to prevent obesity.

13. Sally, an eight-year-old diabetic, is ready to go home from the hospital. Sally's mother should know that
    a.   all of her food must be measured.
    b.   she needs a snack before she exercises.
    c.   she should always carry hard candy with her.
    d.   all of the above.

True/False

Circle T for True and F for False.

14. T F The majority of adult-onset diabetics are underweight at the time the disease is discovered.
15. T F A diabetic diet is a combination of specific special foods that cannot be changed.
16. T F Diabetics should follow a low carbohydrate diet of about 50 grams a day.
17. T F A medium-size fresh peach contains 10 grams carbohydrate and 40 calories.

A diabetic patient in the hospital received insulin in the morning and ate breakfast, but was nauseated at lunch and could not eat. Circle T for the appropriate nursing interventions for this situation and F for the inappropriate ones.

18. T F Remove the lunch tray and tell the patient to let you know when he feels like eating.
19. T F Relieve the nausea by appropriate means.
20. T F Remove the lunch tray, asking the meal preparers to substitute liquids of equal value for the carbohydrate foods on the tray.
21. T F After you observe that the patient is better, offer him or her the liquids you ordered.

Matching

Match the foods in the left column with their nutrient values in the right column.

22. 1 slice bacon
23. 2 tbsp. peanut butter
24. ½ cup oatmeal
25. ½ cup beets

a.   12 g carbohydrate, 8 g protein, 5 g fat
b.   15 g carbohydrate, 3 g protein

26. 1 cup low-fat yogurt (2 percent plain)
    c. 5 g carbohydrate, 2 g protein
    d. 7 g protein, 5 g fat
    e. 5 g fat

27. List five nursing implications for dietary care of a diabetic patient.

    a. _____

    b. _____

    c. _____

    d. _____

    e. _____

28. Describe five of the ten essential factors that a diabetic patient must know to control his or her disease.

    a. _____

    b. _____

    c. _____

    d. _____

    e. _____

Fill-in

29. Calculate the carbohydrate, protein, and fat value of the following day's allowance:

	Carbohydrate (grams)	Protein (grams)	Fat (grams)
Milk (2%), 2 exchanges	___	___	___
Vegetables, 3 exchanges	___	___	___
Fruit, 3 exchanges	___	___	___
Lean meat, 6 exchanges	___	___	___
Medium fat meat, 2 exchanges	___	___	___
Fat, 5 exchanges	___	___	___
Bread, 6 exchanges	___	___	___

30. Arrange the allowances in # 29 into a day's menu:
    Breakfast   Lunch   Dinner   Snack

EXERCISE 16-2
Complete the Chart by Filling In the Information for Each Column

Diet	Disease or Condition	Foods Allowed	Foods Limited	Foods Forbidden	Nursing Implications
Calculated	Weight reduction				

31. The caloric value of this diet is approximately:
    a. 1,250 calories
    b. 1,500 calories
    c. 1,600 calories
    d. 1,850 calories

32. An intake reduction of 1,000 calories daily would enable an obese person to lose weight at which of the following rates?
    a. 1 lb. per week
    b. 2 lb. per week
    c. 3 lb. per week
    d. 4 lb. per week

33. Which two of the following food portions have the lowest caloric values?
    a. 4 oz. lean meat
    b. 1 medium-size potato
    c. 1 slice bread
    d. 1 8-oz. glass of milk

34. Fill out Exercise 16-2 for a calculated diet for weight reduction.

References

American Diabetes Association and American Dietetic Association. 1986. *Exchange lists for meal planning.* Chicago: American Dietetic Association.

American Diabetes Association. 1987. Consensus conference statement on self-monitoring of blood glucose. *Diabetes Care* 10:95.

American Dietetic Association. 1987. Position of the American Dietetic Association: Appropriate use of nutritive and nonnutritive sweeteners. *Journal of the American Dietetic Association* 87(12):689.

Anderson, J. W. 1988. Nutrition management of diabetes mellitus. In *Modern nutrition in health and disease,* 7th ed. M. E. Shils and V. R. Young (eds.). Philadelphia: Lea & Febiger.

Anderson, J. W. et al. 1987. Dietary fiber and diabetes: A comprehensive review and practical application. *Journal of the American Dietetic Association* 87(9):1189.

Barrett-Conner, E. et al. 1985. Diabetes and heart disease. In *Diabetes in America.* Department of Health and Human Services Publication No. (NIH) 85-1468.

Beebe, C. A. (ed.). 1988. Obesity management in people with diabetes. *Diabetes Spectrum* 1(1):17.

Berdanier, C. R. 1986. You are what you inherit. *Nutrition Today* 21(5):18.

Berg, K. E. (ed.). 1986. *Diabetic's guide to health and fitness: An authoritative approach to leading an active life.* Champaign, IL: Human Kinetics.

Franz, M. J. 1987. Exercise and the management of diabetes mellitus. *Journal of the American Dietetic Association* 87(7):872.

Gabbe, S. G. 1986. Gestational diabetes mellitus. *New England Journal of Medicine* 315:1025.

Green, J. et al. 1987. *Meal planning approaches in the nutrition management of the person with diabetes.* Chicago: American Dietetic Association.

Jornsay, D. L. et al. 1988. Diabetes and the traveler. *Clinical Diabetes* 6(3):49.

Jovanovic, L., and C. M. Peterson (eds.). 1985. *Contemporary issues in clinical nutrition.* Vol. 8. *Nutrition and diabetes.* New York: Alan R. Liss.

Livingston, J. N. 1988. Getting the message. *Diabetes Forecast.* 41(6):56.

McBride, J. 1987. Starch goes straight to help diabetes victims. *Journal of the American Dietetic Association* 87(7):871.

Metz, R., and E. B. Larson (eds.). 1985. *Blue book of endocrinology.* Philadelphia: Saunders.

Powers, M. A. (ed.). 1987. *Handbook of diabetes nutritional management.* Rockville, MD: Aspen.

Vahouny, G. V. et al. (eds.). 1986. *Dietary fiber: Basic and clinical aspects.* New York: Plenum Press.

Wheeler, M. L. et al. 1987. Diet and exercise in noninsulin-dependent diabetes mellitus: Implications for dietitians from the NIH Consensus Development Conference. *Journal of the American Dietetic Association* 87(4):480.

Williams, G. M. (ed.). 1988. *Sweeteners: Health effects.* Princeton, NJ: Princeton Scientific.

Module 17

Diet and Disorders of the Gallbladder and Pancreas

Time for completion
Activities: _____1_____ hour
Optional examination: ½ hour

Academic credit
Semester units: ²⁄₁₀
Quarter units: ³⁄₁₀

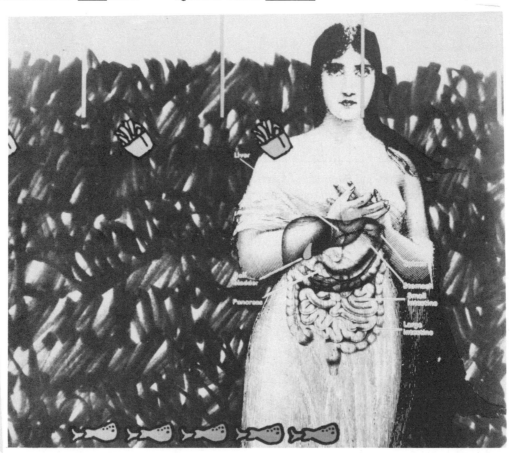

Outline

Objectives

Upon completion of this module, the student should be able to:

1. Discuss the causes of gallbladder and pancreatic disorders and describe how they affect food metabolism.

2. Identify the sequence of physiological events in which bile assists in the absorption and metabolism of foods.

3. Differentiate between cholecystitis, cholelithiasis, and cholecystectomy in relation to their effects on the digestion and metabolism of foods.

4. Describe and give examples of the diet therapy used for gallbladder disease.

5. Discuss appropriate nursing interventions.

6. Identify the major causes of pancreatitis.

7. Relate the association between pancreatitis and gallbladder disease.

8. Describe the diet therapy for pancreatitis and the reasons for its use.

Glossary

Calculi ("stones"): an abnormal concretion, usually of mineral salts, occurring in the body in hollow organs or passages.

Cholecystectomy: removal of the gallbladder by surgical procedure.

Cholecystitis: inflammation of the gallbladder, acute or chronic.

Cholecystokinin: a hormone secreted in the small intestine that stimulates gallbladder contraction and secretion of pancreatic enzymes.

Cholelithiasis: calculi in the common bile duct.

Cholesterol: a steroid alcohol found in animal fats, bile, blood, brain tissue, whole milk, egg yolk, liver, kidneys, adrenal gland, and the myelin sheath of nerve fibers.

Emulsify: to mix together two immiscible liquids. One is dispersed into the other in small drops.

Gallbladder (GB): the pear-shaped organ located below the liver which serves as a storage place for bile.

Pancreas: a large elongated gland located transversely behind the stomach between the spleen and duodenum.

Background Information

The gallbladder (GB) is an accessory organ to the gastrointestinal (GI) tract. The emulsification of fats by bile salts from the GB is an important contribution to the overall efficiency of the GI functioning. Gallbladder disease is a common but potentially serious disorder. The most common disorder is cholelithiasis, or formation of gallstones. It develops in 10 to 20 percent of the Western world's population. Nearly 80 to 90 percent of gallstones are composed primarily of cholesterol.

Some population groups are more susceptible to GB disease, such as older men and women, and especially women who have borne children. Others include American Indians and individuals using oral contraceptives and drugs that lower blood cholesterol levels. Heredity appears to have a major influence in the development of gallstones. Diet plays a role, but a minor one. For example, excess use of polyunsaturated fats can increase the incidence.

Other contributing factors include obesity and intestinal diseases that involve the malabsorption of bile salts. Occasionally, the stress of pregnancy is responsible. Populations with a low intake of total fat appear to be less vulnerable to cholelithiasis.

Medical management of GB disease includes temporary use of drugs to dissolve the stones and surgery, if the patient is not undernourished or obese. An undernourished patient can be replenished, while an obese one can lose weight. The actual surgery (cholecystectomy) has less nutritional implication than previously believed. The procedure allows bile to enter the small intestine on a continuous basis. With time, the bile ducts may enlarge and store bile. Because of this adaptation, many clients resume a normal diet one to two months after surgery.

Since the pancreas is an important accessory organ of the GI tract and a major producer of digestive enzymes, any pancreatic disorder can seriously impair the body's ability to digest food. Reduced production of pancreatic enzymes may occur in cystic fibrosis, chronic pancreatitis, pancreatic cancer, or protein calorie malnutrition. The pancreas may become inflamed and/or obstructed by chronic alcohol abuse or GB disease. Food eaten during these conditions becomes the source of excruciating pain, and the client will avoid eating. Consequently, the person's nutritional status is very poor. Determining the type of pancreatic disorder is of major importance when planning nutritional care for patients with pancreatitis.

ACTIVITY 1: Diet and Gallbladder Disorders

Background Information

The normal function of the gallbladder is to concentrate and store the bile derived from the liver. The liver produces 600 to 800 milliliters of bile per day, and the gallbladder concentrates and stores 40 to 70 milliliters. When fat enters the duodenum, it stimulates the secretion of a hormone, cholecystokinin, which is carried by the blood to the gallbladder. This hormone directs the gallbladder to contract, so that bile is released into the common duct and then travels to the duodenum. The function of bile is to emulsify fats so that they can be broken down or digested by fat-splitting enzymes, the lipases. Any interference with the flow of bile impairs fat digestion.

Gallbladder Disorders

The three major disorders of the gallbladder are

Cholecystitis. Cholecystitis usually results from a low-grade chronic infection. The major component of bile is cholesterol. When the gallbladder mucosa becomes inflamed or infected, the cholesterol may precipitate, forming gallstones of almost pure cholesterol crystals.

Cholelithiasis. Cholelithiasis is an end result of cholecystitis, but a high fat intake over a long period of time also predisposes people to gallstone formation. The body will produce more cholesterol to make more bile to assist in the metabolism of fat.

Cholecystectomy. Cholecystectomy is the surgical removal of the gallbladder. When a person with cholecystitis or cholelithiasis eats a meal, especially if fat content is high, the gallbladder contracts in response to cholecystokinin stimulation. This causes severe pain, fullness, distention, nausea, and vomiting. Surgery is usually the treatment of choice. However, surgery may be postponed for two reasons: until the inflammation subsides or until the patient loses weight, if he or she is obese, which many are. In these cases, supportive therapy is largely dietary.

Diet Therapy

Dietary fat is reduced to diminish gallbladder contraction, which is responsible for pain and associated symptoms. Fat modification involves only its quantity, approximately 40 to 50 grams intake per day. Protein comprises only 10 to 12 percent of the daily calories, since most protein foods also contain fats. The remainder of the day's calories should be derived from carbohydrates.

If weight loss is indicated, calories will be reduced accordingly. Use of both the weight reduction diets discussed in other modules and the food Exchange System is recommended. Caloric intake should not be less than 1,200 calories per day. These diets are used only before surgery. Otherwise, a patient can be placed on these diets after he or she has completely recovered from surgery. Another consideration is to provide such patients with vitamin K to reduce bleeding.

Restriction of foods that can cause abdominal discomfort, such as gas, is individualized and not implemented randomly.

Because the body manufactures its own cholesterol in amounts several times more than are present in the daily diet, restricting dietary cholesterol to reduce gallstone formation has been questioned. Since cholesterol is manufactured from fat in the diet, lowering total fat intake may prove more effective. Table 17-1 describes a low-fat diet, indicating foods to be avoided. Table 17-2 presents a sample meal plan for one caloric level.

Nursing Implications

Responsibilities for nurses treating patients with gallbladder disorders are listed below.

1. Evaluate the low-fat diet for adequacy of fat-soluble vitamins and substitute alternate sources of the vitamins, if necessary.
2. Provide instructions on correct methods of food preparation. Discourage use of fats and oils for seasoning and frying foods.
3. Assess the patient's tolerance for foods that cause discomfort and flatulence. Omit those from the diet.
4. Assure nutritional adequacy of a diet with removal of foods not tolerated and substitution of alternate sources as needed.
5. Implement adequate patient education regarding tissue repair after a cholecystectomy.

PROGRESS CHECK ON ACTIVITY 1

Fill-in

1. Fill in the sheet marked Exercise 17-1 for a low-fat diet.
2. Alter the following day's menu to make it suitable for a patient on a low-fat diet (50 grams). Calories are not restricted. Do not change more than is necessary to meet the diet's restriction.

   Breakfast
   Orange juice

   _____

   Oatmeal with half-and-half and sugar

   _____

   Fried egg

   _____

   Toast with butter and jelly

   _____

   Coffee

   _____

(continued on p. 246)

TABLE 17-1
Permitted and Prohibited Foods in a Fat-Restricted Diet

Food Group	Foods Permitted	Foods Prohibited
Milk and milk products	Skim milk (fortified with vitamins A and D): fluid, dry powder, and evaporated; yogurt and buttermilk made from skim milk (fortified with vitamins A and D).	Whole milk and all products made from it; low-fat and 2 percent milk and all products made from them; heavy cream, half-and-half, sour cream; cream sauces, nondairy cream substitutes.
Breads and equivalents	Enriched or whole-grain bread; plain buns and rolls; crackers; graham crackers, matzo, melba toast; other varieties not specifically excluded; all cereals that are tolerated by the patient; potatoes except those specifically excluded; rice (brown or white); spaghetti, noodles, macaroni; barley; grits; wild rice; flours (all varieties).	Biscuits, dumplings, corn bread, waffles, pancakes, nut breads, doughnuts, spicy snack crackers, sweet rolls, popovers, French toast, corn chips, muffins, all items made with a large quantity of fat; cereals with nuts and 100 percent bran may be omitted if not well tolerated; fried potatoes, creamed potatoes, potato chips, hash-browned potatoes and potato salad, scalloped potatoes; fried rice, egg noodles, casseroles prepared with cream or cheese sauce; chow mein noodles, bread stuffing; Yorkshire pudding; Spanish rice; fritters; spaghetti with strongly seasoned sauce.
Meats and equivalents	Limited to 4 to 6 oz. daily; all lean fresh meat, fish, or poultry (no skin) with fat trimmed; shellfish, salmon, and tuna canned in water; foods may be pan-broiled, broiled, baked, roasted, boiled, stewed, or simmered; soybeans, peas, and meat analogues if tolerated.	Fried, creamed, breaded, or sauteed items; sausage, bacon, frankfurters, ham, luncheon meats, meats with gravy, many processed and canned meats; any seafood packed in oil; nuts, peanut butter, pork and beans.
Cheese and eggs	Any variety not specifically prohibited (2 oz. cheese equivalent to 3 oz. meat); 1 egg yolk a day, any style, with no fat used in cooking; egg whites may be used as desired; 1 egg yolk equals 1 oz. meat.	Any cheese made from whole milk, including cream cheese; any egg that is creamed, deviled, or fried.
Beverages	Most nonalcoholic beverages except those specifically excluded.	All beverages containing chocolate, cream, or whole milk; for example, milk shakes and eggnog, alcoholic beverages if not permitted by doctor.
Fruits and vegetables	All varieties not excluded and tolerated by the patient.	Avocado and any not tolerated by the patient; fried and creamed vegetables, vegetables with cream sauces or fat added; any variety not tolerated.
Soups	Broth, bouillon, or consommé with no fat; fat-free soup stocks; all homemade soups or cream soups made with allowed ingredients; soups made with skim milk, clear soups with permitted vegetables and meats with fat skimmed off; packaged dehydrated soup varieties.	Most commercial soups; any soup made with cream, fat, or whole milk.
Fats	Limited to 2 to 3 tsp. per day; all fats and oils (e.g., margarine, butter, shortening, lard); heavy cream (1 tbsp. = 1 tsp. fat); sour cream or light cream (2 tbsp. = 1 tsp. fat); cream substitute (4 tsp. = 1 tsp. fat); salad dressing (1 tbsp. = 1 tsp. fat); low-calorie dressing in small amounts not counted in fat allowances.	All fats exceeding the 2- to 3-tsp. limit, including bacon drippings.
Sweets	Plain sweets, honey, syrup, sugar, molasses, jams, jellies, plain sugar candies, chewing gum, hard candy, marshmallows, gum drops, jelly beans, sour balls, preserves, marmalade, tutti-frutti.	Any candies or sweets made with nuts, coconut, chocolate, cream, whole milk, margarine, butter.

(continues)

TABLE 17-1 (Continued)

Food Group	Foods Permitted	Foods Prohibited
Desserts	Sherbet, Jell-O, water ice, fruit-flavored Popsicles and ices; rice, bread, cornstarch, tapioca puddings; plain gelatin, gelatin with fruit added; fruit whips, puddings and custards made with skim milk and egg whites; cookies made with skim milk or egg whites; arrowroot cookies, vanilla wafers, angelfood cake, sponge cake.	Any products made with whole milk, cream, chocolate, butter, margarine, nuts, egg yolks.
Miscellaneous	All herbs and spices tolerated and not specifically excluded; artificial sweetener, baking soda, baking powder.	Any sauces made with fat, oil, cream, or milk; olives, pickles, garlic, chili sauce, chutney, horseradish, relish, Worcestershire sauce.

Lunch
Pork chop with dressing
_____

Buttered green beans
_____

Corn on the cob
_____

Roll
_____

Butter
_____

Milk and tea with sugar
_____

Dinner
Spaghetti with meat sauce
_____

Tossed green salad/Italian dressing
_____

French bread/butter
_____

Ice cream with fudge sauce
_____

Red wine
_____

Coffee
_____

TABLE 17-2
Sample Menu Supplying 40 to 45 g of Fat, with 80 to 90 g of Protein, 260 to 280 g of Carbohydrate, and 1,700 to 2,000 kcal

Breakfast	Lunch	Dinner
Orange juice, ½ c.	Beef broth and noodles, ½ c.	Tomato juice, ½ c.
Oatmeal, cooked, ½ c.	Chicken, broiled, 2 oz.	Beef, lean, broiled, 3 oz.
Egg, poached, 1	Saltines, 4	Potato, baked, small, 1
Raisin toast, 1 slice	Margarine, 1 tsp.	Green beans, ½ c.
Jam, 2 tsp.	Green salad with lemon juice, ½ c.	Roll, hard, small, 1
Margarine, 1 tsp.	Orange, 1	Butter, 1 tsp.
Milk, skim, 1 c.	Cola, 8 oz.	Gelatin or fruit cocktail, ½ c.
Sugar, 2 tsp.	Sugar, 2 tsp.	Milk, skim, 1 c.
Coffee or tea	Coffee or tea	Sugar, 2 tsp.
Salt, pepper	Salt, pepper	Coffee or tea
		Salt, pepper

EXERCISE 17-1
Complete the Chart by Filling In the Columns with Appropriate Information

Diet	Disease or Condition	Foods Allowed	Foods Limited	Foods Forbidden	Nursing Implications
Low-fat diet	Gallbladder disease				

ACTIVITY 2: Diet Therapy for Pancreatitis

Background Information

Because gallstones may enter the common bile duct and block the flow of the pancreatic juice and enzymes, pancreatitis is a common complication of gallbladder disease. Pancreatitis is a severe disorder, since the enzymes in the immobile juice can cause the pancreas to digest itself. Acute pain and tenderness result, and in critical cases the pancreas may hemorrhage. The treatment of choice is to inhibit the secretion of the enzymes and to treat for shock and renal shutdown. In this case, diet therapy is useful only after the crisis has subsided.

Another causative factor for pancreatitis, especially a chronic condition, is alcoholism, which will be discussed in the module for diseases of the liver. Irrespective of the cause of pancreatitis, dietary treatment and nursing implications are the same.

Diet Therapy

The aim of diet therapy is to prevent the secretion of pancreatic enzymes. Both food and alcohol stimulate pancreatic secretions. The clinical management procedures of severe pancreatitis are listed below.

1.   Initial measures are lifesaving. These include intravenous (IV) or total parenteral nutrition (TPN) feedings, replacement of fluid and electrolytes, blood transfusions, and drugs for pain and inhibiting gastric secretions. Nasogastric suction may also be used to remove gastric contents. Nothing is given by mouth.

2.   As healing progresses, the first oral diet is usually made up of clear liquid with amino acids, predigested fats, and other commercial preparations added gradually. The patient progresses to a bland diet given in six small feedings. It is low in fat and foods that stimulate pancreatic secretion. Examples of stimulants include caffeine (coffee, cola) and alcohol. Pancreatic enzymes may be given.

Diet therapy for chronic pancreatitis is usually a bland diet of soft or regular consistency in small meals at frequent intervals (six feedings) and contains no stimulant in foods (see above). Pancreatic enzymes may be given orally with food.

Nursing Implications

1.   The patient should be taught that no alcohol or caffeine can be tolerated in his or her diet. Sources of caffeine include coffee, tea, and cola beverages.

2.   The patient can develop diabetes if the islet cells of the pancreas become malfunctioning. Evaluate frequently for symptoms. If diabetes develops, a calculated diet will be used.

3.   Pancreatic enzymes come in capsule and tablet form and should be swallowed whole. They should not be given with hot food or liquids to avoid breaking their protective coating. They are given only with meals.

4.   The patient with pancreatitis has a poor appetite and may not eat well enough to repair damage done. The patient may not enjoy the type of modifications required. Extra support, encouragement, and counseling are necessary.

PROGRESS CHECK ON ACTIVITY 2

Fill-in

Use a separate sheet of paper for your answer.

Write a one-day menu for a patient who has chronic pancreatitis and has lost 20 pounds since the onset two months ago.

References

Enloe, C. F., Jr. 1982. "The pancreas." *Nutrition Today* 17:20–23.

Gracie, W. A., and D. F. Ransohoff. 1982. "The natural history of silent gallstones: The innocent gallstone is not a myth." *New England Journal of Medicine* 307:798.

Hui, Y. H. 1985. *Essentials of nutrition and diet therapy.* Monterey, CA: Wadsworth Health Sciences.

Hurley, R. S., and H. S. Mekjijian. 1987. Dietary habits of patients with cholelithiasis. Do we need to instruct? *Journal of the American Dietetic Association* 87(2):209.

Jeejeebhoy, K. N. 1988. *Current therapy in nutrition.* Philadelphia: B. C. Dekker.

Makhouf, G. M. 1982. "Function of the gallbladder." *Nutrition Today* 17(1):10.

Mayo Clinic. 1988. *Mayo Clinic diet manual.* Philadelphia: B. C. Dekker.

Morris, D. L., et al. 1978. "Gallbladder disease and gallbladder cancer among American Indians in Tricultural New Mexico." *Cancer* 42:2472–77.

Palmer, R. H., and M. C. Carey. 1982. An optimistic view of the national cooperative gallstone study. *New England Journal of Medicine* 306:1171.

Roslyn, J. J. et al. 1983. Gallbladder disease in patients on long-term parenteral nutrition. *Gastroenterology* 84:148.

Sedaghat, A., and S. M. Grundy. 1980. Cholesterol crystals and the formation of cholesterol gallstones. *New England Journal of Medicine* 302:1274.

Tangedahl, T. 1979. Dissolution of gallstones—when and how. *Surg. Clin. M. A.* 59:797.

Thorpe, C. J., and J. A. Caprini. 1980. Gallbladder disease: Current trends and treatments. *American Journal of Nursing* 80:2181.

Tokes, P. P., and N. J. Greenberger. 1983. Acute and chronic pancreatitis. *DM* 29:1.

Tucker, L. 1979. Identification of gallstone disease. *Postgrad. Med.* 66:163.

Tucker, L., and T. N. Tangedahl. 1979. Manifestations of gallstone disease. *Postgrad. Med.* 66:179.

Diet Therapy for Disorders of the Liver

Time for completion

Activities: _____1_____ hour

Optional examination: __½__ hour

Academic credit

Semester units: __²⁄₁₀__

Quarter units: __³⁄₁₀__

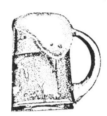
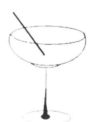
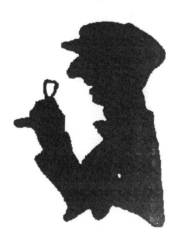
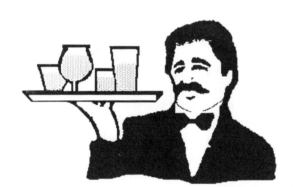

Outline

Objectives

Upon completion of this module, the student should be able to:

1. Describe the major functions of the normal liver.
2. Identify the appropriate diet therapy for treating liver diseases and state the rationale for its use in treating: hepatitis, cirrhosis, hepatic coma and liver failure, and cancer.
3. Evaluate nursing interventions to promote optimal nutrition in a patient with liver disease.

Glossary

Ascites: abnormal accumulation of serous fluid within the peritoneal cavity (the space between the abdominal walls and the pelvic cavity).

Edema: abnormal accumulation of fluid in the intercellular spaces of the body.

Esophageal varices: varicose veins in the esophagus which occur most often as a result of obstruction of the portal circulation.

Hepatic: pertaining to the liver.

Jaundice: yellowness of the skin, mucous membranes, and excretions (jaundice is not a disease, but is a symptom of numerous disorders of the liver, gallbladder, and blood—it occurs when pigment in the blood is destroyed).

Marasmus: protein-calorie malnutrition, causing growth retardation and wasting of muscle.

Portal (circulation): circulation of blood through layer vessels from the capillaries of one organ to those of another (applies here especially to passage of blood from the GI tract and spleen through the portal vein to the liver).

Psychotropic: capable of modifying mental activity; a drug that affects the mental state.

Background Information

A normal liver regulates the proper digestion, metabolism, and absorption of food. An outline of the liver's major functions is listed below.

A. Storage. The liver stores
   1. approximately one pound of glycogen, the body's emergency energy supply; this supply lasts 12 to 36 hours when used as the only energy source.
   2. more fat- than water-soluble vitamins.
   3. more iron than any other part of the body.
B. Circulation. The liver regulates
   1. blood volume.
   2. blood transfer from the portal to systemic circulation.
   3. fluid transfers.
C. Metabolism. The liver participates in
   1. carbohydrate metabolism by interconverting glucose and glycogen as needed; it also converts amino acids to glucose in the presence of excess protein or low carbohydrate level.
   2. fat metabolism by providing bile salts for emulsifying fat, cholesterol, and lipoproteins; and by converting excess amino acid and carbohydrate to fats.
   3. protein metabolism by forming plasma proteins, prothrombin, and urea.
D. Detoxification. The liver detoxifies all ingested
   1. drugs.
   2. poisons.

From the functions of the liver listed, it should be obvious that a diseased liver adversely affects gastrointestinal function and the use of food.

ACTIVITY 1: Diet Therapy for Hepatitis

Hepatitis, an inflammation of the liver, can result in the destruction of liver cells. In most cases, proper medical management, including optimal nutrition, permits destroyed liver cells to regenerate. However, an extensive destruction of liver cells may lead to liver failure and death. Hepatitis interferes with the liver's major functions.

Medical management for hepatitis includes: (a) optimum nutrition for healing; (b) complete bed rest to reduce inflammation and metabolism; and (c) a high fluid intake to prevent dehydration and improve appetite. Alcohol and all other drugs are prohibited to avoid further liver damage. All such considerations permit speedy recovery. An acceptable diet for hepatitis is

1. 75 to 100 grams protein per day. High protein permits liver cell regeneration.
2. 300 to 400 grams carbohydrate per day. This replenishes glycogen storage, meets caloric needs, and spares protein for liver cell repair.
3. 100 to 150 grams fat per day. Hepatitis patients have poor appetites, and fats make the diet more appealing. Dietary fats should be those that are easily utilized, such as oil, butter, cream, margarine, and whole milk.
4. 2,500 to 3,000 calories per day. This meets the increased energy demands of fever, tissue repair, and strength renewal.
5. Two to three times the RDAs for vitamins per day to

replace losses and to aid in liver cell regeneration. Supplements may be required.

6. Fluid intake should be high—3,000 to 3,500 milliliters per day.

7. Multiple feedings—three meals and three snacks to increase tolerance.

Table 18-1 presents a daily food plan for a high-carbohydrate, high-protein, high-vitamin, and moderate-fat diet.

ACTIVITY 2: Diet Therapy for Cirrhosis

Cirrhosis is the final stage of certain liver injuries, including alcoholism, untreated hepatitis, biliary obstruction, and drug and poison ingestion. The liver is unable to regenerate cells, which are replaced with fibrous, nonfunctioning tissue.

Stages of Cirrhosis

Cirrhosis has early and late stages. The early stages affect the digestive system, and cause such symptoms as nausea, vomiting, distention, diarrhea, and anorexia. These symptoms are managed by a dietary plan similar to that for hepatitis. The rationale also is the same: to support residual liver function and prevent further cell destruction. Compliance with dietary and other medical recommendations will delay development of the late stages of the disease for years for some patients.

In the later stages of cirrhosis, the patient is severely malnourished. Edema, ascites, anemia, infections, intestinal bleeding, jaundice, and esophageal varices may be present. Renal failure also may occur. The patient is in critical condition. Primarily, a diet high in protein, carbohydrate, vitamins, and calories, and moderate in fat is preferred for advanced cirrhosis. However, other dietary changes are prescribed according to the patient's condition.

1. *Protein.* If hepatic coma is not indicated, protein remains at 75 to 100 grams daily. If, however, the patient shows signs of impending coma, the physician should reduce protein intake to lessen the chance of coma.

2. *Sodium.* Edema and/or ascites is countered by a 500 to 1,000 mg sodium (daily) diet. Fluid intake may be limited.

3. *Texture.* Esophageal varices, if present, are managed by semisolid or liquid diets to avoid potential rupture and hemorrhage. Tube feedings are not advised for patients with this complication. These patients should avoid coffee, tea, pepper, chili powder, and other irritating seasonings.

4. *Appetite.* For patients with poor appetite, other measures are used to provide adequate nutrients and calories. These include oral formulas high in nutrients and calories; vitamin/mineral supplements; electrolyte replacements; hepatic aids; and parenteral feedings.

If the cirrhosis is alcohol-induced, deficiency of magnesium and vitamin B complex is often present. Alcohol reduces vitamin absorption and increases mineral excretion.

TABLE 18-1
**Sample Menu for a Diet Containing Approximately 2,500 kcal,
90 g of Protein, 300 g of Carbohydrate, and 100 g of Fat**

Breakfast	Lunch	Dinner
Orange juice 1 c.	Grape juice, ½ c.	Lamb chop, 1
Eggs, scrambled	Tuna salad, ½ c.	Carrots, cooked, 1 c.
Muffin, whole wheat, 2	Lettuce leaves, 4	Cole slaw, with mustard and vinegar, 1 c.
Margarine, 1 pat	Tomato, 2 slices	Potato, baked, 1 med.
Coffee, tea	Bread, whole wheat, 2 slices	Margarine, 1 tbsp.
Sugar	Milk, 1 c., skim	Milk, skim, 1 c.
Salt, pepper	Coffee, tea	Fresh peach
Jelly	Sugar	Coffee, tea
	Salt, pepper	Sugar
		Salt, pepper
	Snack	
	8 oz. low-fat yogurt	**Snack**
		4 sugar cookies
		Apple juice, 1 c.

Hepatic Coma

Hepatic coma is caused by brain damage resulting from the inability of a damaged liver to metabolize ammonia compounds. Irritability, confusion, drowsiness, apathy, and irrational behavior precede the coma. Other signs are motor dysfunction and fecal breath odor. Ammonia accumulates because the liver cannot convert it to urea. Ammonia is formed from protein in the intestines by bacterial action. The protein may be ingested or derived from blood (bleeding into the intestine). Treatment includes antibiotics, psychotropic drugs, enemas to remove blood and protein from the bowel, and diet therapy. Diet therapy in impending hepatic coma is as follows.

1. Protein intake is limited to 0 to 50 grams daily, depending on the blood ammonia level. Note that dietary protein is derived chiefly from milk and meats and is of high biological value. It produces minimal ammonia because it is used optimally without waste—that is, it is not metabolized for energy.
2. The diet provides 1,500 to 2,000 calories per day, mainly derived from carbohydrates and fat. This reduces tissue breakdown and ammonia formation.
3. Vitamins are given intravenously; vitamin K is especially needed to reduce bleeding.
4. Fluid output is balanced by equal intake. Urine voided and other fluid lost is recorded.

Liver Cancer

The diet for a patient with liver cancer is high in carbohydrate, protein, fluid, vitamins, and calories, and moderate in fat. Alternate intervals of feeding (other than three meals a day) are indicated for all cancer patients, but especially when the liver is involved and the utilization of nutrients is compromised. The diet will be individualized to fit the patient's tolerance. For instance, when cancer patients develop an aversion to meat, meat substitutes are offered to satisfy the high protein need.

The type of protein-calorie malnutrition that develops during advanced liver disease and hepatic cancer is very severe and is accompanied by the many complications common to marasmus. This malnourishment only adds to other clinical problems, making the restoration and maintenance of optimum nutrition difficult.

All liver disorders present a challenge to the nurse to provide adequate nutrition for the patient.

Nursing Implications

Responsibilities for the nurse in treating cirrhosis are as follows:

A. Dietary plans
   1. The dietary plan for each patient should be individualized according to clinical conditions, appetite, and so on. For example, a patient with advanced cirrhosis may be very hungry in the morning and a large breakfast should be provided.
   2. Many patients with ascites prefer frequent, small meals to large ones, which can cause discomfort by raising portal pressure.
   3. Any meal planning must consider gastrointestinal disorders such as diarrhea, nausea, vomiting, and anorexia. Such conditions interfere, both physically and psychologically, with eating.
   4. Low-sodium milk is more acceptable if flavoring such as honey or vanilla is added.
   5. Patients do not like most oral nutrition formulas with medium-chain triglycerides (MCT) added. Experience confirms better acceptance by some patients when the beverage is served chilled.
B. Patient monitoring
   1. A careful record of food intake is useful.
   2. Be alert to signs of impending coma.
   3. Always balance fluid intake and output.
C. Team work
   1. Team work is mandatory. The team includes the nurse, physician, dietitian, patient, and family members.
   2. Conferences and strategy sessions with members of the team assure that the patient will be encouraged to eat.
D. Alcoholism
   1. The nurse should refrain from judging the patient's drinking habits.
   2. The patient should be provided with assistance, including such therapy as Alcoholics Anonymous meetings and rehabilitation centers.
   3. The patient should be given intense education on the disease and its complications and treatment.
E. Drugs
   1. No alcoholic beverage is permitted in the hospital. Abstinence at home is strongly encouraged.
   2. The patient should comply with specific usage for any prescription drugs and avoid all others.

PROGRESS CHECK ON ACTIVITIES 1 AND 2

Fill-in

Use a separate sheet of paper for your answers.

1. Fill in the sheet marked Exercise 18-1 for a high-carbohydrate, protein, and vitamin diet with moderate fat.
2. Plan a breakfast menu for a diet that is high in calories,

EXERCISE 18-1
Complete the Chart by Filling In the Appropriate Information for Each Column

Diet	Disease or Condition	Foods Allowed	Foods Limited	Foods Forbidden	Nursing Implications
High-carbohydrate, protein, and vitamin; moderate fat	Hepatitis Early cirrhosis Cancer Marasmus Uncomplicated postoperative convalescence				

carbohydrate, protein, and vitamins, and moderate in fat.

3. Alter this breakfast menu to meet the needs of a client who daily requires: (a) 40 grams protein and (b) 2 grams sodium.

Situation

4. Mrs. J. is admitted to the hospital with a diagnosis of infectious hepatitis and is placed in isolation. Her diet prescription is 350 grams carbohydrate, 100 grams protein, and 100 grams of easily digested fat. She will receive Theragran M Multiple Vitamin Supplement. Answer the following questions about her diet:

a. What is the caloric value of her diet? _____

b. Why were the extra calories ordered? _____

c. Compare the ordered protein intake with the RDAs for an adult nonpregnant woman. _____

d. Why is the extra protein needed? _____

e. What is the role of the extra carbohydrate?

f. What is the rationale for the extra vitamins?

g. What foods should be avoided? _____

h. If Mrs. J. develops ascites, what additional restrictions should be placed on her diet? _____

i. What precautions with the eating utensils will the nurse observe with this patient? _____

j. What other diseases require the diet prescribed for hepatitis? _____

References

American Dietetic Association. 1988. *Manual of clinical dietetics*. Chicago: American Dietetic Association.

Blackburn, G. L. et al. (eds.). 1989. *Nutritional medicine: A case management approach*. Philadelphia: Saunders.

Chopra, S. 1988. *Disorders of the liver*. Philadelphia: Lea & Febiger.

Food and Nutrition Board, National Research Council, National Academy of Sciences. 1989. *Recommended dietary allowances*. 10th ed. Washington, DC: National Academy Press.

Fraser, C. L., and A. I. Arieff. 1985. Hepatic encephalopathy. *New England Journal of Medicine* 313:865.

Gitlin, N., and M. B. Heyman. 1984. Nutritional support in liver disease. *Nutr. Supp. Serv.* 4(6):14.

Hiyama, D. T., and J. E. Fischer. 1988. Nutritional support in hepatic failure. *Nutr. Clin. Pract.* 3(3):96.

Jeejeebhoy, K. N. 1988. *Current therapy in nutrition*. Philadelphia: B. C. Dekker.

Mayo Clinic. 1988. *Mayo Clinic diet manual*. Philadelphia: B. C. Dekker.

Mezitis, N. H. 1988. Nutritional management in liver disease. *Nutr. Clin. Pract.* 3(3):108.

Millikin, W. J., and M. A. Hooks. 1988. Nutritional support in hepatic failure. *Nutr. Clin. Pract.* 3(3):96.

Shaw, S., and C. S. Lieber. 1988. Nutrition and diet in alcoholism. In *Modern nutrition in health and disease*, 7th ed. M. E. Shils and V. R. Young (eds.). Philadelphia: Lea & Febiger.

Shronts, E. P. 1988. Nutrition assessment of adults with end-stage hepatic failure. *Nutr. Clin. Pract.* 3(3):113.

Shronts, E. P. et al. 1987. Nutrition support of the adult liver transplant candidate. *Journal of the American Medical Association* 87:441.

Diet Therapy for Renal Disorders

Time for completion
Activities: _____1_____ hour
Optional examination: ½ hour

Academic credit
Semester units: ²⁄10
Quarter units: ³⁄10

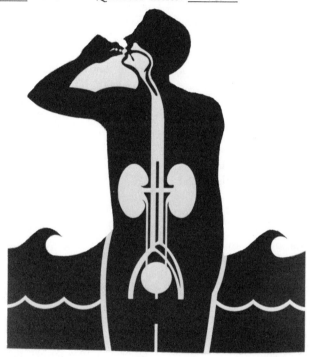

Outline

Objectives
Glossary
Background Information

ACTIVITY 1: Kidney Function and Diseases
Acute Nephrotic Syndrome
Nephrotic Syndrome
Acute Renal Failure
Chronic Renal Failure
Progress Check on Background Information and
    Activity 1

ACTIVITY 2: Chronic Renal Failure
Description and Symptoms
Dietary Management

Nursing Implications for Activities 1 and 2
Progress Check on Activity 2

ACTIVITY 3: Kidney Dialysis
Definitions and Descriptions
Nursing Implications
Progress Check on Activity 3

ACTIVITY 4: Diet Therapy for Renal Calculi
Causes of Kidney Stones
Dietary Management
Nursing Implications
Progress Check on Activity 4
References

Objectives

Upon completion of this module, the student should be able to:

1. Discuss the use of diet therapy in renal disorders.
2. Describe the therapeutic diets used in renal disorders and the rationale for their use.
3. List appropriate nursing interventions to promote adequate nutrition in a patient with renal disease.

Glossary

Albuminuria: albumin in the urine.

Antigen-antibody response: antigens are those substances that induce an immune response (the foreign invaders); they react with antibodies, which are the immune bodies that destroy the invaders.

Azotemia: nitrogenous compounds in the blood.

BUN: blood urea nitrogen.

CNS: central nervous system.

CRF: chronic renal failure.

Dialysis: the passing of molecules in a solution through the semipermeable membrane, passing from the side with the higher concentration of molecules to the side with the lower concentration (a method used in cases of defective renal function to remove from the blood those elements that are normally excreted).

Diaphoresis: perspiration (sweating), especially profuse perspiration.

Filtration: the process of eliminating certain particles from a solution.

GI: gastrointestinal tract.

Glomerulus: a small cluster of capillaries encased in a capsule in the kidney; a part of the nephron.

Hematuria: blood in the urine.

Hyperphosphatemia: high blood phosphate level.

Hypocalcemia: low blood calcium level.

Nephron: the basic unit of the kidney. Each nephron can form urine by itself, and each kidney has approximately one million nephrons. Each glomerulus brings blood and waste products to the nephron, which filters it continuously and produces urine, which carries the wastes to be eliminated. Excess sodium, potassium, and chloride are also eliminated in urine, and blood is reabsorbed.

Oliguria: diminished urine secretion in relation to fluid intake (less output than intake).

Oxalate: a salt of oxalic acid. A poisonous acid found in various fruits, vegetables, and metabolism of ascorbic acid. It combines with calcium and is excreted in urine. High concentration may cause urinary calculi.

Proteinuria: presence of proteins in the urine.

Pyuria: presence of pus in the urine.

Renal: pertaining to the kidney.

Renal calculi: formation of mineral stones, usually calcium, in the renal tubules.

S.O.B.:   shortness of breath.

Uremia: presence of urinary constituents in the blood.

Background Information

The kidney is an organ of excretion, conversion, secretion, reabsorption, manufacture, and regulation. Its structural and functional unit is the nephron. The nephron has a glomerulus attached to a long tube that empties into collecting ducts. Urine enters via the ureter and leaves at the rate of 1,000 to 1,500 ml per day. The convoluted tubule, known as Henle's loop, filters blood that circulates through it. It excretes nitrogenous waste: ammonia, urea, uric acid, and creatinine, as well as toxic substances ingested or formed from body metabolism. These substances are excreted in water that is not reabsorbed at the time. The glomerulus holds back in circulation large molecules such as blood proteins. Another function of the kidney is the manufacture of erythropoietin, which stimulates the formation of red blood cells in bone marrow. The kidney also converts inactive vitamin D to the active form the body uses and releases into the blood stream, but does not excrete, thus maintaining the calcium to phosphorus ratio in the bone.

The kidney, along with the lungs, regulates the blood pH by restoring neutrality. This is accomplished by secreting hydrogen ions when there is too much acid and excreting bicarbonate when it is too alkaline. Electrolytes and other substances such as amino acids, glucose, sodium chloride, and vitamin C are either excreted or reabsorbed, depending upon what the blood needs to maintain homeostasis. The kidney also helps regulate blood pressure.

Each kidney contains over a million nephrons. Loss of half of these, such as donation of a kidney or loss of one in an accident, does not affect kidney function. Kidney function diminishes with age, and the elderly person may have only a ½ to ⅔ filtration rate compared to a young adult. However, kidney function is still adequate unless disease occurs.

Mechanisms of kidney function and the role of nutrition in maintaining them are discussed in the following activities.

ACTIVITY 1: Kidney Function and Diseases

Since the kidney is such a major factor in the maintenance of body homeostasis, there is little doubt that the consequences are extremely serious any time disease occurs and the kidneys fail. Renal disease can be caused by damage to the kidneys themselves or by other diseases such as diabetes, atherosclerosis, or hypertension.

The most common terms used in describing kidney malfunctioning are *hematuria, proteinuria, pyuria, albuminuria, oliguria, azotemia,* and *uremia.* These conditions are dangerous to health.

In addition to excretory functions for maintenance of chemical homeostasis, balancing of body fluids, and maintenance of normal pH, the kidney controls blood pressure. Changes in sodium balance affect blood pressure as well as the rise in renin levels. Renin is a proteolytic enzyme secreted by the kidneys, which acts in blood plasma to form angiotensive II, a powerful vasoconstrictor. This further elevates blood pressure. Most patients with renal disease have hypertension.

The damaged kidney also decreases its production of erythropoietin, which is a critical determinant of erythroid activity. This deficiency results in the severe anemia present in chronic renal disease.

The diseased kidneys will cease to produce the active vitamin D hormone so necessary to maintain the calcium-phosphorus ratio in the bone. Serum phosphorus levels rise as the kidneys are no longer able to excrete phosphorus. Hyperphosphaturia occurs and lowers serum calcium levels. Also, calcium is not absorbed from the gut because calcitrol is not present. Renal osteodystrophy is the result of these imbalances. Osteodystrophy is the condition whereby the bones become soft and calcium is deposited in the soft tissues. Osteodystrophy is a common, complex, and usually inevitable outcome of renal disease.

Diseases of the kidney, whether acute or chronic, have many causes. The origin of the disease and the portion of the nephron it affects will determine the symptoms and subsequent treatment. Depending upon the type, kidney disease may produce a nephrotic syndrome with significant protein loss, decreased overall renal function, or a combination of these. Objectives of nutritional care will depend upon the abnormality to be treated. Causes, symptoms, and dietary management of various disorders are described in the following sections.

Acute Nephrotic Syndrome _____

An example of the acute nephrotic syndrome is glomerulonephritis, caused by poststreptococcal infection, which may occur in tonsil, pharynx, or skin. It is most common in children and adolescents. Symptoms vary from mild to severe: fever, discomfort, headache, slight edema, decreased urine volume, mild hypertension, hematuria, proteinuria, and salt and water retention. Prognosis ranges from complete recovery to renal failure.

Dietary management of acute nephrotic syndrome is controversial. Some clinicians prefer restriction of protein, fluid, and sodium intakes, while others do not. Diet therapy may be similar to the initial management of acute renal failure, e.g., 25 grams of protein (70 to 80 percent HBV) and 500 milligrams of sodium. Fluid permitted varies with the patient.

Note: HBV refers to the high biological value of protein. Protein foods in a restricted diet such as this must be from those foods furnishing the greatest amount of essential amino acids. Milk and eggs are the standard, with meat, fish, and poultry following.

Nephrotic Syndrome _____

This disorder covers a group of symptoms resulting from certain kidney disorders (infection, chemical poisoning, etc.). Causes are unknown in some patients. The symptoms are edema, proteinuria, and body wasting. Dietary management covers the restoration of fluid and electrolyte balance, reversal of body wasting, and correction of hyperlipidemia, if present.

Acute Renal Failure _____

Acute renal failure includes an abrupt renal malfunction because of infection, trauma, injury, chemical poisoning, or pregnancy. The symptoms are nausea, lethargy, and anorexia. Oliguria may be present at first, followed by diuresis. Azotemia may also be present.

Dietary management includes the restoration of fluid and electrolyte balance, elimination of azotemia, and implementation of nutritional rehabilitation. The dietary treatment is similar to that for acute glomerulonephritis. Many patients need dialysis, especially if they are progressing to chronic renal failure.

Chronic Renal Failure _____

Chronic renal failure results from a slow destruction of kidney tubules and may be due to infection, hypertension, hereditary defect, or drugs. Dietary management involves the balancing of fluid and electrolytes, correction of metabolic acidosis, minimization of the toxic effect of uremia, and implementation of nutritional rehabilitation.

PROGRESS CHECK ON BACKGROUND INFORMATION AND ACTIVITY 1

Multiple Choice

1. The functional unit of the kidney is the
   a. tubule.
   b. glomerulus.
   c. nephron.
   d. ureter.

2. Approximately how many ml of water leave the body via the kidney per day?
   a. 1,000–1,500
   b. 2,000–2,500
   c. 500–1,000
   d. ≥ 3,000

3. Neutrality is restored to the body by the kidney in which of these ways?
   a. reabsorption of electrolytes
   b. secretion of hydrogen ions
   c. excretion of bicarbonate
   d. all of these

4. The vitamin whose activity depends upon efficient kidney function is
   a. ascorbic acid.
   b. B_{12}.
   c. D.
   d. retinol.

5. When a person loses one kidney through accident or donation, kidney function is altered by
   a. ¼.
   b. ½.
   c. ⅔.
   d. 0.

6. An elderly person's kidney function may be altered by
   a. 0–¼.
   b. ¼–½.
   c. ½–⅔.
   d. ¾–1.

Fill-in

The kidney performs six major functions. Name them and give one example of each function.

	Function	Example
7.	_____	_____
8.	_____	_____
9.	_____	_____
10.	_____	_____
11.	_____	_____
12.	_____	_____

Name five of the most common terms used in kidney malfunctioning and define the term.

	Term	Definition
13.	_____	_____
14.	_____	_____
15.	_____	_____
16.	_____	_____
17.	_____	_____

Define:

18. Renin _____

_____

_____

19. osteodystrophy _____

_____

_____

20. HBV protein _____

_____

ACTIVITY 2: Chronic Renal Failure

Description and Symptoms

Chronic renal failure (CRF) occurs because of progressive degenerative changes in renal tissue. The nephrons gradually deteriorate until they no longer function. The end stage symptom of this disease is uremia.

Renal failure may be the result of diseases that involve the nephron, such as untreated glomerulonephritis, insulin dependent diabetes, infectious renal vascular disease, or congenital abnormalities. The clinical symptoms result from the loss of functioning nephrons and decreased renal blood flow, as well as inability of the kidney to concentrate urine, to maintain acid base and electrolyte balance. Dehydration or water toxicity may occur if the amount of ingested fluid is not carefully controlled.

Metabolic acidosis occurs in advanced stages due to reduced excretion of phosphate sulfates and organic acids from food metabolism. These substances increase in body fluids, displacing the bicarbonates.

Sodium balance cannot be maintained by the failing kidney. Any increase in sodium intake will result in edema, as the sodium is not excreted.

Renal osteodystrophy, as previously discussed, is a result of chronic kidney disease. The metabolism of calcium and phosphorus and the activation of vitamin D is greatly disturbed in CRF, giving rise to hyperphosphatemia and hypocalcemia as well as osteodystrophy.

Nitrogen retention and anemia, as well as increasing hypertension, are all a direct result of advancing deterioration of the nephrons. Laboratory findings indicate azotemia and elevated BUN, serum creatine, and uric acid levels.

CRF progression leads to acute malnutrition with its myriad symptoms. The health professional will observe weakness, lethargy, fatigue, S.O.B., oral and GI bleeding, diarrhea, vomiting, CNS involvement, ulceration in the mouth, fetid breath, and increased susceptibility to any infection, as well as the aching and pain in bones and joints due to the osteodystrophy.

Dietary Management

The general principles of dietary management in renal disease are

1. to achieve a balance between intake and output.
2. to alleviate symptoms.
3. to maintain adequate nutrition.
4. to retard progression of renal failure in order to postpone dialysis.

Diet therapy is focused on controlling five nutrients: protein, sodium, potassium, phosphate, and fluids. Levels of each nutrient will need to be individually adjusted according to progression of the illness, type of treatment being used, and the patient's response to treatment.

Generally the following dietary restrictions apply:

1. Sodium: 1,500 mg to 2,000 mg.
2. Potassium: generally no restriction from food sources. Potassium chloride (salt substitutes) may not be used in renal patients.
3. Phosphorus: restriction varies. Whenever protein is reduced in the diet, the dietary source of phosphorus falls. Further restriction is usually unwarranted unless serum phosphorus is elevated.
4. Protein: 0.4–0.6 g/kg body weight plus 24-hour urinary protein loss. At least 75 percent of protein should come from HBV protein; the use of eggs should be encouraged because of their high biological quality: high protein foods should be distributed over 24 hours.
5. Calories: adjusted for slow weight gain, maintenance of weight, or slow weight loss as necessary. Calories should be from carbohydrate and fat.
6. Fluid: intake to be calculated. Urine output is useful as a basis for estimating daily fluid needs. Five hundred ml for insensible water loss added to 24-hour urine output is the usual pattern for determining fluid intake.

Individual needs vary. Each person's weight, blood pressure, and urine output must be monitored to determine exact needs. Body weight and blood pressure will increase if the person is retaining sodium (and fluid). The person's weight and blood pressure will fall if sodium intake is too low. Calcium carbonate supplements are sometimes ordered by the doctor.

Nursing Implications for Activities 1 and 2

Caloric Intake

1. Be aware that adequate caloric intake is an important health requirement for renal patients.
2. Plan menus knowing that high caloric intake is difficult to accomplish if grains and starchy vegetables are excluded or severely limited.
3. Use caloric-dense items such as heavy cream, sweets, and carbonated beverages to provide calories when they are needed.

Fluid

1. Apportion the limited fluid intake equally throughout the waking hours.
2. Keep the patient's mouth clean and moist when fluids are restricted.
3. Compensate for diarrhea or diaphoresis by prescribing additional fluid intake.
4. Be aware that proper eating posture is needed for patients with edema and ascites. For example, sitting upright causes discomfort and anorexia for this group of patients.

Diet Compliance

1. Plan diets with the knowledge that patients dislike a diet with little bread, potato, and other low-biological value protein foods. Such diets are unpalatable and will be further rejected by patients with nausea, vomiting, and anorexia.
2. Realize that when a patient does not comply with a diet, treatment is handicapped and prolonged.
3. Through patient education, help the patient understand the problems and make an effort to comply with the dietary prescription.

PROGRESS CHECK ON ACTIVITY 2

Multiple Choice

1. Chronic renal failure usually occurs over a long period of time from diseases that affect the nephron. Included are all except which of these diseases?
    a. renal osteodystrophy
    b. congenital abnormalities
    c. untreated glomerulonephritis
    d. insulin dependent diabetes

2. Reduced secretion of phosphate, sulfates, and organic acids from ingested foods results in
    a. metabolic alkalosis.
    b. metabolic acidosis.
    c. edema.
    d. ascites.

3. Hypertension in CRF is usually the result of
    a. sodium retention.
    b. calcium excretion.
    c. metabolic acidosis.
    d. erythrocyte reduction.

4. General dietary restrictions include which of these nutrients?
    a. calcium, phosphorus, vitamin D
    b. calcium, phosphorus, potassium
    c. sodium, protein, and water
    d. all of the above

5. There is an increase in _____ if a patient is retaining sodium.
    a. blood pressure and weight
    b. fluid and acidosis
    c. calcium and appetite
    d. pulse and respiration

Short Answer

List six nursing implications for patients on a renal diet (two from each category of fluid, calorie, and compliance).

6. _____

7. _____

8. _____

9. _____

10. _____

11. _____

List the four general principles of dietary management in renal disease.

12. _____

13. _____

14. _____

15. _____

ACTIVITY 3: Kidney Dialysis

Definitions and Descriptions _____

Dialysis refers to the diffusion of dissolved particles (solutes) from one side of the semipermeable membrane to the other. Kidney dialysis was started in 1960 and has helped many uremic patients since then. Basically, two kinds of dialysis are used to treat the end stage of renal failure: hemodialysis and peritoneal dialysis.

Hemodialysis, sometimes known as extracorporeal dialysis, uses a machine (artificial kidney) outside the body. Blood is drawn or pumped out of the body and made to circulate through a special machine equipped with a synthetic semipermeable membrane. The dialysate in this case also contains glucose and electrolytes, which resemble concentrations of blood plasma found in the body. Much nitrogenous waste from the patient's blood plasma diffuses into the dialysate. The cleansed blood is returned to the patient's body and the used dialysate is replaced with fresh. The patient undergoes hemodialysis two to four times a week for three to six hours at a time in the hospital or at a dialysis center. Between dialysis treatments, nitrogenous waste products, potassium and sodium, and fluids accumulate, and dietary modifications are necessary to control them. Serum amino acids and water-soluble vitamins are lost in the dialysate, and water-soluble vitamin supplements are necessary.

Peritoneal dialysis may be intermittent or continuous. With intermittent dialysis a catheter is placed in the abdominal cavity and one to two liters of dialysis fluid introduced into the abdominal cavity and removed every hour. This process is repeated until the blood urea drops to normal levels. Loss of blood protein and amino acids are greater in peritoneal dialysis than in hemodialysis.

With continuous ambulatory peritoneal dialysis (CAPD), the patient does his or her own dialysis and the process is continuous. The fluid (dialysate) is introduced into the peritoneal cavity and remains there for four to six hours, allowing waste products to diffuse into the dialysate. The dialysate is then drained and replaced with fresh fluid. With CAPD no dietary restriction of fluid, sodium, or potassium is necessary. However, calcium supplements may be needed, and phosphorus is restricted. No phosphate binding antacids are used. The dialysate contains dextrose, which is absorbed by the body. Calorie control and an exercise program may be needed to prevent excess weight gain. In addition, the extra dextrose can lead to elevated triglycerides and a lower level of high density lipoproteins (HDLs), increasing the risk of coronary heart diseases. Protein and amino acid losses are minimal and are easily replaced by diet.

Nursing Implications

Reluctant Patients

Be aware that patients being transferred from hemodialysis to CAPD are often reluctant to give up their restrictive diets. Explain clearly the possible effects of a restricted diet while on CAPD:

1. Hypotension and dizziness from sodium depletion.
2. Nausea, vomiting, irregular heartbeat, and muscle weakness from potassium depletion.
3. Dehydration due to rapid fluid removal.

Dietary Regime

The following counseling plan is used with success at many clinics as a guide for patients on peritoneal dialysis:

1. High protein: 1.2–1.5 g/kg body weight.
2. Limit phosphorus intake to 1,200 mg/day.
   a. Nuts and legumes—one serving/week.
   b. Dairy products—½ cup daily.
   c. Eggs—not more than one.
3. High potassium—eat a wide variety of fruits and vegetables daily.
4. High fluid intake to prevent dehydration.
5. Limit or avoid sweets and fats.
6. Control weight. Incorporate extra calories from dialysate into total calories for the day.
7. Encourage adequate consumption. CAPD patients are often anorectic.

PROGRESS CHECK ON ACTIVITY 3

Fill-in

Define or describe fully:

1. dialysis _____

   _____

2. hemodialysis _____

   _____

3. peritoneal dialysis _____

   _____

4. dialysate _____

   _____

5. CAPD _____

   _____

6. Name the four waste products from the patient's blood that are diffused into the dialysate.

   a. _____

   b. _____

   c. _____

   d. _____

Multiple Choice

7. Which of these nutrients should be restricted in the diet of the person on CAPD?
   a. sodium
   b. potassium
   c. fluid
   d. phosphorus

8. The amount of protein needed for a patient on peritoneal dialysis is
   a. .4–.6 gm/kg/bw.
   b. 1.0–1.2 gm/kg/bw.
   c. 1.2–1.5 gm/kg/bw.
   d. .8 gm/kg/bw.

9. Effects of a severely restricted diet on a patient with CAPD include all of these except
   a. hemorrhagic shock.
   b. nausea and vomiting.
   c. heart arrythmias.
   d. dehydration.

10. Caloric control and exercise is necessary for CAPD patients because
    a. they gain excess weight from being immobilized.
    b. fluid is more easily excreted in this way.
    c. the dialysate contains absorbable dextrose.
    d. amino acids are converted to energy.

Matching

Match the food item on the left with its recommendation on the right. Do not draw lines.

11. eggs
12. oranges/bananas
13. nuts and legumes
14. water
15. milk

a. increase potassium intake
b. decrease phosphorus intake
c. increase to prevent dehydration
d. limited to one
e. limited to ½ cup serving

ACTIVITY 4: Diet Therapy for Renal Calculi

Causes of Kidney Stones

Although the basic cause of kidney stones is unknown, there are many direct and indirect contributing factors. These factors include the chemistry of the urine and/or the conditions of the urinary tract.

Calcium Stones

By far the majority of kidney stones—about 96 percent—are composed of calcium compounds. The calcium usually combines with phosphates or oxalates. Excessive urinary calcium may result from prolonged use of high-calcium foods such as milk and dairy products, from alkali therapy for peptic ulcer, or from continued use of a hard water supply. Also, excess vitamin D may cause increased calcium absorption from the intestine, as well as increased calcium extraction from the bone. Prolonged immobilization such as occurs in body casting, long-term illness, or disability may lead to withdrawal of calcium from the bones and increased calcium in the urine.

Uric Acid Stones

Uric acid stones comprise 3 percent of kidney stones, while cystine stones average only 1 percent (cystine is an amino acid that accumulates in urine from an hereditary disorder). Uric acid stones may come from rapid tissue breakdown (body wasting), prolonged use of high-protein and low-carbohydrate fad diets, and purine breakdown (purine is a body by-product).

Urinary Tract and Stone Formation

Stone formation is facilitated by

1. concentrated urine (examples include not drinking enough fluid, excessive sweating).
2. favorable urine acidity (the lower the acidity of the urine, the higher the calcium stone formation; high-acid urine favors uric acid stone formation).
3. vitamin A deficiency (the resulting changes in the urinary tract tissue favor stone formation).
4. recurrent urinary tract infections.

Dietary Management

Using diet therapy to manage kidney stones is only part of the medical regimen. The overall dietary treatment is based on the type of stone. Dietary recommendations to treat kidney stones are the following:

1. Drink a lot of fluid. This will dilute the urine and flush out the stones in some patients. It is ineffective for other patients.

2. Reduce intake of the components of the stones. For example, a calcium stone may be treated with a low-calcium diet. A stone containing primarily phosphorus may be treated with a low-phosphorus diet. The same applies to stones with oxalic acid. When the stone component changes, these therapeutic diets simultaneously change the pH (acidity or alkalinity) of the urine as indicated:

Stone Chemistry	Diet Modification	Urinary pH
Calcium	low-calcium (200–600 mg)	acid ash
Phosphate	low-phosphate (1,000 mg)	acid ash
Oxalate	low-oxalate	acid ash
Uric acid	low-purine	alkaline ash
Cystine	low-methionine	alkaline ash

3. Change the acidity or alkalinity of the urine by eating certain foods.

To illustrate the use of a low-calcium diet, Tables 19-1 and 19-2 show meal plan and menu, respectively, for a 200 mg calcium diet. Table 19-3 classifies foods according to their acid-base reactions in the body. The acidity or alkalinity of the urine can be modified by consuming more of the appropriate type of foods.

Nursing Implications

Calcium Intake

1. Although milk can increase an acid urinary pH, it is high in calcium.
2. A low-calcium diet should include foods fortified with vitamin D, which promotes absorption of calcium.
3. Ascertain calcium content of drinking water. If necessary, use packaged beverages or distilled water for drinking and food preparation.

Fluid Intake

1. Warn the patient about dehydration. Prescribe more fluids if the patient perspires heavily or is losing fluid for other reasons.
2. Ascertain the reasons for withholding fluid: for example, for scheduled medical tests. Check the validity of the official request.

TABLE 19-1
Daily Meal Planning for a 200 mg Calcium Diet

Food Group	Example	Approximate Calcium Content (mg)
Milk, cheese, eggs	None	0
Breads and equivalents	3 slices bread made without milk	30
Cereals, flours	1 c. Puffed Rice	7
Meat, poultry, fish	3 oz. chicken; 4 oz. lamb; 1½ oz. shad, baked	30
Vegetables	½ c. beets, cooked; ½ c. eggplant, cooked	30
Fruits	½ c. applesauce; 2 medium nectarines; 1 med. apple	20
Fats	5–6 servings bacon fat, salad dressings, and others	5
Potatoes and equivalents	½ c. noodles	15
Soup (broth of permitted meats or soups made with permitted ingredients)	No limit	0
Beverages	2–4 servings	10–20
Desserts	1 c. flavored gelatin	5
Miscellaneous (sugar, nondairy creamer, sweets, etc.)	No limit	0

Note: Water used for cooking and drinking should not contain more than 35 mg of calcium per liter. Use distilled water if necessary.

TABLE 19-2
Sample Menu for a 200 mg Calcium Diet

Breakfast
Juice, cranberry, ½ c.
Farina, ¾ c.
Bread, made without milk, 1 slice
Margarine, 2 tsp.
Salt, pepper. Sugar
Imitation cream, nondairy creamer, or coffee whitener
Coffee or tea

Lunch
Soup, tomato, milk-free, ½ c.
Chicken, boneless, canned, 3 oz.
Mushrooms, canned, ½ c.
Bread, made without milk, 1 slice
Butter or margarine, 2 tsp.
Pears, canned, ½ c.
Salt, pepper. Sugar
Imitation cream, nondairy creamer, or coffee whitener
Coffee or tea

Dinner
Fruit cocktail, canned, ½ c.
Veal roast, 3 oz.
Potato, baked, medium, 1
Cauliflower, cooked, ½ c.
Bread, made without milk, 1 slice
Butter or margarine, 2 tsp.
Lemon ice, 1 c.
Imitation cream, nondairy creamer, or coffee whitener
Coffee or tea
Salt, pepper. Sugar

3. All concerned persons must make sure that the patient is getting plenty of fluids during the day and the night.

New Treatment

1. Some clinicians claim that a large dose of vitamin B_6 is beneficial for patients with oxalate stones, since it can reduce the absorption of oxalates.

PROGRESS CHECK ON ACTIVITY 4

Multiple Choice

Circle the letter of the correct answer.

1. The diet therapy indicated for a patient with calcium phosphate kidney stones is
   a. low-calcium and phosphorus, alkaline ash.
   b. high-calcium and phosphorus, acid ash.
   c. low-calcium and phosphorus, acid ash.
   d. high-calcium and phosphorus, alkaline ash.

2. In planning a diet for a patient with calcium phosphate kidney stones, which of the following foods could you use in unlimited amounts?
   a. fruits

TABLE 19-3
Classification of Foods According to Their Acid-Base Reactions in the Body

Alkaline–Ash–Forming or Alkaline–Urine–Producing Foods	Acid–Ash–Forming or Acid–Urine–Producing Foods	Neutral Foods
Milk and cream, all types	Meat, poultry, fish, shellfish, cheese, eggs	Butter, margarine, fats and oils (cooking), salad oil, lard
Fruits except plums, prunes, and cranberries	Plums, prunes, cranberries	Cornstarch, arrowroot, tapioca
Carbonated beverages	Corn, lentils	Sugar, honey, syrup
All vegetables except corn and lentils	Bread (especially whole-wheat bread not containing baking soda or powder)	Nonchocolate candy
Chestnuts, coconut, almonds	Cereals, crackers	Coffee, tea
Molasses	Rice, noodles, macaroni, spaghetti	
Baking soda and baking powder	Peanuts, walnuts, peanut butter	
	Pastries, cakes, and cookies not containing baking soda or powder	
	Fats, bacon	

   b.   meat
   c.   milk
   d.   cheese

Matching

Match the foods on the left to the type of restriction in an acid ash diet:

3. Dried beans   a.   unrestricted
4. Potato   b.   partially restricted
5. Cranberry relish   c.   not allowed
6. Bananas
7. Egg and cheese omelet
8. Milk
9. Carrots
10. Olives

References

Aaron, M. et al. 1989. *Enteral parenteral handbook: A screening tool for nutritional replacement in the hemodialysis patient.* Redwood City, CA: Satellite Dialysis Centers.

American Dietetic Association. 1988. *Manual of clinical dietetics.* Chicago: American Dietetic Association.

Baig, F. et al. 1982. Nutritional implications in CAPD. *Contemp. Dial.* March:37.

Bannister, D. K. et al. 1987. Nutritional effects of peritonitis in continuous ambulatory peritoneal dialysis (CAPD) patients. *Journal of the American Dietetic Association* 87:53.

Boyd, L. M. et al. 1983. How do you deal with a patient who is uncooperative and noncompliant? *Dialysis Transplant.* 12:417.

Brauer, P. M. 1985. Nutritional support of the critically ill. Part I: Review. *Journal of the Canadian Dietetic Association* 46:292.

Brauer, P. M. et al. 1985. Nutritional support of the critically ill, Part II: Guidelines for the clinical dietitian. *Journal of the Canadian Dietetic Association* 46:304.

Carron, D. 1985. A review of vitamin supplements for adults undergoing hemodialysis. *CRN Quarterly* 9:7.

Cleveland Clinic Foundation Department of Nutrition Services, and P. Ellis. 1987. *The Cleveland Clinic Foundation Creative Cooking for Renal Diets* and *The Cleveland Clinic Foundation Creative Cooking for Renal Diabetic Diets.* Chesterland, OH: Senay Publishing.

Feinstein, E. I. 1988. Total parenteral nutritional support of patients with acute renal failure. *Nutr. Clin. Pract.* 3(1):9.

Food and Nutrition Board, National Research Council, National Academy of Sciences. 1989. *Recommended dietary allowances.* 10th ed. Washington, DC: National Academy Press.

Gillit, D. et al. (eds.). 1987. *A clinical guide to nutrition care in end-stage renal disease.* Chicago: American Dietetic Association.

Goldstein, D. J., and C. B. Frederico. 1987. The effect of urea kinetic modelling on the nutrition management of hemo dialysis patients. *Journal of the American Dietetic Association* 87:474.

Hak, L. J. et al. 1988. Use of amino acids in patients with acute renal failure. *Nutr. Clin. Pract.* 3(1):19.

Harum, P. 1984. Renal nutrition for the renal nurse. *Am. Nurse Assoc. J.* 11(5):38.

Hoy, W. E. et al. 1985. Protein catabolism during the postoperative course after renal transplantation. *Am. J. Kidney Dis.* 5:186.

Klahr, S. et al. 1988. The progression of renal disease. *New England Journal of Medicine* 318(25):1657.

Knochel, J. P. 1980. Potassium deficiency: Causes, complications, and treatment. *Consultant* 20:139.

Kopple, J., and M. Blumenkrantz. 1984. Nutrition in

adults on continuous ambulatory peritoneal dialysis. *Perspect. Peritoneal Dialysis* 2:1.

Kopple, J. D. 1988. Nutrition, diet, and the kidney. In *Modern nutrition in health and disease*, 7th ed. M. E. Shils and V. R. Young (eds.). Philadelphia: Lea & Febiger.

Kunin, C. M. 1987. *Detection, prevention, and management of urinary tract infections*, 4th ed. Philadelphia: Lea & Febiger.

Kurtz, S. B. et al. 1983. Continuous ambulatory peritoneal dialysis three-years' experience at the Mayo Clinic. *Mayo Clin. Proc.* 54:633.

Lancaster, L. E. 1984. *The patient with end-stage renal disease*. New York: Wiley.

Lazarus, J. M., and B. M. Brenner. 1983. *Acute renal failure*. Philadelphia: Saunders.

Lingeman, J. E. et al. 1989. *Urinary calculi: Endourology and medical treatment*. Philadelphia: Lea & Febiger.

Mayo Clinic. 1988. *Mayo Clinic diet manual*. Philadelphia: B. C. Dekker.

Metheny, N. 1982. Renal stones and urinary pH. *American Journal of Nursing* 82:1372.

Senekjian, H., and B. J. Koerpel. 1984. CAPD in the diabetic patient. *Dialysis and Transplantation* 13:780.

Shen, Y. S. et al. 1983. Patient profile and effect of dietary therapy on post-transplant hyperlipidemia. *Kidney Int.* 24:147.

Slatopolsky, F. et al. 1986. Calcium carbonate as a phosphate binder in patients with chronic renal failure undergoing dialysis. *New England Journal of Medicine* 315:157.

Whittier et al. 1985. Nutrition in renal transplantation. *Am. J. Kidney Dis.* 6:405.

Wilkins, K. (ed.). 1986. *Suggested guidelines for nutrition care of renal patients*. Chicago: American Dietetic Association.

Wilkins, K. (ed.). 1986. *Renal practice group: Suggested guidelines for nutritional care of renal patients*. Chicago: American Dietetic Association.

Module 20

Diet Therapy for Burns, Cancer, Anorexia Nervosa, and Acquired Immune Deficiency Syndrome

Time for completion
Activities: _____1½_____ hours
Optional examination: _1_ hour

Academic credit
Semester units: _2/10_
Quarter units: _3/10_

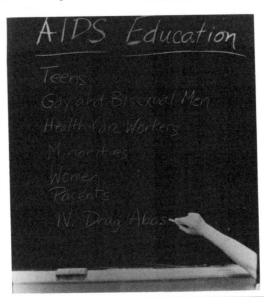

Outline

Objectives

Upon completion of this module, the student should be able to:

Burns

1. Describe the severity of a burn by its degrees.
2. Define the treatment goals of nutritional care of the burn patient.
3. Calculate the nutrient needs of a burn patient.
4. Recognize the teamwork required for efficient nutritional care.
5. Use aggressive nutritional therapy as a major part of the care of the burn patient.

Cancer

1. Assess the metabolic and nutritional changes that occur in cancer patients.
2. Discuss the nutritional problems produced by the three forms of cancer treatment.
3. Determine suitable foods and supplements according to the treatment modes.
4. Analyze the individual's psychological response to cancer and the approved feeding method.
5. Individualize diet therapy for cancer patients.

Anorexia Nervosa

1. Describe the pathophysiological manifestations of anorexia nervosa and bulimia.
2. Discuss the hospital feeding regime suitable for patients with eating disorders.
3. Recognize the necessity of psychological counseling and make arrangements for this procedure to use behavior modification as appropriate.

AIDS

1. Identify the major goals of nutritional intervention for the AIDS patient.
2. Describe the health professional's role in alleviating the nutritional deficits in the AIDS patient.
3. List measures necessary to provide adequate nutritional support to the AIDS patient.
4. Encourage and assist other personnel in maintaining a clean environment.
5. Educate the patient about compliance as a method of prolonging life.

Glossary

AIDS: acquired immune deficiency syndrome.
Hyporalemic: blood volume below normal levels.
Renal calculi: kidney stones.
Asthenia: loss of strength; weakness; debility.
Cachexia: profound and marked state of ill health and malnutrition.
Dysgeusia: impairment of the sense of taste.
Acuity: clearness; acuteness.
Amenorrhea: absence of menstruation.
Dementia: organic loss of intellectual function.
ARC: AIDS-related complex.

Background Information

Space limitation has excluded modules covering diet therapy for a number of other commonly encountered clinical disorders. This module remedies the situation by providing student activities to cover four important clinical subjects not yet addressed. They include burns, cancer, anorexia nervosa, and acquired immune deficiency syndrome or AIDS.

The students should use the references provided at the end of this module to obtain supplemental details.

ACTIVITY 1: Diet and the Burn Patient

Background Information

A severe burn is perhaps one of the most painful injuries a human being can receive. Burn patients undergo many of the physiological changes experienced by surgical patients. The extent of the burn injury partly determines the dietary care recommended. Nutritional principles for treating burn patients can also be applied to treating other forms of trauma, and vice versa.

The terms first-, second-, and third-degree burns are frequently used to describe the severity of a burn. A first-degree burn is the least severe and is considered only a superficial injury. Third-degree burns, on the other hand, are life-threatening, since the skin is totally destroyed and internal organs adversely affected. The degree, or depth, of a burn injury differs from its area, or percentage of the body affected.

The amount of trauma suffered by patients with burns is dependent upon the type of burn (chemical, electrical, and thermal), extent (both depth and area) of the burn injury, and their age. Together these factors determine the likelihood of mortality. Second- and third-degree burns of over 15 percent of the total body surface (10 percent in the elderly and children) can result in burn shock because of the quantity of fluid loss. Burns of more than 50 percent of the body surface are frequently fatal, especially in children and the elderly. Burns that involve the face and respiratory tract are most serious; chemical and electrical burns are more difficult to treat than thermal injuries.

Nutritional and Dietary Care

The goal of treatment is to prevent infection, promote healing, and provide for the body's increased needs for nutrients and fluids. The therapy should continue until an intact skin is achieved and metabolism is normal.

Badly burned patients are extremely unfortunate. They suffer great pain and sometimes face permanent maiming. In addition, they may be extremely anxious about the consequences of plastic surgery and fearful that an altered appearance will alienate their relatives and friends.

In all major burn traumas, body tissues (and thus protein, cells, and protoplasm) are rapidly depleted, as is reserve energy, since the patients usually experience the most severe form of stress experienced by humans. The continuous loss of body tissue and energy may result in death either immediately after the burn or during the "recovery" period. Proper and aggressive nutritional therapy is critical in treating moderately to severely burned patients.

Acute stress rapidly leads to nutritional deficits, which greatly impede the body's efforts to heal damaged tissue and resist bacterial invasion. Proper dietary care can make the difference between life and death. Patients in good nutritional status and with small burns recover because they can eat sufficient food for their needs. However, the survival of an undernourished person suffering a severe burn depends heavily on aggressive nutritional therapy.

The nutritional requirements of burn patients are directly related to the extent and degree of burn. In general, burn patients have more nutritional problems than patients with other kinds of trauma. Since those with large burns have the most difficulty in maintaining an adequate oral intake, they sometimes become debilitated, even in a well-organized and adequately staffed burn center. The nutritional complications of burn victims are worse than those of major surgical patients, since their nutritional therapy is much more than just supportive care.

Many interferences make feeding burn patients difficult. Loss of appetite may occur for many reasons (fear, depression, drug therapy, and so on), making it difficult for patients to eat enough food to meet bodily requirements. An inability to move the head, hands, body, or feet in some patients also makes self-feeding difficult. If pain accompanies any attempt to chew, eat, or swallow, avoidance of food is common. The changing of dressings and skin grafting may also interfere with mealtime. Close supervision and encouragement of the patient are necessary to assure that as many nutrients as possible (especially protein) and optimum calories are ingested.

Calculating Nutrient Needs

A burn patient has a special need for calories and protein in large amounts to replace fat loss, repair and deposit lean

tissues, maintain body functions, and restore water loss. The calorie requirement may be as large as 6,000 to 8,000 kcal/d. This energy expenditure increases with the size of the burn and may be 30 percent to 300 percent above basal levels, and it remains at high levels until grafting is completed. Sources of body weight loss are the breakdown of fat and protein as well as water loss. Food that is consumed provides about 5,000 to 6,000 kcal/d, and the breakdown of body fat provides about 1,000 to 2,000 kcal/d. A formula to calculate the caloric need of a patient with a burn injury is as follows:

> Daily caloric need = 25 kcal/kg body weight + 40 kcal/% body surface with burns.

In the following example, assume that the patient weighs 75 kg and has 50 percent of body surface burned.

> Daily caloric need = 25 kcal/kg body weight
> × 75 kg body weight + 40 kcal/% body surface with burns
> × 50% body surface with burns
> = (25 × 75 + 40 × 50) kcal
> = 1,875 + 2,000 kcal
> = 3,875 kcal (allow 1,000 kcal for margin of safety)
> = 4,500 to 5,000 kcal (approximately).

A burn victim needs more protein to cover skin loss, blood protein loss from the burn, and infection.

A formula used for calculating the protein need of a burn patient follows.

> Total daily protein need = 1 g/kg body weight + 3 g/% body surface with burns

Assume that the patient weights 75 kg and that 50 percent of the body surface has burns. The calculations are as follows:

> Total daily protein need = 1 g/kg body weight ×
> 75 kg body weight + 3 g/% body surface with burns
> × 50% body surface with burns
> = 75 + 150 g protein
> = 225 g protein

A burn patient particularly needs calories and protein. However, in planning menus, fats should provide 30 percent to 40 percent of total calories, and carbohydrates 45 percent to 55 percent. A moderate amount of fat is judicious at the beginning, since a large amount of fat tends to satiate the patient and reduce the patient's appetite.

Most clinicians prescribe two to ten times the RDAs for water-soluble vitamins for burn patients. Vitamin C is given in amounts 20 to 30 times the RDA. However, fat-soluble vitamins are usually prescribed guardedly because of potential risks.

The mineral needs of burn patients require attention even after the fluids and electrolytes have been balanced. Body potassium, iron, calcium, zinc, and copper may have been lowered to unacceptable levels and should be monitored daily and replaced as needed.

It is almost impossible to feed patients three large meals a day that contain up to 6,000 kcal with 200 or more grams of protein. For a patient with moderate to severe burns, it is sometimes necessary to use several feeding methods to supply adequate protein and calories. For example. TPN is used very successfully in restoring balance in and healing severely burned patients.

The nutritional care of a burn patient requires efficient and conscientious teamwork. Many burn centers have established standard guidelines for dietary care. All team members should follow the individualized plans and goals for a particular patient. All personnel should encourage the patients to eat and provide them with psychological support. The entire health team monitors the progress and status of the patient to be certain that nutritional needs are met. Weight status and caloric intake are the two main criteria used. Weighing is done on a daily basis, as is intake and output, and all pertinent information is carefully recorded so that the diet therapy can be adjusted as needed.

Nursing Implications _____

Be aware that aggressive nutrition therapy is the major part of care for a burn patient.

1. A loss of more than 10 percent of preburn body weight places the person at high risk for sepsis and/or death.
2. Peak metabolic needs occur 6–10 days after the injury.
3. Fluid loss is a grave concern immediately after a burn.
4. Replacement of fluid and electrolyte losses is a major concern to prevent hypovolemic shock.
5. Fats, which are calorie dense, help increase caloric intake.
6. The burn patient is thirsty and dehydrated despite the edema that may be present. If N.P.O., good oral hygiene is necessary.
7. IV solutions of electrolytes, glucose, and especially saline may be necessary. Potassium deficit may occur.
8. Schedule dressing changes, pain medications, and other measures far enough in advance of mealtime to not interfere with meals.
9. Foods high in zinc increase wound healing. These include meat, liver, eggs, and seafood.
10. Early ambulation reduces calcium and protein losses due to immobilization.

11. Renal calculi is a common occurrence in the immobilized patient. A generous fluid intake is necessary.
12. "Fast" foods, favorite dishes from home, and any other desired items should be encouraged.
13. Educate the patient and family about the importance of diet to recovery.
14. Tube feedings or TPN, if needed for healing, should be instituted.

PROGRESS CHECK ON ACTIVITY 1 _____

True/False

Circle T for True and F for False.

1. T F Burn patients and surgery patients experience many of the same changes.
2. T F A first-degree burn is the most serious of burns.
3. T F Acute stress leads to nutritional deficits.
4. T F Burn patients have fewer nutritional problems than psychological ones.
5. T F Burn patients have little difficulty in maintaining an adequate diet if it is properly prepared and served.

Multiple Choice

6. The amount of trauma suffered by patients with burns is dependent on
   a. the type of burn.
   b. previous nutritional status.
   c. age of the person.
   d. all of these.

7. Burns of more than _____ of body surface are often fatal.
   a. 15 percent
   b. 25 percent
   c. 50 percent
   d. 10 percent

8. Nutritional requirements of burn patients are directly related to
   a. extent and degree.
   b. type and site.
   c. location and time.
   d. age and previous health.

9. Energy expenditure increases in burn patients range between
   a. 10–20 percent.
   b. 100–1,000 percent.
   c. 500–5,000 percent.
   d. 30–3,000 percent.

Fill-in

10. List five interferences to successful feeding of burn

patients.

a. _____

b. _____

c. _____

d. _____

e. _____

11. Identify three sources of body weight loss of burn patients.

a. _____

b. _____

c. _____

Situation

12. Lenny Lambrusco, age 10, has received second- and third-degree burns over 40 percent of his body in an accident. He weighs 77 pounds. Calculate the amount of protein Lenny will need to repair and replace damaged tissue.

13. List five nursing implications for nutrition that must be observed in caring for a burn patient.

a. _____

b. _____

c. _____

d. _____

e. _____

ACTIVITY 2: Diet and the Cancer Patient

Background Information _____

Nutritional complications are a common consequence of cancer or its treatment. Malnourished individuals are most susceptible to infection and are less likely to tolerate or derive optimal benefits from therapy. In many studies malnutrition has been shown to be an important indicator of survival. Malnutrition is also an important issue in the quality of life of individuals diagnosed with cancer.

When cancer patients undergo treatment and rehabilitation, they face many nutritional problems. They cannot eat well because of a number of factors such as depression, pain, digestive problems, and reaction to drugs. When patients are well nourished, they respond better to treatment, survive longer, and have a greater sense of wellbeing. The situation is a vicious cycle, however. When people have cancer, they are usually malnourished and because they are malnourished, they are more difficult to treat. Without sufficient treatment, the cancer can intensify its devastating effect on their nutritional status. In this section, we will discuss only the dietary treatment.

Certain metabolic and nutritional changes are characteristic of nearly all cancer patients. These include asthenia, cachexia, anorexia, anemia, fluid and electrolyte imbalances, hypogeusia or dysgeusia, an altered metabolic rate, a negative nitrogen balance, and edema. Infection is not uncommon.

Cancer Treatments and Nutritional Disorders _____

Patients invariably suffer some form of nutritional disorder whenever they are subject to one of the three most common forms of cancer treatment. Apart from some localized impairment, their clinical situation may be aggravated by psychological and systemic physiological effects. Table 20-1 summarizes the nutritional problems produced by the three forms of cancer treatment.

Dietary Management _____

If at all feasible, patients should be fed orally with solid foods. The regimen should include between-meal feedings of hospital or commercial nutrient supplements. Otherwise, defined-formula diets and tube feedings may be used. Following is a checklist of considerations in the oral feeding of cancer patients that should assist the health professional in determining suitable foods and supplements.

1. Patient's age and type of cancer
2. Treatment side effects
3. Psychological complications: depression and lack of motivation
4. Food and eating behavior: conditioned responses, overall food acceptance
5. Anorexia
6. Taste and food aversions
7. Swallowing ability and saliva production
8. Nausea and vomiting
9. Ulceration of buccal mucosa
10. Diarrhea
11. Weight and protein loss
12. Pain

One multifaceted problem encountered when attempting to feed cancer patients orally results from psychological complications, conditioned responses, and pain. Many cancer patients develop depressive reactions (anxiety, discomfort, and hyperactivity), especially when informed

TABLE 20-1
Common Nutritional Problems Occurring in Cancer Patients with Three Major Treatment Modes

Radiation Therapy (Effects Depend on Site of Irradiation)
1. Anorexia
2. Impaired taste acuity
3. Reduced food intake
4. Tooth decay and gum diseases
5. Difficulty in swallowing
6. Intestinal obstruction
7. Malabsorption
8. Diarrhea

Surgical Therapy
1. Tube feeding mandatory if food ingestion is impaired
2. Malabsorption and dumping syndrome upon removal of part of the gastrointestinal system; fluid and electrolyte imbalance
3. Possible low blood glucose after gastric resection
4. Insulin deficiency from resection of the pancreas

Chemotherapy
1. Multiple disturbances of nutritional status similar to those that occur with radiation therapy from the use of different categories of drugs
2. Body fluid and electrolyte disturbances from the use of corticosteroids and other hormones
3. Specific intestinal damage from drugs

of the diagnosis or when the disease is not under control. The depression makes them avoid food. If this depression leads to suppressed intestinal activity, digestive problems also occur. If encouragement and support are provided, patients may be motivated to eat, although this does not always occur. Most clinicians disapprove of the use of antidepressive agents to improve eating. In some cancer patients, intestinal obstruction causes pain every time food is eaten. Abdominal pain when eating may continue even after surgical correction of the problem because of a conditioned response. This is a behavioral problem that requires special help. Many patients have general body pain that naturally interferes with eating. Careful use of pain killers before meals helps these patients to eat. In sum, the problem is how to get the patient to eat.

Clinicians sometimes prescribe antiemetcs one-half to one hour before meals, which tends to reduce nausea and vomiting and improve the appetite.

The thresholds for the four taste sensations may change in cancer patients. Patients may complain that food is tasteless or that they have lost their sense of taste. Or, they associate foods that cannot be tolerated with terrible taste sensations, stating that the foods served are either spoiled or rancid. Food texture is compared to sawdust, dry starch,

and leather. Metallic, bitter, sour, or salty taste sensations are emphasized. There is also a tendency to complain about home cooking. Explaining to patients and their families that the patient's taste sensation is altered helps alleviate strained relationships. At present, there is no scientific explanation for this change in the sense of taste.

Taste problems can be managed in a number of ways. First, the patient, doctor, nurse, and dietitian can all provide suggestions on how to make food taste better. Seasoning can be altered to suit the patient. If a patient prefers sweet or salty flavors, these flavors can be emphasized in different foods. Other taste preferences can be satisfied by using a variety of flavorings including sugar, salt, pepper, and lemon juice.

Lunches and main dishes can include cold cuts (such as bologna and salami), cold chicken, and salads. Fresh, cold fruits should be served with the meal to improve the looks of snacks and desserts. All beverages that patients reject should not be served. Those most often liked are cold fruit juices and chocolate drinks, although individual preferences vary. Diet plans should be individualized with the single objective of getting cancer patients to consume as much protein and as many calories as their particular condition requires.

Nursing Implications

I. It is important that cancer patients eat adequately. Measures to tempt their appetite are more successful than verbal reminders that they must eat. Many factors that affect food intake are beyond their control. The nurse should be cognizant of these factors.
1. The effectiveness of both radiation and chemotherapy depends upon adequate nutrition; both affect nutrition intake and use.
2. Fever, stress, and surgical intervention increase body protein catabolism.
3. Use whatever methods and manner of feeding that are most effective for the individual.
    a. TPN provides optimal intake when the patient can't or won't eat. It is not without disadvantages (see Module 12).
    b. Elemental diets require an intact duodenum and jejunum for proper absorption.
    c. The psychological aspects of feeding should be considered despite the feeding method.
    d. Family foods prepared in a blender may be more successful as a tube feeding than a commercial formula.
II. There are no rules for feeding a cancer patient. The diets and methods must be individualized.
1. Some general guidelines may be helpful in feeding:
    a. Alcohol may stimulate appetite; doctors' order required.

b. Common favorite foods include cold foods such as carbonated drinks, ice tea, jello, watermelon, and grapes. Cold meats and eggs are usually better tolerated than warm. All meats are sometimes rejected; cheese, milk, and egg sources of protein should be substituted.

c. Additions of salt, sugar, lemon juice, or spices are often welcome.

d. Food should be offered at a time when the pain is at its lowest level.

e. People who tire easily should be served foods that require little chewing.

f. If there is inflammation in the mouth, cold bland foods and fluids in semisolid form should be offered. Good mouth care is essential.

2. Social eating with visitors may improve intake.
3. Favorite foods brought in are encouraged.
4. Making food trays and the environment attractive and pleasant is important.
5. Assist the patient with eating (cutting, buttering, etc.) as necessary.

PROGRESS CHECK ON ACTIVITY 2

Fill-in

1. Name four psychological problems that interfere with a cancer patient's ability to eat sufficient amounts of food.

   a. _____

   b. _____

   c. _____

   d. _____

2. List four major problems that are characteristic of metabolic and nutritional changes in the cancer patient.

   a. _____

   b. _____

   c. _____

   d. _____

3. Four negative effects occurring with patient receiving radiation therapy include

   a. _____

   b. _____

   c. _____

   d. _____

4. Name the four primary taste sensations.

   a. _____

   b. _____

   c. _____

   d. _____

5. What is a conditioned response to ingested foods?

   _____

   _____

Multiple Choice

6. Individualized diet plans for cancer patients emphasize which of these?
   a. vitamins and minerals
   b. protein and calories
   c. soft, bland foods
   d. carbohydrates and fats

7. Which of these nutritional problems may occur following surgical treatment for cancer?
   a. low blood glucose
   b. insulin deficiency
   c. malabsorption
   d. all of these

8. Tube feedings are best instituted in which of the following situations?
   a. if food ingestion is impaired but digestion and absorption are intact
   b. if fluid and electrolyte imbalance occurs
   c. if malabsorption and diarrhea occur
   d. if the patient has an aversion to food

9. TPN should be the feeding of choice when
   a. the patient refuses to eat.
   b. the GI tract is nonfunctional.
   c. the patient is cachexic.
   d. all of these.

10. Protein catabolism is increased in cancer due to all but which of these factors?
    a. fever and infection
    b. physical and psychological stress
    c. extended use of alcohol and pain medications
    d. treatment modalities

11. List six common favorite foods of cancer patients.

    a. _____

    b. _____

    c. _____

    d. _____

    e. _____

    f. _____

ACTIVITY 3: Anorexia Nervosa

Background Information

Anorexia nervosa refers to the clinical condition in which a person voluntarily eats very little food (self-imposed starvation). As a result, there is a large weight loss with all of its concomitant symptoms. The disorder is more common among females, especially teenage girls, although it has been identified in men and older women. Typically the teenage female patient comes from a middle- to upper-middle-class family. Before the problem occurs, the patient is usually healthy and cooperative and has made good progress in school. All indications point to a "model" student and child. Then, the child develops psychological problems leading her to resent her obesity (which may be real or imagined) and embarks on a self-prescribed starvation diet. She continues to abstain from food even when she has achieved an ideal weight. After that, her health deteriorates.

Clinical Manifestations

The anorexic patient presents several clinical manifestations. Although the desire for food is present, the patient refuses to eat and drink. Occasionally the patient has an uncontrollable urge to gorge, which is followed by self-induced vomiting. Because of this, anorexic patients may lose 25 percent to 35 percent of their body weight and become emaciated and wasted. Electrolyte imbalances occur, and female anorexic patients develop hair over different parts of their body and cease to menstruate. Also present is decreased body metabolism, cold hands and feet, decreased blood pressure, and decreased sensitivity to insulin. Anorexic patients exhibit abnormal behavior such as frequent self-induced vomiting, excessive use of cathartics (laxatives), and overexercise (hyperactivity). In some patients, such actions may lead to death.

A number of events can spark the beginning of a voluntary, continuous reduction of food intake. A worsening mother-daughter relationship may set it off, or a sudden, highly emotional conflict between the patient and someone else may do so. Other possible causes are an abrupt failure in schoolwork and the emotional turmoil over beginning or continuing a sexual relationship.

In-depth studies by psychologists and psychiatrists of anorexic patients have indicated a common psychological profile. These patients show a lack of feeling for hunger, satiety, tiredness, and sometimes even physical pain. They generally have a distorted image of their physical size. Some anorexic patients think that they are 40 percent to 60 percent larger than they, in fact, are. Consequently, they become obsessed with dieting. In addition, these patients commonly feel inadequate in role identity, competence (work or school performance), and effectiveness (in communication, controlling events, etc.). This loss of faith in personal ability leads to an attempt to control the environment by controlling body weight. Food binges, guilt about eating, and a reluctance to admit abnormal food habits are the typical attitudes of anorexic patients toward food.

Treatment for a patient with anorexia nervosa consists of psychotherapy, behavior modification, drug therapy, and hospitalization for refeedings. The treatment objective of diet therapy and hospital feedings is to return the patient to a normal diet and an appropriate, healthy weight. A discussion of rehabilitative measures used in hospitals follows.

Hospital Feeding

Patients with anorexia nervosa are best hospitalized, because the eating environment can be controlled and family involvement is minimized. Some patients eat better in a hospital because they do not have to make any decisions about what and when to eat. In general, satisfactory care requires careful planning, an experienced staff, and a tremendous amount of concern and understanding.

Once anorexia nervosa has been diagnosed, the first major responsibility of the health team is to develop a dietary and nutrition program. There should be complete understanding and communication among the health team members to avoid any inconsistency or friction. This is important, since the patient may try to manipulate health care personnel and parents in order to avoid food intake and secure an opportunity to exercise. Most anorexic patients want to maintain a starved appearance. The nurse can coordinate all activities to assure that the program is implemented. The doctor should describe the treatment procedures to the patient, preferably in the presence of the primary nurse and the dietitian or nutritionist.

Detailed procedures for feeding a hospitalized patient with anorexia nervosa may be obtained from the references at the end of this module. General guidelines are given here.

The attending physician will prescribe a diet after studying the patient's condition. Most practitioners start with a diet containing 1,000 to 3,000 kcal and progressively increase the intake by 200 kcal every three or four days until the daily intake is adequate for an acceptable weight gain. A liquid diet may be more acceptable to the patient; it appears to have fewer calories. To avoid any misunderstandings, any changes in caloric intake must be made by the doctor or an assigned coordinator in the form of a written request. A cooperative patient can be fed three main meals and occasionally a snack. Elimination of privileges followed by a gradual return of them for compliance is a viable approach. The nurse should be fully informed of the patient's condition, including the treatment protocol. Most importantly, the attending nurse should monitor the patient's eating behavior and pay full attention to the following feeding routines.

1. Check that the foods served comply with the meal plan.
2. Pay attention to the patient's hands constantly.
3. Assume a friendly and supportive attitude so that the patient will not feel spied on.
4. Leave the room only in an emergency, since the patient may try to get rid of some foods.
5. Prevent food disposal by keeping any container (such as a facial tissue box, a wastebasket, or a flower pot) away from the patient during the meal and checking the meal tray after he or she has finished eating. The patient may hide food under napkins or smear it under the bed, on the window sill, etc.
6. Permit a maximum of one hour for eating a meal.
7. If feasible, arrange for the patient to eat alone and be monitored by the same nurse.
8. If possible, the patient should wear a pocketless hospital gown while eating.
9. Insist that the patient rest for ½ to 1 hour after a meal and ensure that he or she does not leave the bed, since she may induce vomiting.

Recovery is a long and difficult process that may last from six months to one year or more. About 60 percent to 70 percent of all patients may recover after several years of treatment; the remaining patients may die. Real recovery is extremely important, since most of these patients tend to be mentally unstable, and the condition will tend to recur at other stressful times in their lives.

Nursing Implications

1. All team members must be consistent and caring in their handling of the feeding routines.
2. Patients may not manipulate or dictate food intake.
3. Feeding periods must be closely supervised.
4. Bathroom privileges must be denied for at least 30 minutes after a meal to prevent self-induced vomiting.
5. Major sleep disturbances that occur early in treatment cease as the patient gains weight.
6. Avoid all conversation related to food or weight gain while the patient is hospitalized, except as it relates to an agreed upon contract (i.e., "You have complied with diet goals this week so you may [have] [get] [do] the reward.").
7. Nutrition education for patient and family can begin when the patient is discharged.
8. Psychological counseling takes precedence over nutritional counseling.

PROGRESS CHECK ON ACTIVITY 3

Multiple Choice

1. Clinical manifestations of anorexia nervosa include all except which of these?
   a. disinterest in food
   b. hypotension
   c. hyperactivity
   d. amenorrhea

2. Typical mental attitudes of anorexic patients include
   a. guilt.
   b. denial.
   c. inadequacy.
   d. all of these.

3. Prioritize the following treatment measures for an anorexic patient:
   a. diet therapy, drug therapy, psychotherapy
   b. behavior modification, psychotherapy, diet therapy
   c. psychotherapy, behavior modification, drug therapy, hospitalization
   d. hospitalization, drug therapy, diet therapy, psychotherapy

4. The first responsibility of the health team assigned to care for an anorexic patient is to
   a. remove all sources of stimulation from patient.
   b. develop a satisfactory nutrition program.
   c. implement behavior modification techniques.
   d. assign someone to carefully monitor the patient.

5. The initial diet therapy for an anorexic patient consists of approximately _____ calories.
   a. 1,000–2,000.
   b. 2,000–3,000.
   c. 3,000–4,000.
   d. 4,000–5,000.

Fill-in

Name five feeding routines that should be observed by the nurse attending a patient with anorexia nervosa.

6. _____

7. _____

8. _____

9. _____

10. _____

Name five important nursing implications to observe when caring for persons with anorexia nervosa.

11. _____

12. _____

13. _____

14. _____   15. _____

ACTIVITY 4: Acquired Immune Deficiency Syndrome

The Disease

A report appeared in 1981 that initially drew little attention from infectious disease experts. In that report Dr. Michael Gottleib, of the University of California at Los Angeles, described a rare form of pneumonia occurring in homosexual men. Other reports about the same time indicated that other homosexual men were developing rare forms of cancer. This new set of symptoms (a syndrome in medical terms) was eventually called Acquired Immune Deficiency Syndrome (AIDS) because the symptoms were consistent with damage to the immune system in previously healthy individuals. Moreover, this disease was not congenital or inherited, but appeared to have been acquired. We now know that this resulted from infection by a virus. The acronym AIDS, which is now used to describe the disease, has become a prominent and permanent fixture in our language.

An AIDS patient has many symptoms including severe weight loss, oral lesions, infection, and cancer. While diet therapy cannot change the outcome of the disease, it is important in improving mental attitude and overall status.

Nutrition Care: General Goals and Recommendations

The major goals of nutritional intervention for an AIDS patient are to

1. Stop weight loss.
2. Preserve or rebuild lean body mass.
3. Maintain an adequate diet including nutrient supplements.
4. Minimize malabsorption from various causes.
5. Manage complications and specific problems related to diet and nutritional status.

In order to accomplish these goals, the following measures are recommended for health professionals.

1. Obtain a good assessment of patient's nutritional status.
2. Provide patients with nutrition education.
3. Meet the patient's nutritional needs. An AIDS patient's nutritional requirements resemble those of patients with disabling disease (e.g., cancer), and diet therapy should be directed toward these major goals:

   * Stop further weight loss.

   * Supply the patient with quality and quantity protein. This helps to combat the loss of lean body

mass and preserve the remaining immune system functions.

   * Use prescribed vitamin and mineral supplements with special attention to patients vulnerable to the detrimental effects of drug therapy.

Dietary Management and Support Services

An AIDS patient is a classic example of a clinical situation that cannot be "cured" with any specific diet treatment and that requires the whole spectrum of nutritional support. The health team that provides such support faces a major task full of challenges. Some of the problems of AIDS patients with suggested measures to alleviate them are listed here:

1. Enteral and parenteral feedings. If the oral complications are extensive with severe pain, tube feedings may be needed. If the weight loss is severe with intestinal malfunctions, parenteral feedings are recommended.

2. Anorexia. An AIDS patient suffers a loss or change of appetite resembling that of a cancer patient. Small and frequent feedings are better tolerated than a large meal.

3. Oral and esophageal complications include infection, cancer, side effects of drugs, and lesions. The symptoms can be managed to a certain extent with dietary treatments. For example, a painful mouth is soothed by cold and chilled foods, such as ice cream and cold soft drinks. Acidic juice will cause pain when ingested by a patient with a sore mouth.

4. Nausea and vomiting. The causes are many and treatment procedures must be individualized. Antiemetic and antinausea drugs and rearranging eating schedules so that the patient is comfortable when he or she eats can help.

5. Intestinal problems. Diseases of the small and large intestine vary from mild indigestion to cancer in any part of the tract. Dietary management varies with the type of disorder. Consult Module 15 for more information.

6. Infection and sepsis are inherent in the progression of AIDS. The patient is particularly susceptible to infection and sepsis since his or her immunocompetency is impaired. Various treatments for infections are available. For example, parenteral feedings are ordered by many clinicians for patients with varying degrees of sepsis.

7. Many AIDS patients suffer from respiratory disorders and have difficulty in breathing. This greatly interferes with the ability to eat.

8. Neurological disorders. An AIDS patient may exhibit many of the symptoms of a mental and/or handicapped patient. For example, the patient may need assistance in feeding due to a loss of self-feeding ability.

9. Community resources include feeding programs and food banks, both of which can supplement the nutritional care of nonhospitalized patients. A patient's ability or desire to prepare meals at home may be limited by weakness, depression, or dementia. Community resources can help in many ways (e.g., buying, preparing, and delivering food). Programs such as emergency food box, cooperative buying, Self-Help and Resource Exchange (SHARE), dining rooms for the needy, food banks, and churches can all contribute. This information should be made available.

Food Service and Sanitary Practices

Individuals who serve foods to AIDS patients must be reminded not to discriminate against them. All standard sanitation procedures implemented in the facility against cross-contamination should be complied with whether the patient carries AIDS or any other transmissible disease. For example, articles contaminated with an AIDS patient's emesis, feces, urine, and blood must be decontaminated before being returned for cleaning as would be the case with any other contaminated patient's discharge.

The patients must be protected from infection. Foodborne infections occur more frequently among people with AIDS or ARC (AIDS-related complex) than in other people. If a facility is not practicing sanitary food preparation, service, and storage, it must do so if it is serving AIDS patients. Most facilities that serve food are regulated by state and federal laws to implement acceptable food safety and sanitation practices, and these practices become crucial to those serving patients with AIDS or ARC.

Nursing Implications

1. Multiple disturbances similar to those that occur in cancer patients affect the AIDS patient.
   a. Use whatever feeding methods or type of feeding that is most effective.
   b. Consider the psychological aspects of feeding: Some patients may be willing to fight as long as possible; others are not willing to fight at all.
   c. Foods from outside, favorite foods, attractive foods and surroundings, and social eating with visitors are encouraged to motivate the patient to consume more.
2. Cold foods (carbonated drinks, ice tea, ices, jello), boiled eggs, cooked meats and poultry, all fresh and canned fruits, milk and milk products (such as yogurt, sherbet, cheeses), and any other food that appeals to the patient is encouraged.

3. Assistance with eating (buttering, cutting, dipping, and unwrapping) may be needed. Observe the patient to determine if help is needed or resented.

4. Observe the time that the patient is less tired and feed at that time. Serve foods that require little chewing.

5. Make certain that the environment is free of odors, debris, and clutter and that the tray is attractive and palatable.

6. Encouragement from health personnel is as necessary as encouragement from friends and relatives, so be generous. Educate the patient to gain compliance.

PROGRESS CHECK ON ACTIVITY 4

Fill-in

For each of the goals listed, supply an appropriate nutritional intervention.

1. Stop weight loss. _____

   _____

2. Rebuild lean body mass. _____

   _____

3. Minimize malabsorption. _____

   _____

4. Manage the specific problems related to nutrition.
   a. anorexia _____

   _____

   b. nausea and vomiting _____

   _____

   c. severe weight loss _____

   _____

   d. oral or esophageal lesions _____

   _____

   e. infection and sepsis _____

   _____

5. List five nursing responsibilities pertaining to feeding AIDS patients.

   a. _____

   b. _____

   c. _____

   d. _____

   e. _____

6. Describe the general sanitation techniques to be used by dietary and nursing staff for the protection of staff and patient. _____

_____

_____

_____

References _____

Anorexia Nervosa/Bulimia

Brumberg, J. J. 1988. *Fasting girls: The emergence of anorexia nervosa as a modern disease.* Cambridge, MA: Harvard University Press.

DoCouto, C. et al. 1988. Position of the American Dietetic Association: Nutrition intervention in the treatment of anorexia nervosa and bulimia nervosa. A.D.A. technical support paper. *Journal of the American Dietetic Association* 88(1):69.

Kirkley, B. G. 1986. Bulemia: Clinical characteristics, development, and etiology. *Journal of the American Dietetic Association* 86(4):468.

Lucus, A. R., and D. M. Huse. 1988. Behavioral disorders affecting food intake: Anorexia nervosa and bulemia. In *Modern nutrition in health and disease,* 7th ed. M. E. Shils and V. R. Young (eds.). Philadelphia: Lea & Febiger.

Martin, R. J. et al. 1987. Control of food intake: Mechanisms and consequences. *Nutrition Today* 22(5):4.

Ross Laboratories. 1983. *Understanding anorexia nervosa and bulemia.* Columbus, OH: Ross Laboratories.

Sarker, I. M., and M. A. Zimmer. 1987. *Dying to be thin.* New York: Warren.

Stein, P. M., and B. C. Unell. 1986. *Anorexia nervosa: Finding the life line.* Minneapolis: CompCare Publications.

Story, M. 1986. Nutrition management and dietary treatment of bulemia. *Journal of the American Dietetic Association* 86(4):517.

Bone Marrow Transplants

Aker, S. N., and C. L. Cheney. 1983. The use of sterile and low microbial diets in ultraisolation environments. *Journal of Parenteral and Enteral Nutrition* 7:390.

Barale, K. et al. 1982. Primary taste thresholds in children with leukemia undergoing marrow transplantation. *Journal of Parenteral and Enteral Nutrition* 6:287.

Blume, K. G., and M. D. Lawrence (eds.). 1983. *Clinical bone marrow transplantation.* New York: Churchill-Livingston.

Dezenhall, A. et al. 1987. Food and nutrition services in bone marrow transplant centers. *Journal of the American Dietetic Association* 87(10):1351.

Gauvreau-Stem, J. M. et al. 1989. Food intake patterns and foodservice requirements on a marrow transplant unit. *Journal of the American Dietetic Association* 89(3):367.

Lenssen, P., and S. N. Aker. 1985. *Nutritional assessment and management during marrow transplantation. A resource manual.* Seattle, WA: Fred Hutchinson Cancer Center.

Szeluga, D. J. et al. 1987. Nutritional support of bone marrow transplant recipients: A prospective, randomized clinical trial comparing total parenteral nutrition to an enteral feeding program. *Cancer Research* 47:3309.

Weisdorf, S. A. et al. 1987. Positive effect of prophylactic total parenteral nutrition on longterm outcome of bone marrow transplantation. *Transplantation* 43:833.

Acquired Immune Deficiency Syndrome

Barbaro, D. 1987. Nutrition for AIDS patients. *Direction Appl Nutr* 1(2):4.

Bentler, M. et al. 1987. Nutrition support of the pediatric patient with AIDS. *Journal of the American Dietetic Association* 87(4):488.

Blanchet, K. D. 1988. *Aids: A health care management response.* Rockville, MD: Aspen Publishers.

Collins, C. 1987. AIDS and nutritional care R.D. 7(3):6.

Collins, C. L. 1988. Nutrition care in AIDS. *Dietetic Currents* 15(3):11. Ross Laboratories.

Dwyer, J. T. et al. 1988. Unproven nutrition therapies for AIDS: What is the evidence? *Nutrition Today* 23(2):25.

Garcia, M. E. et al. 1987. The acquired immune deficiency syndrome: Nutritional complications and assessment of body weight status. *Nutr. Clin. Pract.* 2:108.

Gelt, A. et al. 1986. AIDS and gastroenterology. *Am. J. Gastroenterol.* 81:619.

Hyman, C., and S. Kaufmann. 1989. Nutritional impact of acquired immune deficiency syndrome: A unique counseling opportunity. *Journal of the American Dietetic Association* 89(4):520.

O'Sullivan, P. et al. 1985. Evaluation of body weight and nutritional status among AIDS patients. *Journal of the American Dietetic Association* 85:1483.

Piot, P. et al. 1986. AIDS: An international perspective. *Science* 239:573.

Schreiner, J. E. 1988. *Nutrition handbook for AIDS.* Aurora, CO: Carrot Top Nutrition Resources.

Surgeon General's report on acquired immune deficiency syndrome. 1987. U.S. Department of Health and Human Services. Washington, DC: U.S. Government Printing Office.

Traub, B. 1983. The nutritional implications of AIDS. *Environ. Nutr.* 6(8):1.

Cancer

Ames, B. N. et al. 1987. Ranking possible carcinogenic hazards, *Science* 236:271.

Arnold, C. 1986. Nutrition intervention in the terminally ill cancer patient. *Journal of the American Dietetic Association* 86(4):522.

Bishop, J. M. 1987. The molecular genetics of cancer. *Science* 235:305.

Brown, J. 1987. Chemotherapy. In *Cancer nursing: Principles and practices*. S. L. Groenwald (ed.). Boston: Jones and Bartlett.

Cancer. 1986. *Diet and cancer. 58:Supplement.*

Chernoff, R. 1986. The complexities of enteral nutrition. *Nutr. Clin. Pract.* 1(5):239.

Coulston, A. M. et al. 1986. Nutrition management in patients with cancer. *Top. Clin. Nutr.* 1(2):26.

Donaldson, S. S. 1984. Nutritional support as an adjunct to radiation therapy. *Journal of Parenteral and Enteral Nutrition* 8:302.

Eyre, H. J., and J. H. Ward. 1984. Control of cancer chemotherapy-induced nausea and vomiting. *Cancer* 54:2642.

Groenwald, S. L. 1987. Nutritional disorders. In *Cancer nursing: Principles and practices*, S. L. Groenwald (ed.). Boston: Jones and Bartlett.

Hearne, B. E. et al. 1985. Enteral nutrition support in head and neck cancer: Tube vs oral feeding during radiation therapy. *Journal of the American Dietetic Association* 85:669.

Kokal, W. A. 1985. The impact of antitumor therapy on nutrition. *Cancer* 55:273.

Krey, S. H. et al. 1986. Prolonged use of modular enteral hyperalimentation. *Nutr. Clin. Pract.* 1(3):140.

Lingard, C. D. et al. 1986. Planning and implementing a nutrition program for children with cancer. *Top. Clin. Nutr.* 1(2):71.

Little, L. V. et al. 1986. Nutrition and quality of life of cancer patients. *Top. Clin. Nutr.* 1(2):61.

Ota, D. M. et al. 1986. Practical considerations in nutritional management of the cancer patient. *Curr. Probl. Cancer* 10:353.

Reddy, B. R., and L. A. Cohen (eds.). 1986. *Diet, nutrition, and cancer: A critical evaluation. Vol. I. Macronutrients and cancer*. Boca Raton, FL: CRC Press.

Repka, F. J. 1986. Ethical considerations in nutritional support of cancer patients. *Top. Clin. Nutr.* 1(2):50.

Rickard, K. A. et al. 1986. Advances in nutritional care of children with neoplastic diseases: A review of treatment, research, and application. *Journal of the American Dietetic Association* 86(12):1666.

Shils, M. E. 1988. Nutrition and diet in cancer. In *Modern nutrition in health and disease*, 7th ed. M. E. Shils and V. R. Young (eds.). Philadelphia: Lea & Febiger.

Trant, A. S. 1986. Taste and anorexia in cancer patients: A review. *Top. Clin. Nutr.* 1(2):17.

Tryfiates, G. P., and K. N. Prasad (eds.). 1988. *Nutrition, growth, and cancer*. New York: Alan R. Liss.

Burns

Achauer, B. M. (ed.). 1986. *Management of the burned patient*. Norwalk, CT: Appleton and Lange.

Bell, S. J., and J. Wyatt. 1986. Nutrition guidelines for burned patients. *Journal of the American Dietetic Association* 86:648.

Cunningham, J. J. et al. 1988. Nutritional support of the severely burned infant. *Nutr. Clin. Pract.* 3(2):69.

Del Savio, N. 1984. Nutritional support for the thermally injured patient: The role of the dietitian. *Nutr. Supp. Serv.* 4(10):10.

Ireton, C. S. et al. 1986. Evaluation of energy expenditures in burn patients. *Journal of the American Dietetic Association* 86:331.

Jensen, T. G. et al. 1985. Nutritional assessment indications of postburn complications. *Journal of the American Dietetic Association* 85:68.

Luterman, A. et al. 1984. Nutritional management of the burn patient. *Cri. Care Quart.* 7:34.

Matsuda, T. et al. 1985. Use of indirect calorimetry in the nutritional management of burned patients. *Journal of Trauma* 25:32.

O'Neil, C., and J. Roeber. Burn care protocols-nutrition support. *Journal of Burn Care Rehabilitation* 7(6):351.

Williamson, J. 1985. *Standards of care: Nutritional support of adult burn patients*. Seattle, WA: Harborview Medical Center Department of Nutrition and Food Services.

Respiratory Disorders

Armstrong, J. N. 1986. Nutrition and the respiratory patient. *Nutr. Support Serv.* 6(3):8.

Ireton-Jones, C. S. et al. 1987. The use of respiratory quotient to determine the efficacy of nutrition support regimes. *Journal of the American Dietetic Association* 87(2):180.

Keim, N. L. et al. 1986. Dietary evaluation of outpatients with chronic obstructive pulmonary disease. *Journal of the American Dietetic Association* 87(7):902.

Miller, M. A. 1986. A practical approach to eating and breathing in respiratory failure. *Top. Clinc. Nutr.* 1(4):61.

Pingleton, S. K. et al. 1987. Nutritional management in acute respiratory failure. *Journal of the American Medical Association* 257:3094.

Ross Laboratories. 1986. *Monograph: Dietary modification in chronic pulmonary disease*. Columbus, OH: Ross Laboratories.

Part IV

DIET THERAPY
AND CHILDHOOD
DISEASES

* The descriptive contents for Part IV were obtained from Hui, Y. H. "Human Nutrition and Diet Therapy," 1983 Wadsworth Health Sciences, Monterey, Calif. Used with permission. Objectives, Glossaries, Progress checks, Nursing implications, Post-tests, and other materials in these modules were written by the author.

Principles of Feeding a Sick Child

Time for completion
Activities: _____1_____ hour
Optional examination: _½_ hour

Academic credit
Semester units: _²⁄₁₀_
Quarter units: _³⁄₁₀_

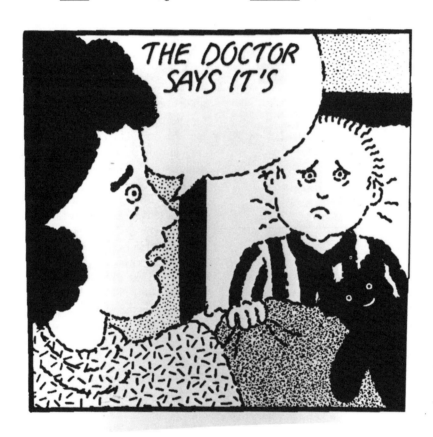

Outline

Objectives
Glossary
Background Information
Progress Check on Background Information

ACTIVITY 1: The Child, the Parents, and the Health Team
Behavioral Patterns of the Hospitalized Child
Teamwork

Nursing Implications
Progress Check on Activity 1

ACTIVITY 2: Special Considerations and Diet Therapy
Special Considerations
Diet Therapy and Dietetic Products
Nursing Implications
Progress Check on Activity 2
References

Objectives

Upon completion of this module, the student should be able to:

1. Describe the principles of diet therapy as they apply to sick children.
2. List the major factors that influence the recovery of a sick child.
3. Identify the causes of inadequate nutrient intake in sick children.
4. Assess the nutritional status of a sick child using the accepted standard guidelines.
5. Identify behavioral patterns of the hospitalized child that may interfere with nutrient intake.
6. Describe the measures by which the health team can facilitate a child's recovery from illness.
7. Discuss ways to involve caregivers in the nutritional treatment of a child who is chronically or terminally ill.
8. Explain ways in which a child and his or her caregivers can be encouraged to comply with a modified diet regime.
9. State measures by which the nutrient intake of a sick child can be improved.
10. Identify the conditions for the use of special dietetic products.

Glossary

Anorexia: lack of appetite.

Casein: milk protein.

Handicap: permanent loss of physical, sensory, or developmental ability (such as mental retardation, behavior disorder, or learning disability).

Lactose: milk sugar.

Medium-chain triglycerides (MCT): a form of fat that is better absorbed than regular fats, and used in diseases where there is malabsorption of ingested foods, especially fat.

Methionine: an amino acid.

Regression: retreat from present level of functioning to past levels of behavior.

Rehabilitation: the restoration of eating abilities to pre-illness levels.

Steatorrhea: a foamy, light colored, foul smelling stool consisting primarily of undigested fats.

Terminal illness: any illness of long or short duration with life threatening outcome.

Background Information

Diseases of infancy and childhood cause distress to all those concerned with the well-being of children. Managing these conditions requires more care than managing similar conditions in adults. Children are particularly vulnerable because their mental and physical development may depend on the proper treatment. Diet and nutritional therapy can play an important role in the full recovery of a sick child.

In spite of advances in pediatric nutrition, we cannot define the absolute nutrient requirements of a child at a particular age. The latest published RDAs serve as convenient guidelines, but they do not necessarily correspond to the optimal quantities for children. However, for practical purposes, it is generally agreed that a diet meeting the RDAs and based on the basic food groups satisfies the nutritional needs of all growing children. The recommendations of the expert panel on blood cholesterol links in children and adolescents, as discussed in Modules 1 and 14, will continue to be important in diet therapy for sick children. The diet should also be appropriate to a child's age and stage of development. This type of diet is satisfactory for normal and sick children. Details on diet planning are presented in Module 1.

Nearly all principles of diet therapy that apply to a sick adult also apply to a young patient. For example, pertinent factors for both groups of patients include personal eating patterns, individual likes and dislikes, and the necessity of frequent diet counseling during a hospital stay. Both children and adults, when ill, encounter the same difficulties in eating well—fatigue, vomiting, nausea, poor appetite, pain from the disease or treatment, drowsiness from medications, fear, anxiety, and so on. Just as with adult patients, the emotional, psychological, social, and physical needs of sick children require careful consideration. In some cases, these may be as important as the attention devoted to the clinical management of the ailment. In general, the principles of feeding a normal child apply more strictly to a sick child.

The nutritional and dietary care of a sick child depends on a number of factors:

1. The disease type, severity, and duration.
2. The management strategy (such as the onset of symptoms, the treatment method).
3. The child's age and growth pattern.
4. The nutritional status of the child before and during hospitalization.
5. The need for rehabilitation.

The major reasons why sick children do not have adequate nutritional intake include the following:

1. A malfunctioning gastrointestinal system.
2. High metabolic demands from stress and trauma such as fever, infection, burns, or cancer.
3. Excessive vomiting and diarrhea.
4. Neurological and psychological disturbances that interfere with eating, such as the inability to chew or the fear of food.
5. Specific nutritionally related diseases such as disorders of the kidney, liver, or pancreas.

Sometimes a child's failure to eat cannot be traced to any specific reason.

As in the case of an adult patient, the evaluation of the nutritional status of a hospitalized child should include the following tools whenever feasible:

1. Anthropometric measurements: height (length), weight, head circumference, appropriate measurements of the arms, chest, and pelvis, and skinfold thickness.
2. General body signs: muscle tone, activity, movement, posture, condition of the hair, mouth (teeth and gums), skin, ears, eyes.
3. Laboratory studies: blood and urine analyses and bone growth assessment using x-rays.

PROGRESS CHECK ON BACKGROUND INFORMATION

Fill-in

1. List five illness factors that interfere with adequate nutrient intake.

   a. _____

   b. _____

   c. _____

   d. _____

   e. _____

2. List the three most commonly used guidelines for evaluating nutritional status.

   a. _____

   b. _____

   c. _____

True/False

Circle T for True and F for False.

3. T F The principles of diet therapy apply to children as well as adults.
4. T F Diet therapy is based upon a balanced normal diet.
5. T F The physical needs of the ill child should take precedence over his or her psychosocial needs.

Multiple Choice

Circle the letter of the correct answer.

6. The major reasons for development of malnutrition in sick children include all of these except
   a. increased metabolism.
   b. interferences with digestion and absorption.
   c. constipation.
   d. refusal to eat.

7. The dietary care of a sick child is formulated by using
   a. the diagnosis of the disease.
   b. the treatment of choice.
   c. evaluation of previous and present nutritional status.
   d. all of the above.

ACTIVITY 1: The Child, the Parents, and the Health Team

Behavioral Patterns of the Hospitalized Child

Problems that adult patients have in adjusting to hospitalization are more acute among children. Children are exposed to a totally new environment without the comfort of their parents, especially the mother, and this emotional stress is superimposed upon that caused by the clinical condition. Children may also be frightened by particular treatments and anxious about their outcome. The presence of strangers may also be confusing. Hospitalized children who become psychologically maladjusted may be unable to express themselves well. They need someone whom they trust and can talk to, especially when they have eating problems. In fact, some sick children develop certain undesirable eating habits. On the other hand, for some children with adjustment problems, food is the principal enjoyment.

Quite often children readopt some elementary feeding practices that do not fit their age or stage of development. For example, an older child may ask for a bottle instead of accepting a cup and may refuse to eat chopped foods, preferring liquid or pureed foods. Although fully capable of self-feeding, the child may want to be fed. Some children find reasons to reject food, even if it is their favorite item and served in a familiar manner. They may complain about the size of the portion or the flavor of the food. Some older children may either refuse to eat or eat too much. To help avoid these problems, new routines and ways of eating should not be forced upon these children. Old eating habits should be accommodated when possible.

The degree of feeding problems depends on the age of the child, the disorder, the child's past experience and nutritional status, and the child's social and emotional makeup. Many young patients are cooperative and eat well.

Teamwork

To provide optimal nutritional and dietary care for a sick child, the health team, especially the nurse, dietitian, or nutritionist, must like children and be willing to work with them. For example, the nurse becomes familiar with a child's eating habits, preferences, reactions, and remarks about food. Conveying this information to the dietary staff helps them to prepare meals that the child will like. Of course, the parents, especially the mother, can provide much useful information about a child's eating habits. The health team must also occasionally yield to children's unreasonable demands, especially those of terminally ill children.

The nurse probably plays the most important role in ensuring that a child eats the foods that are served. When the nurse relates to the child and is considerate and attentive, the child is most likely to eat well The nutritionist, dietitian, and doctor depend on the nurse for coordination and provision of optimal dietary care.

In hospitals where dietitians have many other responsibilities, the suggestions, observations, and opinions of the nurses are especially appreciated. A skillful and considerate nurse can help a child to recover more quickly. Apart from ensuring an adequate intake of food, the nurse monitors the fluid consumption of the child and alerts the doctor and dietitian if the intake is poor.

In caring for a sick child, the health team must be fully aware of the anxiety and concern of the parents. Whenever feasible, members of the team should grant parents' requests for additional visiting hours, thereby helping to fulfill the needs of both the parents and the child. Because their child is ill, both parents have a desire to talk with someone knowledgeable about the illness. The nurse, dietitian, or nutritionist should serve as the contacts. If the parents want to help in the feeding of their child, they should be encouraged to do so and become members of the health team. Further, the team should keep the parents well informed if they are unable to attend to their child. Parents are likely to be depressed when their child is suffering from a terminal illness, and in these instances the team should involve them in the different facets of clinical care, especially the feeding routine.

In sum, the health team shares the problems of the patient with the family and helps the family to overcome psychological and emotional distress. The parents should be taught to care for the child, and it is important that they trust the doctor and other health personnel. Under some circumstances (such as when the child suffers kidney disease, brain damage, or other special disorders) the team, especially the nurse, can assist the family in obtaining applicable financial aid.

It is very important that the child and parents are counseled together on the child's nutrition and dietary care. Sharing information and experience is important—merely instructing the parents without explanation is not sound nutritional education. During hospital feedings, the nurse can make helpful observations about the parent and child; for example, is the parent forcing the child to eat? How extensive are the child's feeding tantrums and food manipulation? While the child is in the hospital, the parents should be fully informed of the child's progress and adjustment especially in regard to nutrition and feeding. The mother should implement recommended changes in eating routines after the child has returned home.

Nursing Implications

These nursing implications are applicable to all types of illness in children. Specific measures may be required for specific disorders.

1. Identify eating patterns: amounts, times, types of food, ethnic, cultural, and religious observances.
2. Make thorough initial physical assessments and monitor height, weight, and other pertinent data regularly.
3. Calculate caloric, fluid, and nutrient intake, and thoroughly document these. Alert health team members of changes as necessary.
4. Involve the child, parents, and caregivers in feeding and care.
5. Explain all modifications of diet.
6. Give emotional support to the parents of ill children.
7. Establish a relationship of trust with both the parents and the child.
8. Allow for regression during periods of illness.
9. Use play as a teaching strategy when a child's condition permits.
10. Encourage interaction with other children.
11. Help the child to feel safe in the strange and new environment of a hospital.
12. Allow expression of feelings.
13. Provide educational opportunities.
14. Realize the stressors of each age group.
15. Provide the assistance needed for coping with illness or injury.
16. Accept the child's (and parents') negative reactions.
17. Allow choices in food whenever possible.
18. Be honest; for example, don't say, "It will make you well," when it won't.
19. Praise the child when the child does the best he or she can.
20. Expect success; convey the impression to the child that you are confident that the child can eat what he or she needs.
21. Assist in securing financial support and referrals when necessary; for example, state and local agencies, social services.

PROGRESS CHECK ON ACTIVITY 1

Fill-In

1. List five factors that may interfere with adequate food intake in hospitalized children.

   a. _____

   b. _____

   c. _____

   d. _____

   e. _____

2. Describe the nurse's primary role as a member of the health team in the feeding of sick children.

   _____

   _____

   _____

   _____

3. List 10 measures that nurses should implement to promote good nutrition in the ill child.

   a. _____

   b. _____

   c. _____

   d. _____

   e. _____

   f. _____

   g. _____

   h. _____

   i. _____

   j. _____

ACTIVITY 2: Special Considerations and Diet Therapy

Special Considerations

When children are required to eat a modified diet, they may have to be reeducated about eating practices. To do this, the health team must first become familiar with the children's normal ways of eating, upon which the appropriate dietary changes must be based. If a child's hospital stay is long, the nutritional education program may be more aggressive and systematic. Depending on the child's age, teaching aids such as movies, slides, and skits may be used. At the beginning of diet modification, children should be given as much freedom as possible in food selection so that they can adjust to the new nutritional environment. Some children like familiar foods such as peanut butter sandwiches, hamburgers, french fries, puddings, milk, soft drinks, and cookies. If a child is expected to be hospitalized for only a short time and has neither a fluid nor electrolyte imbalance, it may be advisable for the child to eat his or her favorite foods even if they are not nutrient dense. When the child is recovering, the missing nutrients can be made up. A sick child should not be forced into new situations at mealtime, such as having to eat new foods or having to eat foods cooked in an unfamiliar way. Using different utensils than the child is accustomed to and serving a combination of new and familiar foods should also be avoided. A child's attitude toward any change in dietary routine should be carefully noted.

As indicated earlier, a sick child's food preferences should be noted by members of the health team and the parents. It is also advisable to put the list in writing. Children of ethnic origins may require special foods and food preparation. However, even when these preferences are taken into account, a child may find all food served in the hospital undesirable. The child is most likely comparing hospital food to food at home, at fast-food chains, or food served in school. Although the food choices for a sick child are invariably limited, it is extremely important to try to select a diet that has familiar foods that the child will readily eat. Whenever a child does not eat, the reasons should be ascertained and new techniques or approaches found for feeding. The child may simply have a poor appetite or be too sick and anxious to eat. Different methods of food serving may be used, including tube and intravenous (IV) feedings. The oral feeding of a hospitalized child should never be forced. Avoid stern commands such as "Drink your milk," "Eat your fruits and vegetables," "There must be no food left on the plate," and "There will be no dessert until you have finished eating your meat and potatoes." When a child does not eat all the food on the plate, it may mean that the serving size was too large.

Regular hospital procedures such as replacing dressings, giving baths, drawing blood, IV adjustments, drainage, or blood pressure measurements should not interfere with mealtimes. The child should not be exposed to pain or physiotherapy while eating.

Whether a child is sick or well, he or she must eat appropriate amounts and kinds of food. Any nutritional problem may become severe if a child is ill for an extended period of time. Ensuring that a child with a lengthy illness eats a proper amount of food is always a problem demanding constant attention.

There are several ways to improve a child's eating and acceptance of foods. The child can become involved in the food selection process by being provided with a selective menu, cafeteria-style food service, fast-food counter food service, or a play-setting food service. Children love to get involved and will eat what they have chosen.

Children generally prefer certain eating practices. First, they like small, frequent meals (especially anorexic children). Second, they like to eat family style or in groups (especially with other sick children of the same age). Sometimes the dietetic staff can save time by serving all young sick children in one place and at one time. Third, children like to be fed by their parents.

A child's food intake may be improved by

1. providing a cheerful eating environment (such as a room having attractive draperies, comfortable chairs and tables, and pleasing paintings), especially when meals are served in a dining room.
2. serving tasty, attractive foods, using creative menu planning and food preparation techniques for children with such preferences.
3. using occasions such as Christmas, Thanksgiving, Halloween, Easter, and birthdays to give surprise parties, which can improve appetites.

Diet Therapy and Dietetic Products

The routine house diets (liquid, soft, and so on) described in Module 12 are also applicable to children. Many therapeutic diets (for treating diabetes, kidney problems, heart problems, and so on) used to treat adult diseases are also used with children, although some modifications may be necessary. There are a number of home and commercial formulas and diets that are used to feed infants, children, and even adults. Table 21-1 presents commercial infant formulas, their manufacturers, and uses. Table 21-2 presents clinical indications for the use of special dietetic products.

Nursing Implications

The responsibilities for nurses treating a sick child are as follows:

1. Educate the parents and the child in the use of a modified diet.
2. Do not change harmless eating habits or lifestyles.
3. Base dietary instruction on the child's developmental stage, ability, readiness to learn, and appropriate teaching aids.
4. Make changes slowly, noting and documenting responses.
5. Understand the role of a nurse as the liaison or activities coordinator among the child, caregiver, physician, dietitian, and other health personnel. Be aware that proper coordination assures a well-nourished child.
6. Document reasons for noncompliance, implementation of new strategies, and any dietary revision.
7. Adjust drug administration and treatment or therapies to avoid interference with mealtimes.
8. Relieve nausea and/or pain before meals are served.
9. Use mealtimes for teaching/socializing with other children.
10. Encourage the child to become involved in his or her own care and selection of foods.
11. Provide a clean and cheerful environment for eating.

PROGRESS CHECK ON ACTIVITY 2

Situation

Allen, age five, is admitted to the hospital with severe burns. He will be in the hospital several weeks. He is withdrawn and eating poorly, and appears very thin. Based on this information, complete the following (use a separate sheet of paper for your responses):

1. Describe data you would collect regarding his eating habits and general nutritional status.
2. Compare nutrient increases needed to the normal growth and development needs of a five-year-old.
3. List the general diet therapy appropriate for Allen and give rationale.
4. Write a one-day menu including snacks that fit the diet therapy requirements.
5. Allen's previous eating habits have not been ideal and hospitalization has made them worse. Discuss several ways to improve his intake.

References

American Dietetic Association. 1987. Position of the American Dietetic Association: Child nutrition services. *Journal of the American Dietetic Association* 87:214.

American Dietetic Association. 1987. Position of the American Dietetic Association: Nutrition in comprehensive program planning for persons with developmental disabilities. *Journal of the American Dietetic Association* 87:1987.

American Dietetic Association. 1988. *Manual of clinical dietetics*. Chicago: American Dietetic Association.

Baer, M. T. (ed.). 1982. *Nutrition services for children with handicaps. A manual for state Title V. programs*. Los Angeles: University Affiliated Training Program, Center for Child Development and Developmental Disorders, Children's Hospital of Los Angeles.

TABLE 21-1
Infant Formulas, Manufacturers, and Uses

Formulas	Manufacturers	Uses
Enfamil with or without iron	Mead Johnson	Infant feeding
Enfamil Premature Formula	Mead Johnson	For growing healthy low birth weights (< 2000 g)
Lofenalac	Mead Johnson	For infants with phenylketonuria
Low Methionine Diet Powder	Mead Johnson	For infants with homocystinuria
Low Phe/Thr Diet Powder	Mead Johnson	For infants with hereditary tyrosinemia
Lytren	Mead Johnson	Electrolyte solutions
Mono- and Disaccharide-Free Diet Powder	Mead Johnson	For children with disaccharidase deficiencies, impaired glucose transport or study of fructose utilization; intractable diarrhea of infancy
MSUD Diet Powder	Mead Johnson	For infants and children with maple syrup urine disease or other disorders in branched chain amino acid metabolism
Nursoy	Wyeth	For infants allergic or sensitive to cow's milk protein or lactose; galactosemia
Nutramigen	Mead Johnson	For infants with sensitivity to intact proteins or severe food allergies; diarrhea, colic, or other gastrointestinal disturbances
Pedialyte	Ross	Electrolyte solutions
Phenyl-Free	Mead Johnson	For children with phenylketonuria
Portagen	Mead Johnson	For infants, children or adults with fat malabsorption such as cystic fibrosis, intestinal resection, steatorrhea, pancreatic insufficiency, celiac disease, bile acid deficiency, lymphatic anomalies
Pregestimil	Mead Johnson	For infants with malabsorption disorders, intractable diarrhea, severe allergies or sensitivity to intact protein, cystic fibrosis, intestinal resection, steatorrhea, lactose or sucrose deficiency
ProSobee	Mead Johnson	For infants allergic or sensitive to cow's milk or lactose; galactosemia; temporary feeding following diarrhea until lactase regenerates; sucrose intolerance
Rehydrate	Ross	Electrolyte solutions
Resol	Wyeth	Electrolyte solutions
Ross Carbohydrate-Free (RCF) Low-Iron Soy Protein Formula Base	Ross	For infants intolerant to all types of carbohydrate; intractable diarrhea
SMA with or without iron	Wyeth	Infant feeding; use for infants with cardiac or renal problems who could benefit from reduced sodium or renal solute load
SMA "Premie"	Wyeth	For growing healthy low birth weight infants (< 2000 g)
Similac with or without iron	Ross	Infant feeding
Similac with Whey + Iron	Ross	Infant feeding
Advance	Ross	Transitional beverage between infant formula and cow's milk for the older infant
Isomil	Ross	For infants allergic or sensitive to cow's milk protein or lactose; galactosemia; temporary feeding following diarrhea until lactase regenerates
Isomil SF	Ross	For infants allergic or sensitive to cow's milk protein lactose or sucrose; temporary feeding following acute diarrhea
Similac LBW	Ross	For rapidly growing healthy low birth weight (< 2500 g) infants
Similac Natural Care	Ross	To fortify human milk for premature infants
Similac PM (60/40)	Ross	For infants whose renal or cardiovascular system might be taxed by a sodium or solute load greater than that of human milk or who have hyperphosphatemia
Similac Special Care	Ross	For growing healthy low birth weight (< 2000 g) infants
Soyalac	Loma Linda	For infants allergic or sensitive to cow's milk protein or lactose; galactosemia
I-Soyalac	Loma Linda	For infants allergic or sensitive to cow's milk protein or lactose; galactosemia

TABLE 21-2
Indications for the Use of Commercial Formulas: A Partial Listing

Indications	Products
For Healthy Normal and Premature Infants	
For normal infants	Enfamil with or without iron, Similac with or without iron, Similac with Whey plus iron
Low-birth weight infants	Enfamil Premature Formula, Similac LBW, Similac Natural Care, Similac Special Care, SMA "Premie"
For Infants with Clinical Disorders	
Allergy	Isomil, Isomil SF, I-Soyalac, Nursoy, Pregestimil, ProSobee, Soyalac
Electrolyte solutions	Lytren, Pedialyte, Rehydrate, Resol
Fat malabsorption	Portagen, Pregestimil
Inborn errors of amino acid metabolism	Lofenalac, Low Methionine Diet Powder, Low Phe/Tyr Diet Powder, MSUD Diet Powder, Phenyl-Free
Inborn errors of metabolism: carbohydrate	Isomil, I-Soyalac, Mono- and Disaccharide-Free Diet Powder, ProSobee, RCF (Ross Carbohydrate-Free), Soyalac
Solute regulated	Similac PM (60/40), SMA with or without iron

Bavin, R., and M. Peck. 1985. Nutritional assessment of the hospitalized child. *Nutr. Support Serv.* 5(11):41.

Brannon, E. 1988. Nutrition training supported by the Office of Maternal and Child Health. *Diet in Pediat Pract Newsletter* 11:3 (Spring).

Brown, L. 1987. Developing a cycle menu for pediatric patients. *Top. Clin. Nutr.* 2(1):55.

Building block for life (pub. of Pediatric Nutrition Practice Group of the American Dietetic Association) 12:2 (Winter).

Caldwell, M. 1989. Public Law 99-457. *An opportunity for nutrition services.*

Cloud, H. H. (ed.).1988. Nutrition and rehabilitation. *Topics Clin. Nutr.* 3 (July).

Crump, I. 1987. *Nutrition and feeding of the handicapped child.* Boston: Little, Brown.

Dwyer, J. et al. (eds.). 1986. *The right to grow: Putting nutrition services for children with special long-term developmental and health needs into action.* Boston: Frances Stern Nutrition Center, New England Medical Center.

Ekvall, S. et al. (eds.). 1987. *Nutritional needs of the child with a handicap or chronic illness. Manual II. Clinical nutrition.* Cincinnati, OH: University Affiliated Cincinnati Center for Developmental Disorders, Children's Hospital Medical Center.

Ekvall, S. et al. (eds.). 1989. *Nutritional needs of the child with a handicap or chronic illness* (Child with special health care needs). *Manual III. Nutritional assessment.* Cincinnati, OH: University Affiliated Cincinnati Center for Developmental Disorders, Children's Hospital Medical Center.

Ekvall, S. M. et al. (eds.). 1987. *Nutritional needs of the handicapped/chronically ill child. Manual I: Nutrition pro-gram planning* (revised). Cincinnati, OH: University Affiliated Cincinnati Center for Developmental Disorders, Children's Hospital Medical Center.

Farnan, S. 1988. Role of nutrition in crippled children's service agencies. *Topics Clin Nutri* 3:33.

Food and Nutrition Board, National Research Council, National Academy of Sciences. 1989. *Recommended dietary allowances.* 10th ed. Washington, DC: National Academy Press.

Forbes, G. B., and C. W. Woodruff (eds.). 1985. *Pediatric nutrition handbook.* Elk Grove, IL: American Academy of Pediatrics.

Gisel, E. G. et al. 1988. Identification of children with cerebral palsy unable to maintain a normal nutritional state. *Lancet* 1:283.

Gortmaker, L. S. 1986. Chronic childhood disorders: Prevalence and impact on planning services, now and in the future. In Dwyer, J. et al. (eds.). *The right to grow.* Boston: Frances Stern Nutrition Center, New England Medical Center Hospital.

Gortmaker, L. S. et al. 1984. Chronic childhood disorders: Prevalence and impact. *Pediatric Clinics of North America* 31:3.

Grant, S. M. 1987. *Pediatric nutrition: Theory and practice.* New York: Butterworth.

Kelts, D. and E. Jones. 1984. *Manual of pediatric nutrition.* Boston: Little, Brown.

Mayo Clinic. 1988. *Mayo Clinic diet manual.* Philadelphia: B. C. Dekker.

Mead Johnson Nutrition. 1990. *Pediatric products handbook.* Evansville, IL: Mead Johnson.

Nelson, W. E. et al. (eds.). 1983. *Textbook of pediatrics,* 12th ed. Philadelphia: W. B. Saunders.

Nutrition programming for the chronically ill handicapped child. 1986. Final Report. Birmingham: Sparks Center for Developmental and Learning Disorders, University of Alabama, Birmingham, and Child Development Center, University of Tennessee Center for the Health Sciences.

Pipes, P. L. (ed.). 1988. *Nutrition in infancy and childhood*, 3rd ed. St. Louis: Mosby.

Ross Laboratory. 1990. *Product handbook*. Columbus, OH: Ross Laboratory.

Tanphaichitr, V. et al. 1988. Principles and practice of nutritional support in diarrhea. *Nutr. Clin. Pract.* 3(1):14.

Walker, W. A., and J. B. Watkins (eds.). 1985. *Nutrition in pediatrics: Basic science and clinical application*. Boston: Little, Brown.

Wodarski, L. A. 1985. Nutrition intervention in developmental disabilities: An interdisciplinary approach. *Journal of the American Dietetic Association* 85:218.

Module 22

Diet Therapy and Cystic Fibrosis

Time for completion
Activities: _____1_____ hour
Optional examination: ½ hour

Academic credit
Semester units: 2/10
Quarter units: 3/10

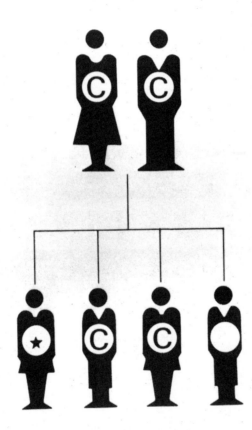

Outline

290

Objectives

Upon completion of this module, the student should be able to:

1. Explain the development of cystic fibrosis:
    a. incidence/organ involvement;
    b. diagnosis;
    c. clinical manifestations;
    d. symptoms;
    e. prognosis; and
    f. treatment.
2. Provide the guidelines for dietary management of cystic fibrosis:
    a. identify the nutritional needs of the patient;
    b. list the nutritional treatment goals;
    c. describe the diet therapy and rationale for the modification;
    d. explain at least three methods of improving nutrient intake;
    e. instruct the child and the family regarding food selection and use of pancreatic enzymes; and
    f. provide adequate support and guidance to the patient's family.

Glossary

Azotorrhea: excess nitrogen in stools.

Etiology: the study of all factors involved in the development of a disease, based on usual course of the disease.

Exocrine: process of externally secreting body substances through a duct to the surface of an organ or tissue or into a vessel.

Meconium: a material that collects in the intestines of the fetus and forms the first stools of a newborn (its texture is normally thick and sticky; in cystic fibrosis it becomes hard, dry, and tenacious, and the infant is unable to pass it).

Mucus: viscous, slippery secretions of mucous membranes and glands.

Prolapse: falling, sinking, or sliding of an organ from its normal position in the body.

Pulmonary: pertaining to the lungs.

Steatorrhea: excess fat in stools.

Tenacious (adjective): grasping, holding, or immobilizing.

Tenacity (noun): process of grasping, holding, or immobilizing.

Villi (pl): short filaments (or hair tufts) on the inside of the intestine through which digested food substances pass.

Viscid: sticky or glutinous.

Background Information

Occurrence and Type of Disorders

Among Caucasian children, cystic fibrosis is one of the more frequent and lethal of inherited diseases. It is estimated that about 1 child per 1,500 to 3,500 live births is affected. Although cystic fibrosis is most common in infants and children, it also occurs in adults. Two major sites of this disease are the exocrine area of the pancreas and the mucous and sweat glands of the body. The mucous glands produce a tenacious and viscid mucous secretion, and an excessive amount of sodium chloride is found in the sweat. The patient may show any or all of the following clinical manifestations:

1. Pulmonary disorder with recurrent infections and other lung trouble
2. Pancreatic insufficiency resulting in a lack of digestive enzymes. Steatorrhea and azotorrhea indicate malabsorption of fat and protein
3. Excessive electrolytes in sweat
4. Malnutrition
5. Failure to thrive

Clinical Symptoms and Diagnosis

If the affected child is not treated, overt symptoms occurring during the first year may include any or all of the following: (1) frequent, large bowel movements with foul odor; (2) substandard weight gain even with good appetite; (3) abdominal bloating; (4) moderate to severe steatorrhea, with stool fat about three to five times normal; (5) frequent and excessive crying; (6) potential sodium deficiency and circulatory collapse resulting from an excessive salt loss in sweat (especially in hot weather); and (7) frequent episodes of pneumonia characterized by coughing and wheezing. This last symptom by itself can indicate cystic fibrosis. At present, the proper diagnosis of a child with cystic fibrosis is determined from clinical symptoms, the level of sodium chloride in the sweat, and x-rays of the chest.

About 8 to 12 percent of cystic fibrosis patients can be diagnosed at birth because of a bowel obstruction (meconium ileus) caused by a thickened meconium. This early diagnosis is helpful, since the proper nutritional and dietary care can be instituted early to prevent suffering from undernourishment. In addition, other appropriate medical treatments can be administered. At the time of this writing, improved medical management has permitted an increasing number of patients to survive to adulthood, especially males.

PROGRESS CHECK ON BACKGROUND INFORMATION

Fill-in

1. List five symptoms of cystic fibrosis that may be observed during the first year of the child's life.

   a. _____

   b. _____

   c. _____

   d. _____

   e. _____

Multiple Choice

Circle the letter of the correct answer.

2. The clinical manifestations of cystic fibrosis include all except

   a. pulmonary infections, malabsorption, and malnutrition.
   b. coronary heart disease, acidosis, and tuberculosis.
   c. failure to thrive, electrolyte imbalance.
   d. steatorrhea, bloating, and circulatory collapse.

3. The three determinations that are made for proper diagnosis of cystic fibrosis are

   a. chest x-rays, stool cultures, anthropometric measures.
   b. clinical symptoms, sweat test, chest x-rays.
   c. saliva test, sweat test, CAT scan.
   d. all of the above.

4. Which of the following indicators, when present at birth, leads to the diagnosis of cystic fibrosis?
   a. excessive sodium chloride in the sweat
   b. excessive crying and wheezing
   c. meconium ileus
   d. steatorrhea

ACTIVITY 1: Dietary Management of Cystic Fibrosis

Nutritional Needs and Goals of Diet Therapy

The nutritional needs of the cystic fibrosis patient must include the following considerations:

1. The problem of recurrent infection is accompanied by defective gastrointestinal functions, increasing the child's nutritional needs.
2. The child needs a working immune defense system for survival. An adequate supply of essential nutrients is necessary to assure sufficient production of antibodies and phagocytic activity of white blood cells.
3. The child suffers from severe malabsorption because of a lack of three pancreatic enzymes: lipase, trypsin, and amylase.

Children with uncontrolled cystic fibrosis have a typical profile. They have a retarded body weight for their age and height, with occasional arrested growth. They are undersized, with a bloated belly and wasted arms and legs, and they appear malnourished. Early diagnosis and management can restore body size and the deposition of muscle and fat. This allows the children to regain a normal appearance, although sexual development may be delayed. However, complete recovery is possible in some cases.

The goals of diet therapy in cases of cystic fibrosis are

1. to improve fat and protein absorption.
2. to decrease the frequency and bulk of stools.
3. to increase the body weight.
4. to control or prevent rectum prolapse.
5. to increase resistance to infection.
6. to control, prevent, or improve associated emotional problems.

General feeding techniques may be used in feeding these children.

Use of Pancreatic Enzymes

Pancreatic enzymes administered to children with cystic fibrosis can greatly improve their condition. As the enzyme extracts are used (Viokase and Cotazym are the most common), the digestive problems abate. The children gain weight and their physical development improves.

Infants and small children should take enzymes in granule or powder form, sometimes just before a meal and sometimes mixed with food. Older children should take tablets or capsules. If too much of the enzyme is given, a child will have difficulty accepting it. There may even be psychological problems if the child is forced to take the enzymes. Therefore, prolonged usage can also cause problems.

The amount of enzyme given depends on the age of the child and the improvement in stool characteristics. A small amount is sufficient initially (for example, ⅕, ¼, or ⅓ tsp. or one tablet). The dosage amount can be increased progressively over one or two months. Progress is monitored by studying the child's fecal waste. If stool conditions do not improve and the child is already taking a large amount of enzyme (for example, 8 tablets or 1 tsp. per treatment), fat intake may need to be restricted. Enzyme replacement does not always work. Malabsorption may remain because of possible mucosal damage, intestinal gland malfunctioning, and viscid mucous coating the intestinal villi.

General Feeding

Feeding a child with cystic fibrosis can be made easier in several ways. Menu planning should be adapted to foods that the child finds acceptable, the clinical condition of the child, and the child's response to enzyme treatment. Generally, the diet should be high in calories and protein with a modified fat content. Details on diet planning for reduced fat intake can be obtained from Module 14. However, the extent of fat restriction varies with the patient. Medium-chain triglycerides (MCTs) and essential fatty acids can be used to advantage when fat restriction is indicated. MCTs facilitate fat absorption, and essential fatty acids prevent linoleic acid deficiency. MCTs used in food preparation can increase energy intake, promote weight gain, and reduce fat malabsorption problems.

Protein malabsorption is mild and usually presents no problem. However, in severe cases the child may lose his or her appetite to the extent that the protein deficiency must be treated. Several procedures can increase the total calorie and protein intake.

One of these involves the addition of dry skim milk powder fortified with fat-soluble vitamins to foods prepared for regular meals. This can be done both at home and in the hospital. It is an inexpensive, easy, and effective way to add calories and protein to the diet. Properly timed snacks at home and in the hospital are also effective, if tolerated. However, the use of pancreatic enzymes must be appropriately scheduled to improve the digestion and absorption of these items.

Apart from a high-protein and modified-fat diet, the child should be given dense nutrient and protein supplements. Supplements are listed below.

1. A mixture of MCTs, oligosaccharides (a carbohydrate chain composed of four to ten glucose segments), beef serum, and protein hydrolysates
2. Commercial nutrient-protein solutions such as Pregestimil, Portagen, and Nutramigen
3. Fat and sugar added to foods if the child can tolerate them
4. Water-miscible vitamins A, D, and E given at one to three times the respective RDAs

If an infant is being treated, nutritional rehabilitation may require 180 to 210 kcal/kg/day, while the caloric need of an older child may be 80 to 110 percent above the norm for that age group.

Foods that are not tolerated by the child (such as raw vegetables and high-fat items) must be identified. Some cystic fibrosis patients get diarrhea when they eat rich carbohydrate foods such as fruit, ice cream, or cookies. They may be suffering a temporary carbohydrate intolerance when this occurs. Lactase deficiency, which occurs in about 1 to 10 percent of the patients, is to blame. Special formulas that are lactose-free can be used for as long as the intolerance persists.

A high ambient temperature may cause a child with cystic fibrosis to lose electrolytes through sweating. Salty foods such as peanuts, potato chips, and other items will alleviate the problem if the foods are tolerated.

Family Involvement and Follow Up

Since the intake of several nutrients must be tightly controlled in a child with cystic fibrosis, the child's family should become involved as early as possible. Merely handing the mother a list of foods that should not be eaten by her child is not sufficient dietary education, since it could result in the child being fed a lopsided diet that omits some major food groups. Without appropriate instruction, family members cannot easily make substitutions for various foods (such as for fat) and they may not assess the nutritional intake correctly. Furthermore, concessions may have to be made to the child's demands occasionally if a restricted diet is to be implemented effectively.

Thus the dietitian, nutritionist, and nurse must work with the family (especially the primary food provider). The essentials of the four food groups should be taught, as well as techniques of substituting acceptable nutritious replacements for high-fat and poorly tolerated food items. It should be emphasized that dietary planning for a cystic fibrosis child takes into consideration the following factors:

1. the food preferences of the child
2. the use of MCTs whenever possible so that the child can occasionally eat favorite foods (such as potato chips, doughnuts, and fried chicken)
3. the preparation of foods that contain little fat (such as low-fat gravy and spreads)
4. maintenance of a food record for reference so that the nutritional status of the child can be assessed and the nurse or dietitian can make suggestions

A prescheduled procedure (weekly, monthly, checkup) should be used to follow up on the progress of a child being treated for cystic fibrosis. An evaluation of nutritional status should be made that includes height, weight, skinfold measurement, and bone age. The information obtained should then be compared with standard values. Some practitioners recommend continuing this evaluation for five years. The child's dietary intake and the nutritional education of the family should also be assessed. If the condition of a child who has been feeling well and who has had a good appetite should suddenly deteriorate, immediate investigation and referral is necessary. Complications such as infection or the ineffectiveness of the diet may cause sudden changes. Arrangements can be made so that such evaluations, assessments, investigations, referrals, and emergency handling can be done by a clinic, family physician, or other health professional (nutritionist, dietitian, nurse, or public health worker).

Nursing Implications

The responsibilities of the nurse for treating a child with cystic fibrosis are listed below.

1. Maintain adequate nutrition.
   a. Provide diet high in carbohydrate and protein: supplement diet to increase intake.
   b. Provide altered forms of fat as necessary.
   c. Assure adequate salt intake.
   d. Administer pancreatic enzymes with meals and snacks.
   e. Administer water-soluble vitamin and iron supplements.
2. Promote growth and development by encouraging optimal nutrition.
3. Provide support to the family: references, resources, support groups, counseling.
4. Educate the child and the family.
   a. Provide accurate information regarding diet and rationale.
   b. Teach the use of and proper administration of pancreatic enzymes.
   c. Promote eating at the table to improve posture and lung expansion.
   d. Encourage good dental hygiene: cystic fibrosis children may have unhealthy teeth because of deficiencies in nutrition.
   e. Encourage high fluid intake to assist in liquefying secretions.
   f. Encourage optimal nutritional status as a means of preventing rectal prolapse.
   g. Employ strategies to improve child's appetite.

PROGRESS CHECK ON ACTIVITY 1

Situation

Susie is a ten-year-old girl with cystic fibrosis who is hospitalized with a severe upper respiratory infection. She has poor muscle development and tires easily. She is 42 inches tall and weighs 50 pounds. Based on your knowledge of growth and development patterns in children and the etiology of cystic fibrosis, answer the following questions:

1. Are Susie's height and weight appropriate for her age? Explain. _____

2. Susie has chronic diarrhea, and is acting lethargically. To what factors would each of these deviations be attributed? _____

3. List the diet modifications and the reasons they are necessary for restoring adequate nutrition to Susie.

4. Susie's appetite is very poor. List several things you can do to tempt her to eat. _____

5. Outline a day's food plan for Susie. Check the amount of protein and calories by calculating the total food values. _____

References

Foster, R. L., Romness, M. M., and J. J. T. Anderson. 1989. *Family-centered nursing care of children*. Philadelphia: Saunders.

Kelleher, J. et al. 1986. Essential element nutritional status in cystic fibrosis. *Human Nutri Applied Nutri* 40A:79.

Lifshitz, F. (ed.). 1985. *Nutrition for special needs in infancy: Protein hydrolysates*. New York: Marcel Dekker.

Listernick, R. et al. 1986. Outpatient oral rehydration in the United States. *Am. J. Dis. Child.* 140:211.

Michel, J. H. et al. 1987. Practical approaches to nutrition care of patients with cystic fibrosis. *Topics Clin. Nutr.* 2(1):10.

Moore, M. C. et al. 1986. Enteral-tube feeding as adjunct therapy in malnourished patients with cystic fibrosis: A clinical study and literature review. *American Journal of Clinical Nutrition* 44:33.

Roberts, L. 1988. Race for the cystic fibrosis gene nears end. *Science* 240:282.

Robertson, L. M. et al. 1987. Promoting oral rehydration therapy for acute diarrhea. *Journal of the American Dietetic Association* 87(4):496.

Rose, M. H., and R. B. Thomas (eds.). 1987. *Children with chronic conditions: Nursing in a family and community context.* New York: Grune & Stratton.

Shepherd, R. W. et al. 1984. Malnutrition in cystic fibrosis: The nature of the nutritional deficit and optimal management. *Nutr. Abst. Rev.* 54:1009.

Tanphaichitr, V. et al. 1988. Principles and practice of nutritional support in diarrhea. *Nutr. Clin. Pract.* 3(1):14.

Vaisman, N. et al. 1987. Energy expenditure of patients with cystic fibrosis. *J. Pediat.* 11:496.

Module 23

Diet Therapy and Celiac Disease

Time for completion
Activities: _____1_____ hour
Optional examination: ½ hour

Academic credit
Semester units: ²⁄₁₀
Quarter units: ³⁄₁₀

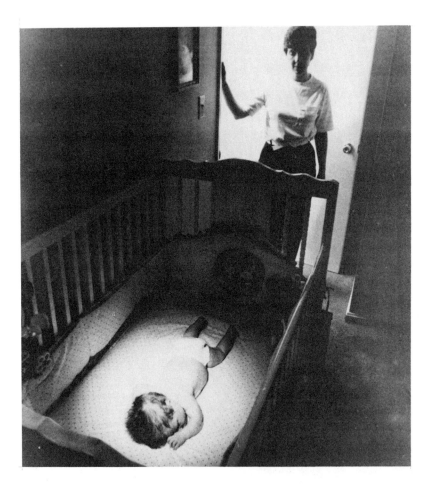

Outline

Objectives

Upon completion of this module, the student should be able to:

1. Describe the etiology of celiac disease.
2. Explain the role of gluten in the pathophysiology of celiac disease.
3. Identify the sources of gluten.
4. Plan a gluten-free diet.
5. Provide adequate substitutes in the diet that enable the individual with celiac disease to meet his or her RDAs.
6. Teach parents or caregivers the specifics of dietary control and methods of dietary compliance.
7. Alert adults with celiac disease of the necessity of strict adherence to the diet and methods of dietary compliance.

Glossary

Atrophy: decrease in size of a developed organ or tissue; wasting.

Cheilosis: cracking open and dry scaling of the lips and angles of the mouth.

Emaciation: a wasted condition of the body; excessively lean.

Enteropathy: any disease of the intestine, such as celiac disease.

Glossitis: inflammation of the tongue.

Hyperosmolarity: abnormally high (increased) concentration of a solution.

Jejunum: part of the small intestine that extends from the duodenum to the ileum of the intestine; *jejunal:* of, or relating to the jejunum.

Lumen: the cavity or channel within a tube or tubular organ, as in blood vessel or intestine.

Macrocytic anemia: anemia marked by abnormally large red blood cells.

Microcytic anemia: anemia marked by abnormally small red blood cells.

Villi: threadlike projections covering the lining of the small intestine and serving as sites for the absorption of nutrients.

Background Information

Celiac disease results from a patient's sensitivity to flour protein (gluten). Flour is made up of about 10 percent protein. This disease tends to run in families. Celiac disease has many names: gluten (or gluten-induced) enteropathy, nontropical sprue, and celiac sprue.

A jejunal biopsy of a patient with celiac disease invariably shows mucosal atrophy of the small intestine. The cells, instead of being columnar, are squamous (flat). These abnormal cells secrete only small amounts of digestive enzymes. Villi are also lacking in the intestine.

Medical records indicate that before the cause of celiac disease was identified, only children were suspected to have this disease. At present, adults with symptoms and positive identification from intestinal biopsy are also classified as having adult celiac disease, especially if they respond to gluten-free diets.

ACTIVITY 1: Dietary Management of Celiac Disease

Symptoms

The symptoms exhibited by a patient with celiac disease are diarrhea, steatorrhea, two to four bowel movements daily, loss of appetite and weight, emaciation, and in children, failure to thrive (such children typically have pot bellies). Children's growth is retarded because of the incompetent mucosa, which causes severe malabsorption. When the fat is not absorbed, it is moved to the large intestine and becomes emulsified by bile and calcium salts. The odor of the stool is caused by large amounts of fatty acids. The unabsorbed carbohydrates are fermented by the bacteria in the large intestine, producing gas and occasional abdominal cramps. Hyperosmolarity induces the colon to secrete water and electrolytes into the lumen. The patient may show many malnutrition symptoms, including bone pain and tetany, anemia, rough skin, and lowered prothrombin time. Most adult patients have iron and folic acid deficiencies, with microcytic and macrocytic anemias. Symptoms such as cheilosis and glossitis, caused by water-soluble vitamin deficiencies, may also be present.

Principles of Diet Therapy

The basic principle of diet therapy for celiac disease is to exclude all foods containing gluten—chiefly buckwheat, malt, oats, rye, barley, and wheat. The patient's response to such a regimen is dramatic. A child shows improvement in one to two weeks, while an adult takes one to three months for visible improvement. In either case, symptoms gradually disappear. With the child patient, there is weight gain and thriving, and diarrhea and steatorrhea clear up. The mucosal changes will also return to normal after a gluten-free diet. The degree of improvement is directly related to the extent the patient adheres to the diet. The therapy can be proven to be curing the disease if symptoms reappear when the patient returns to a regular diet. For some young patients, the treatment lasts at least five years before they can eat wheat and other formerly excluded products. However, some children must exclude gluten from their diet permanently. Adult patients appear to have a lower percentage rate of complete recovery.

Table 23-1 lists those foods that are permitted or prohibited in a gluten-restricted diet. Table 23-2 provides a sample meal plan for such a diet.

Patient Education

After celiac disease has been diagnosed, patients should be educated about its cause and treatment. Patients who understand this illness are much more likely to follow a prescribed diet. They should first be taught that adherence to a gluten-free or gluten-restricted diet is essential. If the patients also have lactose intolerance (as is sometimes the case), the necessity of avoiding milk and milk products must also be emphasized.

Patients should be forewarned of the great difficulty in following a gluten-restricted diet. Buckwheat, malt, oats, barley, rye, and wheat all contain gluten and are extensively used in different food products. Patients must therefore be taught to read all labels on prepared and packaged foods to ascertain if they contain gluten. Gluten-free wheat products are commercially available for those on special diets. In addition, potato, rice, corn, and soybean flours, and tapioca may be substituted.

If a patient is already malnourished when treatment begins, an aggressive nutritional rehabilitation regimen should be instituted. This includes high amounts of calories, protein, vitamins, and minerals. It should also provide fluids and electrolyte compensation (with special attention to potassium, magnesium, and calcium). Medium-chain triglycerides (MCTs) should also be included. A gluten-restricted diet may be deficient in thiamin (vitamin B_1) and should include vitamin supplements.

All patients should be taught to plan their menus in accordance with some food guides to achieve their daily RDAs. Health professionals should help the patient in this planning.

Nursing Implications

The responsibilities of the nurse to patients with celiac disease are listed below.

1. Emphasize to parents and child the importance of complying with diet therapy to treat the disease.
2. Explain the disease etiology to the parents, especially the specific role of gluten in the pathophysiology.
3. Advise the patient and parents regarding the necessity of reading all food labels carefully.
4. Explain the necessity of any other restrictions that may be placed on the diet due to the child's condition, such as low-residue, lactose-free diets.
5. Recommend that the diet be continued indefinitely.

6. Provide a gluten-free diet tailored to the child's appetite and capacity to absorb; emphasize suitable substitutes.
7. Arrange for dietitian-caregiver-child-nurse conferences to coordinate care.
8. Administer aqueous vitamin-mineral supplements as ordered; request prescription for supplements if child's intake is poor.
9. Monitor fluid and food intake carefully, and document well.
10. Teach parents or caregivers specifics of dietary control; provide a written list of common food sources of gluten.
11. Emphasize other dietary principles, such as high-calorie, high-protein, low-residue diets.
12. Stress the importance of good health in preventing infections, the dangers of fasting, and drug and food interactions.
13. Make referrals for financial aid or additional dietary counseling and follow up after patient is discharged.
14. Assist the parents and the child in adjusting to lifelong regimes; be positive about dietary treatment.

PROGRESS CHECK ON ACTIVITY 1

Multiple Choice

Circle the letter of the correct answer.

1. Gluten is found in
   a. wheat, rye, oats, barley.
   b. rice, potato, corn, beans.
   c. milk and meat.
   d. all of the above.

2. Jane has been diagnosed as having celiac disease. Which of the following snacks would be suitable for her to have in nursery school?
   a. malted milk shake
   b. popcorn and apple slices
   c. hot dog with catsup
   d. graham crackers and peanut butter.

3. Diet therapy for celiac disease is continued
   a. indefinitely.
   b. until patient is middle-aged.
   c. through prepubertal growth spurt.
   d. for at least six weeks.

Situation

Mrs. Jones, age 30, was recently diagnosed as having adult celiac disease and her physician ordered a gluten-free diet for her. She recognizes you as a health professional and states that she is quite apprehensive about her diet. Counsel her regarding the following:

TABLE 23-1
Foods Permitted and Prohibited in a Gluten-Restricted Diet

Food Group	Foods Permitted	Foods Prohibited
Meat, poultry	Those prepared without prohibited grains or their flours	All products using prohibited flours, including swiss steak, chili con carne, commercial sausages (e.g., weiners), gravies, sauces, stews, batter, stuffings, croquettes
Fish	All fish and shellfish containing no restricted grains or their flours	Any product made with the restricted grains and flours, e.g., wheat flour breaded fish sticks and shrimp
Cheese	All not specifically prohibited	Processed cheese and cheese spread prepared with gluten as a stabilizer
Eggs	All frozen and fresh eggs and egg substitutes without restricted grains or their flours	All others
Textured vegetable proteins	All those made from soy ingredients	All others
Milk, milk products	All not specifically prohibited	Milk shakes and malted milk
Fats, oils	Butter, margarine, cream and cream substitutes; bacon; olive oil, vegetable oil, salad oil; vegetable (hydrogenated) shortening; mayonnaise	Salad dressings thickened with wheat or rye products; cream, butter, white sauce made with forbidden flour
Cereals	All cereals made from corn and rice, e.g., Sugar Pops, Rice Krispies, Corn Chex, corn flakes, Puffed Rice, Frosted Flakes, Cream of Rice, grits, hominy, and cornmeal	All cereals containing prohibited grains, e.g., Cream of Wheat
Bread	Muffins, pone, and corn bread prepared without wheat flour; rolls, muffins, and breads prepared with cornmeal, cornstarch, lima bean flour, and arrowroot; rice pancakes; products made with low gluten wheat starch	All products made from prohibited grains, e.g., sweet rolls, crackers, muffins, prepared mixes, bread crumbs, commercial yeast breads
Vegetables, vegetable juices	All vegetables and juices; sauces made with potato flour or cornstarch may be used	Vegetables prepared with cracker crumbs, bread, or cream sauces thickened with prohibited flours or cereals
Fruits, fruit juices	All fruits and juices	Fruit sauces thickened with prohibited grains
Potatoes or substitutes	Potatoes, rice, grits, corn, sweet potatoes, dried peas and beans	Pasta
Sweets	All unless specifically prohibited	Candies and chocolate syrup with bases made from prohibited grains
Soups	Cream or vegetable soups thickened with cornstarch or potato flour; meat stock; clear broths	Milk and cream soups; bouillon cubes or powdered soups; canned soups; soups with prohibited grain products; soups thickened with wheat flour
Beverages	Coffee, tea, cocoa, chocolate, carbonated beverages, milk, Kool Aid	Ale, beer, malted milk; instant cocoa, coffee, or tea; cereal beverages; milk shakes; others including Ovaltine, Postum
Desserts	Products made with permitted grains; plain or fruit-flavored gelatin; homemade ice, ice cream, sherbet, Popsicles, cornstarch, rice and tapioca puddings; cakes, pies, and cookies, using water, sugar, and fruits	All products made with prohibited grains, e.g., pastries (cakes), desserts (ice cream cones, sherbet), prepared mixes
Miscellaneous	Herbs, pepper, olives, salt, vinegar, catsup, pickles, relishes, spices, sauces prepared from permitted grains and their flours; peanut butter, nuts, flavoring extracts, popcorn	Creamed and scalloped foods; au gratin dishes, rarebit; fritters, timbales, malt products, prepared mixes of all kinds; condiments prepared with gluten base

TABLE 23-2
Sample Meal Plan for a Gluten-Restricted Diet

Breakfast	Lunch	Dinner
Juice	Meat	Meat, fish, or poultry
Cereal, hot or dry	Potato	Potato
Scrambled egg(s)	Vegetable	Vegetable
Corn bread (special)	Salad with dressing	Juice
Margarine	Fruit or dessert	Fruit or dessert
Jelly	Corn bread	Corn bread
Milk	Margarine	Margarine
Coffee or tea	Milk	Milk
Sugar	Beverage	Beverage
Cream	Cream	Cream
Salt, pepper	Sugar	Sugar
	Salt, pepper	Salt, pepper

4. Explain what gluten is and why it is restricted.

   _____

   _____

   _____

   _____

5. Since Mrs. Jones works outside the home, she will be eating lunch away from home. Provide lunch suggestions that conform to her diet.

   _____

   _____

   _____

   _____

6. Name at least six typical foods containing gluten for Mrs. Jones.

   _____

   _____

   _____

   _____

7. List the cereal grains that can be used on Mrs. Jones's diet.

   _____

   _____

   _____

8. Name at least five hidden food sources of gluten.

   _____

   _____

   _____

   _____

9. Mrs. Jones states that she is also lactose-intolerant. What additional foods must be omitted from her diet?

   _____

   _____

   _____

10. Would you recommend that Mrs. Jones add medium-chain triglycerides to her diet? Explain. _____

   _____

   _____

   _____

   _____

Optional Exercise

Write down all the foods you ate yesterday. Change the menu to make it gluten free.

   _____

   _____

   _____

   _____

   _____

References

Auricchio S. et al. 1985. Toxicity mechanisms of wheat and other cereals in celiac disease and related enteropathies. *J. Pediatr. Gastroenterol. Nutr.* 4:923.

Bayless, T. M. 1986. *Current therapy in gastroenterology and liver disease, vol. 2.* St. Louis: Mosby.

Cashman, M. D. 1986. Principles of digestive physiology for clinical nutrition. *Nutr. Clin. Pract.* 1(5):241.

Desai, M. B. et al. 1988. Nutrition and diet in management of disease of the gastrointestinal tract. In *Modern nutrition in health and disease,* 7th ed. M. E. Shils and V. R. Young (eds.). Philadelphia: Lea & Febiger.

Eastwood, G. L. 1984. *Core textbook of gastroenterology.* Philadelphia: Lippincott.

Food and Nutrition Board, National Research Council, National Academy of Sciences. 1989. *Recommended dietary allowances.* 10th ed. Washington, DC: National Academy Press.

Hattner, J. A. T. 1987. The dietitian's role in the treatment of common gastrointestinal problems. *Topics in Clinical Nutrition* 2(1):62.

Heatley, R. V. et al. (eds.). 1986. *Clinical nutrition in gastroenterology.* London: Churchill.

Hunter, J. O., and V. A. Jones (eds.). 1985. *Food and the gut.* London: Bailliere Tindall.

Kern, F., Jr., and A. Blum (eds.). 1986. *The gastroenterology annual, No. 3.* New York: Elsevier.

Moore, F. D. 1986. Current thoughts on malabsorption: Parenteral, enteral, and oral feeding. *Journal of the American Dietetic Association* 86(9):1169.

Rawcliffe, P., and R. Rolph (eds.). 1985. *The gluten-free diet book.* New York: Arco.

Shiner, M. 1984. Present trends in celiac disease. *Postgrad. Med.* 60:773.

Sleisenger, M. H., and J. S. Fordtran (eds.). 1983. *Gastrointestinal disease pathophysiology, diagnosis, management,* 3rd ed. New York: W. B. Saunders.

Wilson, P. C., and H. L. Greene. 1988. The gastrointestinal tract: Portal to nutrient utilization. In *Modern nutrition in health and disease,* 7th ed. M. E. Shils and V. R. Young (eds.). Philadelphia: Lea & Febiger.

Module 24

Diet Therapy and Congenital Heart Disease

Time for completion
Activities: _____1_____ hour
Optional examination: ½ hour

Academic credit
Semester units: 2/10
Quarter units: 3/10

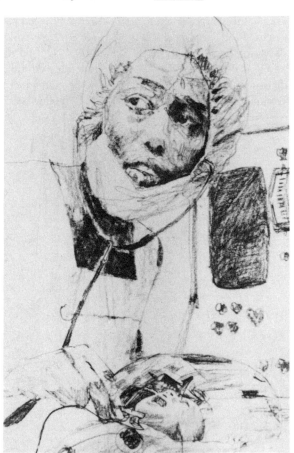

Outline

Objectives

Upon completion of this module, the student should be able to:

1. Describe the effects of congenital heart disease upon the nutritional status of children.
2. List three reasons for growth retardation in a child with congenital heart disease.
3. Identify the four major nutritional problems to be considered for patients with congenital heart disease.
4. Explain the appropriate diet therapy for congenital heart disease and give supporting rationale.
5. Describe formulas and supplements used for infants with congenital heart disease.
6. Evaluate the introduction of solid foods and precautions used when feeding.
7. Compare the feeding problems encountered in a child with a defective heart to those of normal children.
8. Describe methods of maintaining optimum nutritional status in the hospitalized child.
9. Teach parents and the child the principles of feeding and eating when congenital heart disease is present.
10. Describe appropriate discharge procedures.

Glossary

Congenital: present at birth

Cyanotic: condition exhibiting bluish discoloration of the skin and mucous membranes due to excessive concentrations of reduced hemoglobin or extensive oxygen extraction.

Dehydration: excessive loss of water from body tissue, accompanied by imbalance of electrolytes, especially sodium, potassium, and chloride (dehydration is of particular concern among infants and young children).

Diuretic: a drug or other substance that promotes the formation and excretion of urine.

Milliequivalent (mEq): the number of grams of solute dissolved in one milliliter of normal solution.

Milliliter: a metric unit of measurement of volume.

Milliosmol (mosm): a unit of measure representing the concentration of an ion in solution.

Renal: of or pertaining to the kidney.

Respiration (breathing): exchange of carbon dioxide and oxygen in the lungs.

Respiratory distress: inability of the infant to make the exchange, characterized by rapid breathing, grunting on expiration, and other severe symptoms.

Solute: any substance dissolved in a solution.

Background Information

It is currently believed that about 10 out of 100 newborns with birth defects have congenital heart disease. This disorder, which may not be identified at birth, involves a heart that is structurally defective. The causes are unknown, although the presence of German measles during pregnancy may be a factor. The disorder can result in a multitude of complications, especially respiratory distress and heart failure. It is also responsible for height and weight retardation.

Congenital heart disease can retard a child's growth in a number of ways. First, it can cause the child to eat too little. The child may voluntarily reduce food intake in order to reduce the workload of the heart. Or, the child can become listless because of rapid respiration and a lack of oxygen, thus reducing the child's ability to eat an adequate amount of food. A second reason for growth retardation is a high body metabolic rate due to the increased nutrient needs of the organs and tissues and elevated body temperature and thyroid activity. A third reason for growth retardation is a high loss of body nutrients due to inadequate intestinal absorption, excessive urine output, and the presence of hemorrhages or open wounds. It is not known how a heart defect can cause all these clinical problems.

The only cure for congenital heart disease is successful surgery, performed during early or late infancy.

Although corrective surgery can be successful, the mortality rate is high for small children. However, if death is imminent because of heart failure, high-risk surgery is indicated. It is therefore of paramount importance that the infant with heart disease is provided adequate nutrition so that the infant weighs 30 to 50 pounds when surgery is performed. This must be accomplished despite the diminished nutrient supply to cells due to the decreased oxygen supply that results from a defective heart.

ACTIVITY 1: Dietary Management of Congenital Heart Disease

Major Considerations in Dietary Care

There are four major considerations in feeding children with congenital heart disease. One is caloric need. Because of the expected retardation of growth caused by the clinical condition, the child's caloric need is higher than the RDAs. For example, if the RDA of calories for a normal child is 100 kcal/pound, the need for a patient with congenital heart disease may be 130 to 160 kcal/pound.

A second concern is renal load. The child may have difficulty handling any large renal load of solutes. A large renal load may be caused by excessive electrolytes or dehydration, which can result from an insufficient fluid intake.

The third consideration is food intolerance. A large amount of simple sugars may produce diarrhea, the fat in regular milk and food may cause steatorrhea, and food ingestion may cause abdominal discomfort.

The fourth major consideration is vitamin and mineral need. Vitamin and mineral deficiencies have been documented in infants with congenital heart disease. Because of the small quantity of food consumed, the child's intake of these nutrients must be carefully monitored.

Formulas and Regular Foods

An infant with congenital heart disease is usually fed a special formula, although regular foods are sometimes used. The formula should be high in calories but contain only the minimal amount of protein and electrolytes needed for growth without causing kidney overload. Some guidelines are as follows: 8 to 10 percent of the daily calories should come from protein; 35 to 65 percent from carbohydrate; and 35 to 50 percent from fat. Infants under four months old should get 1.8 to 2.0 grams of protein per 100 kcal, and infants four- to twelve-months-old should get 1.65 to 1.75 grams of protein per 100 kcal.

Some clinicians prefer special low-electrolyte, low-protein formulas supplemented with fat or carbohydrate solution. The preparer adds supplements to these formulas, which are commercially available. Other clinicians recommend using formulas with 25 to 30 kcal per ounce and diluting accordingly. The solute load of such preparations must be calculated, and their effects on the child carefully monitored. Sometimes the prepared formulas are supplemented with a limited amount of solid foods that is not adequate to support growth by itself. Some clinicians have good experience with Wyeth's SMA and Ross's Similac PM 60/40 (Module 21).

If formulas are not used, the calorie and sodium contents, digestibility, and renal solute load of the foods fed to the child must be appropriate. Carbohydrate and fat do not affect the solute load. Clinical practice has established that 1 milliosmol (mosm) of solute is formed by 1 milliequivalent (mEq) of sodium, potassium, and chloride, and that 1 gram (g) of dietary protein provides about 4 mosm of renal solute load. If the infant is given regular food, the diet should begin with easily digested and accepted items such as fruit, with cereal or unsalted vegetables included later.

Certain precautions are important in feeding a child with congenital heart disease. If the child is given any high caloric supplement, small amounts should be used, at least at the beginning, since large portions can produce diarrhea and reduce appetite. If the child is eating moderately to considerably less than the calculated amount, he or she is especially susceptible to folic acid deficiency. Since many nonprescription vitamin supplements for children do not contain folic acid, it is important to obtain a proper preparation. The child may also require iron and calcium supplementation.

Table foods may be introduced when the child is over 5½ to 6½ months old. Very small servings of chopped, mashed, or pureed cereal, fruits, potato, and meat with vegetables can be served, all prepared without salt. The amount of meat should be limited to less than 1 oz. a day if the child's condition is poor.

The sodium intake of the child must be carefully considered. Most commercial strained baby foods, especially meat and vegetable items, contain a large amount of sodium and are usually not suitable. If they are used, their sodium contents must be ascertained and the effects monitored. Home-prepared baby foods must be properly selected and quantified and prepared without salt. The child's need for sodium is a delicate balance between too much, which is bad for the heart, and too little, which affects growth. For example, if the child suffers any clinical symptoms of heart failure, dietetic low-sodium formulas may be indicated. If diuretics are used to remove body sodium, all complications associated with their usage must be monitored and corrected. The child's intake of sodium should be under 8 mEq per day.

The fluid intake of the child should also be carefully monitored because children with heart disease can lose much water from fever, high environmental temperature, diarrhea, vomiting, and rapid respiration. Thus, children with congenital heart disease need more water than normal children of the same age. Both urine and solute level should be monitored to assure that patients drink enough fluid and are not overloaded with solutes. An acceptable urine solute load is 400 mosm per liter.

Managing Feeding Problems

Feeding children with congenital heart disease also poses problems. A child may lose his or her appetite or become tired, thus reducing food intake. Of course, food intake may be inadequate due to the regular feeding problems of normal children. For example, if the parents force a child to eat, the child may stubbornly refuse. The child may cry and become cyanotic, which can frighten some parents. If a child does not enjoy eating and the parents do not know what to do, the child's eating problems can be perpetuated.

Educating parents of children with congenital heart disease is important. The parents should become familiar with the basic eating pattern of a normal child and all associated feeding problems. They should also become familiar with managing a child with feeding problems that are psychological. For example, they can learn to anticipate the problems, to be aware of their child using food as a weapon, to avoid overconcern for their child, to be consistent in their management, and to avoid being manipulated by the child.

In addition to learning how to cope with normal feeding problems, the parents should learn about feeding difficulties related to the heart condition, such as vomiting, gagging, and regurgitation. They should learn such techniques as massaging and stimulation of the child's gums, lips, and tongue to increase the child's sucking ability. They should also learn to evaluate the child's responses such as tiredness, resting, amount of formula consumed over a fixed period, and complexion after eating. At the same time, they should seek professional help to make sure that their child is adequately nourished.

Discharge Procedures _____

When a child with congenital heart disease is discharged from the hospital, certain procedures must be followed by the health professionals. The child's nutritional status must be studied periodically. The child's family background and daily routine, especially the eating pattern of the entire family, should be evaluated, and preparations should be made for meeting the child's nutritional needs (the role of the caretaker, the times when the child can be fed, the frequency of the child's visits to the clinic). The parental food preparer should be completely familiar with the nutritional and dietary care of the child. If the parents are unable to cope with the different methods of combining or preparing formulas, they should be taught easier feeding methods. A list of low-sodium, non-dietetic products such as sugar, cereal, fruits, and vegetables should be provided. If diarrhea and steatorrhea occur, medium-chain triglycerides can be used and the consumption of simple sugars can be reduced.

Nursing Implications _____

Nursing responsibilities for treating a child with congenital heart disease are listed below.

1. Adjust the diet to the child's condition and capabilities.
2. Avoid extremes of temperature in the child's environment.
3. Maintain optimum nutrition with a well-balanced diet.
4. Discourage consumption of food with high salt content; do not add salt to any foods.
5. Encourage potassium-rich foods to prevent depletion.
6. If supplements are used, mix them in juice to hide their taste.
7. Request iron supplements as needed to correct anemia.
8. Provide consistent discipline from infancy to prevent behavior problems such as overdependency and manipulation.
9. Feed the child slowly; administer small and frequent meals.
10. Encourage the anorexic child to eat.
11. Delay self-feeding to minimize exertion.
12. Stay calm.

PROGRESS CHECK ON ACTIVITY 1 _____

Matching

Match the factors in dietary care in the column at the left to the appropriate nutritional alteration at the right:

1.	renal overload/dehydration	a. 130–160 kcal per pound body weight
2.	high metabolic rate	b. high fluid intake
3.	poor food intake	c. low in sugar, moderate-fat
4.	food intolerances/malabsorption	d. vitamin/mineral supplement

Multiple Choice

Circle the letter of the correct answer.

5. The effects of congenital heart disease on the nutritional status of a child include all but
   a. growth retardation.
   b. esophageal varices.
   c. lack of energy.
   d. inadequate absorption.

6. Congenital heart disease can retard a child's growth by
   a. elevating body temperature.
   b. increasing thyroid activity.
   c. decreasing intestinal absorption.
   d. all of the above.

7. Energy supplements suitable for infants with congenital heart defects include
   a. MCT oil and corn oil.
   b. Karo syrup.
   c. pablum and albumin.
   d. a and b.

8. Guidelines for nutrient distribution for the infant with congenital heart disease should be in the range of
   a. 50 percent carbohydrate, 20 percent protein, 30 percent fat.
   b. 35 to 65 percent carbohydrate, 10 percent protein, 35 to 50 percent fat.
   c. 30 percent carbohydrate, 30 percent protein, 60 percent fat.
   d. none of the above.

9. The electrolytes that must be closely monitored in the diet when congenital heart disease is present are

a.   sodium, chloride, and potassium.
b.   calcium, iron, and iodine.
c.   carbohydrate, protein, and fat.
d.   phosphorus, magnesium, and calcium.

10. The child with congenital heart disease is especially susceptible to which of the following vitamin deficiencies?
    a.   ascorbic acid
    b.   linoleic acid
    c.   folic acid
    d.   amino acid

Fill-in

11. Write a one-day menu for a 6-1/2-month-old child with congenital heart disease who has just been introduced to solid foods. _____

    _____

    _____

    _____

    _____

    _____

12. List five feeding problems of children with congenital heart disease and ways to overcome them.

    a.   _____
    b.   _____
    c.   _____
    d.   _____
    e.   _____

13. List five ways the nurse/health care provider can maintain optimal nutrition in a child with congenital heart disease.

    a.   _____
    b.   _____
    c.   _____

d.   _____

e.   _____

14. Name three discharge procedures to be followed when a child with congenital heart disease is going home.

    a.   _____
    b.   _____
    c.   _____

References

American Dietetic Association. 1988. *Manual of clinical dietetics*. Chicago: American Dietetic Association.

Aristimuno, G. G. et al. 1984. Influence of persistent obesity in children on cardiovascular risk factors: The Bogalusa Heart Study. *Circulation* 69:895.

Food and Nutrition Board, National Research Council, National Academy of Sciences. 1989. *Recommended dietary allowances*. 10th ed. Washington, DC: National Academy Press.

Forbes, G. B., and C. W. Woodruff (eds.). 1985. *Pediatric nutrition handbook*. Elk Grove, IL: American Academy of Pediatrics.

Grant, S. M. 1987. *Pediatric nutrition: Theory and practice*. New York: Butterworth.

Kelts, D., and E. Jones. 1984. *Manual of pediatric nutrition*. Boston: Little, Brown.

Mayo Clinic. 1988. *Mayo Clinic diet manual*. Philadelphia: B. C. Dekker.

Mead Johnson Nutrition. 1990. *Pediatric products handbook*. Evansville, IL: Mead Johnson.

Nelson, W. E. et al. (eds.). 1983. *Textbook of pediatrics*, 12th ed. Philadelphia: W. B. Saunders.

Ohio Neonatal Nutritionists. 1985. *Nutritional care for high risk newborns*. Philadelphia: George F. Stickley.

Pipes, P. L. (ed.). 1988. *Nutrition in infancy and childhood*, 3rd ed. St Louis: Mosby.

Ross Laboratory. 1990. *Product handbook*. Columbus, OH: Ross Laboratory.

Walker, W. A., and J. B. Watkins (eds.). 1985. *Nutrition in pediatrics: Basic science and clinical application*. Boston: Little, Brown.

Module 25

Diet Therapy and Food Allergy

Time for completion

Activities: _____1½_____ hours

Optional examination: _1_ hour

Academic credit

Semester units: _²⁄₁₀_

Quarter units: _³⁄₁₀_

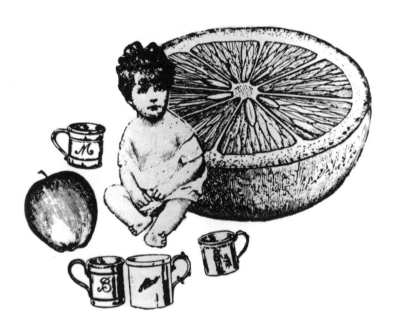

Outline

Objectives

Upon completion of this module the student should be able to:

1. Identify the most common food allergens.
2. Differentiate between food allergy and food intolerance.
3. Describe the symptoms and management of food allergies.
4. Identify testing that is used to diagnose and confirm food allergies.
5. Name the most common food offenders and their expected symptoms.
6. Explain how nutritional status is affected by food allergies.
7. Educate children and their caregivers about the management of allergies while maintaining adequate nutrition.

Glossary

Angioedema: swelling and spasm of the blood vessels, resulting in wheals.

Asthma: "panting," respiratory spasm and wheezing in an attempt to get more air.

Bronchitis: inflammation of the mucous membranes of one of the tubes leading to the lung.

Challenge diet: a diet designed to elicit a reaction by deliberately feeding a person certain ingredients, assuming the person is reactive to them.

Dermatitis: inflammation of the skin with symptoms such as itching, redness, and so on.

Eczema: acute or chronic inflammation of skin and immediately underneath it, with symptoms such as pus, discharge, and itching.

Elimination diet: a diet with certain ingredients removed, assuming a person is reactive to such ingredients. The disappearance of symptoms assumes that the person is reactive to the missing ingredients.

Immunoglobulin (Ig): one of a family of proteins that are capable of forming antibodies.

Mastitis: inflammation of the breasts.

Purpura: a variety of symptoms, e.g., hemorrhage into skin.

Urticaria: eruption of the skin with severe itching.

Wheals: *see* Urticaria.

Background Information

Allergy refers to an excess sensitivity to substances or conditions such as food; hair; cloth; biological, chemical, or mechanical agents; emotional excitement; extremes of temperature; and so on. The hypersensitivity and abnormal reactions associated with allergies produce various symptoms in affected people. The substance that triggers an allergic reaction is called an allergen or antigen, and it may enter the body through ingestion, injection, respiration, or physical contact.

In food allergies, the offending substance is usually, though not always, a protein. After digestion, it is absorbed into the circulatory system, where it encounters the body's immunological system. If this is the first exposure to the antigen, there are no overt clinical signs. Instead, the presence of an allergen causes the body to form immunoglobulins (Ig): IgA, IgE, IgG, and IgM. The organs, tissues, and blood of all healthy people contain antibodies that either circulate or remain attached to the cells where they are formed. When the body encounters the antigen a second time, the specific antibody will complex with it. Because the resulting complexes may or may not elicit clinical manifestations, merely identifying a specific immunoglobulin in the circulatory system will not indicate whether a person is allergic to a specific food antigen.

The human intestine is coated by the antibody IgA, which protects a person from developing a food allergy. However, infants under 7 months old have a lower amount of intestinal IgA. The mucosa thus permits incompletely digested protein molecules to enter. These can then enter the circulation and cause antibodies to form.

Children can also develop a food allergy called the delayed allergic reaction or hypesensitivity. The classic sign of this is the tension-fatigue syndrome. Children with the syndrome have a dull face, pallor, infraorbital circles, and nasal stuffiness. A delayed food allergy symptom is more difficult to diagnose than an immediate one.

Although food allergy is not age-specific, it is more prevalent during childhood. Because a reaction to food can impose stress and interfere with nutrient ingestion, absorption, and digestion, the growth and development of children with food allergies can be delayed. Half of the adult patients with food allergy claim that they had a childhood allergy as well. Apparently, a childhood food allergy rarely disappears completely in an adult. If a newborn baby develops hypersensitivity in the first 5 to 8 days of life, the pregnant mother was probably eating a large quantity of potentially offending foods, such as milk, eggs, chocolate, or wheat. The child becomes sensitized in the womb, and the allergic tendency may either continue into adult life or gradually decrease.

In clinical medicine, it is extremely important to differentiate food allergy from food intolerance. The former relates to the immunosystem of the body, while the latter is the direct result of maldigestion and malabsorption due to a lack of intestinal enzyme(s) or an indirect intestinal reaction because of psychological maladjustment.

ACTIVITY 1: Food Allergy and Children

Symptoms and Management

About 2 percent to 8 percent of all Americans have some form of food allergy. The clinical management of food allergy is controversial and has many problems. For instance, a food allergy is influenced by the amount of allergen consumed, whether the allergen is cooked or raw, and the cumulative effects from successive ingestions of the allergen. A person with a food allergy also tends to be allergic to one or more of the following: pollen, mold, wool, cosmetics, dust, and other inhalable items. Because these substances are so common, they are difficult to avoid.

Other difficulties in allergy management are as follows: (1) If a person is allergic to a food, even a very small amount can produce a reaction. (2) Some patients allergic to an item at one time are not at another. (3) Some patients react to an allergen only when they are tired, frustrated, or emotionally upset. (4) Although protein is suspected to be the substance most likely to cause allergy, people can be allergic to almost any food chemical.

In managing patients with food allergy, there are two basic objectives. First, the offending substance must be identified. Patients should then be placed on a monitored antiallergic diet to assure adequate nutrient intake, especially young patients whose growth and development may be adversely affected by the allergy.

The clinical reactions of patients allergic to a food vary from relatively mild ones such as skin rash, itchy eyes, or headache to more severe ones such as abdominal cramps, diarrhea, vomiting, and loss of appetite. Other symptoms include cough, asthma, bronchitis, purpura, urticaria, dermatitis, and various problems affecting the digestive tract (vomiting, colic, ulceration of colon, etc.). In children, undernutrition and arrested development may occur.

Milk Allergy

Many individuals of all ages develop an allergy as well as an intolerance to milk and milk products. The reaction may occur when a person is sick (e.g., with infection, alcoholism, surgery, or trauma). Thus, dietitians and nurses should always check to see whether a patient can tolerate milk. If the intolerance is due to a reduced activity of lactase, proper dietary therapy can be implemented.

Someone allergic to milk must also avoid many foods containing milk products. Ingesting regular homogenized fresh milk can damage the digestive mucosa of some susceptible individuals, especially children. The damaged cells bleed continuously but only minute amounts of blood are lost. The result is occult blood loss in the stool and iron-deficiency anemia. Professionals do not agree about whether this phenomenon is an allergic reaction. In rare cases, penicillin used in cows to prevent or control mastitis may leave a residue in milk. Consequently, some individuals who are allergic to the penicillin may have an allergic reaction to the inoculated cow's milk.

Breast milk is much preferred over cow's milk for feeding a baby in a family whose members have allergies. Cow's milk contains the protein Beta-lactoglobulin, which may trigger an allergic reaction, while breast milk does not. If an infant has symptoms of milk allergy, special formulas with soy or another protein source as a base can be safely substituted for milk.

However, breast-feeding does have one major problem when it is used to prevent an infant from having an allergic reaction to cow's milk. If the child is also allergic to substances such as cheese, crab, or chocolate, the mother can in effect feed them to her child via breast milk if she ingests them herself. Therefore, the breast-fed child may show allergic reactions.

Testing and Treatment

Food allergies are difficult to test for and subsequently to diagnose and confirm. Furthermore, patients with an allergic reaction to one food may in reality be allergic to many others that contain a common ingredient. Or, when an infant is allergic to a formula, it is usually assumed that the protein is responsible. In reality, it could be the vegetable oil base.

When food allergy is suspected in a child, the parents, nurse, and dietitian or nutritionist should work together to identify the culprit. The child's reactions to food coloring and additives (which are found in many processed foods) and salicylate-related chemicals should also be noted. Allergens are likely to be found in some of these items. Also, for a defined period, the parents should keep a complete record of food eaten by the child. Unless the culprit is one of the common offenders, it is difficult for the physician to make an accurate diagnosis because of the many different components in a child's diet.

Currently, two types of tests are available for diagnosing food allergy in children. None of them is guaranteed to identify an offending substance, although they can provide some information about the patient's reaction toward different foods. These two procedures are skin testing and elimination diets.

Skin testing for food allergy involves exposing the skin to the suspected offending chemical (from a food). If the patient is allergic, local swelling and inflammation develop from within a few minutes to a day after application. However, some clinicians use this test for preliminary diagnosis while others consider it useless and unreliable.

One method of diagnosing food allergy that has been somewhat successful is the use of elimination diets. Suspected items in the child's diet are removed one at a time. When symptoms disappear with the removal of the food and reappear with its reintroduction, this particular food is the likely offender. Unfortunately, it is not so simple in practice. Experiments like this with a child must take into consideration the nutritional adequacy of the diet when one item is removed. Nutrient supplements, especially vitamins and minerals, may be needed if the diet is long-term. This is especially important for children.

Consultation with a nurse, dietitian, or nutritionist is important, especially when such a diet is first implemented. At least one family member should also be involved. If the diet is to succeed, the diet instructions and implementation must be completely understood. Although a progressive elimination diet does not always yield positive results, total compliance is mandatory to maximize its effectiveness.

Food allergies can generally be determined by diet control. The suspected offender or offenders can be removed from the diet until all symptoms disappear. Then, the suspected foods can be reintroduced to the list one at a time. This process, known as elimination and challenges, can lead to identification of an offender. Treatment consists of avoiding the offender.

Nursing Implications _____

The nurse should be aware of the following principles when caring for children with allergies:

1. Diet therapy is used to identify allergic reactions and also to avoid these reactions.
2. Newborns of parents with allergies should be protected from potential allergens in breast milk.
3. Breast milk is the best food for a potentially allergic infant.
4. Pregnant women with a family history of allergies should avoid foods known to be allergens to reduce the risk of sensitizing the infant.
5. Solid foods should be introduced one at a time and evaluated over several days before adding another.
6. Delay introduction of solid foods in an infant's diet to reduce absorption of potential allergens in an immature GI tract.
7. Appropriate substitutions or supplementation of an allergic child's diet is essential to prevent malnutrition created by gaps in permitted foods.
8. Children who are allergic to eggs should never be immunized with vaccines grown on chick embryo.
9. Diabetic children allergic to pork are unable to use insulin made from hog pancreas.
10. Children with allergens should wear med alert tags.
11. Allergens are usually (though not always) proteins.
12. Raw foods are more likely to be allergens than cooked ones.
13. Parents and children should read all labels carefully and be taught to look for hidden sources of the allergen.
14. Foods that cause immediate allergic reactions in susceptible individuals are eggs, seafood, nuts, especially peanuts, and berries.
15. Foods that cause delayed reactions are wheat, milk legumes, corn, white potatoes, chocolate, and oranges (citrus).
16. Patients who are allergic to a specific food will react to other foods in the same family.
17. Foods that cause allergic responses may be reintroduced at a later time because children tend to outgrow food allergies.
18. Differentiate between food allergies and food intolerance. The treatments are very different.

PROGRESS CHECK ON BACKGROUND INFORMATION AND ACTIVITY 1

Fill-in

1. Define allergy. _____
   _____

2. Name the substance(s) that trigger allergic reactions. _____

3. Describe how IgA, IgE, IgG and IgM are formed in the body. _____
   _____

4. What is the delayed allergic reaction syndrome?
   _____
   _____

5. Describe the difference between a food allergy and a food intolerance. _____
   _____

6. Identify six major problems that arise in regard to management of food allergies.
   a. _____
   b. _____
   c. _____
   d. _____
   e. _____
   f. _____

7. Name the two basic diet objectives in allergy management.
   a. _____

b. _____

8. Why is breast milk preferred over cow's milk for feeding infants? _____
_____

9. Identify the two types of tests available for diagnosing children.

a. _____

b. _____

ACTIVITY 2: Common Offenders

Although food allergy rarely constitutes a serious, life-threatening concern, it results in chronic illness for many sufferers. This problem can be significantly eliminated if one is alert to the most common allergens and the manifestations of allergic reaction.

Cow's Milk

The allergen in cow's milk is probably the most common. A susceptible person may be allergic to whole, skimmed, evaporated, or dried milk, as well as to milk-containing products such as ice cream, cheese, custard, cream and creamed foods, and yogurt. If exquisite milk allergy exists, even butter and bread can create a reaction. Symptoms can include either or both constipation and diarrhea, abdominal pain, nasal and bronchial congestion, asthma, headache, foul breath, sweating, fatigue, and tension.

Kola Nut Products

Chocolate (cocoa) and cola are products obtained from the kola nut. An allergy to one almost always means an allergy to the other as well. Symptoms most commonly include headache, asthma, gastrointestinal allergy, nasal allergy, and eczema.

Corn

Because corn syrup is widely used commercially, corn allergy can result from a wide variety of foods. Candy, chewing gum, prepared meats, cookies, rolls, doughnuts, some breads, canned fruits, jams, jellies, some fruit juices, ice cream, and sweetened cereals all utilize corn syrup. Additionally, whole corn, cornstarch, corn flour, corn oil, and cornmeal can cause allergic reactions to such foods as cereals, tortillas, tamales, enchiladas, soups, beer, whiskey, fish sticks, and pancake or waffle mixes.

Symptoms can be bizarre, ranging from allergic tension to allergic fatigue. Headache can take the form of migraine.

Eggs

Those with severe allergy to eggs can react to even their odor. Egg allergy can also cause reaction to vaccines, since they are often grown on chicken embryo. Allergic reactions are generally to such foods as eggs themselves, baked goods, candies, mayonnaise, creamy dressings, meat loaf, breaded foods, and noodles.

Symptoms can be widely varied, as with milk. Egg allergy often results in urticaria (hives) though, like chocolate, larger amounts are usually necessary to produce that symptom. Other symptoms include headache, gastrointestinal allergy, eczema, and asthma.

Peas (Legumes)

The larger family of plants that are collectively known as peas include peanuts, soybeans, beans, and peas. Peanuts tend to be the greatest offender, and dried beans and peas cause more difficulties than fresh ones. Products that can cause selected allergy reaction are honey (made from the offending plants) and licorice, a legume. Soybean allergy presents a problem similar to corn owing to its widespread use in the form of soybean concentrate or soybean oil.

Legume allergies can be quite severe, even resulting in shock. They commonly cause headache and can be especially troublesome for asthma patients, urticaria patients, and angioedema sufferers.

Citrus Fruits

Oranges, lemons, limes, grapefruit, and tangerines can cause eczema and hives and often, asthma. They commonly cause canker sores (aphthous stomatitis). Although citrus fruit allergy does not cause allergy to artificial orange and lemon-lime drinks, if patients are allergic to citric acid in the fruits then they will also react to tart artificial drinks and may also react to pineapple.

Tomatoes

This fruit, commonly called a vegetable, can cause hives, eczema, and canker sores. It can also cause asthma. In addition to its natural form, it can be encountered in soups, pizza, catsup, salads, meat loaf, and tomato paste or tomato juice.

Wheat and Other Grains

Wheat, rice, barley, oats, millet, and rye are known allergens, with wheat the commonest of the group. Wheat occurs in many dietary products. All common baked goods, cream sauce, macaroni, noodles, pie crust, cereals, chili, and breaded foods contain wheat.

Reaction to wheat and its related grains can be severe. Asthma and gastrointestinal disturbances are the most common reactions.

Spices

Of various spices that can cause allergic reaction, cinnamon is generally the most potent. It can be found in catsup, chewing gum, candy, cookies, cakes, rolls, prepared meats, and pies. Bay leaf allergy generally occurs as well, since this spice is related to cinnamon. Pumpkin pie reactions are common owing to their high cinnamon content. Other spices most frequently mentioned as allergens are black pepper, white pepper, oregano, the mints, paprika, and cumin.

Artificial Food Colors

Although various artificial food colors have been implicated in such problems as hyperactive syndrome in children, as allergens the two most common offenders are amaranth (red dye) and tartrazine (yellow dye). Amaranth is most often encountered, but reactions to tartrazine tend to be more severe. Food colors occur in carbonated beverages, some breakfast drinks, bubble gum, flavored ice foods, gelatin desserts, and such medications as antibiotic syrups.

Other Food Allergens

Any food is capable of producing an allergic reaction. However, those offenders often mentioned after the top ten are pork and beef, onion and garlic, white potatoes, fish, coffee, shrimp, bananas, and walnuts and pecans.

Vegetables, other than those already mentioned, rarely cause allergic reactions. Fruits that usually are safe include cranberries, blueberries, figs, cherries, apricots, and plums. Chicken, turkey, lamb, and rabbit have proven to be the safest meats. Tea, olives, sugar, and tapioca are also relatively safe foods, although some herbal teas can cause unique difficulties.

PROGRESS CHECK ON ACTIVITY 2

Multiple Choice

1. The most common offender to trigger allergies is
   a. wheat.
   b. cow's milk.
   c. corn.
   d. eggs.

2. The most common artificial food colors to trigger allergies in susceptible children include
   a. amaranth and tantrazine.
   b. tyrosine and amaranth.
   c. chlorophyll and rubella.
   d. melanine and xanthine.

3. Egg allergies can cause reaction to vaccines because
   a. egg yolk is a very common allergen in children.
   b. egg forms a complex with the drug causing the reaction.
   c. the vaccine is grown on a chicken embryo.
   d. all of the above.

True/False

4. T F Allergic reactions to chocolate include asthma and eczema.
5. T F Corn allergies do not develop from ingestion of corn syrup.
6. T F People with severe allergies to eggs can react to their odor.
7. T F Legume allergies are not usually as severe as milk allergies.
8. T F Citrus allergy sufferers usually do not react to artificial citrus flavors.
9. T F The most common grain allergen is wheat.
10. T F The most potent spice allergen is ginger.

References

Bahna, S. I., and D.C. Heiner. 1980. Allergies to milk. New York: Grune & Stratton.

Breneman, J. C. (ed.). 1987 *Handbook of food allergies*. New York: Marcel Dekker.

Brostoff, J., and S. J. Challacombe (eds.). 1987. *Food allergy and intolerance*. Philadelphia: Saunders.

Butkus, S. N. et al. 1986. Food allergies: Immunological reactions to food. *Journal of the American Dietetic Association* 85(5):601.

Cant, A. J. 1985. Food allergy in childhood. *Human Nutrition: Applied Nutrition* 39A:277.

Chandra, R. K. (ed.). 1987. *Food allergy*. St. John's, Newfoundland: Nutrition Research Foundation.

Chandra, R.K. 1988. Food allergy. In *Modern nutrition in health and disease*, 7th ed. M.E. Shils and V. R. Young (eds.). Philadelphia: Lea & Febiger.

Clinical pocket manual: Pediatric care. 1987. Springhouse Corp.

Dong, F. M. 1984. *All about food allergy*. Philadelphia: George F. Stickley.

Kempe, C. H., H. K. Silver, D. O'Brien, and V. A. Fulginiti (eds.). 1987. *Current pediatric diagnosis and treatment*. East Norwalk, CT: Appleton & Lange.

May, C. D. 1980. Food allergy: Perspective, principles,

practical management. *Nutrition Today* 15:28.

Pillitteri, Adele. 1987. *Child health nursing: Care of the growing family*, 3rd ed. Boston: Little, Brown.

Sly, R. M. 1981. *Pediatric allergy*. New York: Medical Examination Publishing.

Thomas, L. L. 1980. *Caring and cooking for the allergic child*. New York: Sterling.

Module 26

Diet Therapy
and Phenylketonuria

Time for completion
Activities: _____1_____ hour
Optional examination: _½_ hour

Academic credit
Semester units: _²⁄₁₀_
Quarter units: _³⁄₁₀_

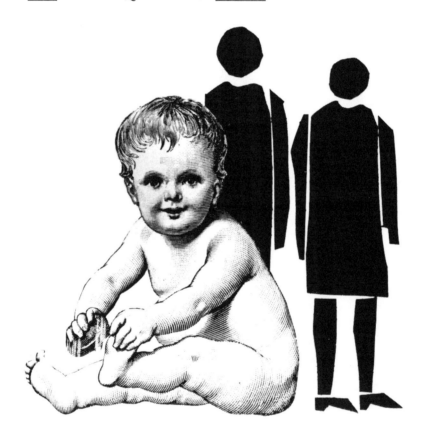

Outline

Objectives

Upon completion of this module, the student should be able to:

1. Explain the etiology of phenylketonuria (PKU).
2. Identify the method of diagnosing PKU.
3. Relate the symptoms of untreated PKU.
4. Describe the dietary management of PKU:
   a. requirements
   b. restrictions
   c. appropriate supplements
5. Evaluate the controversies regarding terminating diet therapy and restricted diet during pregnancy.
6. Discuss the responsibilities of the health team for follow-up care in monitoring the progress of a PKU child.
7. List health team interventions appropriate to successful dietary management of PKU children.
8. Provide information to caregivers on diet management, resources, and counseling as necessary.

Glossary

Casein hydrolysate: principal protein of milk, partially digested.

Eczema: a superficial inflammatory process of the skin, marked by redness, itching, scaling, sometimes weeping and oozing.

Electroencephalogram (EEG):   the recording of changes in the electrical potential of the brain by evaluating the brain waves.

Fibrinogen: a protein in the blood necessary for clotting.

Mental retardation: significantly subaverage general intellectual functioning existing along with deficits in adaptive behavior, which manifests itself during the developmental period.

Phenylketonuria (PKU):   an inborn error of amino acid metabolism.

Plasma: fluid portion of the blood in which corpuscles are suspended.

Reticulosarcoma: a type of malignant tumor; a lymphoid neoplasm; also called stem cell lymphoma and undifferentiated malignant lymphoma.

Serum: plasma from which fibrinogen has been removed in the process of clotting.

Background Information

Each of the eight to ten essential amino acids in the human body is metabolized via a unique pathway. Some infants are born with a defect in one of the enzyme systems that regulate one or more of these pathways. As a result, if the amino acid is not metabolized properly, certain products may accumulate in the blood or urine. If this occurs, an inborn error of metabolism for that particular amino acid results.

One example of faulty protein metabolism involves phenylalanine and tyrosine. Although both substances are essential amino acids, the body derives part of its tyrosine needs from phenylalanine with the help of a certain enzyme (phenylalanine hydroxylase). A newborn may have no or very low activity of this enzyme, and as a result the body is unable to change phenylalanine to tyrosine. Consequently, the chemicals phenylalanine, phenylpyruvic acid, and other metabolites accumulate. If they exceed certain levels in the blood, they cross the brain barriers (membranes) and the child suffers mental retardation. It is currently believed that about 1 in 10,000 newborns inherit this disorder, commonly referred to as phenylketonuria (PKU), which causes a high level of phenylpyruvic acid in the urine. Immediately after birth the baby appears normal, but the child soon becomes slightly irritable and hyperactive. The urine has a musty odor.

If the disorder is not diagnosed and treated, the child will develop aggressive behavior, unstable muscular and nervous systems, eczema, convulsions, and seizures. Since tyrosine is responsible for making pigments, its decreased supply results in decreased coloration, with such effects as decreased body pigmentation, blue eyes, a fair complexion, and blond hair in Caucasian patients. Some patients develop reticulosarcoma-like skin lesions. Severe mental retardation may result. The accumulation of chemicals in the blood interferes with the normal development of the central nervous system and the brain. Some young children show abnormal electroencephalograms. In spite of all these adverse symptoms, the child shows a normal birth weight.

Since a method of diagnosing PKU in newborns was developed in the 1960s, its use has become widespread. The method, known as the Guthrie test, involves analyzing blood drawn from the child's heel. A normal infant's blood contains about 1 to 2 mg of phenylalanine/100 mL of plasma, while that of a PKU child is about 15 to 30 mg/100 mL plasma. However, a positive Guthrie test does not necessarily indicate PKU, because transient high blood phenylalanine may occur in some infants. Thus, additional tests are required for confirmation. Forty-six states now mandate that all newborns be screened for PKU. The remaining states practice voluntary screening.

The Guthrie test is normally done before the baby is removed from the nursery, two to five days after birth. At one month of age, the test is repeated, especially for babies who show high blood phenylalanine during the first blood screening. A blood level of over 4 mg phenylalanine/100 mL plasma may indicate that additional tests are needed. A level of 20 mg/100 mL positively indicates PKU.

PROGRESS CHECK ON BACKGROUND INFORMATION

Multiple Choice

Circle the letter of the correct answer.

1. PKU may be defined as an inborn error of metabolism because
   a. amino acids have a separate pathway from other nutrients.
   b. there is a defect in the enzyme system that regulates certain amino acids.
   c. the amino acids accumulate in the urine.
   d. the mother's diet was very low in amino acids.

2. The absent or limited enzyme that causes the symptoms of PKU to develop is
   a. lactase-galactase.
   b. gliadin.
   c. phenylalanine hydroxylase.
   d. phenylpyruvic acid.

3. The level of phenylalanine in a normal baby's blood is _____/100 mL plasma, while in that of a PKU baby it is _____/100 mL plasma.

   a. 1–2 mg; 15–30 mg
   b. 12–15 mg; 30–40 mg
   c. 30–40 mg; 65–75 mg
   d. 10–20 mg; 50–100 mg

4. The most prominent symptom of untreated PKU is
   a. aggressive behavior.
   b. decreased skin coloration/skin lesions.
   c. convulsions.
   d. severe mental retardation.

5. The diagnostic test for PKU is done
   a. one month after birth.
   b. two to five days after birth.
   c. at birth.
   d. any time before the first year.

True/False

Circle T for True and F for False.

6. **T F** A positive reaction to a Guthrie test always indicates that a baby has PKU.

7. **T F** It is mandatory in the United States that all states screen new babies for PKU.

ACTIVITY 1: Phenylketonuria and Dietary Management

Treatment and Requirement

The dietary management for PKU children consists of rigidly restricting phenylalanine intake. For most patients, if treatment starts one to two months after birth, mental and physical development is likely to be normal. If treatment starts after retardation has already occurred, normal mental ability may not return completely, but there will be no further deterioration and no recurrence of symptoms. Although the intake of phenylalanine must be restricted, these children still need a minimal amount of the amino acid for growth and development, in addition to an adequate supply of all other essential nutrients.

A newborn child needs about 65 to 90 mg of phenylalanine per kilogram of body weight, while a two-year-old needs 20 to 25 mg. Thus, an infant should be provided with enough phenylalanine to maintain a level of 3 to 10 mg per 100 mL of blood. If a particular level of intake raises serum levels to abnormally high concentrations, the level must be lowered. Conversely, the serum level must not be allowed to fall below acceptable limits.

Lofenalac and Phenylalanine Food Exchange Lists

Since phenylalanine is an essential amino acid, it is found in most animal products, including milk, which is the main nutritional component of an infant's diet. Thus, milk has to be specially processed to remove part or all of the phenylalanine. For a number of years most practitioners have used the commercial powder Lofenalac (Mead Johnson). It is a special low-protein powder containing casein hydrolysate with about 95 percent of the phenylalanine removed. It is also supplemented with vitamins and minerals.

Because Lofenalac contains less than 1 percent phenylalanine, it cannot support normal growth and development of a child. As a result, specified amounts of natural foods are commonly provided to increase the child's phenylalanine intake, such as evaporated or whole milk. As the child grows, additional solid foods are given. Close monitoring of the child's nutrient intake is essential. Table 26-1 compares the phenylalanine, calorie, and protein content of Lofenalac with that of evaporated and whole milk. Table 26-2 describes the phenylalanine, energy, and protein intake for a PKU patient under one year old.

To provide the PKU child with regular food, the phenylalanine, protein, and calorie contents of regular foods must be known. As a result, young children's foods are grouped into exchange lists, each of which contains food items that contribute equivalent amounts of phenylalanine.

The Division of Medical Genetics at the Children's Hospital of Los Angeles and the Public Health Service developed and coordinated the currently used dietary

TABLE 26-1
Calorie, Phenylalanine, and Protein Contents of Lofenalac and Milk

Food	Amount	Kilocalories	Protein (g)	Phenylalanine (g)
Lofenalac	10 g	45.4	1.5	0.008
Milk				
evaporated	29–30 g (1 oz.)	44	2.2	106
whole	29–30 g (1 oz.)	19.7	1.1	51

guidelines for management of PKU. Dietary management has two purposes: an appropriate substitute for milk (especially for the infant) and guidelines for adding solid foods. Lofenalac is the milk substitute most generally used in the United States. It contains approximately 5 percent phenylalanine. Other products that are phenylalanine-free can be used by older children and pregnant mothers. This allows them a bigger variety of foods before they reach the limits of the phenylalanine allowance in their diet.

Caregivers, nurses, and physicians must bear the primary responsibility for providing and continuing care so that the child with PKU will grow and develop normally. This requires a coordinated effort of understanding the absolute necessity of following the diet carefully. Patience is very important as counseling, guidance, and education are provided. Teaching guides and materials are available to help in planning and follow-up. Home health nurses may provide follow-up care and reinforcement. Social services and support groups are also good adjuncts to assist in the vigilance required.

Special Considerations

When feeding a patient with PKU, several considerations should be kept in mind. First, calories and taste should be varied. Second, special low-protein products are available and can also be used to advantage. Request a list from dietitians or nurses. Third, patients should avoid meat and dairy products (except the permitted milk). Fourth, the feeding regimen must be consistent with the age and development of the child, and the food quantity and texture must be adjusted to the child's eating ability. Fifth, the nutritional adequacy of the child's diet should be constantly evaluated, using the RDAs as a guide.

One of the most controversial issues in treating a child with PKU is the uncertainty about when to terminate dietary restrictions. Some children are put on a normal diet at the age of five, when further mental progress may require additional phenylalanine. Other clinicians keep the child on a phenylalanine-restricted diet indefinitely. For some children, these restrictions may necessitate the

TABLE 26-2
Suggested Phenylalanine, Energy, and Protein Intakes per Day for PKU Patients under One Year Old

Age (months)*	Amount of Nutrient Needed per Kilogram Body Weight			Lofenalac		Milk (oz.)	
	Phenyl-alanine (mg)	Protein (g)	Kilocalories	Protein provided by product to child's need (%)	Measures[†] permitted per kilogram body weight	Whole	Evaporated
0–2½	85	4.4	125	85	2½–3	2–4	1–3
2½–6½	65	3.3	115	85	2–2½	2–4	1–2½
6½–9½	45	2.5	105	90	1½–2	1½–2½	½–1½
9½–12	32	2.5	105	90	1½–2	½–1½	½–1

Note: the child may or may not need additional foods. See text.
*The separation between age groups is not exact.
[†]One measure equals 1 tbsp., containing about 10 g of powder.
An example: a one-month-old child is permitted 2 to 4 oz. whole milk (or 1 to 3 oz. evaporated milk) and 2½ to 3 measures of Lofenalac per kilogram body weight per day.

TABLE 26-3
Contents of Calories, Protein, and
Phenylalanine in Some Selected Foods

Food	Phenyl-alanine (mg)	Protein (g)	Kilo-calories
Gerber's strained and junior vegetables			
carrots, 5 tbsp.	15	0.5	21
sweet potatoes, 1½ tbsp.	15	0.3	15
Gerber's strained and junior fruits			
applesauce, 7 tbsp.	10	0.2	81
apricots with tapioca, 8 tbsp.	10	0.5	88
orange-pineapple juice, 11 tbsp.	10	0.8	41
peaches, 3 tbsp.	10	0.3	35
Gerber's baby cereals			
barley cereal, 1¼ tbsp.	18	0.4	11
rice with mixed fruit (in jar), 1¾ tbsp.	18	0.3	13
rice with strawberries, 2¼ tbsp.	18	0.5	21
Total	124	3.8	326

use of vitamin and mineral supplements. More research is needed to resolve this issue.

It should be noted that if a restrictive diet is discontinued, the child and family go through a very important transition period. The parents and the child will need time and patience to adapt to this sudden exposure to meat and a whole variety of other foods.

It was recently discovered that some babies are born with only a transient form of hyperphenylalaninemia. These children also require medical attention. The infants must be identified and treated to prevent possible mental retardation.

Successful management of PKU babies over the years has allowed them to attain normal growth and develop into healthy adults. Now the young women are having babies of their own. The pregnant woman with PKU is at high risk, but the fetal risks are even higher. The major hazards to the fetus are congenital deformities and mental retardation. Untreated PKU during a pregnancy also leads to higher rates of stillbirth and/or prematurity.

Careful screening and counseling is necessary for identified PKU potential mothers. Their pregnancies should be carefully planned and they should go on a restricted phenylalanine diet. Since PKU diets are low in protein, their diet must be strictly constructed and monitored by a clinical dietitian throughout the pregnancy. Low-phenylalanine formulas and food products become the mainstay of the diet.

Many authorities strongly recommend that PKU children, especially girls, remain on their diets throughout life. In this way, some of the dangers of pregnancy can be minimized.

TABLE 26-4
Sample Menu Plan for a
9-Month-Old Child with PKU

Breakfast
Lofenalac formula, 6 oz.
Rice with strawberries, Gerber's baby cereal, 2¼ tbsp.
Carrots, Gerber's strained and junior vegetables, 5 tbsp.

Mid-Morning Feeding
Peaches, Gerber's strained and junior fruit, 3 tbsp.

Lunch
Lofenalac formula, 6 oz.
Cereal, barley, Gerber's baby cereal, 1¼ tbsp.
Apricots with tapioca, Gerber's strained and junior fruit, 8 tbsp.
Orange-pineapple juice, Gerber's strained and junior fruit, 5 tbsp.

Mid-Afternoon Feeding
Applesauce, 7 tbsp.

Dinner
Lofenalac formula, 6 oz.
Rice with mixed fruit (in jar), Gerber's baby cereal, 1¾ tbsp.
Sweet potatoes, Gerber's strained and junior vegetables, 1½ tbsp.

Bedtime Feeding
Lofenalac formula, 6 oz.
Orange-pineapple juice, Gerber's strained and junior fruit, 6 tbsp.

Follow-Up Care

The health team must monitor progress after a child is placed on a phenylalanine-restricted diet. During the first few weeks of the diet, the child's blood should be tested twice. After the child has been on the diet for a brief period and his or her clinical condition has improved and stabilized, blood tests should be performed weekly until the child is one year old. Later, the toddler's blood should be tested once every two to three weeks. When all symptoms have disappeared and the child has adapted to the diet, the blood tests can be done monthly.

The dietary supply and blood levels of phenylalanine are strongly correlated with the height and weight gains of the child. If children get an insufficient amount of phenylalanine, they will become lethargic, have stunted growth, and lose their appetite. More severe effects include mental retardation, clinical deterioration (fever, coma), and even death. Also, when children with PKU become sick or have infections, blood phenylalanine may rise to unacceptable levels.

Nursing Implications

Nursing responsibilities for treating a child with PKU are as follows:

1. Be aware that dietary management is the only treatment for children with PKU.
2. The diet for PKU must meet two criteria.
   a. It must meet the child's nutritional needs for growth and development.
   b. It must maintain phenylalanine levels within a safe range.
3. The diet therapy is very strict and presents difficulties to the families or caregivers.
4. Lofenalac and Phenyl Free are very expensive; financial aid may be required. Funding sources should be furnished to the parents.
5. Frequent monitoring of urinary and blood levels of phenylalanine are necessary.
6. Careful dietary records as well as height and weight records must be maintained to monitor diet adequacy.
7. While brain damage is irreversible, diet therapy will limit its progress.
8. Restricting phenylalanine in older children with PKU may be beneficial in improving behavior and motor ability, as well as decreasing eczema.
9. The meaning of the treatment must be explained to the health team and the parents. Successful control of PKU requires that the family learn to
   a. plan the baby's diet.
   b. monitor food intake.
   c. take blood samples.
   d. keep accurate records of intake and state of health.
   e. cope with normal developmental stages.
10. Therapeutic communication is necessary to allow parents to voice feelings of guilt, fear, and frustration and to attain a healthy outlook.
11. Provide information on
   a. signs of inadequate phenylalanine intake: anorexia, vomiting, listlessness.
   b. situations that require increased amounts of phenylalanine, such as during periods of rapid growth and during febrile illnesses.
   c. possible deficiencies in other nutrients: intake of manganese, zinc, and niacin may be low when the primary protein source is synthetic.
12. Closely monitor hemoglobin levels, since protein is severely restricted.
13. Lofenalac provides 454 calories, 15 grams protein, 60 grams carbohydrate, and 18 grams fat per 100 mg powder.
14. Special products such as low-protein flour, cookies, pasta, and other bakery items can be purchased to augment this severe diet and increase carbohydrate intake.
15. Recognize that primary diet teaching may require the services of a specialist, and the nurse may prefer to reinforce the teaching and encourage compliance.

PROGRESS CHECK ON ACTIVITY 1

Multiple Choice

Circle the letter of the correct answer.

1. The objectives of dietary management of the child with phenylketonuria (PKU) include
   a. lowering phenylalanine content to the minimum requirement for growth by calculating the diet for phenylalanine content.
   b. removing all milk and milk products from the diet.
   c. removing all protein foods from the diet.
   d. all of the above.

2. From the following list of lunch menus, choose the one most appropriate for a PKU youngster who is 2½ years old:
   a. 2 tbsp. roast beef, ½ slice bread, ¼ c. green beans, ½ banana, ½ c. Lofenalac
   b. 1 hard boiled egg, raw carrot sticks, 2 Ritz crackers, 1 pear half, ½ c. Lofenalac
   c. ¼ c. sliced beets, ¼ c. green beans, 3 tbsp. boiled potato, ½ c. Lofenalac vanilla pudding with whipped topping, apple juice
   d. 4 potato chips, 1 graham cracker with butter, ½ c. Lofenalac vanilla pudding, 8 oz. cola

3. In which of the following persons with PKU could the diet be safely liberalized?
   a. pregnant female
   b. 20-year-old male
   c. 4-year-old female
   d. 2-year-old male

4. The young parents of an infant consistently forget to give the child the required milk allowance in addition to his Lofenalac. The following may be expected:
   a. the child will become allergic to milk
   b. the child's growth and development will be retarded
   c. the child will develop a lactose intolerance
   d. the child will become hyperactive

5. If dietary treatment starts after mental retardation occurs, the following may be expected:
   a. the brain will continue its deterioration
   b. no further deterioration will take place
   c. the mental retardation will be reversed and the child will become normal
   d. physical growth will be retarded

6. Phenylalanine may not be omitted from the infant's diet because
   a. as an essential amino acid, it must be supplied by diet or the infant will fail to develop.
   b. the electrolytes of the body will be in negative balance.
   c. it must be in the diet to produce tyrosine.
   d. the child will get bradycardia.

7. The diet of the PKU child must be calculated for
   a. phenylalanine, tyrosine, and histamine.
   b. protein, carbohydrate, and fat.
   c. phenylalanine, protein, and calories.
   d. calcium, iron, and ascorbic acid.

8. Techniques that promote compliance when feeding a PKU child include
   a. varying taste by using allowed flavorings and seasonings.
   b. using low-protein grain products for variety.
   c. adjusting quantity and texture to child's eating ability.
   d. all of the above.

9. Insufficient phenylalanine will result in which of the following symptoms?
   a. stunted growth
   b. anorexia, lethargy
   c. mental retardation
   d. all of the above

True/False

Circle T for True and F for False.

10. T F Feeding must be consistent with age and development.
11. T F Nutritional adequacy must be constantly evaluated.
12. T F Meat and milk are not used in the diet plan for PKU, except for a small quantity of evaporated milk daily.
13. T F PKU is a self-limiting disorder: the child will "grow out of it" as he or she grows up.

Fill-in

14. List five steps necessary to the planning of an adequate diet for PKU.
   a. _____
   b. _____
   c. _____
   d. _____
   e. _____

15. Describe three ways to vary calories and taste in a PKU diet without unbalancing it.
   a. _____
   b. _____
   c. _____

References

Acosta, P. B. et al. 1985. *Protocol for nutrition support of maternal PKU*. Bethesda, MD: U.S. Department of Health and Human Services, National Institutes of Health, National Institute of Child Health and Human Development.

American Academy of Pediatrics. 1985. *Final report, task force on the dietary management of metabolic disorders*. Chicago: American Academy of Pediatrics.

Betz, C. L., and E. C. Poster. 1989. *Mosby's pediatric nursing reference*. St. Louis: Mosby.

Caballero, B. 1985. Dietary management of inborn errors of amino acid metabolism. *Clin. Nutr.* 4(3):85

Elsas, L. J., and P. B. Acosta. 1988. Nutrition support of inherited metabolic diseases. In *Modern nutrition in health and disease*, 7th ed. M. E. Shils and V. R. Young (eds.). Philadelphia: Lea & Febiger.

Friedman, E. G. et al. 1988. Report from the Maternal PKU Collaborative Study. *Metabolic Currents* 1(1):4.

Kennedy, B. et al. 1985. Nutrition support of inborn errors of amino acid metabolism. *Int. J. Biomed. Comput* 17:69.

Martin, S. B. et al. 1987. Nutrition support of phenylketonuria and maple syrup urine disease. *Top. Clin. Nutr.* 2(3):9.

Schuett, V. E. 1987. Inborn errors of metabolism in the United States: An overview. *Top. Clin. Nutr.* 2(3):1.

Schuett, V. E. 1988. *Low protein food list, low protein cookery for phenylketonuria*, 2nd ed. Madison: University of Wisconsin Press.

Stanbury, J. B. et al. (eds.). 1983. *The metabolic basis of inherited disease*, 5th ed. New York: McGraw Hill.

Module 27

Diet Therapy for Constipation, Diarrhea, and High-Risk Infants

Time for completion
Activities: _____1_____ hour
Optional examination: ½ hour

Academic credit
Semester units: 2/10
Quarter units: 3/10

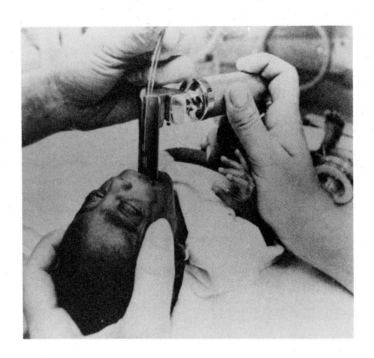

Outline

Objectives

Upon completion of this module the student should be able to:

1. Describe the normal patterns and characteristics of bowel movements in infants and young children.
2. Identify deviations from normal when
   a. constipation is the problem.
   b. diarrhea is the problem.
3. Identify the major causes of constipation and diarrhea.
4. List the major purposes of diet therapy for constipation and diarrhea in infants and children.
5. Identify the types of feedings necessary to meet the goals of diet therapy in these disorders.
6. Describe the strategies the health professional would teach caregivers to prevent further problems.
7. Name the categories of high-risk infants requiring specialized nutritional therapy.
8. Describe the types of feedings necessary to meet the individual needs of each infant.
9. Exhibit proficiency in the selection of formulas and recommended feeding methods.
10. Teach all caregivers the pertinent facts they must know in order to adequately nourish their high-risk infant.

Glossary

Benign: not malignant, not recurrent.
Electrolyte: a chemical substance, which, when dissolved in water or melted, dissociates into electrically charged particles (ions).

Fiber (dietary): that portion of undigested foods that cannot be broken down by enzymes, so it passes through the intestine and colon undigested.
Immune (immunological): highly resistant to a disease because of developed antibodies or development of immunologically competent cells or both.
Meconium: mucilagenous material in the intestine of the full-term fetus.
Mucilage: aqueous solution of a gummy substance.
Osmolarity: concentrating a solution in terms of osmoles of solutes per liter of solution (osmolality).
Osmosis: passage of a solvent from a solution of lesser to one of greater solute concentration when separated by a membrane.
Prematurity: underdevelopment; born or interrupted before maturity or occurring before the proper time.
Residue: that which remains in the intestine after the removal of other substances; a remainder.
Suppository: a medicated mass used for introduction into the rectum, urethra, or vagina.

Background Information

Space limitation has excluded modules covering diet therapy for a number of other clinical disorders of infancy and childhood. This module remedies the situation by providing student activities to cover three important clinical subjects not yet discussed. They include: constipation, diarrhea, and high-risk infants.

The student should use the references provided at the end of this module to obtain more details to supplement the activities provided.

ACTIVITY 1: Constipation

Background Information

Patterns of bowel movements among children and infants vary. If a child is active, passes a soft to slightly compact stool, gains weight progressively, shows normal development, and is free from any known clinical disorder, the mother has no reason to worry.

A newborn may have a constipation problem that is most likely the result of plugging by meconium. Constipation in an older infant is usually due to a change in the type of feeding. An anatomical defect may also be a cause, but this is rare. There are several ways to recognize the presence of constipation in a young infant:

1. A change in the stool (number, consistency, texture, appearance).
2. Pain in the infant when defecating.

3. Distended abdomen with or before every bowel movement.
4. Very black or bloody stools.

The constipation of many newborns disappears shortly after discharge from the hospital. If this does not occur, the mother should consult her pediatrician.

Infants

Constipation in a baby may be caused by a change in diet. Some babies develop constipation when breast-feeding is replaced with formula (homemade or commercial). Characteristic signs include the face turning red, straining, and the legs turned upward while defecating, even though the child may pass a soft stool. The doctor will evaluate the child after being informed of the symptoms. The doctor first looks for any obstruction that may require special medical attention. If no obstruction is found, the mother should be advised of the benign nature of the constipation and told that the child's bowel habits will return to normal after it adapts to the new formula. Actually, the stools of some infants change from soft to hard even if they are not constipated.

Other babies develop constipation when they are switched from liquid or strained food to solid food. The signs of such constipation vary. In some infants, a day with normal bowel movements is followed by one with none. In others, the passing of hard stools is accompanied by crying and intense straining. Many of these cases are of unknown origin. A typical cause is excessive water absorption (reabsorption) by the colon, resulting in dry stools and constipation. The anal passage may be stretched, causing pain and bleeding if there is an open wound. The child passes red stools, which are easily observed on toilet paper. The management of this form of constipation consists of a reduction in milk intake and an increased intake of juices, fruits, and fluids. Some clinicians may prescribe enemas, laxatives, and suppositories, such as a glycerine suppository. The dosage and frequency of application of these drugs must be determined with care.

Simple home remedies have proven effective in managing constipated infants, making a visit to the doctor unnecessary. Because of the high osmotic effect of sugars, adding 1 teaspoon of table sugar to 4 to 5 ounces of formula or water can help some infants to defecate. If the child can eat solid foods, the use of prune juice, apricots, and baby cereals containing bran or fiber is also beneficial, although the amount used should not be excessive, for example, under ½ ounce in any one feeding. Some foods appear more likely to cause constipation than others, such as bananas, barley, and rice cereal, but this claim is presently being debated. Sick babies may also develop constipation if they do not take in an adequate amount of formula or if they have a fever.

Young Children

Constipation in children under 4 or 5 years old is of two types: psychological and anatomical. The latter refers to a defect in the muscles regulating the defecation process. In some children under 2 years old, any initial sign of constipation can create a psychological barrier to defecation. When children start passing hard stools, they experience some pain, so they subsequently strain to retain the stools in order to reduce the pain. The accumulated feces become larger and harder, causing more pain in subsequent defecations. Some parents report that their children turn red in the face, strain, and arch their backs during bowel movement. Though toilet trained, they soil their pants fre-

quently and are reluctant to go to the bathroom. Some parents complain that these children are lazy. In this case, the parental attitudes make the constipation problem worse. This psychological barrier to bowel movement can be difficult to overcome.

On the other hand, constipation in some children results from fecal impaction, which may develop for a number of reasons. For instance, children between the ages of five and eight may develop constipation because they consider visiting the bathroom a waste of time. How are older children with a constipation problem managed? The basic principles are similar to those for an adult. If the parents consult a physician, the doctor may need to study the problem and advise the parents about what actions to take.

As a start, the parents may help the child initiate a good bowel movement by using an enema. The dose, which may be large at the beginning, may be used until a defecation pattern of three to five times a day is established. However, if a laxative such as mineral oil is used, care must be taken to avoid the potential loss of fat-soluble vitamins. Next, the child should be put on a conditioning schedule, such as 10 to 20 minutes daily on the toilet. The child should also be encouraged to have bowel movements as frequently as possible. At the same time, milk intake may be reduced to 60 percent to 80 percent of normal, and the intake of fruits, juices, and bran cereals increased. A diet high in fiber and fluid should be designed for future use to aid in regulation.

Nursing Implications

Health care personnel should

1. Be aware of the signs and symptoms of constipation in the infant.
2. Be prepared to counsel parents about the possible reasons for constipation in their child.
3. Consult the physician regarding the diagnosis of constipation in any given infant before educating the parents.
4. Expect that signs of constipation may be different for individual infants.
5. Teach the caregivers the necessity of precision of dosage and monitoring of any drugs prescribed by a physician.
6. If the infant is on solid food, food sources that relieve constipation in adults will also, in smaller proportions, help the child to defecate.
7. Be alert for psychological problems that prevent defecation in the young child.
8. Assist the caregivers to help the child initiate regular bowel habits.

PROGRESS CHECK ON ACTIVITY 1

Multiple Choice

1. All except which of these characteristics indicate that a child is not constipated?
   a. steady weight gain
   b. good appetite
   c. one to three bowel movements daily
   d. active

2. Newborns' constipation problems are most likely the result of a(n)
   a. change in feeding.
   b. anatomical defect.
   c. clinical disorder.
   d. change in routine.

3. Safe food(s) that may be used to combat constipation in infants include
   a. prune juice.
   b. 1 teaspoon sugar/4 ounces of formula.
   c. strained apricots.
   d. all of the above.

4. Recommended treatment for dry, hard stools in an infant is to
   a. increase formula feedings.
   b. increase fluids.
   c. increase laxative intake.
   d. increase activity level.

5. Two types of constipation common in children under 5 years old are
   a. physiological and psychological.
   b. anatomical and environmental.
   c. psychological and anatomical.
   d. environmental and physiological.

Fill-in

6. Fecal impaction in children is usually the result of

   _____

   _____

7. Name three ways a parent may assist the child to initiate regular elimination habits.

   a. _____

   b. _____

   c. _____

8. Name five nursing responsibilities in dealing with the problem of constipation in the infant and young child.

   a. _____

   b. _____

   c. _____

   d. _____

   e. _____

ACTIVITY 2: Diarrhea

Fecal Characteristics and Causes of Diarrhea _____

The stools of infants change with age and development, as indicated in Table 27-1. It is important for parents to recognize a child's normal feces. Children with diarrhea have an abnormally frequent evacuation of watery (and sometimes greasy and/or bloody) stools. Diarrhea is frequent among infants and children and can be a very distressing condition. In chronic cases, it may last for weeks or months, while the child continues to grow normally. Chronic diarrhea may be a symptom of a disease. In general, diarrhea is classified as acute or chronic according to its stool, profile, cause, or site of clinical defect. There are a number of common causes of diarrhea in infants and children:

1. It can be due to a specific clinical disorder.
2. Bacterial contamination of formulas or foods can cause food poisoning.
3. Some youngsters develop diarrhea because of intesti-

nal reactions to certain foods such as sugars, fats (too little or too much), milk, and eggs.

Treatment and Caution _____

The initial management of diarrhea in children involves two steps. The clinician's first and major objective is to restore fluid and electrolyte balance by oral or IV therapy, since a child is highly susceptible to dehydration. Subsequently, the clinician determines if the child can be managed adequately by oral nourishment without parenteral feeding, which requires hospitalization.

If a child's diarrhea is accompanied by mild to moderate dehydration with persistent vomiting, hospitalization for parenteral fluid therapy is indicated. In general, it is feasible to provide oral fluids and electrolytes for children with mild diarrhea or children recovering from severe diarrhea. If diarrhea is mild to moderate and the patient shows normal clinical signs otherwise and is not dehydrated, most physicians prescribe out-patient therapy con-

TABLE 27-1
Fecal Characteristics of Infants

| Age (months) | Diet | Fecal Characteristics | | | Number of Bowel Movements Daily |
		pH	Color	Texture	
0–4	Home or commercial formulas	6–8	Pale yellow to light brown	Compressed, solid	2–3
4–12	Breast milk	< 6	Yellow to golden	Like cream or ointment	2–4
	Regular foods and/or milk	Variable	Intensified yellow	Harder	1–3
Over 12	Regular foods and/or milk	Variable	Similar to adult, i.e., highly variable (yellow to black)	Similar to adult, i.e., highly variable (soft to very hard)	Similar to adult, i.e., highly variable (1–4)

sisting of an oral hypotonic solution of glucose and electrolytes.

In caring for an infant with diarrhea, the major concern is supplying an adequate supply of fluid and electrolytes. Some readily available regular and commercial solutions are listed in Table 27-2. Because milk contains too many electrolytes, especially sodium, most clinicians do not recommend it at the beginning of treatment. All other solutions listed in the table may be initially fed to a child with diarrhea. To prevent gas from being trapped and the accompanying discomfort, some soda drinks can be decarbonated. Gelatin should be made in half strength to avoid aggravating dehydration. Kool-Aid and unflavored gelatin should not be used, since they contain few electrolytes.

After about two days of fluid and electrolyte support as described, the diarrhea should subside somewhat. At this stage, the child should be given a diluted regular infant formula, for example, one-fourth, one-third, or even one-half of normal strength. Additional calories are supplied by adding corn syrup (1 teaspoon per 3 ounces of formula) or using a supplemental feeding of strained baby cereals and fruits.

Recent concern has been expressed about the common practice of eliminating milk, eggs, and wheat to reduce diarrhea in a young patient. Although some pediatric patients benefit from this treatment, the attending physician must be alert to (1) potential undernutrition that may occur if the elimination diet is prolonged and (2) the possibility that the child has celiac disease (see Module 23). An elimination diet may mask this disorder.

The initial treatment for diarrhea in children over one year old consists of giving clear liquids such as diluted

TABLE 27-2
Calorie, Sodium, and Potassium Contents of Some Preparations for Treating Diarrhea

Beverage	mg Sodium/100 mL	mg Potassium/100 mL	kcal/100 mL
Milk, whole	50	144	62
Milk, skim	52	145	36
Apple juice, canned or bottled	1	101	47
Grape juice, canned or bottled	2	116	66
Orange juice, from concentrate	1	202	49
7-Up	10	Trace	40
Coca-Cola	1	52	44
Pepsi-Cola	15	3	46
Ginger ale	8	Trace	35
Root beer	13	2	41
Flavored gelatin	54	Trace	59
Pedialyte	69	78	20
Lytren	69	98	30

broth, fruit juices, soft drinks, gelatin dessert, and popsicles. After the diarrhea has subsided, a low-residue diet may be used. Subsequent management is the same as that for an adult (see Module 15). Once the condition has stabilized, a regular diet appropriate to the child's age can be implemented.

Nursing Implications

Health care personnel should

1. Be able to recognize normal fecal characteristics of infants.
2. Differentiate between acute and chronic diarrhea.
3. Develop care plans to meet the individual child's problems.
   a. Replace fluid and electrolytes.
   b. Restore adequate nutrition orally or parenterally.
4. Be familiar with common beverages and foods that can be used for treating diarrhea.
5. Alert the physician to observed potential problems if the child is on an elimination diet for a prolonged period.
6. A low-residue diet is the diet therapy of choice after acute symptoms have subsided.

PROGRESS CHECK ON ACTIVITY 2

Fill-in

1. On what three bases is diarrhea classified as acute or chronic?

   a. _____

   b. _____

   c. _____

2. Name three common causes of diarrhea in children.

   a. _____

   b. _____

   c. _____

3. Describe the two steps in the dietary management of children with diarrhea.

   a. _____

   b. _____

4. Name three beverages with a high sodium content suitable for the treatment of diarrhea.

   a. _____

   b. _____

   c. _____

5. Name three beverages with a high potassium content suitable for the treatment of diarrhea.

   a. _____

   b. _____

   c. _____

6. Name two well-known commercial preparations suitable for the treatment of diarrhea. _____

   _____

7. Describe three ways to increase caloric content of a recovering child's food intake. Assume the child is 6 months old.

   a. _____

   b. _____

   c. _____

ACTIVITY 3: High-Risk Infants

Background Information

Five major categories of infants are considered high risk at birth: those of low birth weight, those born prematurely with complications, those delivered by diabetic mothers, those who are critically ill, and those with birth defects. These newborns are unable to function properly as normal infants and need special help. One of the major criteria for survival is proper nutrition, without which the child may die.

There is considerable controversy over what constitutes a low birth weight or prematurity. In this text, a premature infant is defined as one born before the 37th or 38th week of gestation. Standard charts show the expected infant weight at different gestational ages (GA). If weight is unacceptably low for gestational age, the infant is small for date (SFD) or small for gestational age (SGA). These infants have suffered intrauterine retardation but may be either full-term or premature. A low birth weight (LBW) infant weighs 2,500 g (5½ pounds) or less. These infants may be premature, small for gestational age, and/or small for date. They account for 60 percent to 70 percent of all cases of newborn mortality after birth; about 5 percent to 10 percent of live births are of low birth weight. Infants weighing less than 1,500 g (3.3 pounds) at birth are considered to have very low birth weight (VLBW).

Nutrient Needs

The caloric need of the high-risk infant is definitely higher than that of a normal infant: about 100 to 130 kcal/kg/d. This is about three to four times that of an adult and twice that of a normal infant.

The estimated protein need of high-risk child is 3 to 4 g/kg/d. Excessive protein is undesirable, since it can increase blood amino acids and nitrogen. However, a premature infant may require the essential amino acids tyrosine and cystine.

A high-risk infant needs a large amount of fluid for a number of reasons. It has a high body water content. Its ambient temperature may be too high, causing increased evaporation. Vomiting or diarrhea, if present, may result in a loss of intestinal fluid. The child's kidney is unable to concentrate urine, resulting in more fluid loss. If the child undergoes any form of treatment that causes body evaporation, such as photo or radiant heat therapy, its need for fluid will be further increased.

One way to assure that a child gets enough fluid is to measure the intake and output of fluid, monitor overt clinical signs of dehydration, and analyze urine osmolality, using blood sodium and nitrogen levels as guides. Extra fluid may be given orally (water, milk, or 10 percent glucose) or intravenously (10 percent glucose).

High-risk infants have special needs for calcium, iron, and vitamin K. If the intake of these nutrients is inadequate, appropriate supplementation is needed.

Initial Feedings

The first feeding should be given to a high-risk infant several hours after birth, when the child is given fluid and calories. A normal-term infant receives the first feeding two to four hours after birth, as does a baby weighing at least 1,500 g with a gestational age of 33 or 34 weeks and without any complications such as respiratory difficulty and infection. In general, this latter baby receives smaller but more frequent feedings than a normal child.

If an infant has complications, weighs less than 1,500 g, and has a gestational age of less than 33 weeks, the feeding practice is more cautious and varies with the infant and the doctor's evaluation. Depending on the practitioner, the child may be fed in one of two ways. In one, only 10 percent glucose is given intravenously with no other nourishment until the infant stabilizes, usually 3 days later, at which time oral or tube feedings or total parenteral nutrition is used. Some practitioners prefer direct oral feeding within the first 12 to 24 hours. If oral feeding is not feasible, total parenteral nutrition is started at the beginning of the second day.

Use of Breast Milk or Formulas

The decision of whether to nurse or formula-feed a high-risk infant depends partly on the degree of risk. Babies of nearly normal size may respond well to breast milk. Breast milk permits satisfactory growth for infants weighing more than 1,500 g, especially because of the quality of fat and protein, the solute load, and immunological protection provided. In some circumstances, breast milk produces less necrotizing enterocolitis than formulas. The mother should be actively encouraged to breast-feed if the child can suck and weighs over 2,000 g. If the child is unable to breast-feed, the mother can provide milk by manually squeezing her breasts. The milk is then given to the child by tube, gavage, bottle, or dropper. This procedure can also strengthen the mother's emotional attachment to the child. The milk should be fresh, unheated, unrefrigerated, and less than 8 to 10 hours old.

Although breast milk has certain advantages, it does not provide enough protein to enable some high-risk infants to grow. To supplement the low supply of protein in breast milk, a breast-fed child can be given some concentrated or standard formulas. Neither regular formulas nor breast milk alone is adequate for growth for most high-risk infants.

There are no readily available "standard" formulas for low-birth-weight or high-risk infants, since their requirements for nutrients are unknown. The best guide is to use the estimated nutrient needs as described earlier. However, most standard formulas are high in protein, calories, and calcium. The smaller the child, the more unsatisfactory these formulas are. Some clinicians propose that the formula should contain 80 to 100 kcal/100 mL and 2.6 to 3.0 g of protein/100 kcal (ideally 2.8 g).

Some clinics and hospitals use defined formula diets containing glucose, amino acids, minerals, vitamins, and medium-chain triglycerides (or no fat). Some infants respond favorably when fed these diets, while others do not. The major problems with these defined-formula diets are their high solute load and excessive nitrogen. Since infant response to any method of feeding varies, the high-risk baby's growth must be closely monitored. In addition to the type of formula chosen, its dilution must be carefully considered. The concentration, calories, protein, and fluid of a high-risk baby's formula should all be sufficient but within the eating and digestive capacity of the child. Whereas a normal child is usually provided about 67 kcal/ 100 mL (20 kcal/oz) of milk, a high-risk infant needs about 80 to 100 kcal/100 mL (25 to 30 kcal/oz) of milk. And although a normal child drinks about 100 mL milk/kg, a high-risk infant may need as much as 200 mL/kg. If the formula is too concentrated, the excessive osmotic load can be harmful to the gastrointestinal tract and the kidney.

Nursing Implications _____

Health personnel should

1. Be alert to the five major categories of infants at risk at birth and be prepared to provide the specialized nutrition needed on an individual basis.
2. Recognize the physiological feeding problems of a high-risk infant:
    a. protein deficit and risk of overload
    b. increased fluid needs: fluctuating body temperature, inability to concentrate urine
    c. need for increased calories
    d. graduated vitamin and mineral needs
3. Be proficient in the use of feeding methods recommended by the practitioner.
4. Encourage mothers of high-risk infants to breast feed unless mother or baby has medical problems.
5. Be familiar with the types and dilutions of formulas suitable for high-risk infants, depending upon their size/weight.
6. Closely monitor infant response to feedings.
7. Be prepared to teach all caregivers the proper feeding techniques, prescribed formulas, signs, and symptoms of acceptance and any other pertinent facts.
8. Follow up for further evaluation.

PROGRESS CHECK ON ACTIVITY 3

Multiple Choice

1. The SGA infant is
    a. full-term but underweight.
    b. premature but small for date.
    c. either full-term or premature.
    d. any child who weighs less than 6 lb.

2. LBW infants account for _____ percent of all live births.
    a. 60–70
    b. 20–30
    c. 1–2
    d. 5–10

3. Caloric needs of the high-risk infant are
    a. twice those of a normal infant.
    b. three to four times those of a normal infant.
    c. approximately six times those of a normal infant.
    d. the same as those of the normal infant; they have little movement.

4. High-risk infants need large amounts of fluid for all except which of these reasons?
    a. They require extra essential amino acids.
    b. They have a larger body water content than normal infants.
    c. Their kidneys can't concentrate urine.
    d. They have increased water evaporation.

5. First feedings for high-risk infants include
    a. TPN.
    b. fluid with extra calories.
    c. 10 percent glucose IVs.
    d. no food or fluid until stabilized.

Fill-in

6. What are the criteria for breast feeding a high-risk infant?

    a. _____

    b. _____

7. Describe the procedure for feeding breast milk to an infant who cannot nurse.

    a. _____

    b. _____

    c. _____

8. Describe the four most appropriate guides for meeting nutrient needs of high-risk infants.

    a. _____

    b. _____

    c. _____

    d. _____

9. What is a defined formula? _____

    _____

    _____

References _____

Bercowitz, C. D. et al. 1984. Environmental failure to thrive: The need for intervention. *American Family Physician* 29:191.

Carrazza, F. et al. 1984. Oral hydration and feeding of the child with diarrhea. *Clinical Nutrition.* 3(1):18.

Epstein, L. H. et al. 1986. Family-based behavioral weight control in obese young children. *Journal of the American Dietetic Association* 86(4):481.

Farrell, P. M. et al. 1987. Predigested formula for infants with cystic fibrosis. *Journal of the American Dietetic Association* 87(10):1353.

Gracey, M. 1985. *Diarrheal disease and malnutrition.* New York: Churchill Livingstone.

Greene, H. L. and F. K. Ghishan. 1983. Excessive fluid intake as a cause of chronic diarrhea, in young children. *Journal of Pediatrics* 102:836.

Hattner, J. T. 1987. The dietitian's role in the treatment of common gastrointestinal problems. *Topics in Clinical Nutrition* 64:62.

Johns, C. 1985. Encopresis. *American Journal of Nursing* 85:153.

Kilars, J. C. et al. 1984. Yogurt: An autodigesting source of lactase. *New England Journal of Medicine.* 310:1

Newcomer, A. D. and D. B. McGill, 1984. Clinical importance of lactase deficiency. *New England Journal of Medicine* 310:42.

Ohio Neonatal Nutritionists. 1985. *Nutritional care for high risk newborns.* Philadelphia: George F. Stickley.

Paige, D. M. and T. M. Bayless (eds.). 1981. *Lactose digestion: Clinical and nutritional implications.* Baltimore: Johns Hopkins.

Patterson, R. E. et al. 1986. Factors related to obesity in preschool children. *Journal of the American Dietetic Association.* 86(10):1376.

Powell, G. F. 1985. Nutrition in nonorganic failure to thrive. *Clinical Nutrition* 4(2):54.

Pugliese, M. T. et al. 1987. Parental health beliefs as a cause of nonorganic failure to thrive. *Pediatrics* 80:175.

Risenberg, D. 1986. Progress in research, therapy of Prader-Willi Syndrome. *Journal of the American Medical Association.* 255:3211.

Robinson, N. B. et al. 1987. TWIGS—a weight control program designed for children. *Journal of the American Dietetic Association.* 87(4):500.

Sorenson, T. I. A. et al. 1988. Risk in childhood of development of severe adult obesity: Retrospective population-based case-cohort study. *American Journal of Epidemiology* 127:104.

Tsang, R. C. 1985. *Vitamin and mineral requirements in preterm infants.* New York: Marcel Dekker.

Villar, J. et al. 1986. Nutritional factors associated with low birth weight and short gestational age. *Clinical Nutrition* 5(2):28

Warman, N. L. et al. 1987. Nonorganic failure to thrive: Etiology, evaluation, and treatment. *Topics in Clinical Nutrition* 2(1):31.

APPENDICES

Appendix A

Dietary Standards

1989 TABLE 1
Food and Nutrition Board, National Academy of Sciences–National Research Council
Recommended Dietary Allowances,[a] Revised 1989

Category	Age (years) or Condition	Weight[b] (kg)	(lb)	Height[b] (cm)	(in)	Protein (g)	Fat-Soluble Vitamins Vitamin A (μg RE)[c]	Vitamin D (μg)[d]	Vitamin E (mg α-TE)[e]	Vitamin K (μg)
Infants	0.0–0.5	6	13	60	24	13	375	7.5	3	5
	0.5–1.0	9	20	71	28	14	375	10	4	10
Children	1–3	13	29	90	35	16	400	10	6	15
	4–6	20	44	112	44	24	500	10	7	20
	7–10	28	62	132	52	28	700	10	7	30
Males	11–14	45	99	157	62	45	1,000	10	10	45
	15–18	66	145	176	69	59	1,000	10	10	65
	19–24	72	160	177	70	58	1,000	10	10	70
	25–50	79	174	176	70	63	1,000	5	10	80
	51+	77	170	173	68	63	1,000	5	10	80
Females	11–14	46	101	157	62	46	800	10	8	45
	15–18	55	120	163	64	44	800	10	8	55
	19–24	58	128	164	65	46	800	10	8	60
	25–50	63	138	163	64	50	800	5	8	65
	51+	65	143	160	63	50	800	5	8	65
Pregnant						60	800	10	10	65
Lactating	1st 6 months					65	1,300	10	12	65
	2nd 6 months					62	1,200	10	11	65

Source: Reprinted with permission from *Recommended Dietary Allowances*, 10th Edition, © 1989 by the National Academy of Sciences. Published by Nationl Academy Press, Washington, D.C.

[a]The allowances, expressed as average daily intakes over time, are intended to provide for individual variations among most normal persons as they live in the United States under usual environmental stresses. Diets should be based on a variety of common foods in order to provide other nutrients for which human requirements have been less well defined.

[b]Weights and heights of Reference Adults are actual medians for the U.S. population of the designated age, as reported by NHANES II. The median

1989   TABLE 1 (Continued)

Water-Soluble Vitamins							Minerals						
Vitamin C (mg)	Thiamin (mg)	Riboflavin (mg)	Niacin (mg NE)^f	Vitamin B_6 (mg)	Folate (μg)	Vitamin B_{12} (μg)	Calcium (mg)	Phosphorus (mg)	Magnesium (mg)	Iron (mg)	Zinc (mg)	Iodine (μg)	Selenium (μg)
30	0.3	0.4	5	0.3	25	0.3	400	300	40	6	5	40	10
35	0.4	0.5	6	0.6	35	0.5	600	500	60	10	5	50	15
40	0.7	0.8	9	1.0	50	0.7	800	800	80	10	10	70	20
45	0.9	1.1	12	1.1	75	1.0	800	800	120	10	10	90	20
45	1.0	1.2	13	1.4	100	1.4	800	800	170	10	10	120	30
50	1.3	1.5	17	1.7	150	2.0	1,200	1,200	270	12	15	150	40
60	1.5	1.8	20	2.0	200	2.0	1,200	1,200	400	12	15	150	50
60	1.5	1.7	19	2.0	200	2.0	1,200	1,200	350	10	15	150	70
60	1.5	1.7	19	2.0	200	2.0	800	800	350	10	15	150	70
60	1.2	1.4	15	2.0	200	2.0	800	800	350	10	15	150	70
50	1.1	1.3	15	1.4	150	2.0	1,200	1,200	280	15	12	150	45
60	1.1	1.3	15	1.5	180	2.0	1,200	1,200	300	15	12	150	50
60	1.1	1.3	15	1.6	180	2.0	1,200	1,200	280	15	12	150	55
60	1.1	1.3	15	1.6	180	2.0	800	800	280	15	12	150	55
60	1.0	1.2	13	1.6	180	2.0	800	800	280	10	12	150	55
70	1.5	1.6	17	2.2	400	2.2	1,200	1,200	320	30	15	175	65
95	1.6	1.8	20	2.1	280	2.6	1,200	1,200	355	15	19	200	75
90	1.6	1.7	20	2.1	260	2.6	1,200	1,200	340	15	16	200	75

weights and heights of those under 19 years of age were taken from Hamill et al. (1979) (see pages 16–17). The use of these figures does not imply that the height-to-weight ratios are ideal.

[c]Retinol equivalents. 1 retinol equivalent = 1 μg retinol or 6 μg β-carotene. See text for calculation of vitamin A activity of diets as retinol equivalents.

[d]As cholecalciferol. 10 μg cholecalciferol = 400 IU of vitamin D.

[e]α-Tocopherol equivalents. 1 mg d-α-tocopherol = 1 α-TE. See text for variation in allowances and calculation of vitamin E activity of the diet as α-tocopherol equivalents.

[f]1 NE (niacin equivalent) is equal to 1 mg of niacin or 60 mg of dietary tryptophan.

1989   TABLE 2
Estimated Safe and Adequate Daily Dietary
Intakes of Selected Vitamins and Minerals[a]

Category	Age, years	Vitamins		Trace Elements[b]				
		Biotin, μg	Pantothenic Acid, mg	Copper, mg	Manganese, mg	Fluoride, mg	Chromium μg	Molybdenum, μg
Infants	0–0.5	10	2	0.4–0.6	0.3–0.6	0.1–0.5	10–40	15–30
	0.5–1	15	3	0.6–0.7	0.6–1.0	0.2–1.0	20–60	20–40
Children and Adolescents	1–3	20	3	0.7–1.0	1.0–1.5	0.5–1.5	20–80	25–50
	4–6	25	3–4	1.0–1.5	1.5–2.0	1.0–2.5	30–120	30–75
	7–10	30	4–5	1.0–2.0	2.0–3.0	1.5–2.5	50–200	50–150
	11+	30–100	4–7	1.5–2.5	2.0–5.0	1.5–2.5	50–200	75–250
Adults		30–100	4–7	1.5–3.0	2.0–5.0	1.5–4.0	50–200	75–250

Reproduced with permission from *Recommended Dietary Allowances*, 10th edition, © 1990, by the National Academy of Sciences, National Academy Press, Washington, DC.
[a]Because there is less information on which to base allowances, these figures are not given in the main table of RDA and are provided here in the form of ranges of recommended intakes.
[b]Since the toxic levels for many trace elements may be only several times usual intakes, the upper levels for the trace elements given in this table should not be habitually exceeded.

1989   TABLE 3
Median Heights and Weights and Recommended Energy Intake

Category	Age (years) or Condition	Weight		Height		REE[a] kcal/day	Average Energy Allowance, kcal[b]		
		kg	lb	cm	in		Multiples of REE	Per kg	Per day[c]
Infants	0.0–0.5	6	13	60	24	320		108	650
	0.5–1.0	9	20	71	28	500		98	850
Children	1–3	13	29	90	35	740		102	1,300
	4–6	20	44	112	44	950		90	1,800
	7–10	28	62	132	52	1,130		70	2,000
Males	11–14	45	99	157	62	1,440	1.70	55	2,500
	15–18	66	145	176	69	1,760	1.67	45	3,000
	19–24	72	160	177	70	1,780	1.67	40	2,900
	25–50	79	174	176	70	1,800	1.60	37	2,900
	51+	77	170	173	68	1,530	1.50	30	2,300
Females	11–14	46	101	157	62	1,310	1.67	47	2,200
	15–18	55	120	163	64	1,370	1.60	40	2,200
	19–24	58	128	164	65	1,350	1.60	38	2,200
	25–50	63	138	163	64	1,380	1.55	36	2,200
	51+	65	143	160	63	1,280	1.50	30	1,900
Pregnant	1st trimester								+0
	2nd trimester								+300
	3rd trimester								+300
Lactating	1st 6 months								+500
	2nd 6 months								+500

[a]Calculation based on FAO equations (Table 3-1), then rounded.
[b]In the range of light to moderate activity, the coefficient of variation is ± 20%.
[c]Figure is rounded.

1989   TABLE 4
Estimated Sodium, Chloride, and Potassium
Minimum Requirements of Healthy Persons[a]

Age	Weight (kg)[a]	Sodium (mg)[a,b]	Chloride (mg)[a,b]	Potassium (mg)[c]
Months				
0–5	4.5	120	180	500
6–11	8.9	200	300	700
Years				
1	11.0	225	350	1,000
2–5	16.0	300	500	1,400
6–9	25.0	400	600	1,600
10–18	50.0	500	750	2,000
> 18[d]	70.0	500	750	2,000

Reproduced with permission from *Recommended Dietary Allowances*, 10th edition, © 1990, by the National Academy of Sciences, National Academy Press, Washington, DC.
[a]No allowance has been included for large, prolonged losses from the skin through sweat.
[b]There is no evidence that higher intakes confer any health benefit.
[c]Desirable intakes of potassium may considerably exceed these values (~ 3,500 mg for adults).
[d]No allowance included for growth. Values for those below 18 years assume a growth rate at the 50th percentile reported by the National Center for Health Statistics (Hamill, P.V.V., Drizd, T.A., Johnson, C.L., Reed, R.B., Roche, A.F., and Moore, W.M. Physical growth: National Center for Health Statistics percentiles. *Am. J. Clin. Nutr.* 32:607, 1979).

TABLE 5
Recommended Nutrient Intakes for Canadians[a]

Age	Sex	Weight (kg)	kcal/kg[b]	Protein (g/day)[c]	Vitamin A (RE/day)[d]	Vitamin D (μg/day)[e]	Vitamin E (mg/day)[f]	Vitamin C (mg/day)	Folacin (μg/day)[c,g]	Vitamin B$_{12}$ (μg/day)	Calcium (mg/day)	Magnesium (mg/day)[c]	Iron (mg/day)	Iodine (μg/day)	Zinc (mg/day)
					Fat-Soluble Vitamins			Water-Soluble Vitamins			Minerals				
Months															
0–2	Both	4.5	120–100	11[h]	400	10	3	20	50	0.3	350	30	0.4[i]	25	2[j]
3–5	Both	7.0	100–95	14[h]	400	10	3	20	50	0.3	350	40	5	35	3
6–8	Both	8.5	95–97	17[h]	400	10	3	20	50	0.3	400	50	7	40	3
9–11	Both	9.5	97–99	18	400	10	3	20	55	0.3	400	50	7	45	3
Years															
1	Both	11	101	19	400	10	3	20	65	0.3	500	55	6	55	4
2–3	Both	14	94	22	400	5	4	20	80	0.4	500	70	6	65	4
4–6	Both	18	100	26	500	5	5	25	90	0.5	600	90	6	85	5
7–9	M	25	88	30	700	2.5	7	35	125	0.8	700	110	7	110	6
7–9	F	25	76	30	700	2.5	6	30	125	0.8	700	110	7	95	6
10–12	M	34	73	38	800	2.5	8	40	170	1.0	900	150	10	125	7
10–12	F	36	61	40	800	2.5	7	40	180	1.0	1,000	160	10	110	7
13–15	M	50	57	50	900	2.5	9	50	150	1.5	1,100	210	12	160	9
13–15	F	48	46	42	800	2.5	7	45	145	1.5	800	200	13	160	8
16–18	M	62	51	55	1,000	2.5	10	55	185	1.9	900	250	10	160	9
16–18	F	53	40	43	800	2.5	7	45	160	1.9	700	215	14	160	8
19–24	M	71	42	58	1,000	2.5	10	60	210	2.0	800	240	8	160	9
19–24	F	58	36	43	800	2.5	7	45	175	2.0	700	200	14	160	8
25–49	M	74	36	61	1,000	2.5	9	60	220	2.0	800	250	8	160	9
25–49	F	59	32	44	800	2.5	6	45	175	2.0	700	200	14[k]	160	8
50–74	M	73	31	60	1,000	2.5	7	60	220	2.0	800	250	8	160	9
50–74	F	63	29	47	800	2.5	6	45	190	2.0	800	210	7	160	8
75+	M	69	29	57	1,000	2.5	6	60	205	2.0	800	230	8	160	9
75+	F	64	23	47	800	2.5	5	45	190	2.0	800	220	7	160	8
Pregnancy (additional)															
1st trimester			100	15	100	2.5	2	0	305	1.0	500	15	6	25	0
2nd trimester			300	20	100	2.5	2	20	305	1.0	500	20	6	25	1
3rd trimester			300	25	100	2.5	2	20	305	1.0	500	25	6	25	2
Lactation (additional)			450	20	400	2.5	3	30	120	0.5	500	80	0	50	6

Adapted from *Recommended Nutrient Intakes for Canadians*. Ottawa: Canadian Government Publishing Centre, 1983. Reproduced with permission of The Minister of Supply and Services Canada 1992.
[a]Recommended intakes during periods of growth are taken as appropriate for individuals representative of the midpoint in each age group. All recommended intakes are designed to cover individual variations in essentially all of a healthy population subsisting upon a variety of common foods available in Canada.
[b]Figures for energy are estimates of average requirements for expected patterns of activity. For nutrients not shown, the following amounts are recommended: thiamine, 0.4 mg/1,000 kcal (0.48 mg/5,000 kJ); riboflavin, 0.5 mg/1,000 kcal (0.6 mg/5,000 kJ); niacin, 7.2 NE/1,000 kcal (8.6 NE/5,000 kJ); vitamin B$_6$, 15 μg, as pyridoxine, per gram of protein; phosphorus, same as calcium.

cThe primary units are expressed per kilogram of body weight. The figures shown here are only examples.
dOne retinol equivalent (RE) corresponds to the biological activity of 1 μg of retinol, 6 μg of beta-carotene, or 12 μg of other carotenes.
eExpressed as cholecalciferol or ergocalciferol.
fExpressed as d-alpha-tocopherol equivalents, relative to which beta- and gamma-tocopherol and alpha-tocotrienol have activities of 0.5, 0.1, and 0.3, respectively.
gExpressed as total folate.
hAssumption that the protein is from breast milk or is of the same biological value as that of breast milk and that between 3 and 9 months adjustment for the quality of the protein is made.
iIt is assumed that breast milk is the source of iron up to 2 months of age.
jBased on the assumption that breast milk is the source of zinc for the first 2 months.
kAfter the menopause the recommended intake is 7 mg day.

337

1983 TABLE 6
Canada's Food Guide

Variety	Choose different kinds of foods from within each group in appropriate numbers of servings and portion sizes.
Energy balance	Needs vary with age, sex, and activity. Balance energy intake from foods with energy output from physical activity to control weight. Foods selected according to the Guide can supply 1000–1400 kilocalories. For additional energy, increase the number and size of servings from the various food groups and/or add other foods.
Moderation	Select and prepare foods with limited amounts of fat, sugar, and salt. If alcohol is consumed, use limited amounts.

Food Group	Recommended Number of Servings (adults)	Some Examples of One Serving
Milk and milk products	2[a]	1 cup milk; ¾ cup yogurt; 1½ oz. cheddar or processed cheese
Meat, fish, poultry, and alternates	2	2–3 oz. cooked lean meat, fish, poultry, or liver; 4 T peanut butter, 1 cup cooked dried peas, beans, or lentils; ½ cup nuts or seeds; 2 oz. cheddar cheese; ½ cup cottage cheese; 2 eggs
Breads and cereals[b]	3–5	1 slice bread; ½ cup cooked cereal; ¾ cup ready-to-eat cereal; 1 roll or muffin; ½–¾ cup cooked rice, macaroni, spaghetti, or noodles; ½ hamburger or wiener bun
Fruits and vegetables	4–5[c]	½ cup vegetables or fruits—fresh, frozen, or canned; ½ cup juice—fresh, frozen, or canned; 1 medium-sized potato, carrot, tomato, peach, apple, orange, or banana

Source: Adapted from "Canada's Food Guide," Health and Welfare Canada, 1983 with permission of the Canadian Communications Group Publishing Department of Supply and Services, Ottawa, Ontario, Canada K1A 0S9.
[a]For children up to 11 years, 2–3 servings; adolescents, 3–4 servings; pregnant and nursing women, 3–4 servings.
[b]Whole grain or enriched whole grain products are recommended.
[c]Include at least two vegetables. Choose a variety of both vegetables and fruits—cooked, raw, or their juices. Include yellow, green, or green leafy vegetables.

Weight and Height

TABLE 7
Heights and Weights for Men and Women*†

Men					Women				
Height		Small Frame	Medium Frame	Large Frame	Height		Small Frame	Medium Frame	Large Frame
Feet	Inches	(pounds)**			Feet	Inches	(pounds)#		
5	2	128–134	131–141	138–150	4	10	102–111	109–121	118–131
5	3	130–136	133–143	140–153	4	11	103–113	111–123	120–134
5	4	132–138	135–145	142–156	5	0	104–115	113–126	122–137
5	5	134–140	137–148	144–160	5	1	106–118	115–129	125–140
5	6	136–142	139–151	146–164	5	2	108–121	118–132	128–143
5	7	138–145	142–154	149–168	5	3	111–124	121–135	131–147
5	8	140–148	145–157	152–172	5	4	114–127	124–138	134–151
5	9	142–151	148–160	155–176	5	5	117–130	127–141	137–155
5	10	144–154	151–163	158–180	5	6	120–133	130–144	140–159
5	11	146–157	154–166	161–184	5	7	123–136	133–147	143–163
6	0	149–160	157–170	164–188	5	8	126–139	136–150	146–167
6	1	152–164	160–174	168–192	5	9	129–142	139–153	149–170
6	2	155–168	164–178	172–197	5	10	132–145	142–156	152–173
6	3	158–172	167–182	176–202	5	11	135–148	145–159	155–176
6	4	162–176	171–187	181–207	6	0	138–151	148–162	158–179

*Metropolitan Life Insurance Company, New York, 1983. Data from 1979 Build Study. Society of Actuaries and Associates of Life Insurance Medical Directors of America, 1980.
†Weight at ages 25 to 59 based on lowest mortality.
**Weight in indoor clothing weighing 5 pounds, shoes with 1-inch heel.
#Weight in indoor clothing weighing 3 pounds, shoes with 1-inch heel.

Appendix C

Growth Grids

**GIRLS: BIRTH TO 36 MONTHS
PHYSICAL GROWTH
NCHS PERCENTILES***

NAME_____ RECORD #_____

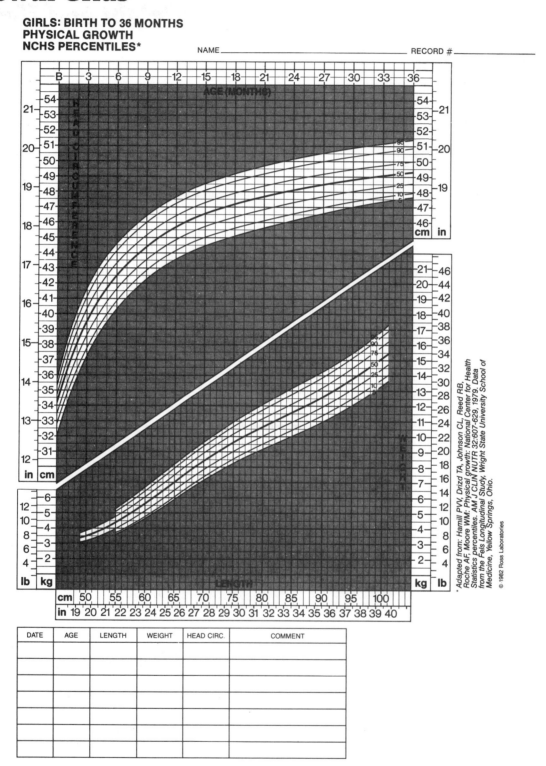

DATE	AGE	LENGTH	WEIGHT	HEAD CIRC.	COMMENT

* Adapted from: Hamill PVV, Drizd TA, Johnson CL, Reed RB, Roche AF, Moore WM: Physical growth: National Center for Health Statistics percentiles. AM J CLIN NUTR 32:607-629, 1979. Data from the Fels Longitudinal Study, Wright State University School of Medicine, Yellow Springs, Ohio.

© 1982 Ross Laboratories

GIRLS: BIRTH TO 36 MONTHS
PHYSICAL GROWTH
NCHS PERCENTILES*

NAME_____   RECORD #_____

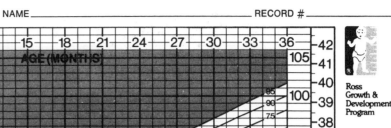
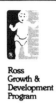

Ross
Growth &
Development
Program

DATE	AGE	LENGTH	WEIGHT	HEAD CIRC.	COMMENT
	BIRTH				

MOTHER'S STATURE _____   GESTATIONAL
FATHER'S STATURE _____   AGE _____ WEEKS

* Adapted from: Hamill PVV, Drizd TA, Johnson CL, Reed RB, Roche AF, Moore WM: Physical growth: National Center for Health Statistics percentiles. AM J CLIN NUTR 32:607-629, 1979. Data from the Fels Longitudinal Study, Wright State University School of Medicine, Yellow Springs, Ohio.

© 1982 Ross Laboratories

GIRLS: 2 TO 18 YEARS
PHYSICAL GROWTH
NCHS PERCENTILES*

NAME_____ RECORD #_____

MOTHER'S STATURE _____		FATHER'S STATURE _____		
DATE	AGE	STATURE	WEIGHT	COMMENT

Ross
Growth &
Development
Program

AGE (YEARS)

STATURE

WEIGHT

AGE (YEARS)

*Adapted from: Hamill PVV, Drizd TA, Johnson CL, Reed RB, Roche AF, Moore WM: Physical growth: National Center for Health Statistics percentiles. AM J CLIN NUTR 32:607-629, 1979. Data from the National Center for Health Statistics (NCHS), Hyattsville, Maryland.

**GIRLS: PREPUBESCENT
PHYSICAL GROWTH
NCHS PERCENTILES***

NAME _____   RECORD # _____

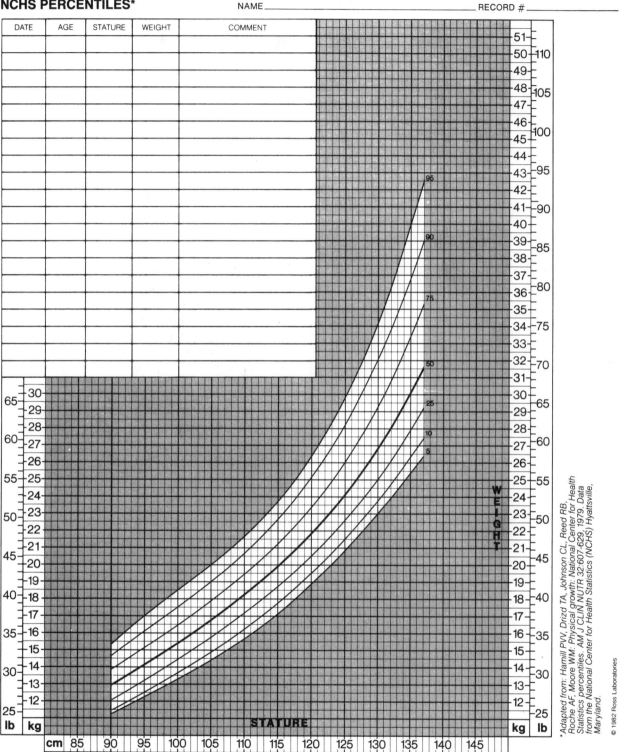

DATE	AGE	STATURE	WEIGHT	COMMENT

STATURE

cm 85 90 95 100 105 110 115 120 125 130 135 140 145

in 34 35 36 37 38 39 40 41 42 43 44 45 46 47 48 49 50 51 52 53 54 55 56 57 58

*Adapted from: Hamill PVV, Drizd TA, Johnson CL, Reed RB, Roche AF, Moore WM: Physical growth: National Center for Health Statistics percentiles. AM J CLIN NUTR 32:607-629, 1979. Data from the National Center for Health Statistics (NCHS) Hyattsville, Maryland.

© 1982 Ross Laboratories

**BOYS: BIRTH TO 36 MONTHS
PHYSICAL GROWTH
NCHS PERCENTILES***

NAME_____ RECORD #_____

*Adapted from: Hamill PVV, Drizd TA, Johnson CL, Reed RB, Roche AF, Moore WM: Physical growth: National Center for Health Statistics percentiles. AM J CLIN NUTR 32:607-629, 1979. Data from the Fels Longitudinal Study, Wright State University School of Medicine, Yellow Springs, Ohio.

© 1982 Ross Laboratories

DATE	AGE	LENGTH	WEIGHT	HEAD CIRC.	COMMENT

**BOYS: BIRTH TO 36 MONTHS
PHYSICAL GROWTH
NCHS PERCENTILES***

NAME _____   RECORD # _____

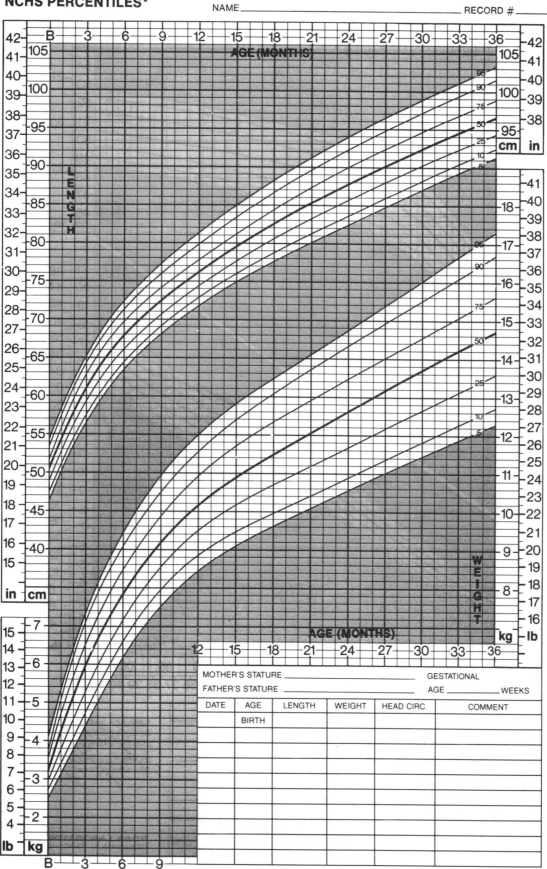

Ross
Growth &
Development
Program

MOTHER'S STATURE _____   GESTATIONAL
FATHER'S STATURE _____   AGE _____ WEEKS

DATE	AGE	LENGTH	WEIGHT	HEAD CIRC.	COMMENT
	BIRTH				

*Adapted from: Hamill PVV, Drizd TA, Johnson CL, Reed RB, Roche AF, Moore WM: Physical growth: National Center for Health Statistics percentiles. AM J CLIN NUTR 32:607-629, 1979. Data from the Fels Longitudinal Study, Wright State University School of Medicine, Yellow Springs, Ohio.

© 1982 Ross Laboratories

BOYS: 2 TO 18 YEARS
PHYSICAL GROWTH
NCHS PERCENTILES*

NAME_____ RECORD #_____

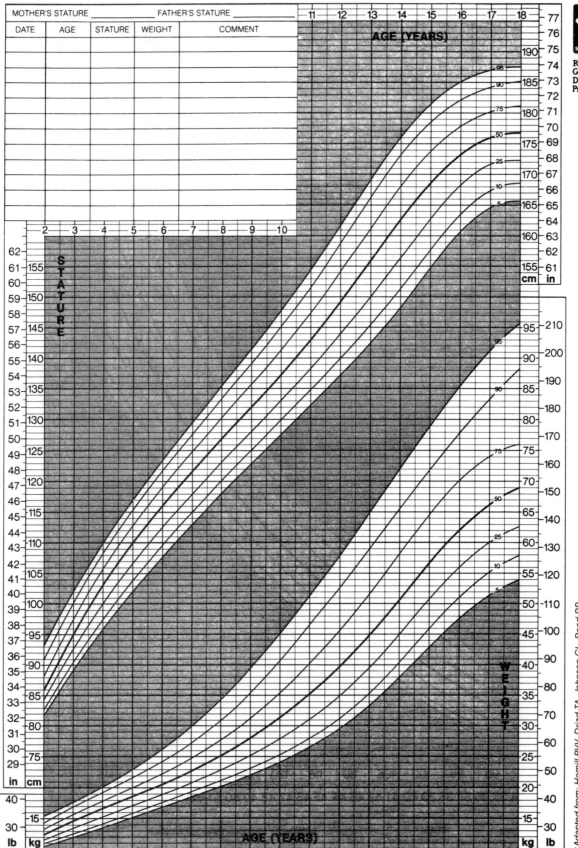

Ross
Growth &
Development
Program

*Adapted from: Hamill PVV, Drizd TA, Johnson CL, Reed RB, Roche AF, Moore WM: Physical growth: National Center for Health Statistics percentiles. AM J CLIN NUTR 32:607-629, 1979. Data from the National Center for Health Statistics (NCHS), Hyattsville, Maryland.

© 1982 Ross Laboratories

BOYS: PREPUBESCENT
PHYSICAL GROWTH
NCHS PERCENTILES*

NAME_____   RECORD #_____

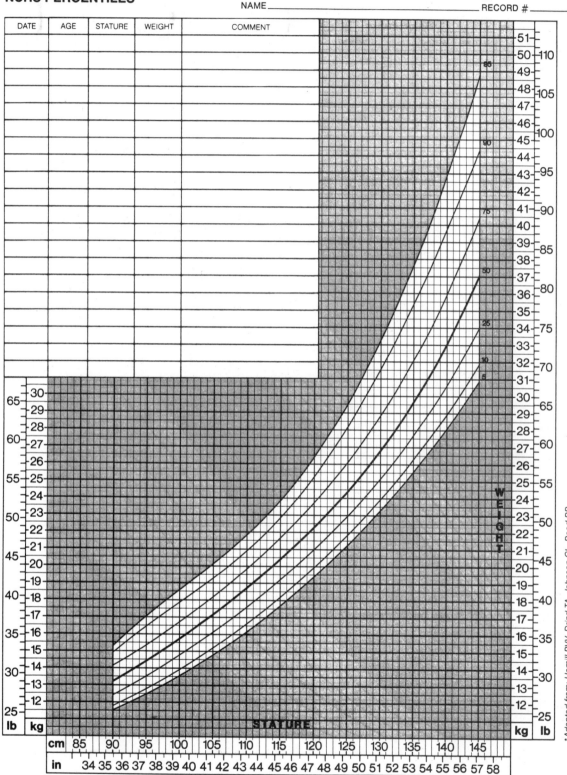

Appendix D

Weights and Measures

TABLE 8
Common Weights and Measures

Measure	Equivalent	Measure	Equivalent
3 tsp.	1 tbsp.	1 fl oz.	28.35 g
2 tbsp.	1 oz.	½ c.	120 g
4 tbsp.	¼ c.	1 c.	240 g
8 tbsp.	½ c.	1 lb.	454 g
16 tbsp.	1 c.		
		1 g	1 ml
2 c.	1 pt.	1 tsp.	5 ml
4 c.	1 qt.	1 tbsp.	15 ml
4 qt.	1 gal.	1 fl oz.	30 ml
1 tsp.	5 g	1 c.	240 ml
1 tbsp.	15 g	1 pt.	480 ml
1 oz.	28.35 g	1 qt.	960 ml
		1 L	1,000 ml

TABLE 9
Weights and Measures Conversions

U.S. System to Metric		Metric to U.S. System	
U.S. Measure	Metric Measure	Metric Measure	U.S. Measure
Length		Length	
1 in.	25.0 mm	1 mm	0.04 in.
1 ft.	0.3 m	1 m	3.3 ft.
Mass		Mass	
1 g	64.8 mg	1 mg	0.015 g
1 oz.	28.35 g	1 g	0.035 oz.
1 lb.	0.45 kg	1 kg	2.2 lb.
1 short ton	907.1 kg	1 metric ton	1.102 short tons
Volume		Volume	
1 cu. in.	16.0 cm^3	1 cm^3	0.06 in.^{3}
1 tsp.	5.0 ml	1 mL	0.2 tsp.
1 tbsp.	15.0 ml	1 mL	0.07 tbsp.
1 fl oz.	30.0 ml	1 mL	0.03 oz.
1 c.	0.24 L	1 L	4.2 c.
1 pt.	0.47 L	1 L	2.1 pt.
1 qt. (liq)	0.95 L	1 L	1.1 qt.
1 gal.	0.004 m^3	1 m^3	264.0 gal.
1 pk.	0.009 m^3	1 m^3	113.0 pk.
1 bu.	0.04 m^3	1 m^3	28.0 bu.
Energy		Energy	
1 cal.	4.18 J	1 J	0.24 cal.

Temperature
To convert Celsius degrees into Fahrenheit, multiply by ⅘ and add 32.
To convert Fahrenheit degrees into Celsius, subtract 32 and multiply by ⅝. For example:

$$30\ °C = (30 \times \frac{9}{5} + 32)\ °F = (54 + 32)\ °F = 86\ °F \qquad 90\ °F = (90 - 32) \times \frac{5}{9}\ °C = 58 \times \frac{5}{9}\ °C = 32.2\ °C$$

Food Exchange Lists

The Exchange Lists are the basis of a meal planning system designed by a committee of the American Diabetes Association and The American Dietetic Association. While designed primarily for people with diabetes and other people who must follow special diets, the Exchange Lists are based on principles of good eating that apply to everyone. *Exchange Lists for Meal Planning* © 1989 American Diabetes Association, Inc., The American Dietetic Association.

Symbols appear on some foods in the exchange groups. Foods that are high in fiber (3 grams or more per exchange) have an [F] symbol. Foods that are high in sodium (400 milligrams or more of sodium per exchange) have an [S] symbol; foods that have 400 mg or more of sodium if two or more exchanges are eaten have a * symbol.

TABLE 10
Outline of the 1986 American Diabetes Association Exchange Lists

Exchange List	Carbohydrate (grams)	Protein (grams)	Fat (grams)	Calories
Starch/Bread	15	3	trace	80
Meat				
Lean	–	7	3	55
Medium-Fat	–	7	5	75
High-Fat	–	7	8	100
Vegetable	5	2	–	25
Fruit	15	–	–	60
Milk				
Skim	12	8	trace	90
Lowfat	12	8	5	120
Whole	12	8	8	150
Fat	–	–	5	45

LIST 1: STARCH/BREAD LIST**

Cereals/Grains/Pasta

Bran cereals, concentrated (such as Bran Buds®, All Bran®)[F]	⅓ cup
Bran cereals, flaked[F]	½ cup
Bulgur (cooked)	½ cup
Cooked cereals	½ cup
Cornmeal (dry)	2½ Tbsp.
Grape-Nuts®	3 Tbsp.
Grits (cooked)	½ cup
Other ready-to-eat unsweetened cereals	¾ cup
Pasta (cooked)	½ cup
Puffed cereal	1½ cup
Rice, white or brown (cooked)	⅓ cup
Shredded wheat	½ cup
Wheat germ[F]	3 Tbsp.

Dried Beans/Peas/Lentils

Beans and peas (cooked) (such as kidney, white, split, blackeye)[F]	⅓ cup
Lentils (cooked)[F]	⅓ cup
Baked beans[F]	¼ cup

Starchy Vegetables

Corn[F]	½ cup
Corn on cob, 6 in. long[F]	1
Lima beans[F]	½ cup
Peas, green (canned or frozen)[F]	½ cup
Plantain[F]	½ cup
Potato, baked	1 small (3 oz.)
Potato, mashed	½ cup
Squash, winter (acorn, butternut)[F]	1 cup
Yam, sweet potato, plain	⅓ cup

(continues)

LIST 1: STARCH/BREAD LIST (Continued)

Bread

Bagel	½ (1 oz.)
Bread sticks, crisp, 4 in. long x ½ in.	2 (⅔ oz.)
Croutons, lowfat	1 cup
English muffin	½
Frankfurter or hamburger bun	½ (1 oz.)
Pita, 6 in. across	½
Plain roll, small	1 (1 oz.)
Raisin, unfrosted	1 slice (1 oz.)
Rye, pumpernickel	1 slice (1 oz.)
Tortilla, 6 in. across	1
White (including French, Italian)	1 slice (1 oz.)
Whole wheat	1 slice (1 oz.)

Crackers/Snacks

Animal crackers	8
Graham crackers, 2½ in. square	3
Matzoh	¾ oz.
Melba toast	5 slices
Oyster crackers	24
Popcorn (popped, no fat added)	3 cups
Pretzels	¾ oz.
Rye crisp, 2 in. x 3½ in.[F]	4
Saltine-type crackers	6
Whole-wheat crackers, no fat added (crisp breads, such as Finn®, Kavli®, Wasa®)[F]	2–4 slices (¾ oz.)

Starch Foods Prepared with Fat

Biscuit, 2½ in. across	1
Chow mein noodles	½ cup
Corn bread, 2 in. cube	1 (2 oz.)
Cracker, round butter type	6
French fried potatoes, 2 in. to 3½ in. long	10 (1½ oz.)
Muffin, plain, small	1
Pancake, 4 in. across	2
Stuffing, bread (prepared)	¼ cup
Taco shell, 6 in. across	2
Waffle, 4½ in. square	1
Whole-wheat crackers, fat added (such as Triscuit®)[F]	4–6 (1 oz.)

Source: American Diabetes Association, American Dietetic Association, 1989.
**Each item in this list contains approximately 15 gms of carbohydrate, 3 gms of protein, a trace of fat, and 80 calories.
[F]3 grams or more of fiber per exchange.

LIST 2: MEAT LIST***

Lean Meat and Substitutes
(One exchange is equal to any one of the following items.)

Beef: USDA Select or Choice grades of lean beef, such as round, sirloin, and flank steak; tenderloin; and chipped beef[S]	1 oz.
Pork: lean pork, such as fresh ham; canned, cured, or boiled ham[S]; Canadian bacon[S]; tenderloin	1 oz.
Veal: all cuts are lean except for veal cutlets (ground or cubed). Examples of lean veal are chops and roasts.	1 oz.
Poultry: chicken, turkey, Cornish hen (without skin)	1 oz.
Fish:	
all fresh and frozen fish	1 oz.
crab, lobster, scallops, shrimp, clams (fresh or canned in water)	2 oz.
oysters	6 medium
tuna* (canned in water)	¼ cup
herring* (uncreamed or smoked)	1 oz.
sardines (canned)	2 medium
Wild game:	
venison, rabbit, squirrel	1 oz.
pheasant, duck, goose (without skin)	1 oz.
Cheese:	
any cottage cheese*	¼ cup
grated parmesan	2 Tbsp.
diet cheeses[S] (with less than 55 calories per ounce)	1 oz.

Other

95% fat-free luncheon meat[S]	1½ oz.
egg whites	3 whites
egg substitutes with less than 55 calories per ½ cup	½ cup

Medium-Fat Meat and Substitutes
(One exchange is equal to any one of the following items.)

Beef: most beef products fall into this category. Examples are: all ground beef, roast (rib, chuck, rump), steak (cubed, Porterhouse, T-bone), and meatloaf	1 oz.
Pork: most pork products fall into this category. Examples are: chops, loin, roast, Boston butt, cutlets	1 oz.
Lamb: most lamb products fall into this category. Examples are: chops, leg, and roast.	1 oz.
Veal: cutlet (ground or cubed, unbreaded)	1 oz.
Poultry: chicken (with skin), domestic duck or goose (well drained of fat), ground turkey	1 oz.
Fish:	
tuna* (canned in oil and drained)	¼ cup
salmon* (canned)	¼ cup
Cheese:	
skim or part-skim milk cheeses, such as:	
ricotta	¼ cup

(continues)

LIST 2: MEAT LIST (Continued)

mozzarella	1 oz.	Lamb: patties (ground lamb)	1 oz.
diet cheeses^S (with 56–80 calories per ounce)	1 oz.	Fish: any fried fish product	1 oz.
		Cheese: all regular cheeses, such as American^S, blue^S, cheddar*, Monterey Jack*, Swiss	1 oz.

Other
  86% fat-free luncheon meat*   1 oz.
  egg (high in cholesterol, limit to 3 per week)   1
  egg substitutes with 56–80 calories per ¼ cup   ¼ cup
  Tofu (2½ in. x 2¾ in. x 1 in.)   4 oz.
  Liver, heart, kidney, sweetbreads (high in cholesterol)   1 oz.

Other:
  luncheon meat^S, such as bologna, salami, pimento loaf   1 oz.
  sausage^S, such as Polish, Italian smoked   1 oz.
  knockwurst^S   1 oz.
  bratwurst*   1 oz.
  frankfurter^S (turkey or chicken)   1 frank (10/lb.)
  peanut butter (contains unsaturated fat)   1 Tbsp.

High-Fat Meat and Substitutes
(Remember, these items are high in saturated fat, cholesterol, and calories, and should be used only three (3) times per week. One exchange is equal to any one of the following items.)
  Beef: most USDA Prime cuts of beef, such as ribs, corned beef*   1 oz.
  Pork: spareribs, ground pork, pork sausage^S (patty or link)   1 oz.

Count as one high-fat meat plus one fat exchange:
  frankfurter^S (beef, pork, or combination)   1 frank (10/lb.)

Source: American Diabetes Association, American Dietetic Association, 1989.
**This list is divided into three parts based on the amount of fat and calories.
^S400 mg or more of sodium per exchange.
*400 mg or more of sodium if two or more exchanges are eaten.

	Carbohydrate (grams)	Protein (grams)	Fat (grams)	Calories
Lean	0	7	3	55
Medium-Fat	0	7	5	75
High-Fat	0	7	8	100

LIST 3: VEGETABLE LIST**

Artichoke (½ medium)
Asparagus
Beans (green, wax, Italian)
Bean sprouts
Beets
Broccoli
Brussels sprouts
Cabbage, cooked
Carrots
Cauliflower
Eggplant
Greens (collard, mustard, turnip)
Kohlrabi
Leeks
Mushrooms, cooked
Okra

Onions
Pea pods
Peppers (green)
Rutabaga
Sauerkraut^S
Spinach, cooked
Summer squash (crookneck)
Tomato (one large)
Tomato/vegetable juice^S
Turnips
Water chestnuts
Zucchini, cooked
Starchy vegetables such as corn, peas, and potatoes are found on the Starch/Bread List.
For free vegetables, see Free Food List on pages 353–354.

Source: American Diabetes Association, American Dietetic Association, 1989.
**Each vegetable serving on this list contains about 5 g carbohydrate, 2 g protein, and 25 calories. Unless otherwise noted, the serving size for vegetables (one exchange) is: 1/2 c. cooked or juice, 1 c. raw.
^S400 mg or more of sodium per exchange.

LIST 4: FRUIT LIST**

Fresh, Frozen, and Unsweetened Canned Fruit

Apple (raw, 2 in. across)	1
Applesauce (unsweetened)	½ cup
Apricots (medium, raw)	4
Apricots (canned)	½ cup, or 4 halves
Banana (9 in. long)	½
Blackberries (raw)^F	¾ cup
Blueberries (raw)^F	¾ cup
Cantaloupe (5 in. across)	⅓ melon
(cubes)	1 cup
Cherries (large, raw)	12
Cherries (canned)	½ cup
Figs (raw, 2 in. across)	2
Fruit cocktail (canned)	½ cup
Grapefruit (medium)	½
Grapefruit (segments)	¾ cup
Grapes (small)	15
Honeydew melon (medium)	⅛ melon
(cubes)	1 cup
Kiwi (large)	1
Mandarin oranges	¾ cup
Mango (small)	½
Nectarine (2½ in. across)^F	1
Orange (2½ in. across)	1
Papaya	1 cup
Peach (2¾ in. across)	1, or ¾ cup
Peaches (canned)	½ cup, or 2 halves
Pear	½ large, or 1 small
Pears (canned)	½ cup, or 2 halves
Persimmon (medium, native)	2
Pineapple (raw)	¾ cup
Pineapple (canned)	⅓ cup
Plum (raw, 2 in. across)	2
Pomegranate^F	½
Raspberries (raw)^F	1 cup
Strawberries (raw, whole)^F	1¼ cup
Tangerine (2½ in. across)^F	2
Watermelon (cubes)	1¼ cup

Dried Fruit

Apples^F	4 rings
Apricots^F	7 halves
Dates	2½ medium
Figs^F	1½
Prunes^F	3 medium
Raisins	2 Tbsp.

Fruit Juice

Apple juice/cider	½ cup
Cranberry juice cocktail	⅓ cup
Grapefruit juice	½ cup
Grape juice	⅓ cup
Orange juice	½ cup
Pineapple juice	½ cup
Prune juice	⅓ cup

Source: American Diabetes Association, American Dietetic Association, 1989.
**Each item on this list contains approximately 15 g of carbohydrate and 60 calories.
^{F}3 or more grams of fiber per exchange.

LIST 5: MILK LIST**

Skim and Very Lowfat Milk

Skim milk	1 cup
½% milk	1 cup
1% milk	1 cup
Lowfat buttermilk	1 cup
Evaporated skim milk	½ cup
Dry nonfat milk	⅓ cup
Plain nonfat yogurt	8 oz.

Lowfat Milk

2% milk	1 cup fluid
Plain lowfat yogurt (with added nonfat milk solids)	8 oz.

Whole Milk

Whole milk	1 cup
Evaporated whole milk	½ cup
Whole plain yogurt	8 oz.

Source: American Diabetes Association, American Dietetic Association, 1989.
**This list is divided into three parts based on the amount of fat and calories one serving (one exchange) of each contains:

	Carbohydrate (grams)	Protein (grams)	Fat (grams)	Calories
Skim/Very Lowfat	12	8	trace	90
Lowfat	12	8	5	120
Whole	12	8	8	150

*LIST 6: FAT LIST***

Unsaturated Fats		Salad dressing, mayonnaise type, reduced-calorie	1 Tbsp.
Avocado	⅛ medium	Salad dressing (oil varieties)*	1 Tbsp.
Margarine	1 tsp.	Salad dressing, reduced-calorie^S	2 Tbsp.
Margarine, diet*	1 Tbsp.		
Mayonnaise	1 tsp.	(Two tablespoons of low-calorie salad dressing is a free food.)	
Mayonnaise, reduced-calorie*	1 Tbsp.		
Nuts and Seeds:		**Saturated Fats**	
almonds, dry roasted	6 whole	Butter	1 tsp.
cashews, dry roasted	1 Tbsp.	Bacon*	1 slice
pecans	2 whole	Chitterlings	½ ounce
peanuts	20 small or 10 large	Coconut, shredded	2 Tbsp.
walnuts	2 whole	Coffee whitener, liquid	2 Tbsp.
other nuts	1 Tbsp.	Coffee whitener, powder	4 tsp.
seeds, pine nuts, sunflower (without shells)	1 Tbsp.	Cream (light, coffee, table)	2 Tbsp.
pumpkin seeds	2 tsp.	Cream, sour	2 Tbsp.
Oil (corn, cottonseed, safflower, soybean, sunflower, olive, peanut)	1 tsp.	Cream (heavy, whipping)	1 Tbsp.
		Cream cheese	1 Tbsp.
Olives*	10 small or 5 large	Salt pork*	¼ ounce
Salad dressing, mayonnaise-type	2 tsp.		

Source: American Diabetes Association, American Dietetic Association, 1989.
**Each serving (one exchange) contains about 5 g fat and 45 calories.
^S400 mg or more of sodium per exchange.
*400 mg or more of sodium if two or more exchanges are eaten.

FOODS FOR OCCASIONAL USE

Food	Amount	Exchanges
Angel food cake	¹⁄₁₂ cake	2 starch
Cake, no icing	¹⁄₁₂ cake, or a 3" square	2 starch, 2 fat
Cookies	2 small (1¾" across)	1 starch, 1 fat
Frozen fruit yogurt	⅓ cup	1 starch
Gingersnaps	3	1 starch
Granola	¼ cup	1 starch, 1 fat
Granola bars	1 small	1 starch, 1 fat
Ice cream, any flavor	½ cup	1 starch, 2 fat
Ice milk, any flavor	½ cup	1 starch, 1 fat
Sherbet, any flavor	¼ cup	1 starch
Snack chips*, all varieties	1 oz.	1 starch, 2 fat
Vanilla wafers	6 small	1 starch

*400 mg or more of sodium if two or more exchanges are eaten.

*FREE FOODS***

Drinks
Bouillon^S or broth without fat
Bouillon, low-sodium
Carbonated drinks, sugar-free
Carbonated water
Club soda
Cocoa powder, unsweetened (1 Tbsp.)
Coffee/tea
Drink mixes, sugar-free

Tonic water, sugar-free

Nonstick pan spray

Fruit
Cranberries, unsweetened (½ cup)
Rhubarb, unsweetened (½ cup)

Vegetables (raw, 1 cup)
Cabbage

(continues)

FREE FOODS (Continued)

Celery
Chinese cabbage[F]
Cucumber
Green onion
Hot peppers
Mushrooms
Radishes
Zucchini[F]

Salad greens
Endive
Escarole
Lettuce
Romaine
Spinach

Sweet substitutes
Candy, hard, sugar-free
Gelatin, sugar-free
Gum, sugar-free
Jam/jelly, sugar-free (less than 20 cal/2 tsp.)
Pancake syrup, sugar-free (1–2 Tbsp.)
Sugar substitutes (saccharin, aspartame)
Whipped topping (2 Tbsp.)

Condiments
Catsup (1 Tbsp.)
Horseradish
Mustard
Pickles[S], dill, unsweetened
Salad dressing, low-calorie (2 Tbsp.)
Taco sauce (3 Tbsp.)
Vinegar

Seasonings can be very helpful in making food taste better. Be careful of how much sodium you use. Read the label, and choose those seasonings that do not contain sodium or salt.
Basil (fresh)
Celery seeds
Chili powder
Chives
Cinnamon
Curry
Dill
Flavoring extracts (vanilla, almond, walnut, peppermint, butter, lemon, etc.)
Garlic
Garlic powder
Herbs
Hot pepper sauce
Lemon
Lemon juice
Lemon pepper
Lime
Lime juice
Mint
Onion powder
Oregano
Paprika
Pepper
Pimento
Spices
Soy sauce[S]
Soy sauce[S], low-sodium ("lite")
Wine, used in cooking (¼ cup)
Worcestershire sauce

Use up to three servings per day of a food with a specified size. Use as much as you want of those foods with no specified size.
**Each item contains less than 20 kcal/serving.
[F]3 grams or more of fiber per exchange.
[S]400 mg or more of sodium per exchange.

SELECTED COMBINATION FOODS

Combination foods do not fit into only one exchange list. This is a list of average values for some typical combination foods.

Food	Amount	Exchanges
Casseroles, homemade	1 cup (8 oz.)	2 starch, 2 medium-fat meat, 1 fat
Cheese pizza[S], thin crust	¼ of 15 oz. or ¼ of 10"	2 starch, 1 medium-fat meat, 1 fat
Chili with beans[F,S] (commercial)	1 cup (8 oz.)	2 starch, 2 medium-fat meat, 2 fat
Chow mein[S] (without noodles or rice)	2 cups (16 oz.)	1 starch, 2 vegetable, 2 lean meat
Macaroni and cheese[S]	1 cup (8 oz.)	2 starch, 1 medium-fat meat, 2 fat
Soup		
Bean[F,S]	1 cup (8 oz.)	1 starch, 1 vegetable, 1 lean meat
Chunky, all varieties[S]	10¾ oz. can	1 starch, 1 vegetable, 1 medium-fat meat
Cream[S] (made with water)	1 cup (8 oz.)	1 starch, 1 fat
Vegetable[S] or broth-type[S]	1 cup (8 oz.)	1 starch
Spaghetti and meatballs[S] (canned)	1 cup (8 oz.)	2 starch, 1 medium-fat meat, 1 fat
Sugar-free pudding (made with skim milk)	½ cup	1 starch
If beans are used as a meat substitute		
Dried beans[F], peas[F], lentils[F]	1 cup (cooked)	2 starch, 1 lean meat

[F]3 grams or more of fiber per exchange.
[S]400 mg or more of sodium per exchange.

Appendix F

Food Composition Tables

The food composition table in this appendix contains approximately 7,500 foods which are divided into 20 categories as indicated in Table F-1. As noted in this table, baby foods, fast foods, and commercial prepared foods are not included. Their exclusion is based on the following factors:

1. The frequent changes in nutrient contents of these foods.
2. The infrequent use of these foods in patient care.
3. Space limitation to assure a reasonable price for the book.

There are various abbreviations used in the food composition table including:
1. Abbreviations used in the heading as described in Table F-2.
2. Abbreviations used in the description for each food as described in Table F-3.

3. The numerical values for certain nutrients in some foods are represented by "—." This means any one of the following:
   a. The nutrient occurs in a trace amount.
   b. The nutrient level is unknown.
   c. The nutrient level is extremely variable and no one particular value is selected.
   d. Other situations in which the original sources of the data have been unable to provide the appropriate values.

Table F-4 presents the food composition table. The data in the food composition are copyrighted by and used by the courtesy of CAMDE Corporation (P.O. Box 2006, Chandler, AZ 85244-2006) which markets three nutrition software programs (**Nutri-Calc, Nutri-Calc HD, and Nutri-Calc Plus**).

TABLE F-1
The 20 Categories of Food Products

Category	Food Products	Category	Food Products
1	Baked goods	11	Lamb, veal, game
2	Beef products	12	Legumes
3	Beverages and drinks	13	Nuts and seeds
4	Breakfast cereals	14	Pork products
5	Dairy products and milk	15	Poultry products
6	Eggs	16	Snacks
7	Fats, oils, and related products	17	Soups, sauces, gravies
8	Fish and shellfish products	18	Sugars and sweets
9	Fruits and fruit products	19	Vegetables and vegetable products
10	Grain and bread products	20	Miscellaneous

TABLE F-2
Abbreviations Used in the Headings for the Table

PRO	Protein	B_{12}	Vitamin B_{12}
TFAT	Total fat	Fol	Folacin
SFAT	Saturated fat	PA	Pantothenic acid
PFAT	Polyunsaturated fat	C	Vitamin C
MFAT	Monounsaturated fat	Ca	Calcium
Chol	Cholesterol	Fe	Iron
CHO	Carbohydrate	Mg	Magnesium
CFib	Crude fiber	P	Phosphorus
DFib	Dietary fiber	K	Potassium
Alc	Alcohol	Na	Sodium
A	Vitamin A	Zn	Zinc
B_1	Thiamine	Cu	Copper
B_2	Riboflavin	Mn	Manganese
NI	Niacin	Wt	Weight
B_6	Pyridoxine	RE	Retinol equivalent

TABLE F-3
Abbreviations Used in the Description for Each Food

BBQ	Barbeque	MG	Milligram
BRAIS	Braised	ML	Milliliter
CALIF	California	OZ	Ounce
CAL	Calories	PAST	Pasteurized
CAN	Canned	PEP.FARM	Pepperidge Farm
CC	Cubic Centimeter	PLN	Plain
CHOC	Chocolate	PREP	Prepared
COND	Condensed	PTS	Parts
CTR	Center	RED	Reduced
DBL	Double	REG	Regular
DEHY	Dehydrated	RND	Round
DIA	Diameter	RSTD	Roasted
DNR	Dinner	R-T-S	Ready to Serve
F.A.	Franco-American	S.C.	Soft Crumb
F.C.	Firm Crumb	SL	Slice
FL	Fluid	SQ	Square
FRZN	Frozen	SUB	Substitute
GAL	Gallon	SUG	Sugar
GM	Gram	SULP	Sulphur
GR	Grain	TBSP	Tablespoon
HVY	Heavy	TSP	Teaspoon
HYDROG	Hydrogenated	TSTD	Toasted
IMIT	Imitation	UNSWT	Unsweetened
INST	Instant	VEG	Vegetable
JR	Junior	W/	With
KSL	Kitchens of Sara Lee	WAT	Water
LB	Pound	WHL	Whole
LN	Lean	WHT	White
LT	Light	X-	Extra
MED	Medium		

TABLE F-4
Food Composition Table

Food description; serving; item number	Energy (kcal)	Water (g)	PRO (g)	TFAT (g)	SFAT (g)	PFAT (g)	MFAT (g)	Chol (mg)	CHO (g)	CFib (g)	DFib (g)	Alc (g)	A (RE)
Category 1: Baked Goods													
Brownies, Commercial, Large; each; #186	227	7.6	2.7	9.1	2.42	1.44	4.73	10	35.8	0.4	1.34	—	11
Cake, Angelfood, 1/12 Piece; Slices; #217	73	9.4	1.7	0.2	0.03	0.1	0.02	0	16.4	—	0.43	—	0
Cake, Boston Cream Pie, 1/6 Piece; Slices; #218	217	45.7	2.2	7.8	2.33	0.93	4.08	18	35.5	—	1.29	—	21
Cake, Carrot w/Cream Cheese, Recipe; 1/2 Pc; #219	484	22.9	5.1	29.3	5.43	15.1	7.24	60	52.4	0.6	—	—	427
Cake, Choc. w/Choc. Icing, Commerci; 1/8 Pc; #220	235	14.7	2.6	10.5	2.97	1.22	5.76	—	34.9	0.3	1.79	—	18
Cake, Choc., Mix, Plain; 1/12 Pc; #221	198	20.8	3.6	7.6	1.75	2.3	3.07	35	31.8	0.1	—	—	5
Cake, Fruitcake; Pieces; #225	139	10.9	1.3	3.9	0.48	1.39	1.79	2	26.5	—	1.59	—	8
Cake, Gingerbread, Mix, Prep.; 1/9 Pc; #227	205	22.2	2.7	6.4	1.64	0.84	3.53	24	34.4	0.1	1.94	—	4
Cake, KSL, Iced 1 Layer, Banana; Slices; #229	170	—	1	6	—	—	—	—	28	—	—	—	20
Cake, KSL, Iced 1 Layer, Carrot; Slices; #230	250	—	3	13	—	—	—	25	30	—	—	—	400
Cake, Pineapple Upside-Down, Recipe; 1/9 Pc; #233	367	37.1	4	13.9	3.35	3.77	5.97	25	58	0.01	—	—	75
Cake, Pound, Made w/But, Commercial; 1/10 Pc; #235	117	7.4	1.6	6	3.34	0.32	1.67	66	14.7	0.1	—	—	47
Cake, Spongecake, 1/12 Piece; Slices; #237	110	11.3	2	1	0.31	0.17	0.36	39	23.2	0	—	—	18
Cake, White, Mix, Plain; 1/12 Pc; #239	190	19.1	2.5	4.8	0.72	1.8	1.99	0	34.4	0.1	—	—	0
Cake, Yellow, Mix, Plain; 1/12 Pc; #241	202	18.8	3	5.9	1.02	2.02	2.44	87	34.3	0.1	—	—	12
Cheesecake, Commercial, Plain; 1/6 Pc; #298	256	36.5	4.4	18	9.21	1.1	6.2	44	20.4	0.4	1.68	—	129
Cinnamon Rolls, KSL, All Butter Pln; each; #356	230	—	3	11	—	—	—	—	31	—	—	—	40
Coffeecake, Cinn w/Crumb Top, Mix; 1/8 Pc; #394	159	15.3	2.7	4.8	1.33	0.62	2.49	25	26.4	0.1	—	—	7
Cookies, Animal Crackers; 11 each; #409	126	1.1	1.9	3.9	0.98	0.52	2.19	0	21	0.1	—	—	0
Cookies, Butter, Commercial, 2" Dia; each; #411	23	0.2	0.3	0.9	0.54	0.05	0.26	4	3.4	0	0.12	—	8
Cookies, Chocolate Chip, Commercial; each; #416	48	0.4	0.5	2.3	0.78	0.22	1.15	0	6.7	0.1	0.25	—	0
Cookies, Chocolate Chip, Recipe; each; #417	78	0.9	0.9	4.5	1.29	1.35	1.66	5	9.3	0.2	—	—	26
Cookies, Chocolate Chip, Refrig Bkd; each; #418	59	0.4	0.6	2.7	0.93	0.28	1.35	3	8.2	0	—	—	2
Cookies, Coconut Macaroons, Recipe; each; #421	97	2.5	0.9	3	2.7	0.03	0.13	0	17.3	0.2	—	—	0
Cookies, Fig Bars; each; #422	56	2.6	0.6	1.2	0.21	0.2	0.64	0	11.3	0.4	0.74	—	1
Cookies, Gingersnaps; each; #423	29	0.4	0.4	0.7	0.12	0.1	0.39	0	5.4	—	—	—	0
Cookies, Hydrox, Chocolate Sandwich; 3 Each; #424	160	—	2	7	—	—	—	0	21	—	—	—	—
Cookies, Nabisco, Fig Newtons; each; #427	60	—	1	1	—	—	—	0	11	—	—	—	—
Cookies, Nabisco, Lorna Doone; 3 Each; #428	70	—	1	4	—	—	—	0	9	—	—	—	—
Cookies, Nabisco, Mallomars Choc Ca; each; #429	60	—	1	3	—	—	—	0	9	—	—	—	—

B₁ (mg)	B₂ (mg)	NI (mg)	B₆ (mg)	B₁₂ (μg)	Fol (μg)	PA (mg)	C (mg)	Ca (mg)	Fe (mg)	Mg (mg)	P (mg)	K (mg)	Na (mg)	Zn (mg)	Cu (mg)	Mn (mg)	Wt (g)
0.14	0.12	0.96	0.02	—	—	0.31	—	16	1.26	17	57	84	175	0.4	0.13	—	56
0.03	0.14	0.25	0.01	0	—	0.06	0	40	0.15	3	189	26	212	0.02	0.02	0.02	28.35
0.38	0.25	0.18	0.02	0.15	7	0.28	—	21	0.35	6	46	36	132	0.15	—	0.05	92
0.15	0.17	1.13	0.08	0.12	14	0.25	1.2	27	1.39	20	78	124	273	0.54	0.15	0.38	111
0.02	0.09	0.37	—	—	—	—	—	28	1.41	22	78	128	213	0.44	0.16	0.2	64
0.06	0.1	0.63	0.02	0.07	7	0.14	0	70	2.08	22	132	153	370	0.45	0.18	0.32	65
0.02	0.04	0.34	—	—	1	0.1	—	14	0.89	7	22	66	116	0.12	0.02	0.09	43
0.13	0.13	1.05	0.03	0.04	6	0.15	0.1	46	2.22	11	113	162	307	0.27	0.11	0.24	67
0.03	0.07	0.4	—	—	—	—	—	—	0.72	—	—	—	160	—	—	—	48.6
—	0.07	0.8	—	—	—	—	—	—	0.72	—	—	—	240	—	—	—	67.3
0.18	0.18	1.37	0.04	0.09	8	0.23	1.4	137	1.7	15	95	129	367	0.36	0.1	0.4	115
0.04	0.07	0.39	—	—	—	—	—	11	0.41	3	41	36	119	0.14	0.01	0.03	30
0.09	0.1	0.73	0.02	0	5	0.18	0	26	1.03	4	52	38	93	0.19	0.02	0.08	38
0.08	0.1	0.43	0.01	0.05	3	0.08	0.1	85	0.61	6	149	59	301	0.21	0.04	0.13	62
0.07	0.12	0.71	0.04	0.12	6	0.2	0.1	64	0.78	6	150	46	299	0.22	0.03	0.09	63
0.02	0.16	0.16	0.04	0.14	12	0.46	—	40	0.51	8	75	72	165	0.41	0.02	0.11	80
0.09	0.1	0.8	—	—	—	—	—	—	0.36	—	—	—	220	—	—	—	56.7
0.08	0.09	0.76	0.03	0.07	6	0.13	0.1	68	0.71	9	107	56	211	0.23	0.07	0.16	50
0.1	0.09	0.98	0.01	0.01	4	0.11	0.4	12	0.78	5	32	28	112	0.18	0.05	0.12	28.35
0.02	0.02	0.16	0	0.01	0	0.02	0	1	0.11	1	5	6	18	0.02	0.01	0.01	5
0.02	0.03	0.27	0.01	0	1	0.02	0	2	0.28	3	11	14	32	0.06	0.02	0.05	10
0.03	0.03	0.22	0.01	0.01	2	0.04	0	6	0.39	9	16	36	58	0.15	0.06	0.11	16
0.02	0.02	0.24	—	—	—	—	0	3	0.3	3	9	24	28	0.07	0.02	—	12
0	0.03	0.03	0.02	0.01	1	0.06	0	2	0.18	5	10	38	50	0.17	0	0.23	24
0.03	0.04	0.3	0.01	—	2	0.06	—	10	0.46	4	10	33	56	0.06	0.02	0.05	16
0.01	0.02	0.23	—	0	—	—	—	5	0.45	3	6	24	46	0.04	0.02	0.11	7
—	0.03	0.8	—	—	—	—	—	—	1.08	—	—	—	140	—	—	—	28.35
0.03	0.03	—	—	—	—	—	—	—	0.36	—	—	—	60	—	—	—	14.2
0.03	0.03	0.4	—	—	—	—	—	—	0.36	—	—	—	65	—	—	—	14.2
—	—	—	—	—	—	—	—	—	0.36	—	—	—	20	—	—	—	14.2

Food description; serving; item number	Energy (kcal)	Water (g)	PRO (g)	TFAT (g)	SFAT (g)	PFAT (g)	MFAT (g)	Chol (mg)	CHO (g)	CFib (g)	DFib (g)	Alc (g)	A (RE)
Cookies, Nabisco, Nilla Wafers 3 1/2 Ea.; #430	60	—	1	2	—	—	—	1	11	—	—	—	—
Cookies, Oatmeal, Commercial; each; #433	81	1	1.1	3.3	0.6	0.49	1.87	0	12.4	0	0.56	—	0
Cookies, Oreo, Chocolate Sandwich; each; #435	50	—	1	2	—	—	—	1	8	—	—	—	—
Cookies, Peanut Butter, Recipe; each; #436	95	1.2	1.8	4.6	0.89	1.45	2.17	6	11.8	0.1	0.36	—	31
Cookies, Shortbread, Commercial; each; #437	40	0.3	0.5	1.9	0.49	0.25	1.08	2	5.2	—	0.14	—	1
Cookies, Sugar Wafers w/Filling, Lg; each; #438	46	0.1	0.4	2.2	0.4	0.29	1.29	0	6.3	—	—	—	0
Cookies, Vanilla Sandwich; each; #447	48	0.2	0.4	2	0.36	0.28	1.18	0	7.2	—	0.15	—	0
Cookies, Vanilla Wafers; 10 Each; #448	185	1.12	2.2	6.7	1.7	1.7	2.8	20	29.8	—	—	—	10
Cream Puffs, Custard Filled, Recipe; each; #542	336	69.6	8.7	20.1	4.78	5.4	8.48	174	29.8	0	—	—	258
Custard, Baked; Cups; #561	305	204.58	14.3	14.6	6.8	—	—	—	29.4	—	—	—	—
Danish Pastry, Cinnamon, 4 1/4" Dia; each; #572	262	15.8	4.5	14.5	3.73	1.86	8.1	38	29	0.3	0.85	—	12
Danish, KSL, Cheese; each; #575	130	—	2	8	—	—	—	—	13	—	—	—	20
Doughnuts, Cake, Plain, Medium; each; #598	198	9.8	2.3	10.8	1.76	3.83	4.53	18	23.4	0.1	0.8	—	8
Doughnuts, Cake, Sugared or Glazed; each; #599	192	8.8	2.4	10.3	2.4	1.16	5.38	14	22.9	0.1	0.41	—	1
Doughnuts, Yeast, Glazed; each; #600	242	15.2	3.9	13.7	3.49	1.72	7.74	17	26.6	0.2	1.26	—	6
Doughnuts, Yeast, Jelly Filled; each; #601	289	30.2	5	15.9	4.05	1.99	8.98	22	33.2	—	—	—	7
Eclairs, Custard Filled, Recipe; each; #605	262	52.4	6.4	15.7	4.12	3.95	6.48	127	24.2	0.1	—	—	191
Muffins, KSL, Apple-Spice; each; #977	220	—	4	8	—	—	—	0	36	—	—	—	250
Muffins, KSL, Blueberry; each; #978	220	—	3	12	—	—	—	25	25	—	—	—	—
Muffins, KSL, Raisin Bran; each; #979	220	—	4	7	—	—	—	0	37	—	—	—	250
Pie, Apple, Commercial, 1/8 Piece; Slices; #1106	370	81.4	3	17.2	3.21	3.46	9.06	7	53	0.6	2.65	—	47
Pie, Apple, Recipe, 1/8 Piece; Slices; #1107	411	73.3	3.7	19.3	4.73	5.17	8.36	0	57.5	0.6	—	—	19
Pie, Cherry, Commercial, 1/8 Piece; Slices; #1109	406	72.1	3.2	17.1	3.18	3.44	9.09	0	62.1	—	1.25	—	78
Pie, Cherry, Recipe, 1/8 Piece; Slices; #1110	486	82.5	5	21.9	5.37	5.84	9.57	0	69.4	0.2	—	—	86
Pie, Coconut Creme, Commercial; 1/6 Pc; #1112	329	48.4	3.3	16.8	7.59	1.49	6.82	6	43.7	—	—	—	0
Pie, Egg Custard, Commercial; 1/6 Pc; #1113	197	57.2	5.1	10.9	3.08	1.32	5.73	31	19.5	0.2	1.5	—	49
Pie, Lemon Meringue, Commercial; 1/6 Pc; #1114	303	47.1	1.7	9.8	1.75	3.27	4.1	27	53.3	—	1.36	—	59
Pie, Peach, 1/6 Piece; Slices; #1116	244	59.3	2	10.9	2.02	2.3	5.72	0	35.8	—	—	—	24
Pie, Pecan, Commercial, 1/8 Piece; Slices; #1117	452	21.8	4.6	20.9	4.25	3.36	12.14	36	64.7	1.2	3.95	—	53
Pie, Pumpkin, Commercial, 1/8 Piece; Slices; #1118	229	63.3	4.3	10.4	2.17	1.91	5.34	22	29.8	0.4	2.94	—	524
Pie, Pumpkin, Recipe, 1/8 Piece; Slices; #1119	316	90.7	7	14.4	4.91	2.81	5.73	65	41	1	—	—	1213

B₁ (mg)	B₂ (mg)	NI (mg)	B₆ (mg)	B₁₂ (μg)	Fol (μg)	PA (mg)	C (mg)	Ca (mg)	Fe (mg)	Mg (mg)	P (mg)	K (mg)	Na (mg)	Zn (mg)	Cu (mg)	Mn (mg)	Wt (g)
0.03	0.03	0.4	—	—	—	—	—	—	0.36	—	—	—	45	—	—	—	14.2
0.05	0.04	0.4	—	0	—	—	—	7	0.46	6	25	26	69	0.14	0.02	0.15	18
—	—	—	—	—	—	—	—	—	0.36	—	—	—	75	—	—	—	14.2
0.04	0.04	0.7	0.02	0.02	4	0.07	0	8	0.45	8	23	46	104	0.16	0.04	0.11	20
0.03	0.03	0.27	—	—	1	—	—	3	0.22	1	9	8	36	0.04	0.01	0.03	8
0.01	0.02	0.22	—	—	—	—	0	2	0.18	1	5	5	13	0.03	0.01	0.03	9
0.03	0.02	0.27	—	0	1	0.04	0	3	0.22	1	8	9	35	0.04	0.01	0.03	10
0.01	0.03	0.1	—	—	—	—	0	16	0.2	—	25	29	101	—	—	—	40
0.16	0.36	1.09	0.08	0.47	20	0.67	0.4	86	1.52	16	141	149	444	0.77	0.05	0.15	130
0.11	0.5	0.3	—	—	—	—	1	297	1.1	—	310	387	209	—	—	—	265
0.16	0.13	1.4	—	0	—	—	0	46	1.22	12	70	81	241	0.47	0.06	0.24	65
0.09	0.07	0.4	—	—	—	—	—	—	0.36	—	—	—	130	—	—	—	36.5
0.1	0.11	0.87	0.03	0	4	0.13	0	21	0.92	9	127	60	257	0.26	0.05	0.16	47
0.1	0.09	0.68	0.01	—	—	—	—	27	0.48	8	53	46	181	0.2	0.05	0.15	45
0.22	0.13	1.71	0.03	—	13	0.28	—	26	1.22	13	56	65	205	0.46	0.1	0.16	60
0.26	0.12	1.82	—	—	—	—	—	21	1.5	17	72	67	249	0.64	0.12	—	85
0.12	0.27	0.8	0.06	0.34	14	0.49	0.3	63	1.18	15	107	117	337	0.61	0.06	0.13	100
0.38	0.43	5	—	—	—	—	4.8	150	4.5	—	—	—	280	—	—	—	71
0.06	0.1	0.4	—	—	—	—	0	20	0.36	—	—	—	140	—	—	—	64
0.38	0.43	5	—	—	—	—	2.4	150	4.5	—	—	—	400	—	—	—	71
0.04	0.04	0.41	0.06	—	6	0.19	4.9	16	0.7	11	37	102	415	0.25	0.07	0.28	156
0.23	0.17	1.91	0.05	0	7	0.14	2.7	11	1.74	10	44	123	327	0.29	0.08	0.29	155
0.04	0.05	0.31	0.06	—	12	0.5	—	19	0.74	12	45	127	384	0.28	0.06	0.22	156
0.27	0.23	2.3	0.06	0	12	0.22	1.8	18	3.34	15	55	138	343	0.37	0.14	0.36	180
0.06	0.09	0.23	—	—	—	—	—	33	0.9	—	—	73	288	—	—	—	113
0.04	0.2	0.28	0.05	0.4	18	0.62	—	75	0.55	10	105	100	225	0.49	0.02	0.06	94
0.07	0.24	0.73	0.03	—	10	0.9	3.6	63	0.69	16	119	100	165	0.55	0	0.07	113
0.07	0.04	0.22	0.03	—	—	—	—	9	0.54	—	—	136	294	0.1	—	—	109
0.1	0.14	0.28	0.02	—	7	0.48	1.3	19	1.17	20	87	84	480	0.65	0.22	0.89	113
0.06	0.17	0.2	0.07	0	17	0.55	2	66	0.87	16	77	168	308	0.5	0.05	0.26	109
0.14	0.31	1.21	0.07	0.14	16	0.69	2.7	145	1.97	29	152	289	349	0.72	0.1	0.31	155

Food description; serving; item number	Energy (kcal)	Water (g)	PRO (g)	TFAT (g)	SFAT (g)	PFAT (g)	MFAT (g)	Chol (mg)	CHO (g)	CFib (g)	DFib (g)	Alc (g)	A (RE)
Shortcake, Biscuit-Type, Recipe; each; #1349	225	18.5	4	9.2	2.45	2.36	3.93	2	31.5	0.1	—		11
Strudel, Apple; each; #1457	195	30.9	2.3	8	2.08	1.01	4.38	—	29.2	—	1.56	—	6
Sweet Rolls, Cinn-Raisin Commercial; each; #1472	223	14.9	3.7	9.9	2.53	1.27	5.46	4	30.5	0.3	0.78	—	38

Category 2: Beef Products

Food description; serving; item number	Energy (kcal)	Water (g)	PRO (g)	TFAT (g)	SFAT (g)	PFAT (g)	MFAT (g)	Chol (mg)	CHO (g)	CFib (g)	DFib (g)	Alc (g)	A (RE)
Beef and Vegetable Stew, Canned; cups; #71	194	202.13	14.2	7.6	—	—	—	—	17.4	—	—	—	476
Beef Jerky; each; #72	38	—	4.2	1.7	—	—	—	—	1.4	—			
Beef, Brisket, Whole, Lean, Braised; 3 Oz; #76	205	47.3	24.97	10.91	3.91	0.33	4.91	79	0	0	—	—	—
Beef, Chuck, Arm, Prime, Lean, Brsd; 3 Oz; #77	222	45.86	28.07	11.35	4.31	0.46	4.95	85	0	0	—	—	—
Beef, Ground, Lean, Broiled, Med.; 3 Oz; #80	231	47.38	21.01	15.69	6.16	0.58	6.87	74	0	0	—	—	—
Beef, Ground, Reg, Broiled, Med.; 3 Oz; #82	246	46.1	20.46	17.59	6.91	0.66	7.7	76	0	0	—	—	—
Beef, Ground, X-Lean, Broiled, Med.; 3 Oz; #84	217	48.67	21.59	13.88	5.45	0.52	6.08	71	0	0	—	—	—
Beef, Liver, Pan Fried; 3 Oz; #86	184	47.32	22.71	6.8	2.27	1.45	1.38	410	6.67	0	—	—	9119
Beef, Porterhouse, Broiled; 3 Oz; #87	254	44.5	21.33	18.03	7.46	0.68	7.77	70	0	0	—	—	—
Beef, Rib, Whole, Roasted; 3 Oz; #90	304	40.37	19.12	24.66	9.94	0.88	10.6	72	0	0	—	—	—
Beef, Ribeye, 0" Fat, Ln, Chc, Brld; 3 Oz; #92	191	49.89	23.83	9.94	4.02	0.28	4.2	68	0	0	—	—	0
Beef, Round, Bottom, Braised; 3 Oz; #93	234	44.32	24.36	14.36	5.42	0.55	6.25	81	0	0	—	—	0
Beef, Round, Bottom, Lean, Braised; 3 Oz; #94	178	48.96	26.85	6.97	2.35	0.27	3.05	82	0	0	—	—	0
Beef, Round, Tip, Roasted; 3 Oz; #98	199	51.15	22.87	11.26	4.27	0.44	4.69	70	0	0	—	—	0
Beef, Round, Top, Lean, Broiled; 3 Oz; #99	153	52.7	26.93	4.16	1.43	0.19	1.62	71	0	0	—	—	0
Beef, Shank, Lean, Choice, Simmered; 3 Oz; #100	171	49.48	28.63	5.41	1.94	0.18	2.43	66	0	0	—	—	0
Beef, Shortribs, Lean, Choice, Brsd; 3 Oz; #101	251	42.63	26.14	15.41	6.58	0.47	6.78	79	0	0	—	—	—
Beef, Sirloin, Broiled; 3 Oz; #102	219	48.05	23.63	13.1	5.22	0.5	5.63	76	0	0	—	—	0
Beef, T-Bone, Choice, Broiled; 3 Oz; #104	253	44.84	21.24	17.99	7.25	0.68	7.56	70	0	0	—	—	0
Beef, T-Bone, Lean, Choice, Broiled; 3 Oz; #105	182	51.22	23.91	8.81	3.53	0.33	3.54	68	0	0	—	—	0
Beef, Tenderloin, Broiled; 3 Oz; #106	247	45.09	21.47	17.22	6.76	0.65	7.06	73	0	0	—	—	0
Beef, Tenderloin, Roasted; 3 Oz; #109	282	40.56	20.07	21.76	8.61	0.88	9.11	73	0	0	—	—	0
Beef, Top Loin, Broiled; 3 Oz; #110	244	44.87	21.73	16.79	6.65	0.6	7.06	67	0	0	—	—	0
Bologna, Beef, 4 1/2" Dia.; Ounces; #125	88	15.7	3.5	8.1	3.42	0.31	3.91	16	0.2	0	—	—	—
Breakfast Strips, Beef, Cooked; 3 Slices; #175	153	8.91	10.64	11.7	4.88	0.54	5.73	40	0.48	0	—	—	—
Corned Beef, Brisket, Cured, Cooked; 3 Ounces; #467	213	50.82	15.44	16.13	5.39	0.57	7.83	83	0.4	0	—	—	—
Hot Dog, Beef, Cured; each; #759	142	24.62	5.41	12.84	5.42	0.62	6.13	27	0.81	0	—	—	—
Pastrami, Beef, Cured; Ounces; #1059	99	13.25	4.89	8.27	2.95	0.28	4.1	26	0.86	0	—	—	—

B₁ (mg)	B₂ (mg)	NI (mg)	B₆ (mg)	B₁₂ (μg)	Fol (μg)	PA (mg)	C (mg)	Ca (mg)	Fe (mg)	Mg (mg)	P (mg)	K (mg)	Na (mg)	Zn (mg)	Cu (mg)	Mn (mg)	Wt (g)
0.2	0.18	1.67	0.02	0.05	7	0.16	0.1	133	1.65	10	93	69	329	0.31	0.05	0.22	65
0.03	0.02	0.23	—	—	—	—	1.2	11	0.3	6	24	—	191	0.13	0.02	0.14	71
0.19	0.16	1.43	0.06	—	14	—	1.2	43	0.96	10	46	67	229	0.36	0.05	0.18	60
0.07	0.12	2.5	—	—	—	—	7	29	2.2	—	110	426	1007	—	—	—	245
0.02	0.08	0.8	—	—	—	—	—	—	0.6	4	—	—	—	—	—	—	10
0.06	0.19	3.19	0.26	2.17	7	0.3	0	5	2.36	20	203	244	61	5.85	0.1	0.01	85
0.07	0.25	3.16	0.28	2.89	9	0.33	0	7	3.22	21	228	246	56	7.36	0.14	0.02	85
0.04	0.18	4.39	0.22	2	8	0.32	0	9	1.79	18	134	256	65	4.56	0.06	0.01	85
0.03	0.16	4.91	0.23	2.49	8	0.28	0	9	2.07	17	144	248	70	4.4	0.07	0.01	85
0.05	0.23	4.22	0.23	1.84	8	0.3	0	6	2	18	137	266	59	4.63	0.06	0.01	85
0.18	3.52	12.27	1.22	95.03	18	75.03	19	9	5.34	20	392	309	90	4.63	3.8	0.36	85
0.08	0.19	3.48	0.3	1.83	6	0.26	0	7	2.26	21	161	303	52	4	0.11	0.01	85
0.06	0.15	2.9	0.2	2.16	6	0.26	0	9	1.99	17	149	256	54	4.55	0.07	0.01	85
0.09	0.18	4.08	0.34	2.82	7	0.29	0	11	2.18	23	177	335	59	5.94	0.09	0.01	85
0.06	0.2	3.17	0.28	2	8	0.33	0	5	2.66	19	208	239	42	4.17	0.1	0.01	85
0.06	0.22	3.47	0.31	2.1	9	0.36	0	4	2.94	21	231	262	43	4.66	0.11	0.01	85
0.08	0.21	2.99	0.32	2.35	6	0.37	0	5	2.34	21	192	305	53	5.53	0.1	0.01	85
0.1	0.23	5.13	0.48	2.11	10	0.42	0	5	2.45	26	632	376	52	4.73	0.1	0.01	85
0.12	0.18	5.01	0.31	3.22	8	0.35	0	27	3.28	25	224	380	54	8.92	0.15	0.02	85
0.05	0.17	2.73	0.24	2.94	6	0.29	0	9	2.86	19	199	266	50	6.63	0.09	0.01	85
0.1	0.23	3.34	0.35	2.29	8	0.3	0	10	2.6	24	189	311	53	4.98	0.11	0.01	85
0.08	0.19	3.47	0.29	1.83	6	0.26	0	7	2.25	21	157	302	52	3.98	0.11	0.01	85
0.09	0.21	3.94	0.33	1.93	7	0.28	0	6	2.55	25	177	346	56	4.59	0.12	0.01	85
0.1	0.22	2.99	0.33	2.05	5	0.29	0	7	2.68	22	179	313	50	4.15	0.13	0.01	85
0.07	0.22	2.52	0.21	2.08	6	0.21	0	8	2.6	19	170	277	48	3.38	0.1	0.01	85
0.07	0.15	3.99	0.32	1.65	6	0.28	0	8	1.9	20	165	297	54	3.89	0.08	0.01	85
0.01	0.03	0.68	0.04	0.4	1	0.08	6	3	0.47	3	25	44	278	0.61	0.01	0.01	28.35
0.03	0.09	2.2	0.11	1.17	—	—	12.2	—	1.07	9	80	140	766	2.17	—	—	34
0.02	0.14	2.58	0.2	1.39	—	0.36	13.6	7	1.58	11	106	123	964	3.89	0.13	0.02	85
0.02	0.05	1.09	0.05	0.69	2	0.13	10.8	9	0.64	2	39	75	462	0.98	0.03	0.01	45
0.03	0.05	1.44	0.05	0.5	—	—	0.9	2	0.54	5	43	65	348	1.21	—	—	28.35

Food description; serving; item number	Energy (kcal)	Water (g)	PRO (g)	TFAT (g)	SFAT (g)	PFAT (g)	MFAT (g)	Chol (mg)	CHO (g)	CFib (g)	DFib (g)	Alc (g)	A (RE)
Salami, Beef, Cured, Smoked, 4" Dia; Slices; # 1296	60	13.36	3.46	4.76	2.07	0.24	2.17	15	0.65	0	—	—	—
Smoked Sausage, Beef, Cured; Ounces; # 1358	89	15.18	4	7.63	3.24	0.3	3.68	19	0.69	0	—	—	—
Summer Sausage, Beef, Cured; Ounces; # 1469	95	14.39	4.47	8.37	3.41	0.34	3.68	21	0.07	0	—	—	—

Category 3: Beverages and Drinks

Food description; serving; item number	Energy (kcal)	Water (g)	PRO (g)	TFAT (g)	SFAT (g)	PFAT (g)	MFAT (g)	Chol (mg)	CHO (g)	CFib (g)	DFib (g)	Alc (g)	A (RE)
Beer, Light; 12 Fl Oz; #112	100	337	0.7	0	0	0	0	0	4.8	—	—	11.33	0
Beer, Regular; 12 Fl Oz; #113	146	328.8	0.9	0	0	0	0	0	13.2	—	1.78	12.82	0
Club Soda, Carbonated, Can; 12 Fl Oz; #363	0	354.8	0	0	0	0	0	0	0	0	—	—	0
Coca-Cola; 6 Fl Oz; #364	77	—	—	—	—	—	—	—	20	—	—	—	—
Cocktail, Bloody Mary, 5 Fl Oz; Each; #366	116	127.3	0.8	0.1	0.01	0.04	0.02	0	4.8	—	—	13.91	51
Cocktail, Bourbon/Soda, 4 Fl Oz; Each; #367	105	100.8	0	0	0	0	0	0	0	—	—	15.08	0
Cocktail, Daiquiri, 2 Fl Oz; Each; #368	111	41.9	0	0	0	0.01	0	0	4.1	—	—	13.92	0
Cocktail, Gin & Tonic, 7.5 Fl Oz; Each; #369	171	193	0	0	0	0.01	0	0	15.8	—	—	15.98	0
Cocktail, Manhattan, 2 Fl Oz; Each; #370	128	37.7	0	0	0	0	0	0	1.8	—	—	17.44	—
Cocktail, Martini, 2.5 Fl Oz; Each; #371	156	47.3	0	0	0	0	0	0	0.2	—	—	22.4	—
Cocktail, Pina Colada, 4.5 Fl Oz; Each; #372	262	91.7	0.6	2.6	1.23	0.49	0.23	0	39.9	—	—	13.96	0
Cocktail, Screwdriver, 7 Fl Oz; Each; #373	174	178.6	1.2	0.1	0.01	0.02	0.02	0	18.4	—	—	14.06	13
Cocktail, Tequila Sunrise, 5.5 Fl O; Each; #374	189	137.2	0.6	0.2	0.02	0.04	0.03	0	14.7	—	—	18.75	17
Cocktail, Tom Collins, 7.5 Fl Oz; Each; #375	121	202.9	0.1	0	0.01	0.01	0	0	3	—	—	15.98	0
Cocktail, Whiskey Sour, 3 Fl Oz; Each; #376	123	69.3	0.2	0.1	0.02	0.04	0	0	5	—	—	15.12	1
Coffee, Brewed; 6 Fl Oz; #388	4	175.7	0.1	0	0	0	0	0	0.8	—	—	—	—
Coffee, Inst, Reg, Powder w/ Water; 6 Fl Oz; #391	4	177.2	0.2	0	0	0	0	0	0.7	—	—	—	0
Cola, Carbonated, Can; 12 Fl Oz; #398	151	330.8	0.1	0.1	—	—	—	0	38.5	0	—	—	0
Cranberry Juice Cocktail, Bottled; Cups; #530	147	215.05	0.08	0.13	—	—	—	0	37.65	—	—	—	—
Eggnog, Dairy, Nonalcoholic; Cups; #622	342	188.9	9.68	19	11.29	0.86	5.67	149	34.39	0	—	—	203
Fruit Punch Drink, Canned; 6 Fl Oz; #662	87	163.7	0.1	0	0	0.01	0	0	22.1	—	—	—	3
Gin, 90 Proof, 1 Fl Oz; Svg; #673	73	17.2	0	0	0	0	0	0	0	—	—	10.5	0
Ginger Ale, Carbonated, Can; 12 Fl Oz; #674	124	333.9	0.1	0	—	—	—	0	31.9	0	—	—	0
Grape Juice, Canned or Bottled; Cups; #690	155	212.81	1.41	0.19	0.06	0.06	0.01	0	37.85	—	—	—	2
Grape Soda, Carbonated, Can; 12 Fl Oz; #692	161	330.3	0	0	0	0	0	0	41.7	0	—	—	0
Hawaiian Punch, Juicy-Red; 6 Fl Oz; #731	90	—	0	0	—	—	—	—	22	—	—	—	—
Kool-Aid, Sugar-Free; 8 Oz.; #807	3	236.8	0.1	0	0	0	—	0	0.3	—	0	—	0
Kool-Aid, Sugar/Powder/Water; 8 Oz.; #808	80	220	0	0	0	0	—	0	20.4	—	0	—	0
Lemon-Lime Soda, Carbonated Can; 12 Fl Oz; #841	149	329.4	0	0	0	0	0	0	38.4	0	—	—	0

B₁ (mg)	B₂ (mg)	NI (mg)	B₆ (mg)	B₁₂ (µg)	Fol (µg)	PA (mg)	C (mg)	Ca (mg)	Fe (mg)	Mg (mg)	P (mg)	K (mg)	Na (mg)	Zn (mg)	Cu (mg)	Mn (mg)	Wt (g)
0.02	0.04	0.75	0.04	0.7	0	0.27	4	2	0.5	3	26	51	271	0.5	0.04	0.01	23
0.01	0.04	0.9	0.03	0.53	—	—	3.4	2	0.5	4	30	50	321	0.79	—	—	28.35
0.04	0.94	1.22	0.07	1.56	—	—	5.7	4	0.72	4	31	77	352	0.72	0.04	—	28.35
0.03	0.11	1.39	0.12	0.02	14.7	0.13	0	18	0.12	17	43	64	10	0.11	0.09	0.06	354
0.02	0.09	1.61	0.18	0.06	21.4	0.21	0	18	0.11	23	44	89	19	0.06	0.03	0.04	356
0	0	0	0	0	0	0	0	17	—	4	0	6	75	0.36	—	—	355
—	—	—	—	—	—	—	0	—	—	—	27	—	4	—	—	—	185
0.05	0.03	0.64	0.11	0	19.6	0.24	20.4	10	0.55	11	21	216	332	0.14	0.1	0.07	148
0	0	0.02	0	0	0	0	0	4	—	1	2	2	16	0.09	—	—	116
0.01	0	0.03	0	0	1.2	0.01	1	2	0.09	1	4	13	3	0.04	0.03	—	60
0	0	0.03	0	0	1.2	0.01	1	4	—	2	2	12	10	—	—	—	225
0.01	0	0.05	0	0	0.1	0	0	1	0.05	1	4	15	2	0.03	0.02	0.02	57
0	0	0.01	0	0	0.2	0	0	1	0.06	1	2	13	2	0.01	0	—	70
0.04	0.02	0.17	—	0	14.4	—	6.7	11	0.31	—	10	100	9	0.19	0.12	—	141
0.14	0.03	0.34	0.08	0	74.8	0.27	66.5	16	0.17	17	29	325	2	0.09	0.08	0.02	213
0.06	0.03	0.33	0.09	0	—	—	33.2	10	0.47	12	17	178	7	0.11	0.07	—	172
0.01	0	0.03	0.01	0	1.5	0.01	3.8	10	—	3	1	18	39	0.17	—	—	222
0.19	0	0.11	0.02	0	4.6	0.04	11.4	5	0.07	4	6	48	10	0.05	0.03	0.01	90
0	0	0.39	0	0	0.3	—	0	3	0.08	10	2	96	4	0.03	0.01	0.05	177
0	0	0.51	0	0	0	0	0	6	0.09	8	6	64	6	0.05	0.01	0.03	179
0	0	0	0	0	0	0	0	9	0.13	3	46	4	14	0.05	0.04	0.13	370
0.01	0.04	0.13	—	0	0.5	0.17	107.8	8	0.4	8	3	61	10	0.05	0.03	0.4	253
0.09	0.48	0.27	0.13	1.14	2	1.06	3.81	330	0.51	47	278	420	138	1.17	—	—	254
0.04	0.04	0.04	0	0	2.3	0.03	55.1	14	0.38	4	2	47	41	0.23	0.09	0.37	186
0	0	0	0	0	0	0	0	0	0	0	0	0	1	0	0	—	27.7
0	0	0	0	0	0	0	0	12	0.66	3	1	5	25	0.18	0.07	—	366
0.07	0.09	0.66	0.16	0	6.5	0.1	0.2	22	0.6	24	27	334	7	0.13	0.07	0.91	253
0	0	—	0	0	0	0	0	12	0.31	4	0	3	57	0.26	0.08	—	372
—	—	—	—	—	—	—	60	—	—	—	—	30	20	—	—	—	170.1
0	0	0	0	0	0	0	7	27	—	—	26	4	8	0	—	—	238
0	0	0	0	0	0	0	6	26	—	—	9	1	8	0	—	—	241
0	0	0.05	0	0	0	0	0	9	0.25	2	1	4	41	0.18	0.04	0.05	368

Food description; serving; item number	Energy (kcal)	Water (g)	PRO (g)	TFAT (g)	SFAT (g)	PFAT (g)	MFAT (g)	Chol (mg)	CHO (g)	CFib (g)	DFib (g)	Alc (g)	A (RE)
Lemonade, Frozen Concentrate, w/Wtr; Cups; #842	100	221.6	0.1	0.1	0.01	0.03	0	0	26	0.1	—	—	5
Limeade, Frozen Concentrate, w/Wtr; Cups; #857	102	219.6	0.1	0.1	0	0.01	0	0	27.1	—	—	—	—
Orange Drink, Canned; 6 Fl Oz; #1028	94	161.6	0	0	0	0.01	0	0	24	—	—	—	3
Orange Soda, Carbonated, Can; 12 Fl Oz; #1034	177	325.9	0	0	0	0	0	0	45.8	0	—	—	0
Pepper Type Soda, Carbon., Can; 12 Fl Oz; #1088	151	328.9	0	0.4	—	—	—	0	38.2	0	—	—	0
Pineapple/Grapefruit Drink, Canned; Cups; #1131	117	219.7	0.6	0.2	0.01	0.07	0.03	0	29	0.1	—	—	9
Root Beer, Carbonated, Can; 12 Fl Oz; #1277	152	330.4	0.1	0	0	0	0	0	39.2	0	—	—	0
Rum, 80 Proof, 1 Fl Oz; Svg; #1279	64	18.5	0	0	0	0	0	0	0	—	—	9.29	0
Shake, Fast Food, Chocolate; 10 Fl Oz; #1340	360	202.3	9.6	10.5	6.55	0.4	3.04	37	57.9	0.2	—	—	64
Shake, Fast Food, Strawberry; 10 Fl Oz; #1341	319	209.7	9.5	8	—	—	—	31	53.4	0.2	—	—	83
Shake, Fast Food, Vanilla; 10 Fl Oz; #1342	314	211.5	9.8	8.4	5.26	0.31	2.44	32	50.8	0.3	—	—	90
Sprite Soda; 6 Fl Oz; #1444	71	—	—	—	—	—	—	—	18	—	—	—	—
Tea, Brewed; 6 Fl Oz; #1506	2	177.4	0	0	0	0.01	0	0	0.4	—	—	—	0
Tea, Herb, Brewed; 6 Fl Oz; #1507	1	177.5	0.1	0	0	0.01	0	0	0.3	0	—	—	0
Tea, Instant, Sweet, Lemon, Powder; 3 Tsps; #1509	87	0.1	0.1	0.1	0.01	0.02	0	0	22.1	0	—	—	0
Tea, Instant, Unsweetened, w/Water; Cups; #1510	2	236.2	0.1	0	0	0	0	0	0.4	0	—	—	0
V8 Vegetable Juice Cocktail; 6 Oz; #1574	35	—	1	0	—	—	—	—	8	—	—	—	450
Vodka, 80 Proof, 1 Fl Oz; Svg; #1607	64	18.5	0	0	0	0	0	0	0	—	—	9.29	0
Whiskey, 86 Proof, 1 Fl Oz; Svg; #1637	69	17.8	0	0	0	0	0	0	0	—	—	10	0
Wine, Table, Red, 3.5 Fl Oz; Svg; #1641	74	91.1	0.2	0	0	0	0	0	1.8	—	—	9.58	0
Wine, Table, Rose, 3.5 Fl Oz; Svg; #1642	73	91.6	0.2	0	0	0	0	0	1.5	—	—	9.58	—
Wine, Table, White, 3.5 Fl Oz; Svg; #1643	70	92.3	0.1	0	0	0	0	0	0.8	—	—	9.58	0

Category 4: Breakfast Cereals

Food description; serving; item number	Energy (kcal)	Water (g)	PRO (g)	TFAT (g)	SFAT (g)	PFAT (g)	MFAT (g)	Chol (mg)	CHO (g)	CFib (g)	DFib (g)	Alc (g)	A (RE)
All-Bran Cereal; 1/3 Cups; #4	71	0.9	4	0.5	—	—	—	—	21.1	2	10.02	—	375
Bran Buds Cereal; Cups; #129	217	2.4	11.7	2	—	—	—	—	63.9	6	23.3	—	1112
Bran Chex Cereal; Cups; #130	156	1.1	5.1	1.4	—	—	—	—	39	2.23	7.9	—	11
Bran Flakes, 40%, Kelloggs; Cups; #131	127	1.2	4.9	0.7	—	—	—	—	30.5	1.4	7.33	—	516
Bran Flakes, 40%, Post; Cups; #132	152	1.4	5.3	0.8	—	—	—	—	37.3	1.8	8.84	—	622
C.W. Post Cereal w/Raisins; Cups; #209	446	4	8.9	14.7	10.97	1.38	1.67	—	73.9	1.2	2	—	1364
Cheerios Cereal; 1 1/4 Cups; #263	111	1.4	4.3	1.8	0.34	0.75	0.64	—	19.6	0.4	3.01	—	375
Corn Chex Cereal; Cups; #450	111	0.5	2	0.1	—	—	—	—	24.9	0.1	0.5	—	14
Corn Flakes, Kelloggs; 1 1/4 Cups; #455	110	0.7	2.3	0.1	—	—	—	—	24.4	0.1	0.57	—	375
Corn Flakes, Low Sodium; Cups; #456	100	0.8	1.9	0.1	—	—	—	—	22.2	0.2	—	—	—

B_1 (mg)	B_2 (mg)	NI (mg)	B_6 (mg)	B_{12} (µg)	Fol (µg)	PA (mg)	C (mg)	Ca (mg)	Fe (mg)	Mg (mg)	P (mg)	K (mg)	Na (mg)	Zn (mg)	Cu (mg)	Mn (mg)	Wt (g)
0.01	0.05	0.04	0.01	0	5.5	0.03	9.8	8	0.41	5	5	38	8	0.09	0.05	0.01	248
0	0	0.05	—	—	—	—	6.6	7	0.06	2	3	33	6	0.05	0.01	0	247
0.01	0.01	0.06	0.02	0	—	0.03	63.5	12	0.53	3	3	33	31	0.16	0.01	0.03	186
0	0	—	0	0	0	0	0	19	0.23	4	4	9	46	0.38	0.06	—	372
0	0	0	0	0	0	0	0	12	0.14	1	41	2	38	0.15	0.02	—	368
0.08	0.04	0.67	0.1	0	26.2	0.13	114.9	18	0.77	15	14	154	34	0.15	0.11	1.03	250
0	0	0	0	0	0	0	0	19	0.18	4	2	3	49	0.26	0.03	—	370
0	0	0	0	0	0	0	0	0	0.03	0	1	1	0	0.02	0.01	—	27.8
0.16	0.69	0.46	0.14	0.97	9.9	1.1	1.3	319	0.88	47	288	567	273	1.15	0.18	0.11	283
0.13	0.55	0.5	0.13	0.88	8.5	1.39	2.1	320	0.3	36	283	516	234	1	0.06	0.04	283
0.13	0.51	0.52	0.15	1.01	9.2	1.18	2.2	344	0.26	35	289	492	232	1.01	0.14	0.04	283
—	—	—	—	—	—	—	0	—	—	—	—	—	23	—	—	—	184
0	0.03	0	0	0	9.2	—	0	0	0.04	5	1	66	5	0.04	0.02	—	178
0.02	0.01	0	0	0	1	0.02	0	4	0.14	2	0	15	2	0.06	0.03	0.08	178
0	0.05	0.09	—	0	9.6	—	0	1	0.04	3	3	49	—	0.02	0.01	0.67	22.7
0	0	0.09	0	0	0.7	0.03	0	5	0.04	5	3	47	8	0.08	0.02	0.52	237
0.03	0.03	1.2	—	—	—	—	30	20	0.72	—	—	—	560	—	—	—	170.4
0	0	0	0	0	0	0	0	1	0	0	0	0	0	0	0	0	27.8
0	0	0.01	0	0	0	0	0	0	0.01	0	2	1	0	0.01	0.01	0	27.8
0	0.03	0.08	0.04	0.01	2.1	0.04	0	8	0.44	13	14	115	6	0.1	0.02	0.62	103
0	0.02	0.08	0.03	0.01	1.1	0.03	0	9	0.39	10	15	102	5	0.06	0.05	0.11	103
0	0	0.07	0.01	0	0.2	0.02	0	9	0.33	11	14	82	5	0.07	0.02	0.47	103
0.4	0.4	5	0.5	—	100	0.49	15	23	4.5	106	264	350	320	3.7	0.32	—	28.4
1.1	1.3	14.8	1.5	—	297	1.63	45	56	13.4	267	729	1404	516	11.1	0.89	—	84
0.6	0.26	8.6	0.9	2.60	173	0.5	26	29	7.8	126	327	394	455	2.14	0.39	—	49
0.5	0.6	6.9	0.7	2.10	138	—	—	19	11.2	71	192	248	363	5.1	0.29	—	39
0.6	0.7	8.3	0.8	2.50	166	—	—	21	7.5	102	296	251	431	2.5	0.32	—	47
1.3	1.5	18.1	1.9	5.50	364	—	—	51	16.4	74	232	260	160	1.64	0.4	—	103
0.4	0.4	5	0.5	1.5	6	0.29	15	48	4.5	39	134	101	307	0.79	0.14	0.76	28.4
0.4	0.07	5	0.5	1.50	100	0.05	15	3	1.8	4	11	23	271	0.1	0.02	0.02	28.4
0.4	0.4	5	0.5	—	100	0.05	15	1	1.8	3	18	26	351	0.08	0.02	0.02	28.4
0	0.05	0.11	—	—	—	—	—	11	0.56	3	12	18	3	0.07	0.02	—	25

Food description; serving; item number	Energy (kcal)	Water (g)	PRO (g)	TFAT (g)	SFAT (g)	PFAT (g)	MFAT (g)	Chol (mg)	CHO (g)	CFib (g)	DFib (g)	Alc (g)	A (RE)
Corn Grits, Cooked; Cups; #457	146	206.5	3.5	0.5	0.06	0.2	0.11	0	31.4	0.2	—	—	—
Corn Grits, Inst, Plain Prepared; Pkt; #458	82	116.4	2.1	0.2	—	—	—	—	17.8	0.1	—	—	—
Cracklin' Oat Bran, Kellogg's; 1/2 Cups; #528	110	—	3	4	—	—	—	0	20	—	5	—	—
Cream of Rice, Cooked; Cups; #536	126	213.5	2.1	0.1	—	—	—	—	28.1	0.1	—	—	—
Cream of Wheat, Instant, Cooked; Cups; #538	153	203.5	4.4	0.6	—	—	—	—	31.6	—	—	—	—
Cream of Wheat, Mix'n Eat, Flavored; Pkt; #539	132	117.2	2.5	0.4	—	—	—	—	28.9	—	—	—	375
Cream of Wheat, Regular, Cooked; Cups; #541	134	218.7	3.8	0.5	—	—	—	—	27.7	—	—	—	—
Farina, Cooked; Cups; #627	116	204.7	3.4	0.2	0.02	0.07	0.02	0	24.6	0.1	3.26	—	—
Frosted Mini-Wheats Cereal; 4 Biscuits; #659	111	1.6	3.2	0.3	—	—	—	—	25.6	0.5	2.3	—	410
Granola, Homemade; Cups; #688	595	4	15	33.1	5.84	17.21	9.37	—	67.3	1.7	12.81	—	—
Grape-Nuts Cereal; 1/4 Cups; #693	101	0.9	3.3	0.1	—	—	—	—	23.2	0.5	1.85	—	375
Honey and Nut Corn Flakes Cereal; 3/4 Cups; #741	113	1.1	1.8	1.5	—	—	—	—	23.3	0.1	0.3	—	375
Malt-O-Meal, Plain/Choc, Cooked; Cups; #879	122	210.2	3.5	0.3	—	—	—	—	25.8	0.2	—	—	—
Maypo Cereal, Cooked; Cups; #907	170	198.6	5.8	2.4	—	—	—	—	31.8	0.4	—	—	702
Mueslix 5 Grain Cereal, Kellogg's; 1/2 Cups; #972	150	—	4	2	—	—	—	0	31	—	3	—	—
Product 19 Cereal; Cups; # 1222	126	1.1	3.2	0.2	—	—	—	—	27.4	0.2	0.4	—	1748
Quaker Oats, Apple/Cinnamon, Prep.; Pkt; # 1234	135	115.9	3.9	1.6	—	—	—	—	26.3	0.4	—	—	435
Quaker Oats, Bran/Raisin, Prep.; Pkt; # 1235	158	155.7	4.9	1.9	—	—	—	—	30.4	0.9	—	—	479
Quaker Oats, Inst, Plain, Cooked; Pkt; # 1236	104	151.8	4.4	1.7	—	—	—	—	18.1	0.3	—	—	455
Quaker Oats, Maple/Brown Sugar Prep; Pkt; # 1237	163	115.3	4.6	1.9	—	—	—	—	31.9	0.3	—	—	451
Raisin Bran Cereal, Kellogg's; 3/4 Cups; # 1242	115	3.1	4	0.7	—	—	—	—	27.9	1.1	4.95	—	375
Raisin Bran Cereal, Post; 1/2 Cups; # 1243	87	2.6	2.6	0.5	—	—	—	—	21.4	0.9	3.81	—	375
Ralston Cereal, Cooked; Cups; # 1248	134	217.7	5.5	0.8	—	—	—	—	28.2	0.8	4.2	—	—
Rice Chex Cereal; 1 1/8 Cups; # 1262	112	0.7	1.5	0.1	—	—	—	—	25.3	0.1	0.2	—	—
Rice Krispies Cereal; Cups; # 1263	112	0.7	1.9	0.2	—	—	—	—	24.8	0.1	0.34	—	375
Rice, Puffed Cereal; Cups; # 1266	56	0.4	0.9	0.1	—	—	—	—	12.6	0	0.1	—	—
Special K Cereal; 1 1/3 Cups; # 1436	111	0.6	5.6	0.1	—	—	—	—	21.3	0.1	0.2	—	375
Sugar Frosted Flakes, Kellogg's; Cups; # 1463	133	0.9	1.8	0.1	—	—	—	—	31.7	0.1	0.78	—	463
Total Cereal; Cups; # 1541	116	1.3	3.3	0.7	0.1	0.34	0.07	—	26	0.6	2.97	—	1748
Wheat Chex Cereal; Cups; # 1627	169	1.1	4.5	1.1	—	—	—	—	37.8	1	3.4	—	—
Wheat Germ, Toasted, BrownSug/Honey; Cups; # 1629	426	6.3	24.7	9.1	1.57	5.5	1.32	—	68.7	1.9	—	—	—
Wheat Germ, Toasted, Plain; Cups; # 1630	431	6.3	32.9	12.1	2.07	7.48	1.7	0	56.1	2.6	—	—	—
Wheat, Puffed, Plain; Cups; # 1632	44	0.4	1.8	0.1	—	—	—	—	9.5	0.2	0.4	—	—
Wheat, Shredded, Large Biscuit; Each; # 1633	83	1.5	2.6	0.3	—	—	—	—	18.8	0.5	2.2	—	—
Wheatena, Cooked; Cups; # 1635	135	207.5	5	1.1	—	—	—	—	28.7	0.7	—	—	—
Wheaties Cereal; Cups; # 1636	101	1.3	2.8	0.5	0.07	0.24	0.05	—	23.1	0.6	2.61	—	384
Whole Wheat, Hot Nat. Cereal, Prep; Cups; # 1640	151	202.3	4.9	4.9	—	—	—	—	33.2	0.9	—	—	—

B₁ (mg)	B₂ (mg)	NI (mg)	B₆ (mg)	B₁₂ (μg)	Fol (μg)	PA (mg)	C (mg)	Ca (mg)	Fe (mg)	Mg (mg)	P (mg)	K (mg)	Na (mg)	Zn (mg)	Cu (mg)	Mn (mg)	Wt (g)
0.24	0.15	1.96	0.06	—	1	—	—	1	1.55	11	29	54	0	0.17	0.03	0.04	242
0.17	0.09	1.3	—	—	1	0.43	—	7	1.02	5	17	29	344	0.09	0.01	—	137
0.38	0.43	5	0.5	—	0.1	—	15	15	1.8	59	166	160	140	1.5	0.19	—	28.4
0.1	0	1	0.07	—	8	—	—	8	0.4	8	42	49	2	0.39	0.08	0.35	244
0.2	0.1	1.8	—	—	11	—	—	59	12	14	43	48	6	0.41	0.09	—	241
0.4	0.2	5	0.5	—	100	—	—	40	8.1	9	20	55	241	0.23	0.06	—	150
0.2	0.1	1.5	—	—	9	0.19	—	51	10.3	10	42	43	2	0.33	0.08	—	251
0.19	0.12	1.28	0.02	—	6	0.13	—	4	1.16	4	28	30	1	0.16	0.03	—	233
0.4	0.5	5.5	0.6	—	109	—	16	10	2	26	81	106	9	1.6	0.14	—	31
0.73	0.31	2.14	0.43	—	99	0.74	1	76	4.84	141	494	612	12	4.47	0.7	—	122
0.4	0.4	5	0.5	1.50	100	0.27	—	11	1.23	19	71	95	197	0.62	0.09	—	28.4
0.4	0.4	5	0.5	—	100	—	15	3	1.8	6	13	36	225	0.11	—	—	28.4
0.4	0.3	5.9	0.02	—	6	0.14	—	5	9.5	—	23	—	2	0.17	0.03	—	240
0.7	0.8	9.4	0.9	2.8	9	0.34	28	125	8.4	51	248	211	9	1.49	0.16	—	240
0.38	0.43	5	0.5	2	0.1	—	—	17	4.5	31	102	170	60	3.75	0.07	—	41.18
1.7	2	23.3	2.3	7	466	0.21	70	4	21	12	47	51	378	0.5	0.09	—	33
0.48	0.28	5.13	0.7	—	137	0.35	—	158	6.07	—	117	107	222	—	—	—	149
0.56	0.63	8.12	0.76	—	155	0.45	—	173	7.61	57	206	236	247	1.35	0.28	1.59	195
0.53	0.29	5.49	0.74	—	150	0.35	—	163	6.32	—	133	100	286	—	—	—	177
0.53	0.32	5.35	0.74	—	145	0.32	—	162	6.35	—	143	102	280	—	—	—	155
0.4	0.4	5	0.5	1.50	100	—	—	13	4.5	48	137	192	269	3.8	0.21	—	36.9
0.4	0.4	5	0.5	1.50	100	—	—	13	4.5	48	119	175	185	1.5	0.16	—	28.4
0.2	0.18	2.05	0.11	0.11	18	0.33	—	14	1.64	59	148	153	4	1.42	0.2	—	253
0.4	—	5	0.5	1.50	100	0.1	15	4	1.8	7	28	33	237	0.39	0.08	—	28.4
0.4	0.4	5	0.5	—	100	0.2	15	4	1.8	10	34	30	340	0.48	0.07	0.28	28.4
0.02	0.01	0.42	0.01	—	3	0.05	—	1	0.15	3	14	16	0	0.14	0.02	0.21	14
0.4	0.4	5	0.5	—	100	0.15	15	8	4.5	16	55	49	265	3.7	0.13	—	28.4
0.5	0.5	6.2	0.6	—	124	—	19	1	2.2	3	26	22	284	0.05	0.07	—	35.4
1.7	2	23.3	2.3	7	466	0.24	70	56	21	37	137	123	409	0.78	0.14	0.5	33
0.6	0.17	8.1	0.8	2.40	162	0.21	24	18	7.3	58	182	174	308	1.23	0.27	—	46
1.41	0.7	4.73	0.83	—	298	1.17	—	38	7.71	272	971	803	3	14.13	0.52	16.91	113
1.89	0.93	6.31	1.11	—	398	1.57	7	50	10.28	362	1294	1070	4	18.83	0.7	22.55	113
0.02	0.03	1.3	0.02	—	4	0.06	—	3	0.57	17	43	42	0	0.28	0.05	—	12
0.07	0.06	1.08	0.06	—	12	0.19	—	10	0.74	40	86	77	0	0.59	0.12	0.73	23.6
0.02	0.05	1.34	0.05	—	17	0.1	—	11	1.36	49	146	187	5	1.68	0.13	2	243
0.4	0.4	5.1	0.5	1.5	9	0.21	15	44	4.6	32	100	108	363	0.65	0.13	0.44	29
0.17	0.12	2.15	—	—	26	0.4	—	17	1.5	54	167	171	1	1.16	0.2	1.41	242

Food description; serving; item number	Energy (kcal)	Water (g)	PRO (g)	TFAT (g)	SFAT (g)	PFAT (g)	MFAT (g)	Chol (mg)	CHO (g)	CFib (g)	DFib (g)	Alc (g)	A (RE)
Category 5: Dairy Products and Milk													
Butter, Regular, 1" Square; Pats; #207	36	0.79	0.04	4.06	2.52	0.15	1.17	11	—	0	—	—	38
Cheese Food, American, Pasteurized; Ounces; #264	93	12.23	5.56	6.97	4.38	0.2	2.04	18	2	0	—	—	—
Cheese Spread, Amer., Past Process; Ounces; #268	82	13.51	4.65	6.02	3.78	0.18	1.76	16	2.48	0	—	—	—
Cheese, American, Pasteurized; Ounces; #269	106	11.1	6.28	8.86	5.58	0.28	2.54	27	0.45	0	—	—	82
Cheese, Blue; Ounces; #270	100	12.02	6.07	8.15	5.3	0.23	2.21	21	0.66	0	—	—	65
Cheese, Brie; Ounces; #271	95	13.73	5.88	7.85	—	—	—	28	0.13	0	—	—	—
Cheese, Camembert; Ounces; #272	85	14.68	5.61	6.88	4.33	0.2	1.99	20	0.13	0	—	—	71
Cheese, Cheddar; Ounces; #273	114	10.42	7.06	9.4	5.98	0.27	2.66	30	0.36	0	—	—	86
Cheese, Colby; Ounces; #274	112	10.83	6.74	9.1	5.73	0.27	2.63	27	0.73	0	—	—	78
Cheese, Feta; Ounces; #275	75	15.66	4.03	6.03	4.24	0.17	1.31	25	1.16	0	—	—	—
Cheese, Goat, Soft Type; Ounces; #276	76	17.22	5.25	5.98	4.13	0.14	1.36	13	0.25	0	—	—	—
Cheese, Gouda; Ounces; #277	101	11.75	7.07	7.78	4.99	0.19	2.2	32	0.63	0	—	—	49
Cheese, Gruyere; Ounces; #278	117	9.41	8.45	9.17	5.36	0.49	2.85	31	0.1	0	—	—	—
Cheese, Lt.Neufchatel, Phil. Brand; Ounces; #285	80	—	3	7	4	0	—	25	1	—	—	—	60
Cheese, Monterey; Ounces; #286	106	11.63	6.94	8.58	—	—	—	—	0.19	0	—	—	—
Cheese, Mozzarella; Ounces; #287	80	15.35	5.51	6.12	3.73	0.22	1.86	22	0.63	0	—	—	68
Cheese, Muenster; Ounces; #289	104	11.84	6.64	8.52	5.42	0.19	2.47	27	0.32	0	—	—	90
Cheese, Parmesan, Grated; Tbsps; #290	23	0.88	2.08	1.50	0.95	0.03	0.44	4	0.19	0	—	—	—
Cheese, Pimento, Past. Process; Ounces; #292	106	11.08	6.27	8.84	5.57	0.28	2.53	27	0.49	—	—	—	—
Cheese, Provolone; Ounces; #293	100	11.61	7.25	7.55	4.84	0.22	2.10	20	0.61	0	—	—	75
Cheese, Ricotta, w/Part Skim; Cups; #294	340	183.05	28.02	19.46	12.12	0.64	5.69	76	12.64	0	—	—	278
Cheese, Romano; Ounces; #295	110	8.76	9.02	7.64	—	—	—	29	1.03	0	—	—	—
Cheese, Roquefort; Ounces; #296	105	11.16	6.11	8.69	5.46	0.37	2.40	26	0.57	0	—	—	—
Cheese, Swiss; Ounces; #297	107	10.55	8.06	7.78	5.04	0.28	2.06	26	0.96	0	—	—	72
Coffee Whitener, Nondairy Powder; Tsps; #387	11	0.04	0.10	0.71	0.65	—	0.02	0	1.10	0	—	—	—
Cottage Cheese, Creamed; Cups; #472	217	165.82	26.23	9.47	5.99	0.29	2.70	31	5.63	0	—	—	101
Cottage Cheese, Low Fat, 2%; Cups; #473	203	179.24	31.05	4.36	2.76	0.13	1.24	19	8.20	0	—	—	45
Cracker Barrel Sharp Cheddar; Ounces; #483	100	—	4	7	4	0	—	20	4	—	—	—	40
Cream Cheese; Ounces; #533	99	15.24	2.14	9.89	6.23	0.36	2.79	31	0.75	0	—	—	124
Cream Cheese, Phil. Brand; Ounces; #534	100	—	2	10	6	0	—	30	1	—	—	—	60
Cream Cheese, Phil. Brand, Light; Ounces; #535	60	—	3	5	3	0	—	10	2	—	—	—	60
Cream, Half and Half; Tbsps; #544	20	12.08	0.44	1.72	1.07	0.06	0.50	6	0.64	0	—	—	16
Cream, Heavy, Whipping, Fluid; Tbsps; #545	52	8.66	0.31	5.55	3.46	0.21	1.60	21	0.42	0	—	—	63
Cream, Light, Coffee or Table; Tbsps; #546	29	11.06	0.40	2.90	1.80	0.11	0.84	10	0.55	0	—	—	27
Cream, Light, Whipping, Fluid; Tbsps; #547	44	9.52	0.32	4.64	2.90	0.13	1.36	17	0.44	0	—	—	44
Eggnog; Cups; #621	342	188.90	9.68	19	11.29	0.86	5.67	149	34.39	0	—	—	203
Ice Cream, French Vanilla, Soft; Cups; #769	377	103.38	7.04	22.52	13.51	0.98	6.68	153	38.28	0	—	—	199

B$_1$ (mg)	B$_2$ (mg)	NI (mg)	B$_6$ (mg)	B$_{12}$ (µg)	Fol (µg)	PA (mg)	C (mg)	Ca (mg)	Fe (mg)	Mg (mg)	P (mg)	K (mg)	Na (mg)	Zn (mg)	Cu (mg)	Mn (mg)	Wt (g)
—	0	0	—	—	—	—	0	1	0.01	—	1	1	41	—	0	0	5
0.01	0.13	0.04	—	0.32	—	0.16	0	163	0.24	9	130	79	337	0.85	—	—	28
0.01	0.12	0.04	0.03	0.11	2	0.19	0	159	0.09	8	202	69	381	0.73	—	—	28
0.01	0.1	0.02	0.02	0.2	2	0.14	0	174	0.11	6	211	46	406	0.85	—	—	28
0.01	0.11	0.29	0.05	0.34	10	0.49	0	150	0.09	7	110	73	396	0.75	0.01	0	28
0.02	0.15	0.11	0.07	0.47	18	0.2	0	52	0.14	—	53	43	178	—	0	0.01	28
0.01	0.14	0.18	0.06	0.37	18	0.39	0	110	0.09	6	98	53	239	0.68	0.01	0.01	28
0.01	0.11	0.02	0.02	0.23	5	0.12	0	204	0.19	8	145	28	176	0.88	0.01	0	28
0	0.11	0.03	0.02	0.23	—	0.06	0	194	0.22	7	129	36	171	0.87	0.01	0	28
—	—	—	—	—	—	—	0	140	0.18	5	96	18	316	0.82	0.01	0.01	28
0.02	0.11	0.12	—	—	—	—	—	40	0.54	4	73	7	104	0.26	0.21	0.03	28.35
0.01	0.09	0.02	0.02	—	6	0.1	0	198	0.07	8	155	34	232	1.11	0.01	0	28
0.02	0.08	0.03	0.02	0.45	3	0.16	0	287	—	—	172	23	95	—	0.01	0	28
—	0.03	—	—	—	—	—	—	20	—	—	0.02	30	115	—	—	—	28
—	0.11	—	-1	—	—	—	0	212	0.20	8	126	23	152	0.85	0.01	0	28
0	0.07	0.02	0.02	0.19	2	0.02	0	147	0.05	5	105	19	106	0.63	0.01	0	28
0	0.09	0.03	0.02	0.42	3	0.05	0	203	0.12	8	133	38	178	0.80	0.01	0	28
0	0.02	0.02	0	—	—	0.03	0	69	0.05	3	40	5	93	0.16	0	0	5
0.01	0.10	0.02	0.02	0.20	2	0.14	—	174	0.12	6	211	46	405	0.84	0.01	0	28
0	0.09	0.04	0.02	0.41	3	0.14	0	214	0.15	8	141	39	248	0.92	0.01	0	28
0.05	0.46	0.19	0.05	0.72	—	—	0	669	1.08	36	449	308	307	3.30	0.01	0	246
—	0.10	0.02	—	—	2	—	0	302	—	—	215	—	340	—	0.01	0.01	28
0.01	0.17	0.21	0.04	0.18	14	0.49	0	188	0.16	8	111	26	513	0.59	0.01	0	28
0.01	0.10	0.03	0.02	0.47	2	0.12	0	272	0.05	10	171	31	74	1.11	0.01	0	28
0	0	0	0	0	0	0	0	—	0.02	—	8	16	4	0.01	0.02	0.03	2
0.04	0.34	0.26	0.14	1.31	26	0.45	—	126	0.29	11	277	177	850	0.78	0.06	0.01	210
0.05	0.42	0.32	0.17	1.61	30	0.55	—	155	0.36	14	340	217	918	0.95	0.06	0.01	226
—	0.14	0.10	—	—	—	—	—	150	—	—	—	120	240	—	—	—	28
0	0.06	0.03	0.01	0.12	4	0.08	0	23	0.34	2	30	34	84	0.15	0	0	28
—	0.03	—	—	—	—	—	—	20	—	—	0.02	25	90	—	—	—	28
—	0.07	—	—	—	—	—	—	40	—	—	0.04	60	160	—	—	—	28
0	0.02	0.01	0.01	0.05	—	0.04	0.13	16	0.01	2	14	19	6	0.08	0	0	15
0	0.02	0.01	0	0.03	1	0.04	0.09	10	—	1	9	11	6	0.03	0	0	15
0	0.02	0.01	0	0.03	—	0.04	0.11	14	0.01	1	12	18	6	0.04	0	0	15
0	0.02	0.01	0	0.03	1	0.04	0.09	10	—	1	9	15	5	0.04	0	0	15
0.09	0.48	0.27	0.13	1.14	2	1.06	3.81	330	0.51	47	278	420	138	1.17	0.03	0.01	254
0.08	0.45	0.18	0.09	1	9	1.07	0.92	236	0.43	25	199	338	153	1.99	0.03	0.01	173

Food description; serving; item number	Energy (kcal)	Water (g)	PRO (g)	TFAT (g)	SFAT (g)	PFAT (g)	MFAT (g)	Chol (mg)	CHO (g)	CFib (g)	DFib (g)	Alc (g)	A (RE)
Ice Cream, Vanilla,Rich,16%Fat,Hard; Cups; #777	349	87.13	4.13	23.68	14.74	0.88	6.84	88	31.95	0	—	—	219
Ice Milk, Vanilla, Hardened; Cups; #778	184	89.89	5.16	5.63	3.51	0.21	1.63	18	28.96	0	—	—	52
Ice Milk, Vanilla, Soft Serve; Cups; #779	223	121.87	8.03	4.62	2.88	0.17	1.33	13	38.38	0	—	—	44
Milk, Chocolate Lowfat, 2% Fat; Cups; #943	179	208.95	8.02	5	3.10	0.18	1.47	17	26	0.15	—	—	142
Milk, Chocolate, Cocoa Home-made; Cups; #944	218	204.05	9.10	9.05	5.61	0.33	2.65	33	25.78	0.20	—	—	85
Milk, Chocolate, Whole, Fluid; Cups; #945	208	205.75	7.92	8.48	5.26	0.31	2.48	30	25.85	0.15	—	—	72
Milk, Cond., Sweetened, Canned; Cups; #946	982	83.11	24.20	26.62	16.79	1.03	7.43	104	166.46	0	—	—	248
Milk, Dry, Non-Fat, Regular; 1/4 Cups; #947	109	0.95	10.85	0.23	0.15	0.01	0.06	6	15.59	0	—	—	2
Milk, Evaporated, Skim, Canned; Fl Oz; #948	25	25.33	2.41	0.06	0.04	0	0.02	1	3.62	0	—	—	37
Milk, Evaporated, Whole, Canned; Fl Oz; #949	42	23.32	2.14	2.38	1.45	0.08	0.74	9	3.16	0	—	—	17
Milk, Human, Whole; Fl Oz; #950	21	26.95	0.32	1.35	0.62	0.15	0.51	4	2.12	0	—	—	20
Milk, Low Sodium, Whole, Fluid; Cups; #952	149	215.21	7.56	8.44	5.26	0.31	2.44	33	10.88	0	—	—	78
Milk, Lowfat, 2% Fat, Fluid; Cups; #953	121	217.67	8.12	4.68	2.92	0.17	1.35	18	11.71	0	—	—	140
Milk, Lowfat, 2%, Protein Fortif.; Cups; #954	137	215.77	9.72	4.87	3.03	0.18	1.41	19	13.5	0	—	—	140
Milk, Skim, Protein Fortified; Cups; #957	100	219.83	9.74	0.62	0.4	0.02	0.16	5	13.68	0	—	—	149
Milk, Whole, 3.3% Fat, Fluid; Cups; #95	150	214.7	8.03	8.15	5.07	0.3	2.35	33	11.37	0	—	—	76
Shake, Chocolate, Thick, 10.6 Oz; Each; # 1339	356	216.6	9.15	8.1	5.04	0.3	2.34	32	63.45	0.75	—	—	—
Shake, Vanilla, Thick, 11 Oz.; Each; # 1343	350	233.03	12.08	9.48	5.9	0.35	2.74	37	55.56	0.19	—	—	88
Sherbet, Orange; Cups; # 1345	270	127.52	2.16	3.82	2.38	0.14	1.1	14	58.73	—	—	—	39
Sour Cream, Cultured; Tbsps; # 1413	26	8.51	0.38	2.52	1.57	0.09	0.73	5	0.51	0	—	—	23
Sour Cream, Imitation, Nondairy; Ounces; # 1414	59	20.17	0.68	5.53	5.04	0.02	0.17	0	1.88	0	—	—	0
Yogurt, Coffee/Vanilla, Lowfat; 8 Ounces; # 1648	194	179.33	11.19	2.84	1.83	0.08	0.78	11	31.33	0	—	—	30
Yogurt, Fruit, Lo-Fat 10gm Protein; 8 Oz; # 1649	231	169.07	9.92	2.45	1.58	0.07	0.67	10	43.24	0.27	—	—	25
Yogurt, Plain, 8 Oz Container; Each; # 1651	139	199.53	7.88	7.38	4.76	0.21	2.03	29	10.58	0	—	—	68
Yogurt, Plain, Low Fat, 8 Oz; Each; # 1652	144	193.11	11.92	3.52	2.27	0.1	0.97	14	15.98	0	—	—	36
Yogurt, Plain, Skim Milk, 8 Oz; Each; # 1653	127	193.47	13.01	0.41	0.26	0.01	0.11	4	17.43	0	—	—	5

Category 6: Eggs

Food description; serving; item number	Energy (kcal)	Water (g)	PRO (g)	TFAT (g)	SFAT (g)	PFAT (g)	MFAT (g)	Chol (mg)	CHO (g)	CFib (g)	DFib (g)	Alc (g)	A (RE)
Egg, Chicken, White, Fresh, Raw; Each; #610	17	29.33	3.52	0	0	0	0	0	0.34	0	—	—	—
Egg, Chicken, Whole, Fresh, Raw; Each; #611	75	37.66	6.25	5.01	1.55	0.68	1.9	213	0.51	0	—	—	95
Egg, Chicken, Whole, Fried; Each; #612	91	31.53	6.23	6.9	1.92	1.28	2.75	211	0.63	0	—	—	114

B$_1$ (mg)	B$_2$ (mg)	NI (mg)	B$_6$ (mg)	B$_{12}$ (µg)	Fol (µg)	PA (mg)	C (mg)	Ca (mg)	Fe (mg)	Mg (mg)	P (mg)	K (mg)	Na (mg)	Zn (mg)	Cu (mg)	Mn (mg)	Wt (g)
0.04	0.28	0.12	0.05	0.54	2	0.56	0.61	151	0.10	16	115	221	108	1.21	0.03	0.01	148
0.08	0.35	0.12	0.09	0.88	3	0.66	0.76	176	0.18	19	129	265	105	0.55	0.03	0.01	131
0.12	0.54	0.18	0.13	1.37	5	1.03	1.17	274	0.28	29	202	412	163	0.86	0.05	0.02	175
0.09	0.41	0.31	0.10	0.85	12	0.75	2.30	284	0.60	33	254	422	150	1.02	0.16	0.19	250
0.10	0.44	0.37	0.11	0.87	12	0.81	2.40	298	0.78	56	270	480	123	1.22	0.29	0.34	250
0.09	0.41	0.31	0.10	0.83	12	0.74	2.28	280	0.60	33	251	417	149	1.02	—	—	250
0.28	1.27	0.64	0.16	1.36	34	2.30	7.96	868	0.58	78	775	1136	389	2.88	0.05	0.02	306
0.13	0.47	0.28	0.11	1.21	15	1.07	2.03	377	0.10	33	290	538	161	1.22	0.01	0.01	30
0.01	0.10	0.06	0.02	0.08	3	0.23	0.40	92	0.09	9	62	106	37	0.29	0	0	31.90
0.01	0.10	0.06	0.02	0.05	2	0.20	0.59	82	0.06	8	64	95	33	0.24	0	0	31.50
0	0.01	0.05	0	0.01	2	0.07	1.54	10	0.01	1	4	16	5	0.05	0.02	0.01	30.80
0.05	0.26	0.10	0.08	0.88	—	0.74	—	246	—	12	209	617	6	—	0.02	0.01	244
0.09	0.4	0.21	0.1	0.89	12	0.78	2.32	297	0.12	33	232	377	122	0.95	0.02	0	244
0.11	0.48	0.25	0.13	1.05	15	0.93	2.76	352	0.15	40	276	447	145	1.11	0.02	0	246
0.11	0.48	0.25	0.12	1.05	15	0.93	2.76	352	0.15	40	275	446	144	1.11	—	—	246
0.09	0.4	0.2	0.1	0.87	12	0.77	2.29	291	0.12	33	228	370	120	0.93	0.02	0.01	244
0.14	0.67	0.37	0.08	0.94	15	.1.09	0	396	0.93	48	378	672	333	1.44	0.19	0.12	300
0.09	0.61	0.46	0.13	1.63	21	—	0	457	0.31	37	361	572	299	1.22	0.16	0.04	313
0.03	0.09	0.13	0.03	0.16	14	0.06	3.86	103	0.31	15	74	198	88	1.33	0.06	0.02	193
0	0.02	0.01	0	0.04	1	0.04	0.1	14	0.01	1	10	17	6	0.03	0	0	12
0	0	0	0	0	0	0	0	1	—	—	13	46	29	—	0.02	0.03	28
0.09	0.46	0.24	0.1	1.2	24	1.25	1.7	389	0.16	37	306	498	149	1.88	0.03	0.01	227
0.08	0.4	0.22	0.09	1.06	21	1.11	1.5	345	0.16	33	271	442	133	1.68	0.18	0.15	227
0.07	0.32	0.17	0.07	0.84	17	0.88	1.2	274	0.11	26	215	351	105	1.34	0.02	0.01	227
0.1	0.49	0.26	0.11	1.28	25	1.34	1.82	415	0.18	40	326	531	159	2.02	0.03	0.01	227
0.11	0.53	0.28	0.12	1.39	28	1.46	1.98	452	0.2	43	355	579	174	2.2	0.03	0.01	227
0	0.15	0.03	0	0.07	1	0.04	0	2	0.01	4	4	48	55	0	0	0	33.4
0.03	0.25	0.04	0.07	0.5	23	0.63	0	25	0.72	5	89	60	63	0.55	0.01	0.01	50
0.03	0.24	0.04	0.07	0.42	18	0.56	0	25	0.72	5	89	61	162	0.55	0.01	0.01	46

Food description; serving; item number	Energy (kcal)	Water (g)	PRO (g)	TFAT (g)	SFAT (g)	PFAT (g)	MFAT (g)	Chol (mg)	CHO (g)	CFib (g)	DFib (g)	Alc (g)	A (RE)
Egg, Chicken, Whole, Hard-Cooked; Each; #613	77	37.31	6.29	5.3	1.63	0.71	2.04	213	0.56	0	—	—	84
Egg, Chicken, Whole, Poached; Each; #615	74	37.51	6.22	4.99	1.54	0.68	1.9	212	0.61	0	—	—	95
Egg, Chicken, Whole, Scrambled; Each; #616	101	44.62	6.77	7.45	2.24	1.31	2.91	215	1.34	0	—	—	119
Egg, Chicken, Yolk, Fresh, Raw; Each; #617	59	8.1	2.78	5.12	1.59	0.7	1.95	213	0.03	0	—	—	97
Egg, Substitute, Liquid; Cups; #619	211	207.7	30.12	8.31	1.66	4.02	2.25	3	1.61	0	—	—	542

Category 7: Fats, Oils, and Related Products

Food description; serving; item number	Energy (kcal)	Water (g)	PRO (g)	TFAT (g)	SFAT (g)	PFAT (g)	MFAT (g)	Chol (mg)	CHO (g)	CFib (g)	DFib (g)	Alc (g)	A (RE)
Margarine, Corn, Hard; Sticks; #884	815	17.8	1	91.3	15.9	27.3	44	—	1	—	—	—	1126
Margarine, Corn, Hard, Tsp; Tsps; #885	33.8	0.7	0	3.8	0.6	0.8	2.2	—	0	—	—	—	47
Margarine, Fleischmann's, Diet; Tbsps; #886	50	—	0	6	1	2	—	0	0	—	—	—	100
Margarine, Imit, Corn, 40% Fat; Tsps; #888	16.6	2.8	0	1.9	0.3	0.8	0.7	—	0	—	—	—	48
Margarine, Soft, Corn, Tub; Tsps; #894	33.7	0.8	0	3.8	0.7	1.5	1.5	—	0	—	—	—	47
Margarine, Soft, Safflower, Tub; Tsps; #895	33.7	0.8	0	3.8	0.4	2.1	1.1	—	0	—	—	—	47
Margarine, Soft, Soy/Safflower; Tsps; #896	33.7	0.8	0	3.8	0.5	1.7	1.5	—	0	—	—	—	47
Mayonnaise, Imit, No Cholest.; Tbsps; #903	67.5	4.8	0	6.7	1.1	3.9	1.5	0	2.2	0	—	—	—
Mayonnaise, Imit, w/Soybean; Tbsps; #904	34.7	9.4	0	2.9	0.5	1.6	0.7	4	2.4	0	—	—	—
Salad Dress. Miracle Whip; Tbsps; #1281	70	—	0	7	1	4	—	5	2	—	—	—	—
Salad Dress. Miracle Whip Free Nonf; Tbsps; #1282	20	—	0	0	0	0	—	0	5	—	—	—	—
Salad Dressing, 1000 Island; Tbsps; #1283	58.9	7.2	0.1	5.6	0.9	3.1	1.3	—	2.4	0.3	—	—	—
Salad Dressing, 1000 Island, Lo-cal; Tbsps; #1284	24.3	10.6	0.1	1.6	0.2	1	0.4	2	2.5	0.2	—	—	—
Salad Dressing, Blue Cheese; Tbsps; #1285	77.1	4.9	0.7	8	1.5	4.3	1.9	—	1.1	0	—	—	—
Salad Dressing, French; Tbsps; #1288	67	5.9	0.1	6.4	1.5	3.4	1.2	—	2.7	0.1	—	—	—
Salad Dressing, French, Lo-cal; Tbsps; #1289	21.9	11.3	0	0.9	0.1	0.5	0.2	1	3.5	0	—	—	—
Salad Dressing, Italian; Tbsps; #1290	68.7	5.6	0.1	7.1	1	4.1	1.7	—	1.5	0	—	—	—
Salad Dressing, Italian Lo-cal; Tbsps; #1291	15.8	12.3	0	1.5	0.2	0.9	0.3	1	0.7	0	—	—	—
Salad Dressing, Mayo-type; Tbsps; #1292	57.3	5.9	0.1	4.9	0.7	2.6	1.3	4	3.5	0	—	—	—
Salad Dressing, Oil/Vinegar; Tbsps; #1293	71.8	7.6	0	8	1.5	3.9	2.4	—	0.4	—	—	—	—
Salad Dressing, Russian; Tbsps; #1294	76	5.3	0.2	7.8	1.1	4.5	1.8	—	1.6	0	—	—	—
Salad Dressing, Russian Lo-cal; Tbsps; #1295	23.1	10.6	0.1	0.7	0.1	0.4	0.2	1	4.5	0.1	—	—	—
Shortening, Household, Tbsp; Tbsps; #1352	113.2	0	0	12.8	3.2	3.3	5.7	—	0	0	—	—	—
Vegetable Oil, Canola; Tbsps; #1590	124	0	0	14	0.99	4.14	8.25	—	0	0	—	—	—

B₁ (mg)	B₂ (mg)	NI (mg)	B₆ (mg)	B₁₂ (µg)	Fol (µg)	PA (mg)	C (mg)	Ca (mg)	Fe (mg)	Mg (mg)	P (mg)	K (mg)	Na (mg)	Zn (mg)	Cu (mg)	Mn (mg)	Wt (g)
0.03	0.26	0.03	0.06	0.56	22	0.7	0	25	0.6	5	86	63	62	0.52	0.01	0.01	50
0.03	0.22	0.03	0.06	0.4	18	0.56	0	25	0.07	5	89	60	140	0.55	0.01	0.01	50
0.03	0.27	0.05	0.07	0.47	18	0.61	0.1	44	0.73	7	104	84	171	0.61	0.01	0.01	61
0.03	0.11	0	0.06	0.52	24	0.63	0	23	0.59	1	81	16	7	0.52	0	0.01	16.6
0.28	0.75	0.28	—	0.75	—	1.27	0	133	5.27	—	304	828	444	3.26	0.06	0.02	251
0.01	0.04	0.03	0.01	0.11	1.34	0.09	0.18	33.91	—	2.95	25.97	48.08	1069.84	—	—	—	113.4
0	0	0	0	0	0.06	0	0.01	1.41	—	0.12	1.08	1.99	44.34	—	—	—	4.7
—	—	—	—	—	—	—	—	—	—	—	—	5	100	—	—	—	15
0	0	0	0	0	0.03	0	0	0.85	—	0.07	0.66	1.21	46.06	—	—	—	4.8
0	0	0	0	0	0.05	0	0.01	1.25	—	0.11	0.95	1.77	50.7	—	—	—	4.7
0	0	0	0	0	0.05	0	0.01	1.25	0	0.11	0.95	1.77	50.7	—	—	—	4.7
0	0	0	0	0	0.05	0	0.01	1.25	—	0.11	0.95	1.77	50.7	—	—	—	4.7
—	—	—	—	—	—	—	—	—	—	—	—	—	49.42	—	—	—	14
—	—	—	—	—	—	—	—	—	—	—	—	—	74.55	0.02	—	—	15
—	—	—	—	—	—	—	—	—	—	—	—	0	85	—	—	—	14
—	—	—	—	—	—	—	—	—	—	—	—	15	210	—	—	—	16
—	—	—	—	—	—	—	—	2	0.1	—	3	18	109	0.02	—	—	15.6
—	—	—	—	—	—	—	—	2	0.1	—	3	17	153	—	—	—	15.3
0	0	0	—	—	—	—	0.3	12.4	0	—	11.3	—	—	—	—	—	15.3
—	—	—	—	—	—	—	—	1.7	0.1	—	2.2	12.3	213.7	0.01	—	—	15.6
—	—	—	—	—	—	—	—	2	0.1	—	2	13	128	0.03	—	—	16.3
—	—	—	—	—	—	—	—	1	0	—	1	2	116	0.02	—	—	14.7
—	—	—	—	—	—	—	—	0	0	—	1	2	118	—	—	—	15
—	—	—	—	—	—	—	—	4	0	0.29	2	1	104.48	—	—	—	14.7
—	—	—	—	—	—	—	—	—	—	—	—	1.2	0.1	—	—	—	15.6
0.01	0.01	0.1	—	—	—	—	1	3	0.1	—	6	24	133	0.07	—	—	15.3
—	—	—	—	—	—	—	—	3	0.1	—	6	26	141	—	—	—	16.3
—	—	—	—	—	—	—	—	—	—	—	—	—	—	—	—	—	12.8
—	—	—	—	—	—	—	—	—	—	—	—	—	—	—	—	—	14

Food description; serving; item number	Energy (kcal)	Water (g)	PRO (g)	TFAT (g)	SFAT (g)	PFAT (g)	MFAT (g)	Chol (mg)	CHO (g)	CFib (g)	DFib (g)	Alc (g)	A (RE)
Vegetable Oil, Corn; Tbsps; # 1591	120.2	0	0	13.6	1.7	8	3.3	—	0	0	—	—	—
Vegetable Oil, Cottonseed; Tbsps; # 1592	120.2	0	0	13.6	3.5	7.1	2.4	—	0	0	—	—	—
Vegetable Oil, Olive; Tbsps; # 1593	119	0	0	13.5	1.8	1.1	9.9	—	0	0	—	—	—
Vegetable Oil, Palm; Tbsps; # 1594	120.2	0	0	13.6	6.7	1.3	5	—	0	0	—	—	—
Vegetable Oil, Safflower, Linoleic; Tbsps; # 1595	120.2	0	0	13.6	1.2	10.1	1.6	—	0	0	—	—	—
Vegetable Oil, Sunflower, Linoleic; Tbsps; # 1596	120.2	0	0	13.6	1.4	5.5	6.2	—	0	0	—	—	—

Category 8: Fish and Shellfish Products

Food description; serving; item number	Energy (kcal)	Water (g)	PRO (g)	TFAT (g)	SFAT (g)	PFAT (g)	MFAT (g)	Chol (mg)	CHO (g)	CFib (g)	DFib (g)	Alc (g)	A (RE)
Abalone, Mixed, Fried; 3 Oz; #1	161	51.09	16.68	5.77	1.4	1.42	2.33	80	9.4	0.11	—	—	—
Anchovy, European, Canned, in Oil; 5 Each; #10	42	10.06	5.78	1.94	0.44	0.51	0.75	—	0	0	—	—	—
Catfish, Channel Breaded/Fried; 3 Ounces; #255	194	49.99	15.37	11.33	2.8	2.83	4.77	69	6.83	0.36	—	—	7
Caviar, Black/Red, Granular; Tbsps; ; #259	40	7.6	3.94	2.86	—	—	—	94	0.64	0	—	—	—
Clams, Mixed, Breaded/Fried; 3 Ounces; #359	171	52.32	12.1	9.48	2.28	2.44	3.86	52	8.78	0.13	—	—	77
Clams, Mixed, Canned; 3 Ounces; #360	126	54.09	21.71	1.65	0.16	0.47	0.15	57	4.36	0	—	—	145
Cod, Pacific, Dry Heat; 3 Ounces; #384	89	64.6	19.51	0.69	0.09	0.27	0.09	40	0	0	—	—	8
Crab, Alaska King, Imit./Surimi; 3 Ounces; #478	87	62.65	10.22	1.11	—	—	—	17	8.69	0	—	—	—
Crab, Alaska King, Moist Heat; 3 Ounces; #479	82	65.92	16.45	1.31	0.11	0.46	0.16	45	0	0	—	—	7
Crab, Blue, Canned; 3 Ounces; #480	84	64.73	17.44	1.04	0.21	0.37	0.19	76	0	0	—	—	—
Crab, Blue, Crab Cakes; Each; #481	93	42.6	12.13	4.51	0.89	1.36	1.69	90	0.29	0.03	—	—	—
Croaker, Atlantic, Breaded/Fried; 3 Ounces; #550	188	50.79	15.47	10.77	2.95	2.48	4.52	71	6.4	0.12	—	—	—
Dolphinfish (Mahimahi), Dry Heat; 3 Ounces; #593	93	60.54	20.16	0.76	0.2	0.18	0.13	80	0	0	—	—	—
Fish Fillets, MSP, Crunchy Batter; 2 Fillets; #633	280	—	12	14	—	—	—	22	26	—	—	—	—
Fish Sticks, Frozen, Reheated; Each; #636	76	12.97	4.38	3.42	0.88	0.89	1.42	31	6.65	0.12	—	—	9
Flounder, MSP, Crunchy Batter; 2 Fillets; #637	220	—	12	9	—	—	—	40	23	—	—	—	—
Flounder/Sole, Dry Heat; 3 Ounces; #638	99	62.18	20.53	1.3	0.31	0.35	0.26	58	0	0	—	—	10
Haddock, Dry Heat; 3 Ounces; #712	95	63.12	20.61	0.79	0.14	0.26	0.13	63	0	0	—	—	16
Halibut, Atl/Pacif, Dry Heat; 3 Ounces; #714	119	60.93	22.68	2.49	0.35	0.8	0.82	35	0	0	—	—	46
Herring, Atlantic, Pickled, 1 3/4"; Each; #736	39	8.28	2.13	2.7	0.36	0.25	1.79	2	1.45	0	—	—	39
Herring, Pacific, Dry Heat; 3 Ounces; #737	213	53.96	17.86	15.13	3.55	2.64	7.49	84	0	0	—	—	29
Lobster, Northern, Cooked, Moist; 3 Ounces; #860	83	64.63	17.43	0.5	0.09	0.08	0.14	61	1.09	0	—	—	22
Mackerel, Pac/Jack, Mixed, Dry Heat; 3 Ounces; #877	1710	52.47	21.87	8.6	2.45	2.11	2.87	51	0	0	—	—	12

B$_1$ (mg)	B$_2$ (mg)	NI (mg)	B$_6$ (mg)	B$_{12}$ (µg)	Fol (µg)	PA (mg)	C (mg)	Ca (mg)	Fe (mg)	Mg (mg)	P (mg)	K (mg)	Na (mg)	Zn (mg)	Cu (mg)	Mn (mg)	Wt (g)
—	—	—	—	—	—	—	—	—	—	—	—	—	—	—	—	—	13.6
—	—	—	—	—	—	—	—	—	—	—	—	—	—	—	—	—	13.6
—	—	—	—	—	´	—	—	0.02	0.05	0	0.16	—	0	0.01	—	—	13.5
—	—	—	—	—	—	—	—	—	0	—	0.02	—	—	—	—	—	13.6
—	—	—	—	—	—	—	—	—	—	—	—	—	—	—	—	—	13.6
—	—	—	—	—	—	—	—	0.03	0	0.03	—	—	0.01	—	—	—	13.6
—	—	—	—	—	4.6	—	—	32	3.23	47	—	—	502	0.8	0.19	—	85
0.02	0.07	3.98	0.04	0.18	—	—	—	46	0.93	14	50	109	734	0.49	0.07	—	20
0.06	0.11	1.94	—	—	—	—	0	37	1.22	23	183	289	238	0.73	0.09	—	85
—	—	—	—	—	—	—	—	—	—	—	—	—	240	—	—	—	16
—	0.21	1.75	—	34.23	—	—	—	54	11.83	12	160	277	309	1.24	0.3	—	85
—	0.36	2.85	—	84.06	—	—	—	78	23.76	16	287	534	95	2.32	0.58	—	85
0.02	0.04	2.11	—	—	—	0.14	—	8	0.28	26	190	439	77	0.44	0.03	0.01	85
0.03	0.02	0.15	—	—	—	—	—	11	0.33	—	—	77	715	—	—	—	85
0.05	0.05	1.14	—	—	—	—	—	50	0.64	—	238	222	911	6.48	1	—	85
—	0.07	1.16	—	0.39	—	—	—	86	0.71	33	221	318	283	3.41	0.65	—	85
—	—	—	—	3.56	—	—	—	63	0.65	20	128	195	198	2.46	0.37	—	60
—	—	—	—	—	—	—	—	27	0.73	35	184	289	296	0.44	0.05	—	85
—	—	—	—	—	—	—	—	—	1.23	—	—	453	96	0.5	0.05	0.02	85
0.06	0.07	1.6	—	—	—	—	—	20	0.36	—	—	—	730	—	—	—	112.5
0.04	0.05	0.6	0.02	0.5	5.1	—	—	6	0.21	7	51	73	163	0.19	0.03	0.07	28
0.06	0.07	0.4	—	—	—	—	—	20	0.36	—	—	—	560	—	—	—	112.5
0.07	0.1	1.85	0.2	2.13	—	—	—	16	0.28	50	246	292	89	0.53	0.02	—	85
0.03	0.04	3.94	0.29	1.18	—	—	—	36	1.14	43	205	339	74	0.41	0.03	—	85
0.06	0.08	6.05	0.34	1.16	—	—	—	51	0.91	91	242	490	59	0.45	0.03	—	85
0	0.02	—	—	0.64	0.4	0.01	—	12	0.18	1	13	10	131	0.08	0.02	0.01	15
—	—	—	—	—	—	—	—	—	1.22	—	—	461	81	0.58	0.09	0.05	85
0.01	0.06	0.91	0.06	2.64	9.4	0.24	—	52	0.33	30	157	299	323	2.48	1.65	0.05	85
12	0.46	9.07	0.32	3.6	2	0.31	—	25	1.26	31	136	442	94	0.73	0.1	0.02	85

Food description; serving; item number	Energy (kcal)	Water (g)	PRO (g)	TFAT (g)	SFAT (g)	PFAT (g)	MFAT (g)	Chol (mg)	CHO (g)	CFib (g)	DFib (g)	Alc (g)	A (RE)
Mussels, Blue, Moist Heat; 3 Ounces; #989	147	51.98	20.23	3.81	0.72	1.03	0.86	48	6.28	0	—	—	—
Ocean Perch, Atlantic, Dry Heat; 3 Ounces; # 1016	103	61.78	20.3	1.78	0.27	0.47	0.68	46	0	0	—	—	12
Octopus, Common, Moist Heat; 3 Ounces; # 1017	140	51.42	25.35	1.77	0.38	0.41	0.28	82	3.74	0	—	—	—
Oysters, Eastern, Breaded/Fried; 6 Medium; # 1042	173	56.96	7.72	11.07	2.81	2.91	4.14	72	10.22	0.13	—	—	—
Oysters, Eastern, Canned; 3 Ounces; # 1043	58	72.37	6	2.1	0.54	0.63	0.21	46	3.33	0	—	—	—
Oysters, Pacific, Moist Heat; 3 Ounces; # 1044	138	54.5	16.06	3.91	0.87	1.52	0.61	—	8.41	0	—	—	—
Oysters, Pacific, Raw; Ounces; # 1045	69	69.75	8.03	1.96	0.43	0.76	0.3	—	4.21	0	—	—	—
Perch, VDK Today's Catch; 5 Oz; # 1099	160	—	25	2	—	—	—	—	5	—	—	—	0
Pike, Northern, Dry Heat; 3 Ounces; # 1123	96	62.02	20.98	0.75	0.13	0.22	0.17	43	0	0	—	—	21
Pollock, Walleye, Dry Heat; 3 Ounces; # 1149	96	62.95	19.98	0.95	0.2	0.44	0.15	82	0	0	—	—	19
Roughy, Orange, Dry Heat; 3 Ounces; # 1278	75	58.74	16.02	0.76	0.02	0.01	0.52	22	0	0	—	—	—
Salmon, Chinook, Dry Heat; 3 Ounces; # 1300	196	55.76	21.86	11.38	2.73	2.26	4.88	72	0	0	—	—	—
Salmon, Pink, Dry Heat; 3 Ounces; # 1302	127	59.23	21.73	3.76	0.61	1.47	1.02	57	0	0	—	—	35
Sardines, Atlantic, Can/Oil/ Bones; 2 Each; # 1307	50	14.31	5.91	2.75	0.37	1.24	0.93	34	0	0	—	—	16
Sardines, Pacific, Can/Tom/ Bones; Each; # 1308	68	25.95	6.21	4.55	1.17	1.63	1.39	23	0	0.01	—	—	26
Scallops, Mixed Breaded/Fried; 2 Large; # 1334	67	18.12	5.6	3.39	0.83	0.88	1.39	19	3.1	0.05	—	—	—
Shrimp, Imitation, Surimi; 3 Ounces; # 1353	86	63.67	10.53	1.25	—	—	—	31	7.76	0	—	—	—
Shrimp, Mixed, Breaded/Fried; 4 Large; # 1354	73	15.86	6.42	3.68	0.63	1.53	1.14	53	3.44	0.04	—	—	—
Shrimp, Mixed, Canned; 3 Ounces; # 1355	102	61.68	19.62	1.67	0.32	0.64	0.25	147	0.88	0	—	—	—
Shrimp, Mixed, Moist Heat; 4 Large; # 1356	22	17	4.6	0.24	0.06	0.1	0.04	43	0	0	—	—	—
Snapper, Mixed, Dry Heat; 3 Ounces; # 1362	109	59.8	22.35	1.46	0.31	0.5	0.27	40	0	0	—	—	—
Swordfish, Dry Heat; 3 Ounces; # 1477	132	58.43	21.58	4.37	1.2	1	1.68	43	0	0	—	—	35
Trout, Rainbow, Dry Heat; 3 Ounces; # 1544	129	53.91	22.39	3.66	0.71	1.31	1.13	62	0	0	—	—	19
Tuna, Canned In Oil, Drained; 3 Ounces; # 1546	169	50.86	24.76	6.98	1.3	2.45	2.51	15	0	0	—	—	20
Tuna, Canned in Water, Drained; 3 Ounces; # 1547	111	60.57	25.14	0.43	0.14	0.11	0.12	—	0	0	—	—	—
Tuna, White, Can/Oil, Drained; 3 Ounces; # 1550	158	54.41	22.55	6.87	—	—	—	26	0	0	—	—	—
Tuna, White, Can/Water, Drained; 3 Ounces; # 1551	116	59.06	22.66	2.09	0.56	0.78	0.55	35	0	0	—	—	—
Whitefish, Mixed, Dry Heat; 3 Ounces; # 1638	146	55.33	20.8	6.39	0.99	2.34	2.17	65	0	0	—	—	—

B$_1$ (mg)	B$_2$ (mg)	NI (mg)	B$_6$ (mg)	B$_{12}$ (µg)	Fol (µg)	PA (mg)	C (mg)	Ca (mg)	Fe (mg)	Mg (mg)	P (mg)	K (mg)	Na (mg)	Zn (mg)	Cu (mg)	Mn (mg)	Wt (g)
—	—	—	—	—	—	—	—	28	5.71	32	242	228	313	2.27	0.13	—	85
—	0.11	2.07	—	0.98	—	—	—	117	1	33	235	298	82	0.52	0.03	—	85
0.05	0.06	3.21	—	—	—	—	—	90	8.11	—	237	—	—	2.86	0.06	0.04	85
—	0.18	1.45	0.06	13.75	12	—	—	54	6.12	51	140	215	367	76.68	3.78	—	88
—	0.14	1.06	0.08	16.26	7.6	—	—	38	5.7	46	118	195	95	77.31	3.79	—	85
0.11	0.38	3.08	—	—	—	—	—	14	7.82	37	207	257	180	28.25	2.28	1.04	85
3 0.06	0.2	1.71	—	—	—	—	—	7	4.34	19	138	143	90	14.13	1.34	0.55	85
0.06	0.25	2	—	—	—	—	0	40	1.8	—	—	—	150	—	—	—	141.75
0.06	0.06	—	0.12	—	—	—	3.3	62	0.6	—	239	282	42	0.73	0.05	—	85
0.06	0.06	1.4	0.06	3.57	3	—	—	5	0.24	—	—	329	98	0.51	0.05	—	85
—	—	—	—	—	—	—	—	—	0.2	—	—	—	69	—	—	—	85
0.04	0.13	8.54	—	—	—	—	3.5	24	0.77	—	—	429	51	0.48	0.05	0.02	85
—	—	—	—	—	—	—	—	—	0.84	—	—	352	73	0.6	0.08	0.02	85
0.02	0.05	1.26	0.04	2.15	2.8	0.15	—	92	0.7	9	118	95	121	0.31	0.05	0.03	24
0.02	0.09	1.6	0.05	3.42	9.2	0.28	0.4	91	0.87	13	139	130	157	0.53	0.1	0.08	38
0.01	0.03	0.47	—	0.41	—	—	—	13	0.25	18	73	103	144	0.33	0.02	—	31
0.02	0.29	0.14	—	—	—	—	—	16	0.51	—	—	76	599	—	—	—	85
0.04	0.04	0.92	0.03	0.56	2.4	—	—	20	0.38	12	65	67	103	0.41	0.08	—	30
0.02	0.03	2.34	0.09	0.95	1.5	—	—	50	2.32	35	198	179	143	1.07	0.25	—	85
0.01	0.01	0.57	0.03	0.33	0.8	—	—	9	0.68	7	30	40	49	0.34	0.04	0.01	22
0.05	0	0.29	—	—	—	—	—	34	0.2	31	171	444	48	0.37	0.04	0.01	85
0.04	0.1	10.02	0.32	1.72	—	—	0.9	5	0.88	29	287	314	98	1.25	0.14	—	85
0.07	0.19	—	—	—	—	—	3.1	73	2.07	33	272	539	29	1.18	0.12	—	85
0.03	—	—	0.09	—	4.5	—	—	11	1.18	26	265	176	301	0.77	0.06	0.01	85
—	—	—	0.32	—	4	—	—	10	2.72	25	158	267	303	0.37	0.01	—	85
0.01	0.07	9.94	—	—	3.9	—	—	4	0.56	29	227	283	336	0.4	0.11	—	85
0	0.04	4.93	—	—	3.5	—	—	—	0.51	—	—	241	333	—	0.16	—	85
—	—	—	—	—	—	—	—	—	0.4	36	—	345	56	1.08	0.08	—	85

Food description; serving; item number	Energy (kcal)	Water (g)	PRO (g)	TFAT (g)	SFAT (g)	PFAT (g)	MFAT (g)	Chol (mg)	CHO (g)	CFib (g)	DFib (g)	Alc (g)	A (RE)
Category 9: Fruits and Fruit Products													
Apple Juice, Canned/Bottled; Cups; #12	116	218.07	0.15	0.28	0.05	0.08	0.01	0	28.96	0.52	—	—	0
Apples, Canned, Sweetened, Sliced; Cups; #13	136	168.01	0.36	1	0.16	0.29	0.04	0	34.07	1.1	—	—	10
Apples, Dried, Sulfured, Cooked; Cups; #14	144	214.53	0.55	0.19	0.03	0.06	0.01	0	39.08	1.7	—	—	4
Apples, Raw, w/Skin; Each; #16	81	115.83	0.27	0.49	0.08	0.14	0.02	0	21.05	1.06	2.43	—	7
Applesauce, Canned, Sweetened; Cups; #18	194	202.92	0.47	0.47	0.08	0.14	0.02	0	50.78	1.17	3.06	—	3
Applesauce, Canned, Unsweetened; Cups; #19	106	215.57	0.4	0.12	0.02	0.03	0	0	27.55	1.3	3.66	—	7
Apricots, Can, Juice Pack, Halves; Cups; #20	119	214.82	1.56	0.09	0.01	0.02	0.04	0	30.6	0.95	—	—	419
Apricots, Can, Lt. Syrup, Halves; Cups; #21	160	208.87	1.35	0.12	0.01	0.03	0.05	0	41.73	1.04	—	—	334
Apricots, Can, Water Pack, Halves; Cups; #22	65	224.43	1.73	0.39	0.03	0.08	0.17	0	15.52	1.03	—	—	314
Apricots, Raw; 3 Each; #24	51	91.53	1.48	0.41	0.03	0.08	1.8	0	11.78	0.06	—	—	277
Avocados, Raw; Each; #42	324	149.28	3.99	30.79	4.9	3.93	19.31	0	14.85	4.24	—	—	123
Banana, Raw; Each; #56	105	84.66	1.18	0.55	0.21	0.1	0.05	0	26.71	0.57	1.82	—	9
Blackberries, Frozen, Unsweetened; Cups; #122	97	124.13	1.78	0.65	—	—	—	0	23.66	4.08	—	—	17
Blackberries, Raw; Cups; #123	74	123.33	1.04	0.56	—	—	—	0	18.38	5.9	—	—	24
Boysenberries, Frozen, Unsweetened; Cups; #128	66	113.38	1.46	0.35	—	—	—	0	16.1	3.56	—	—	9
Cherries, Sour, Red, Can, Lt Syrup; Cups; #306	189	200.63	1.86	0.24	0.05	0.07	0.07	0	48.63	0.25	—	—	183
Cherries, Sweet, Can, Juice Pack; Cups; #308	136	212.38	2.27	0.05	0.01	0.01	0.01	0	34.53	0.56	—	—	31
Cherries, Sweet, Raw; Cups; #310	104	117.09	1.74	1.39	0.31	0.42	0.38	0	24	0.58	—	—	31
Cranberries, Raw, Whole; Cups; #529	46	82.21	0.37	0.19	—	—	—	0	12.05	1.14	—	—	4
Dates, Domestic, Dry, Chopped; 10 Each; #577	228	18.68	1.63	0.37	—	—	—	0	61.01	1.83	—	—	4
Figs, Canned, Lt Syrup Pack; Cups; #628	173	204.78	0.99	0.26	0.05	0.12	0.05	0	45.24	1.41	—	—	9
Figs, Dried, Cooked; Cups; #629	279	180.78	3.33	1.27	0.26	0.61	0.28	0	71.42	5.24	24.09	—	41
Fruit Cocktail, Can, Juice Pack; Cups; #660	113	216.85	1.13	0.03	0	0.01	0	0	29.41	0.87	—	—	76
Fruit Cocktail, Can, Light Syrup; Cups; #661	145	212.6	1.01	0.18	0.03	0.08	0.04	0	37.63	1.14	—	—	52
Grape Juice, Frzn, Sweet, 3 Pts Wtr; Cups; #691	128	217.25	0.47	0.23	0.07	0.06	0.01	0	31.87	—	—	—	2
Grapefruit Juice, Can, Unsweetened; Cups; #695	93	222.55	1.29	0.24	0.03	0.06	0.03	0	22.14	0	—	—	2
Grapefruit, Raw, Red/Pink, All Area; 1/2 Each; #698	37	112.4	0.68	0.12	0.02	0.03	0.02	0	9.45	0.25	0.74	—	32
Grapefruit, Raw, White, All Areas; 1/2 Each; #699	39	106.77	0.81	0.12	0.02	0.03	0.01	0	9.92	0.24	0.71	—	1
Grapes, American, Raw; 10 Fruits; #700	15	19.51	0.15	0.08	0.03	0.02	0	0	4.12	0.18	—	—	2
Grapes, Thompson Seedless Water Pak; Cups; #701	97	217.66	1.23	0.26	0.09	0.08	0.01	0	25.24	0.5	—	—	16
Kiwifruit, Raw, Medium; Each; #803	46	63.12	0.75	0.34	—	—	—	0	11.31	0.84	2.58	—	13
Lime Juice, Canned or Bottled; Tbsps; #855	3	14.25	0.04	0.04	0	0.01	0	0	1.03	—	—	—	0
Lime, Raw; Each; #856	20	59.13	0.47	0.13	0.01	0.04	0.01	0	7.06	0.34	—	—	1
Melons, Cantaloupe, Raw, Pieces; Cups; #937	57	143.64	1.4	0.44	—	—	—	0	13.38	0.58	1.28	—	516

B$_1$ (mg)	B$_2$ (mg)	NI (mg)	B$_6$ (mg)	B$_{12}$ (µg)	Fol (µg)	PA (mg)	C (mg)	Ca (mg)	Fe (mg)	Mg (mg)	P (mg)	K (mg)	Na (mg)	Zn (mg)	Cu (mg)	Mn (mg)	Wt (g)
0.05	0.04	0.25	0.07	0	0.2	—	2.3	16	0.92	8	18	296	7	0.07	0.05	0.28	248
0.02	0.02	0.15	0.09	0	0.6	0.06	0.8	9	0.46	4	11	138	7	0.06	0.11	0.31	204
0.01	0.05	0.33	0.13	0	0	0.14	2.5	8	0.83	9	23	267	52	0.12	0.11	0.05	255
0.02	0.02	0.11	0.07	0	3.9	0.08	7.8	10	0.25	6	10	159	1	0.05	0.06	0.06	138
0.03	0.07	0.48	0.07	0	1.5	0.13	4.4	9	0.89	7	17	156	8	0.1	0.11	0.19	255
0.03	0.06	0.46	0.06	0	1.4	0.23	2.9	7	0.29	7	18	183	5	0.06	0.06	0.18	244
0.05	0.05	0.85	—	0	—	—	12.2	30	0.74	24	50	409	9	0.27	0.13	0.13	248
0.04	0.05	0.77	0.14	0	4.3	0.23	6.9	28	0.99	21	34	349	10	0.27	0.2	0.13	253
0.05	0.06	0.96	0.13	0	4.2	0.22	8.2	19	0.77	17	32	465	7	0.27	0.2	0.13	243
0.03	0.04	0.64	0.06	1	9.1	0.25	10.6	15	0.58	8	21	313	1	0.28	0.09	0.08	106
0.22	0.25	3.86	0.56	0	124.40	1.95	15.9	22	2.05	79	83	1204	21	0.84	0.53	0.45	201
0.05	0.11	0.62	0.66	0	21.8	0.3	10.3	7	0.35	33	22	451	1	0.19	0.12	0.17	114
0.04	0.07	1.82	0.09	0	51.3	0.23	4.7	44	1.21	33	46	211	2	0.37	0.18	1.85	151
0.04	0.06	0.58	0.08	0	—	0.35	30.2	46	0.83	29	30	282	0	0.39	0.2		144
0.07	0.05	1.01	0.07	0	83.6	0.33	4.1	36	1.12	21	36	183	2	0.29	0.11	0.	132
0.04	0.1	0.43	0.11	0	19.4	0.26	5.1	26	3.32	14	24	238	18	0.16	0.17	0.18	252
0.05	0.06	1.01	—	0	—	—	6.2	35	1.46	31	54	326	7	0.25	0.18	0.15	250
0.07	0.09	0.58	0.05	0	6.1	0.18	10.2	21	0.56	16	28	325	1	0.09	0.14	0.13	145
0.03	0.02	0.09	0.06	0	1.6	0.21	12.8	7	0.19	5	8	67	1	0.12	0.05	0.15	95
0.08	0.08	1.83	0.16	0	10.4	0.65	0	27	0.96	29	33	541	2	0.24	0.24	0.25	83
0.05	0.1	1.1	—	0	—	0.17	2.6	69	0.73	26	26	256	3	0.28	0.27	0.22	252
0.03	0.28	1.66	0.34	0	2.6	0.33	11.5	157	2.44	65	75	779	12	0.55	0.34	0.43	259
0.03	0.04	1	—	0	—	—	6.8	20	0.53	17	34	235	9	0.21	0.15	—	248
0.05	0.05	0.96	0.13	0	—	0.15	4.9	16	0.73	14	28	225	15	0.21	0.18	—	252
0.04	0.06	0.31	0.1	0	3.1	0.06	59.7	9	0.26	11	11	53	5	0.1	0.03	0.44	250
0.1	0.05	0.57	0.05	0	25.6	0.32	72	18	0.5	24	27	378	3	0.21	0.09	0.05	247
0.04	0.03	—	0.23	0	15	0.35	46.8	13	0.15	10	11	158	0	0.09	0.05	0.01	123
0.04	0.02	0.32	0.05	0	11.8	0.33	39.3	14	0.07	11	9	175	0	0.08	0.06	0.01	118
0.02	0.01	0.07	0.03	0	0.9	0.01	1	3	0.07	1	2	46	0	0.01	0.01	0.17	24
0.08	0.06	0.32	—	0	—	—	2.5	25	2.39	15	44	262	14	0.13	0.14	0.1	245
0.01	0.04	0.38	—	0	—	—	74.5	20	0.31	23	31	252	4	—	—	—	76
0	0	0.03	0	0	1.2	0.01	1	2	0.03	1	1	12	2	0.01	0	0	15.4
0.02	0.01	0.13	—	0	5.5	0.14	19.5	22	0.4	—	12	68	1	0.07	0.04	—	67
0.06	0.03	0.92	0.18	0	27.3	0.2	67.5	17	0.34	17	27	494	14	0.25	0.07	0.08	160

Food description; serving; item number	Energy (kcal)	Water (g)	PRO (g)	TFAT (g)	SFAT (g)	PFAT (g)	MFAT (g)	Chol (mg)	CHO (g)	CFib (g)	DFib (g)	Alc (g)	A (RE)
Melons, Casaba, Raw, Cubed; Cups; #938	45	156.4	1.53	0.17	—	—	—	0	10.54	0.85	—	—	5
Melons, Honeydew, Raw, Pieces; Cups; #939	60	152.43	0.77	0.17	—	—	—	0	15.61	1.02	—	—	7
Mixed Fruit, Dried; 11 Oz; #961	712	91.36	7.2	1.44	0.12	0.32	0.68	0	187.68	8.48	—	—	715
Nectarines, Raw; Each; #997	67	117.34	1.28	0.62	—	—	—	0	16.03	0.54	2.18	—	100
Olives, Ripe, Canned, Large; Each; # 1022	5	3.52	21	0.04	0.06	0.04	0.35	0	0.28	—	0.1	—	2
Orange Juice, Canned; Cups; # 1031	104	221.63	1.46	0.36	0.05	0.09	0.06	0	24.51	0.25	—	—	44
Orange Juice, Frozen, Conc. w/ Water; Cups; # 1032	112	219.37	1.68	0.14	0.02	0.03	0.03	0	26.83	0.13	0.5	—	19
Orange-Grapefruit Juice, Canned; Cups; # 1036	107	218.93	1.48	0.24	0.03	0.05	0.04	0	25.4	—	—	—	29
Oranges, Raw, Calif. Navels; Each; # 1038	65	121.53	1.44	0.13	0.01	0.03	0.02	0	16.28	0.64	—	—	26
Peaches, Canned, Juice Pack, Sliced; Cups; # 1062	109	216.98	1.57	0.08	0.01	0.04	0.03	0	28.69	0.62	—	—	95
Peaches, Canned, Lt. Syrup Pack; Cups; # 1063	136	212.64	1.13	0.08	0.01	0.04	0.03	0	36.53	0.75	—	—	89
Peaches, Dried Sulf, w/o Sugar,Cooked; Cups; # 1064	198	201.5	2.99	0.63	0.07	0.3	0.23	0	50.81	2.43	—	—	51
Peaches, Raw; Each; # 1065	37	76.26	0.61	0.08	0.01	0.04	0.03	0	9.65	0.56	1.39	—	47
Pears, Can, Juice Pack, Halves; Cups; # 1073	123	214.45	0.85	0.16	0.01	0.04	0.04	0	32.08	1.22	—	—	1
Pears, Raw; Each; # 1075	98	139.13	0.65	0.66	0.04	0.16	0.14	0	25.09	2.32	4.32	—	3
Pineapple Juice, Canned; Cups; # 1127	139	213.82	0.8	0.2	0.01	0.07	0.02	0	34.4	0.25	—	—	1
Pineapple, Can, Juice Pak, Chunks; Cups; # 1128	150	208.77	1.04	0.21	0.01	0.07	0.03	0	39.24	0.87	—	—	9
Pineapple, Raw, Diced; Cups; # 1130	77	134.08	0.6	0.66	0.05	0.23	0.07	0	19.21	0.84	1.86	—	4
Plums, Canned, Purple, Juice Pack; Cups; # 1145	146	211.72	1.3	0.06	0	0.01	0.04	0	38.19	0.66	—	—	254
Plums, Raw; Each; # 1147	36	56.23	0.52	0.41	0.03	0.09	0.27	0	8.59	0.4	—	—	21
Prune Juice, Canned; Cups; # 1223	181	207.96	1.55	0.08	0.01	0.02	0.05	0	44.66	0.03	2.56	—	1
Prunes, Dried, Cooked, w/o Sugar; Cups; # 1224	227	147.83	2.47	0.49	0.04	0.11	0.32	0	59.54	1.94	15.26	—	65
Prunes, Dried, Uncooked; Cups; # 1225	385	52.14	4.2	0.83	0.07	0.18	0.55	0	101	3.29	—	—	320
Raisins, Seedless, Packed; Cups; # 1247	494	25.44	5.32	0.76	0.25	0.22	0.03	0	130.56	2.11	8.74	—	1
Raspberries, Frozen, Sweetened; Cups; # 1250	256	181.88	1.74	0.39	0.01	0.22	0.04	0	65.39	5.53	—	—	15
Raspberries, Raw; Cups; # 1251	61	106.48	1.11	0.68	0.02	0.38	0.06	0	14.24	3.69	—	—	16
Rhubarb, Raw, Diced, Pieces; Cups; # 1258	26	114.2	1.09	0.24	—	—	—	0	5.53	0.85	—	—	12
Strawberries, Frozen, Sweet, Whole; Cups; # 1455	200	199.02	1.31	0.35	0.02	0.17	0.05	0	53.54	1.5	—	—	7
Strawberries, Raw; Cups; # 1456	45	136.44	0.91	0.55	0.03	0.28	0.08	0	10.47	0.79	3.87	—	4
Tangerines, Raw; Each; # 1503	37	73.58	0.53	0.16	0.02	0.03	0.03	0	9.4	0.28	—	—	77
Watermelon, Raw, Diced; Cups; # 1613	50	146.42	0.99	0.68	—	—	—	0	11.49	0.48	0.64	—	58

Category 10: Grain and Bread Products

Bagel, Egg; Each; #46	197	23.2	7.6	1.5	0.3	0.46	0.3	17	37.6	—	—	—	23
Bagel, Plain/Onion/Poppy/ Sesame; Each; #48	202	21.6	7.6	1.1	0.15	0.47	0.09	0	39.6	0.1	1.49	—	0

B₁ (mg)	B₂ (mg)	NI (mg)	B₆ (mg)	B₁₂ (µg)	Fol (µg)	PA (mg)	C (mg)	Ca (mg)	Fe (mg)	Mg (mg)	P (mg)	K (mg)	Na (mg)	Zn (mg)	Cu (mg)	Mn (mg)	Wt (g)
0.1	0.03	0.68	—	0	—	—	27.2	9	0.68	14	12	357	20	—	—	—	170
0.13	0.03	1.02	0.1	0	—	0.35	42.1	10	0.12	12	17	461	17	—	0.07	0.03	170
0.13	0.46	5.65	0.47	0	—	—	11.1	110	7.93	115	226	2332	52	1.47	1.13	0.67	293
0.02	0.06	1.35	0.03	0	5.1	0.22	7.3	6	0.21	11	22	288	0	0.12	0.1	0.06	136
0	0	0	0	0	0	—	0	4	0.15	0	0	0	38	0.01	0.01	0	4.4
0.15	0.07	0.78	0.22	0	—	0.37	45.7	21	1.1	27	36	436	6	0.17	0.14	0.37	249
0.2	0.05	0.5	0.11	0	109.10	0.39	96.9	22	0.24	24	40	474	2	0.13	0.11	0.04	249
0.14	0.07	0.83	0.06	0	—	0.35	71.9	21	1.15	24	34	390	8	0.18	0.19	0.04	247
0.12	0.06	0.41	0.1	0	47.2	0.35	80.3	56	0.17	15	27	250	1	0.08	0.08	0.04	140
0.02	0.04	1.44	—	0	—	—	8.8	15	0.66	18	43	317	11	0.26	0.12	—	248
0.02	0.06	1.49	0.05	0	8.2	0.13	5.9	9	0.9	12	27	244	13	0.22	0.13	0.12	251
0.01	0.05	3.92	0.1	0	0.2	0.47	9.5	23	3.37	35	99	825	6	0.47	0.3	0.25	258
0.01	0.04	0.86	0.02	0	3	0.15	5.7	5	0.1	6	11	171	0	0.12	0.06	0.04	87
0.03	0.03	0.5	—	0	—	—	4	21	0.71	17	29	238	10	0.22	0.13	—	248
0.03	0.07	0.17	0.03	0	12.1	0.12	6.6	19	0.41	9	18	208	1	0.2	0.19	0.13	166
0.14	0.05	0.64	0.24	0	57.7	0.25	26.7	42	0.65	34	20	334	2	0.29	0.22	2.47	250
0.24	0.05	0.71	—	0	—	—	23.8	34	0.7	35	16	304	4	0.24	0.22	—	250
0.14	0.06	0.65	0.14	0	16.4	0.25	23.9	11	0.57	21	11	175	1	0.12	0.17	2.56	155
0.06	0.15	1.19	—	0	—	—	7	25	0.84	20	39	389	3	0.27	0.14	—	252
0.03	0.06	0.33	0.05	0	1.4	0.12	6.3	2	0.07	4	7	113	0	0.06	0.03	0.03	66
0.04	0.18	2.01	—	0	1	—	10.6	30	3.03	36	64	706	11	0.52	0.17	0.39	256
0.05	0.21	1.53	0.46	0	0.1	0.23	6.2	48	2.35	43	75	708	4	0.5	0.41	0.21	212
0.13	0.26	3.16	0.43	0	5.9	0.74	5.4	82	3.99	73	127	1200	6	0.85	0.69	0.35	161
0.26	0.14	1.35	0.41	0	5.5	0.07	5.5	81	3.43	54	159	1239	19	0.44	0.51	0.51	165
0.05	0.11	0.57	0.09	0	65	0.38	41.3	38	1.62	32	42	285	1	0.45	0.26	1.63	250
0.04	0.11	1.11	0.07	0	—	0.29	30.8	27	0.7	22	15	187	0	0.57	0.09	1.25	123
0.02	0.04	0.37	0.03	0	8.7	0.1	0.02	105	0.27	14	17	351	5	0.13	0.03	0.24	122
0.04	0.2	0.75	0.07	0	9.7	0.28	100.7	29	1.21	16	31	249	3	0.14	0.05	0.63	255
0.03	0.1	0.34	0.09	0	26.4	0.51	84.5	21	0.57	16	28	247	2	0.19	0.07	0.43	149
0.09	0.02	0.13	0.06	0	17.1	0.17	25.9	12	0.09	10	8	132	1	—	0.02	0.03	84
0.13	0.03	0.32	0.23	0	3.4	0.34	15.4	13	0.28	17	14	186	3	0.11	0.05	0.06	160
0.38	0.17	2.44	0.06	0.11	16	0.48	0	9	2.83	18	59	48	359	0.55	0.06	0.29	71
0.39	0.23	3.46	0.04	—	16	0.26	0	47	2.45	21	68	72	363	0.62	0.12	0.38	71

Food description; serving; item number	Energy (kcal)	Water (g)	PRO (g)	TFAT (g)	SFAT (g)	PFAT (g)	MFAT (g)	Chol (mg)	CHO (g)	CFib (g)	DFib (g)	Alc (g)	A (RE)
Biscuits, Pln/Buttermilk Refrig Dou; Each; #119	93	7.5	1.8	4	1	0.53	2.22	0	12.8	0	—	—	0
Biscuits, Pln/Buttermilk, Mix, Prep; Each; #120	191	16.5	4.2	6.9	1.59	2.45	2.4	2	27.6	0.1	1.03	—	13
Bread, Banana, Recipe; Slices; #138	203	16.7	2.6	7.1	1.83	1.77	3.02	26	33	0.1	—	—	15
Bread, French/Sourdough 2 1/2"x2"x1; Slices; #139	69	8.6	2.2	0.8	0.16	0.17	0.3	0	13	0	0.68	—	0
Bread, Hollywood Light; Slices; #140	70	—	3	1	—	—	—	—	13	—	0.6	—	0
Bread, Home Pride Butter Top, Wheat; Slices; #141	70	—	3	1	—	—	—	—	13	—	0.8	—	0
Bread, Home Pride Butter Top, White; Slices; #142	70	—	3	1	—	—	—	—	13	—	0.6	—	0
Bread, Italian, 4.5" x 3.25" x .75"; Slices; #143	81	10.7	2.6	1.1	0.26	0.42	0.24	0	15	0.1	0.93	—	0
Bread, Oat Bran; Slices; #144	71	13.2	3.1	1.3	0.21	0.51	0.48	0	11.9	—	1.35	—	0
Bread, Pita, White, 6.50" Dia.; Each; #148	165	19.3	5.4	0.7	0.1	0.32	0.06	0	33.4	0.1	0.96	—	0
Bread, Pumpernickel, 5"x"4x3/8"; Slices; #150	80	12.1	2.8	1	0.14	0.4	0.3	0	15.2	0.2	1.89	—	0
Bread, Raisin; Slices; #151	71	8.7	2.1	1.1	0.28	0.18	0.6	0	13.6	0.2	—	—	0
Bread, Rye, 5" x 4" 1/2"; Slices; #153	83	11.9	2.7	1.1	0.2	0.26	0.42	0	15.5	0.2	—	—	0
Bread, Wheat; Slices; #155	65	9.3	2.3	1	0.22	0.23	0.43	0	11.8	0.2	1.08	—	0
Bread, Wheat Bran; Slices; #156	89	13.6	3.2	1.2	0.28	0.23	0.58	0	13.6	0.2	3.06	—	0
Bread, Wheat Bran, Toasted; Slices; #157	90	10.4	3.2	1.2	0.28	0.23	0.59	0	17.3	0.2	—	—	0
Bread, Wheat, Toasted; Slices; #160	65	7.3	2.3	1	0.22	0.23	0.43	0	11.8	0.2	—	—	0
Bread, White, Commercial; Slices; #161	67	9.2	2.1	0.9	0.2	0.19	0.4	0	12.4	0.1	0.57	—	0
Bread, White, Red. Cal., Toasted; Slices; #165	54	6.1	2	0.6	0.12	0.13	0.24	0	10	1.4	—	—	0
Bread, Whole Wheat, Commercial; Ounces; #166	69	10.9	2.7	1.2	0.26	0.28	0.48	0	12.9	0.4	1.96	—	0
Bread, Wonder Lite, Wheat; Slices; #169	40	—	3	1	—	—	—	0	7	—	2	—	0
Bread, Wonder, 100% Whole Wheat; Slices; #171	70	—	3	1	—	—	—	—	12	—	1.8	—	0
Breadcrumbs, Dry, Grated, Plain; Cups; #174	426	6.7	13.5	5.8	1.36	1.68	2.26	0	78.3	1	4.33	—	0
Bulgur, Cooked; 1/2 Cups; #188	76	70.77	2.81	0.22	0.04	0.09	0.03	0	16.9	0.32	—	—	—
Buns, Hamburger/Hot Dog, Plain; Each; #189	123	14.6	3.6	2.2	0.51	0.39	1.07	0	21.6	—	—	—	0
Cornbread, Mix, Prepared; 1/6 Pc; #465	189	19.2	4.3	6	1.64	0.73	3.08	37	28.9	0.2	1.44	—	27
Cornmeal, Self-Rising, Degermed; 1/4 Cups; #469	121	3.46	2.86	0.58	0.08	0.25	0.15	0	25.43	0.18	—	—	—
Cornmeal, Whole-Grain; 1/4 Cups; #470	109	3.08	2.44	1.08	0.15	0.49	0.28	0	23.07	0.55	3.3	—	14
Cornstarch; 1/3 Cups; #471	164	3.58	0.11	0.02	0	0.01	0.01	0	39.25	—	0.39	—	—
Couscous, Cooked; 1/2 Cups; #474	101	65.31	3.41	0.14	0.03	0.06	0.02	0	20.9	0.12	—	—	—
Crackers, Amer Classic Tstd Poppy; 4 Each; #486	70	—	1	3	—	—	—	0	9	—	—	—	—
Crackers, Cheese 1" Square; Each; #488	5	0	0.1	0.3	0.09	0.05	0	0	0.6	0	—	—	0
Crackers, Cheez/Crack, Handi-Snacks; Pkg; #492	120	—	4	8	5	0	—	20	9	—	—	—	40
Crackers, Graham, Honey Maid; 2 Pieces; #496	60	—	1	1	—	—	—	0	11	—	—	—	—

B$_1$ (mg)	B$_2$ (mg)	NI (mg)	B$_6$ (mg)	B$_{12}$ (µg)	Fol (µg)	PA (mg)	C (mg)	Ca (mg)	Fe (mg)	Mg (mg)	P (mg)	K (mg)	Na (mg)	Zn (mg)	Cu (mg)	Mn (mg)	Wt (g)
0.09	0.06	0.83	0.01	0	1	0.1	0	5	0.7	4	104	42	324	0.1	0.2	0.07	27
0.2	0.2	1.72	0.04	0.12	3	0.31	0.2	105	1.17	14	268	107	544	0.35	0.07	0.14	57
0.1	0.12	0.88	0.09	0.06	7	0.16	1	11	0.84	8	34	78	119	0.21	0.04	0.13	60
0.13	0.08	1.19	0.01	0	8	0.1	0	19	0.63	7	26	28	152	0.22	0.05	0.13	25
0.12	0.1	1.2	—	—	—	—	0	40	1.08	—	—	—	150	—	—	—	28.35
0.12	0.1	1.2	—	—	—	—	0	40	0.72	—	—	—	140	—	—	—	28.4
0.12	0.1	1.2	—	—	—	—	0	40	0.72	—	—	—	140	—	—	—	28.4
0.14	0.09	1.31	0.01	0	9	0.11	0	23	0.88	8	31	33	175	0.26	0.06	0.14	30
0.15	0.1	1.45	—	—	—	—	—	19	0.94	—	—	—	122	—	—	—	30
0.36	0.2	2.78	0.02	0	14	0.24	0	52	1.57	16	58	72	322	0.51	0.1	0.29	60
0.1	0.1	0.99	0.04	0	11	0.13	0	22	0.92	17	57	66	215	0.47	0.09	0.42	32
0.09	0.1	0.9	0.02	0	9	0.1	0	17	0.75	7	28	59	101	0.19	0.05	0.13	26
0.14	0.11	1.22	0.02	0	16	0.14	0	23	0.9	13	40	53	211	0.36	0.06	0.26	32
0.1	0.07	1.03	0.02	0	10	0.11	0	26	0.83	12	38	50	132	0.26	0.05	0.26	25
0.14	0.1	1.59	0.06	0	—	0.19	—	27	1.1	29	67	82	175	0.49	0.08	0.6	36
0.12	0.09	1.44	0.06	0	—	0.13	—	27	1.11	30	67	82	176	0.49	0.08	0.61	33
0.08	0.06	0.93	0.02	0	7	0.07	0	26	0.83	12	38	50	132	0.26	0.05	0.26	23
0.12	0.09	0.99	0.02	0	8	0.1	0	27	0.76	6	23	30	135	0.15	0.03	0.1	25
0.07	0.06	0.74	0.01	—	—	0.07	—	21	0.72	—	—	17	102	0.3	0.08	—	19
0.1	0.06	1.09	0.05	0	14	0.16	0	20	0.94	24	65	71	149	0.55	0.08	0.66	28.35
0.12	0.07	1.2	—	—	—	—	0	40	0.72	—	—	—	120	—	—	—	22.8
0.15	0.03	1.2	—	—	—	—	0	20	1.08	—	—	—	160	—	—	—	28.35
0.83	0.47	7.4	0.11	0	24	0.33	0	245	6.61	50	158	239	930	1.32	0.18	0.88	108
0.05	0.03	0.91	0.08	0	17	0.31	0	9	0.88	29	36	62	5	0.52	0.07	0.55	91
0.21	0.13	1.69	—	0	—	0.23	0	60	1.36	8	—	60	241	0.27	0.05	0.14	43
0.15	0.16	1.23	0.06	0.09	7	0.26	0.1	44	1.14	12	226	77	467	0.38	0.04	0.13	60
0.23	0.13	1.55	0.13	0	11	—	0	119	1.61	17	212	58	458	0.34	0.04	—	34
0.12	0.06	1.09	0.09	0	—	0.13	0	2	1.04	38	72	86	11	0.54	0.06	0.15	30
—	—	—	—	0	—	—	0	1	0.2	1	6	1	4	0.03	0.02	0.02	43
0.06	0.02	0.88	0.05	0	13	0.33	0	8	0.35	8	20	52	4	0.23	0.04	0.08	90
0.06	0.03	0.4	—	—	—	—	—	20	0.72	—	—	—	140	—	—	—	14.2
0.01	0	0.05	0.01	0	0	0	0	2	0.05	0	2	1	10	0.01	0	0.11	1
0.06	0.1	0.4	—	—	—	—	—	80	0.36	—	0.2	55	360	—	—	—	32
0.03	0.03	0.4	—	—	—	—	—	—	0.36	—	—	—	90	—	—	—	14.2

Food description; serving; item number	Energy (kcal)	Water (g)	PRO (g)	TFAT (g)	SFAT (g)	PFAT (g)	MFAT (g)	Chol (mg)	CHO (g)	CFib (g)	DFib (g)	Alc (g)	A (RE)
Crackers, Graham, Plain/Honey; Each; #498	59	0.6	1	1.4	0.35	0.22	0.7	0	10.8	0.1	0.38	—	0
Crackers, Matzo, Plain; Each; #500	112	1.2	2.8	0.4	0.06	0.17	0.04	0	23.7	0.1	0.85	—	0
Crackers, P'But/Cheese, Handi-Snack; Pkg; #505	190	—	6	14	4	3	—	0	11	—	—	—	—
Crackers, Premium Saltines; 5 Pieces; #506	60	—	1	2	—	—	—	0	10	—	—	—	—
Crackers, Premium Saltines Fat Free; 5 Pcs; #507	50	—	1	0	0	0	—	0	12	—	—	—	—
Crackers, Rye Wafers, Plain; Each; #513	84	1.2	2.4	0.2	0.03	0.1	0.04	0	20.1	0.5	—	—	1
Crackers, Saltine/Oyster/Soda; Each; #514	13	0.1	0.3	0.4	0.06	0.05	0.19	0	2.1	0	0.08	—	0
Crackers, Triscuit Wafers; 3 Pieces; #522	60	—	1	2	—	—	—	0	10	—	—	—	—
Crackers, Wheat; Each; #525	9	0.1	0.2	0.4	0.07	0.06	0.23	0	1.3	0	0.11	—	0
Crackers, Wheat Thins Snack; 8 Pieces; #526	70	—	1	3	—	—	—	0	9	—	—	—	—
Crackers, Whole-Wheat; Each; #527	18	0.1	0.4	0.7	0.12	0.11	0.38	0	2.7	0.1	0.42	—	0
Croutons, Pep. Farm, Seasoned; 1/2 Oz; #554	70	—	2	3	—	—	—	—	9	—	—	—	—
Croutons, Seasoned; Cups; #555	186	1.4	4.3	7.3	2.01	1	3.82	1	25.4	0.3	2	—	2
Egg Noodles, Creamettes Enriched; 2 Oz. Dry; #609	220	—	8	3	—	—	—	—	40	—	—	—	—
English Muffins, Plain, Toasted; Each; #625	133	19.3	4.4	1	0.2	0.35	0.27	0	26	0.1	—	—	0
Flour, All-Purpose, Sifted; Cups; #639	419	13.8	12.1	1.2	—	—	—	—	87.5	—	—	—	0
Flour, Buckwheat, Light, Sifted; Cups; #640	340	11.76	6.3	1.2	—	—	—	—	77.9	—	—	—	0
Flour, Wheat, White, All-Purpose; 1/2 Cups; #648	226	7.39	6 4	0.61	0.1	0.26	0.05	0	47.31	0.15	1.67	—	—
Flour, Wheat, White, Tortilla Mix; 1/3 Cups; #650	150	3.73	3.57	3.93	1.52	0.56	1.68	0	24.84	0.07	—	—	—
Flour, Wheat, Whole; Cups; #651	400	14.4	16	2.4	—	—	—	—	85.2	—	—	—	0
Ice Cream Cone, Cake or Wafer Type; Each; #763	17	0.2	0.3	0.3	0.04	0.1	0.11	0	3.2	—	1.16	—	0
Lasagna/Spaghetti, Westbrae, Spinach; Svg; #838	210	—	8.19	2.3	—	—	—	—	40.5	—	6.07	—	25
Macaroni, Cooked; 1/2 Cups; #869	99	46.19	3.34	0.47	0.07	0.19	0.05	0	19.84	0.06	1.12	—	—
Macaroni, Whole-Wheat, Cooked; 1/2 Cups; #873	87	47.01	3.73	0.38	0.07	0.15	0.05	0	18.58	0.69	—	—	—
Muffins, Blueberry, From Mix; Each; #975	150	17.6	2.5	4.4	1.13	0.6	2.34	21	24.7	0	—	—	3
Muffins, Corn, From Mix; Each; #976	160	15.2	3.7	5.1	1.4	0.63	2.63	31	24.6	0.1	—	—	23
Muffins, Oat Bran; Each; #980	154	19.9	4	4.2	0.51	2.6	0.81	0	27.5	—	4.28	—	1
Noodles, Egg, Cooked; 1/2 Cups; #1006	106	54.96	3.8	1.18	0.25	0.33	0.34	26	19.87	0.1	1.76	—	5
Oat Bran, Cooked; 1/2 Cups; #1010	44	92.4	3.53	0.95	0.18	0.37	0.32	0	12.58	0.41	—	—	—
Oat Bran, Quaker; 1/3 Cups; #1011	110	2.6	5.7	2.5	—	—	—	—	16.2	—	—	—	0
Oatmeal or Rolled Oats, Cooked; Cups; #1013	145	199.6	6	2.4	0.42	0.87	0.75	0	25.2	0.4	—	—	—
Pancakes, Buttermilk, Recipe; 4" Each; #1047	86	20	2.6	3.6	0.7	1.71	0.9	22	10.9	0	—	—	12
Pancakes, Hungry Jack, 4" Dia.; 3 Each; #1048	180	—	4.2	1	—	—	—	—	38.2	—	—	—	—

B₁ (mg)	B₂ (mg)	NI (mg)	B₆ (mg)	B₁₂ (µg)	Fol (µg)	PA (mg)	C (mg)	Ca (mg)	Fe (mg)	Mg (mg)	P (mg)	K (mg)	Na (mg)	Zn (mg)	Cu (mg)	Mn (mg)	Wt (g)
0.03	0.04	0.58	0.01	0	2	0.08	0	3	0.52	4	15	19	85	0.11	0.03	0.11	14
0.11	0.08	1.1	0.03	0	4	0.13	0	4	0.9	7	25	32	0	0.19	0.02	0.18	28.35
0.09	0.03	3	—	—	—	—	—	—	0.72	—	0.1	155	180	—	—	—	32
0.09	0.07	0.8	—	—	—	—	—	20	0.72	—	—	—	180	—	—	—	14.2
0.09	0.07	0.8	—	—	—	—	—	—	0.72	—	—	—	115	—	—	—	14.2
0.11	0.07	0.4	0.07	0	11	0.14	0	10	1.48	30	84	124	199	0.7	0.12	—	25
0.01	0.01	0.16	0	0	1	0.01	0	4	0.16	1	3	4	39	0.02	0.01	0.02	3
0.03	—	0.4	—	—	—	—	—	—	0.36	—	—	—	75	—	—	—	14.2
0.01	0.01	0.1	0	0	0	0.01	0	1	0.09	1	4	4	16	0.03	0.01	0.04	2
0.06	0.03	0.8	—	—	—	—	—	—	0.36	—	—	—	120	—	—	—	14.2
0.01	0	0.18	0.01	0	1	0.03	0	2	0.12	4	12	12	26	0.09	0.02	0.09	4
0.06	0.07	0.8	—	—	—	—	—	20	0.36	—	—	—	180	—	—	—	14.2
0.2	0.17	1.86	0.03	0	16	0.33	0	38	1.13	17	56	72	495	0.38	0.07	0.21	40
0.45	0.17	3	—	—	—	—	—	20	1.8	—	—	135	20	—	—	—	56.7
0.2	0.14	1.98	0.02	—	—	0.16	—	99	1.41	12	75	74	262	0.4	0.07	0.2	52
0.51	0.3	4	—	—	—	—	0	18	3.3	—	100	109	2	—	—	—	115
0.08	0.04	0.4	—	—	—	—	0	11	1	—	86	314	—	—	—	—	98
0.49	0.31	3.66	0.03	0	16	0.27	0	9	2.88	13	67	66	1	0.44	0.09	0.42	62
0.27	0.18	2.15	0.01	0	—	—	0	76	2.61	8	78	37	250	—	0.04	—	37
0.66	0.14	5.2	—	—	—	—	0	49	4.4	—	446	444	4	—	—	—	120
0.01	0.01	0.18	0	0	0	0.02	0	1	0.14	1	4	4	6	0.03	0.01	0.02	4
0.3	0.17	3	—	—	—	—	—	40	1.08	—	—	—	3.18	—	—	—	57
0.14	0.07	1.17	0.02	0	5	0.08	0	5	0.98	13	38	22	0	0.37	0.07	0.2	75
0.08	0.03	0.5	0.05	0	3	0.29	0	10	0.74	21	62	30	2	0.57	0.12	0.97	70
0.08	0.16	1.13	0.04	0.04	5	0.2	0.5	13	0.57	6	95	39	220	0.19	0.04	0.11	50
0.13	0.14	1.05	0.05	0.08	6	0.22	0.1	37	0.97	10	192	65	397	0.32	0.03	0.11	50
0.15	0.05	0.24	0.09	—	10	0.58	—	36	2.39	89	214	289	224	1.05	0.19	1.5	57
0.15	0.07	1.19	0.03	0.07	6	0.12	0	10	1.28	15	55	23	5	0.5	0.07	0.21	80
0.18	0.04	0.16	0.03	0	7	0.24	0	11	0.97	44	131	101000	1	0.59	0.07	1.06	110
0.33	0.12	0.23	0.04	0	20	0	—	20	1.63	67	30	31	170	1	0.08	2	28
0.26	0.05	0.3	0.05	—	9	0.47	—	20	1.59	56	178	132	1	1.15	0.13	1.37	234
0.08	0.12	0.47	0.04	0.13	4	0.19	0.2	82	0.49	9	119	76	192	0.28	0.02	0.05	38
0.24	0.2	2.1	—	—	—	—	0	154	2.65	—	368	80	710	—	—	—	113

Food description; serving; item number	Energy (kcal)	Water (g)	PRO (g)	TFAT (g)	SFAT (g)	PFAT (g)	MFAT (g)	Chol (mg)	CHO (g)	CFib (g)	DFib (g)	Alc (g)	A (RE)
Pancakes, Plain, Frzn, 4" Dia.; Each; # 1050	91	16.6	2	3.4	0.79	0.99	1.24	—	13	0	—	—	10
Popcorn, Plain, Popped; Cups; # 1150	23	0.24	0.8	0.3	—	—	—	—	4.6	—	—	—	—
Popcorn, Popped w/Oil, Salt; Cups; # 1151	41	0.28	0.9	2	1.4	—	—	—	5.3	—	0.9	—	—
Rice, Brown, Long-Grained, Cooked; 1/2 Cups; # 1264	109	71.63	2.53	0.88	0.18	0.32	0.32	0	22.5	0.34	1.67	—	—
Rice, Fried; 1/2 Cups; # 1265	159	62.1	3.2	4.8	0.7	1.8	—	0	25.2	—	—	—	—
Rice, White, Long-Grain, Reg, Ckd; 1/2 Cups; # 1268	131	70.1	2.74	0.29	0.08	0.08	0.09	0	28.45	0.11	—	—	—
Rolls, Brown & Serve; Each; # 1271	84	6.99	2.2	1.9	0.5	—	—	—	14.2	—	0.99	—	—
Rolls, Dinner, Plain, Commercial; Each; # 1273	85	9.1	2.4	2.1	0.5	0.34	1.05	0	14.3	0.1	—	—	0
Rolls, Hard or Kaiser, 3 1/2" Dia.; Each; # 1275	167	17.7	5.7	2.4	0.34	0.98	0.65	0	30.1	0.2	—	—	0
Spaghetti, Cooked; 1/2 Cups; # 1429	99	46.19	3.34	0.47	0.07	0.19	0.05	0	19.84	0.06	1.12	—	—
Spaghetti, Spinach, Cooked; 1/2 Cups; # 1431	91	47.7	3.2	0.44	0.06	0.18	0.05	0	18.31	0.83	—	—	—
Spaghetti/Meatballs, Tom Sauce, F.A; 7 3/8 Oz; # 1433	220	—	10	8	—	—	—	—	28	—	—	—	80
Stuffing Mix, Bread, Prepared; 1/2 Cups; # 1458	178	64.8	3.2	8.6	1.73	2.6	3.81	0	21.7	0.2	2.9	—	49
Stuffing, Pep. Farm, Cube; Ounces; # 1460	110	—	3	1	—	—	—	—	22	—	—	—	—
Stuffing, Pep. Farm, Herb Seasoning; Ounces; # 1461	110	—	3	1	—	—	—	—	22	—	—	—	—
Taco Shells; Each; # 1501	61	0.8	0.9	2.9	0.44	1.12	1.23	0	8.1	0.2	1.05	—	5
Tortillas, Ready to Bake/Fry, Flour; 7-8" Dia.; # 1540	114	9.4	3	2.5	0.39	0.98	1.01	0	19.5	0.3	1.09	—	0
Triticale; 1/2 Cups; # 1542	323	10.09	12.52	2	0.35	0.88	0.2	0	69.25	2.5	17.38	—	—
Waffles, Frozen, Ready to Heat; 4" Sq.; # 1608	88	15.7	2.1	2.7	0.48	0.93	1.07	—	13.5	0.1	0.84	—	9
Wheat Germ, Toasted; Ounces; # 1628	108	1.6	8.3	3	0.52	1.88	0.43	0	14.1	0.7	3.66	—	—

Category 11: Lamb, Veal, Game

Lamb, Arm, Braised; 3 Oz; #823	294	37.59	25.84	20.4	8.39	1.45	8.65	102	0	—	—	—	—
Lamb, Blade, Lean, Braised; 3 Oz; #826	245	42.19	27.5	14.15	5.41	1.24	5.73	99	0	—	—	—	—
Lamb, Cubed, Lean, Broiled; 3 Oz; #827	158	54	23.86	6.23	2.23	0.57	2.51	77	0	—	—	—	—
Lamb, Leg of, Lean, Roasted; 3 Oz; #829	162	54.31	24.05	6.58	2.35	0.43	2.88	76	0	—	—	—	—
Lamb, Leg of, Roasted; 3 Oz; #830	219	48.85	21.72	14.01	5.85	1.01	5.92	79	0	—	—	—	—
Lamb, Loin, Broiled; 3 Oz; #831	268	43.84	21.4	19.62	8.36	1.42	8.24	85	0	—	—	—	—
Lamb, New Zealand, Shoulder, Brsd; 3 Oz; #833	304	36.25	23.98	22.33	10.83	1.13	8.69	104	0	—	—	—	—
Lamb, Rib, Broiled; 3 Oz; #834	307	40	18.81	25.15	10.8	2.02	10.3	84	0	—	—	—	—
Lamb, Rib, Lean, Broiled; 3 Oz; #835	200	50.01	23.57	11	3.95	1.01	4.43	78	0	—	—	—	—
Lamb, Shoulder, Lean, Roasted; 3 Oz; #836	173	53.82	21.2	9.16	3.47	0.81	3.71	74	0	0	—	—	—
Rabbit, Domesticated, Roasted; 3 Oz; # 1238	167	51.52	24.7	6.84	2.04	1.33	1.85	70	0	—	—	—	—
Squirrel, Roasted; 3 Oz; # 1453	147	52.76	26.16	3.95	0.47	1.16	1.46	103	0	—	—	—	—
Veal, Cubed, Lean, Braised; 3 Oz; # 1576	160	50.4	29.7	3.66	1.1	0.38	1.18	124	0	—	—	—	—

B₁ (mg)	B₂ (mg)	NI (mg)	B₆ (mg)	B₁₂ (µg)	Fol (µg)	PA (mg)	C (mg)	Ca (mg)	Fe (mg)	Mg (mg)	P (mg)	K (mg)	Na (mg)	Zn (mg)	Cu (mg)	Mn (mg)	Wt (g)
0.14	0.17	1.44	—	—	—	—	—	22	1.25	5	134	53	295	0.24	0.01	—	36
—	0.01	0.1	—	—	—	—	0	1	0.2	—	17	—	—	—	—	—	6
—	0.01	0.2	—	—	—	—	0	1	0.2	—	19	—	175	—	—	—	9
0.09	0.02	1.5	0.14	0	4	0.28	0	10	0.41	42	81	42	5	0.62	0.1	0.89	98
0.16	0.01	1.4	0.02	0	2	0	0	10	1.3	9	37	47	551	0.37	0.04	—	97
0.17	0.01	1.5	0.09	0	3	0.4	0	12	1.12	13	47	40	2	0.47	0.06	0.48	102
0.07	0.06	0.6	—	—	—	—	—	20	0.5	—	23	25	136	—	—	—	26
0.14	0.09	1.14	0.01	0	8	0.14	0	34	0.89	7	33	38	148	0.22	0.04	0.13	28.35
0.27	0.19	2.42	—	0	8	—	0	54	1.87	16	57	61	310	0.54	0.09	0.26	57
0.14	0.07	1.17	0.02	0	5	0.08	0	5	0.98	13	38	22	0	0.37	0.07	0.2	70
0.07	0.07	1.07	0.07	0	8	0.13	0	21	0.73	43	76	41	10	0.76	0.14	1.05	70
0.15	0.1	2	—	—	—	—	—	20	1.8	—	—	—	870	—	—	—	209.45
0.14	0.11	1.48	0.04	0.01	17	0.08	0	32	1.09	12	42	74	543	0.28	0.07	0.17	100
0.15	0.1	1.6	—	—	—	—	—	40	1.44	—	—	—	400	—	—	—	28.4
0.15	0.1	1.6	—	—	—	—	—	40	1.44	—	—	—	380	—	—	—	28.4
0.03	0.01	0.17	0.05	0	1	0.06	0	21	0.33	14	32	23	48	0.18	0.02	0.06	13
0.19	0.1	1.25	0.02	0	4	0.2	0	44	1.15	9	44	46	167	0.25	0.09	0.16	35
0.4	0.13	1.37	0.13	0	70	1.27	0	36	2.46	125	343	318	5	3.32	0.44	3.08	96
0.16	0.18	1.64	0.33	0.83	17	0.21	0	77	1.49	7	139	43	262	0.19	0.03	—	35
0.47	0.23	1.59	0.28	—	100	0.39	2	13	2.58	91	325	269	1	4.73	0.18	5.67	28.4
0.06	0.21	5.66	0.1	2.19	5.16	0.52	—	21	2.03	22	175	260	61	5.16	0.12	0.02	85
0.05	0.19	4.79	0.1	2.5	18	0.52	—	24	.21	22	172	216	67	6.85	0.11	0.03	85
0.09	0.25	5.62	0.12	2.58	19	0.59	—	11	1.99	26	190	285	65	4.9	0.13	0.02	85
0.09	0.25	5.39	0.14	2.24	20	0.6	—	7	1.81	22	175	287	58	4.2	0.1	0.02	85
0.09	0.23	5.6	0.13	2.2	17	0.58	—	9	1.69	20	162	266	56	3.74	0.1	0.02	85
0.09	0.21	6.04	0.11	2.1	16	0.54	—	17	1.54	21	166	278	65	2.96	0.11	0.02	85
0.06	0.27	5.42	0.06	2.89	1	0.44	—	23	1.79	15	167	125	43	3.85	0.09	0.02	85
0.08	0.19	5.95	0.09	2.16	12	0.52	—	16	1.6	20	151	230	64	3.4	0.1	0.02	85
0.09	0.21	5.57	0.12	2.25	18	0.54	—	14	1.88	25	181	266	73	4.48	0.12	0.02	85
0.08	0.22	4.9	0.12	2.3	21	0.62	—	16	1.81	21	170	225	58	5.14	0.1	0.02	85
0.07	0.18	7.17	0.4	7.06	9	0.79	0	16	1.93	18	223	325	40	1.93	0.16	0.03	85
0.05	0.25	3.94	—	—	—	—	—	2	5.79	24	180	300	102	—	—	—	85
0.06	0.34	7.05	0.33	1.42	14	1.01	—	24	1.23	24	203	291	79	5.1	0.13	0.03	85

Food description; serving; item number	Energy (kcal)	Water (g)	PRO (g)	TFAT (g)	SFAT (g)	PFAT (g)	MFAT (g)	Chol (mg)	CHO (g)	CFib (g)	DFib (g)	Alc (g)	A (RE)
Veal, Loin, Braised; 3 Oz; # 1578	242	44.22	25.66	14.63	5.72	0.98	5.72	100	0	—	—	—	—
Veal, Rib, Lean, Roasted; 3 Oz; # 1580	151	54.94	21.89	6.32	1.77	0.57	2.26	97	0	—	—	—	—
Veal, Rib, Roasted; 3 Oz; # 1581	194	50.93	20.37	11.87	4.6	0.81	4.63	94	0	—	—	—	—
Veal, Shoulder, Braised; 3 Oz; # 1582	194	47.94	27.25	8.62	3.19	0.62	3.31	107	0	—	—	—	—
Veal, Sirloin, Braised; 3 Oz; # 1584	214	46.32	26.57	11.17	4.4	0.74	4.38	92	0	—	—	—	—
Veal, Top Rnd, Fried, Not Breaded; 3 Oz; # 1587	179	49.59	26.99	7.1	2.68	0.5	2.75	89	0	—	—	—	—
Veal, Top Rnd, Lean, Roasted; 3 Oz; # 1588	128	56.96	23.86	2.88	1.04	0.25	1.02	88	0	—	—	—	—

Category 12: Legumes

Food description; serving; item number	Energy (kcal)	Water (g)	PRO (g)	TFAT (g)	SFAT (g)	PFAT (g)	MFAT (g)	Chol (mg)	CHO (g)	CFib (g)	DFib (g)	Alc (g)	A (RE)
Baked Beans, Plain/Veg, Canned; Cups; #49	235	184.53	12.17	1.14	0.29	0.49	0.1	0	52.11	2.89	19.56	—	43
Baked Beans, w/Pork/Tom Canned; Cups; #50	247	183.92	13.05	2.6	1	0.33	1.12	17	49.06	2.99	13.91	—	31
Beans, Black, Boiled; Cups; #59	227	113.08	15.24	0.92	0.24	0.4	0.08	0	40.78	3.49	—	—	1
Beans, Great Northern, Boiled; Cups; #61	210	122.13	14.75	0.79	0.25	0.33	0.04	0	37.32	5.27	—	—	0
Beans, Kidney, Boiled; Cups; #62	225	118.47	15.35	0.88	0.13	0.49	0.07	0	40.37	4.98	—	—	0
Beans, Kidney, Red, Canned; 1/2 Cups; #64	108	99.01	6.71	0.44	0.06	0.24	0.04	0	19.96	1.19	—	—	0
Beans, Navy, Boiled; Cups; #65	259	114.99	15.83	1.04	0.27	0.45	0.09	0	47.89	5.72	—	—	0
Beans, Pinto, Boiled; Cups; #66	235	109.9	14.04	0.89	0.19	0.32	0.18	0	43.86	5.16	—	—	0
Beans, Small White, Boiled; Cups; #67	253	113.19	16.05	1.15	0.3	0.49	0.1	0	46.2	4.3	—	—	0
Chili Con Carne with Beans; Cups; #329	339	—	19.1	15.6	—	—	—	—	31.1	—	—	—	150
Falafel, 2 1/4" Dia. Patty; Each; #626	57	5.89	2.26	3.03	0.41	0.71	1.73	0	5.41	0.18	—	—	0
Lentils, Boiled; Cups; #846	231	137.88	17.87	0.74	0.1	0.35	0.13	0	39.87	5.46	—	—	2
Lima Beans, Baby, Boiled; Cups; #853	229	122.22	14.64	0.68	0.16	0.31	0.06	0	42.43	6.54	13.1	—	0
Lima Beans, Large, Boiled; Cups; #854	217	131.2	14.67	0.71	0.17	0.32	0.06	0	39.26	5.8	13.54	—	0
Mung Beans, Boiled; Cups; #983	213	146.77	14.19	0.78	0.23	0.26	0.11	0	38.67	0.93	—	—	5
Peanut Butter, Chunky Style; 2 Tbsps; # 1069	188	0.36	7.7	15.98	3.07	4.59	7.54	0	6.91	0.8	2.11	—	0
Peanut Butter, Smooth Style; 2 Tbsps; # 1070	188	0.45	7.87	15.99	3.07	4.6	7.55	0	6.63	0.77	1.92	—	0
Peanuts, Dry-Roasted, All Types; Ounces; # 1071	164	0.43	6.63	13.9	1.93	4.39	6.9	0	6.02	1.43	2.24	—	0
Peanuts, Oil-Roasted, All Types; Ounces; # 1072	163	0.55	7.38	13.8	1.92	4.36	6.85	0	5.3	1.49	2.46	—	0
Peas, Split, Boiled; Cups; # 1084	231	136.19	16.35	0.76	0.11	0.32	0.16	0	41.37	3.86	—	—	1
Refried Beans, Canned; Cups; # 1255	270	182.86	15.77	2.7	1.04	0.35	1.17	—	46.81	8.03	—	—	0
Soybeans, Roasted; Cups; # 1420	811	3.35	60.58	43.69	6.32	24.66	9.65	0	57.72	7.91	—	—	34
Tofu, Raw, Firm; 1/2 Cups; # 1517	183	87.98	19.88	10.98	1.59	6.2	2.43	0	5.4	0.18	—	—	21
Tofu, Raw, Regular; 1/2 Cups; # 1518	94	104.84	10.02	5.93	0.86	3.35	1.31	0	2.33	0.09	1.49	—	11

B₁ (mg)	B₂ (mg)	NI (mg)	B₆ (mg)	B₁₂ (μg)	Fol (μg)	PA (mg)	C (mg)	Ca (mg)	Fe (mg)	Mg (mg)	P (mg)	K (mg)	Na (mg)	Zn (mg)	Cu (mg)	Mn (mg)	Wt (g)
0.04	0.26	7.68	0.22	1.03	12	0.67	—	24	0.92	21	187	238	68	3.09	0.08	0.03	85
0.05	0.25	6.37	0.23	1.34	12	1.17	—	10	0.82	20	176	264	82	3.81	0.09	0.03	85
0.05	0.23	5.93	0.21	1.24	11	1.08	—	10	0.82	19	167	251	78	3.48	0.08	0.03	85
0.05	0.29	5.46	0.21	1.57	13	1.3	—	29	1.21	23	213	263	80	5.6	0.13	0.03	85
0.04	0.3	5.6	0.3	1.25	12	0.86	—	15	1.02	23	207	273	67	3.67	0.11	0.03	85
0.06	0.3	10.24	0.41	1.23	13	1	—	5	0.75	26	237	362	64	2.75	0.05	0.03	85
0.05	0.28	8.57	0.26	1	13	0.85	—	5	0.77	24	201	334	58	2.62	0.11	0.03	85
0.39	0.15	1.09	0.34	0	60.7	0.24	—	128	0.74	82	264	752	1008	3.55	0.52	0.88	254
0.13	0.12	1.26	0.17	0.03	56.8	1.34	7.8	141	8.3	88	297	759	1113	14.83	0.64	1.24	253
0.42	0.1	0.87	0.12	0	255.90	0.42	0	47	3.6	121	241	611	1	1.92	0.36	0.76	172
0.28	0.1	1.21	0.21	0	180.90	0.47	2.3	121	3.77	88	293	692	4	1.55	0.44	0.92	177
0.28	0.1	1.02	0.21	0	229.40	0.39	2.1	50	5.2	80	252	713	4	1.89	0.43	0.84	177
0.13	0.11	0.58	0.03	0	64.7	0.19	1.5	31	1.61	36	120	329	437	0.7	0.19	0.19	128
0.37	0.11	0.97	0.3	0	254.60	0.46	1.6	128	4.51	107	285	669	2	1.93	0.54	1.01	182
0.32	0.16	0.68	0.26	0	294.10	0.49	3.5	82	4.47	95	273	800	3	1.85	0.44	0.95	171
0.42	0.11	0.49	0.23	0	245	0.45	0	131	5.09	122	302	828	4	1.96	0.27	0.91	179
0.08	0.18	3.3	—	—	—	—	—	82	4.3	—	321	594	1354	—	—	—	255
0.03	0.03	0.18	0.02	0	13.2	0.05	0.3	9	0.58	14	33	99	50	0.26	0.04	0.12	17
0.34	0.14	2.1	0.35	0	357.90	1.26	2.9	37	6.59	71	356	731	4	2.5	0.5	0.98	198
0.29	0.1	1.2	0.14	0	272.80	0.86	0	52	4.36	97	231	729	5	1.87	0.39	1.07	182
0.3	0.1	0.79	0.3	0	156.30	0.79	0	32	4.5	82	208	955	4	1.79	0.44	0.97	188
0.33	0.12	1.17	0.14	0	320.70	0.83	2	55	2.83	97	201	536	4	1.7	0.31	0.6	202
0.04	0.04	4.38	0.14	0	29.4	0.31	0	13	0.61	51	101	239	156	0.89	0.17	0.6	32
0.04	0.03	4.19	0.12	0	25	0.29	0	11	0.53	50	103	231	153	0.8	0.18	0.49	32
0.12	0.03	3.79	0.07	0	40.7	0.39	0	15	0.63	49	100	184	228	0.93	0.19	0.58	28
0.07	0.03	4	0.07	0	35.2	0.39	0	25	0.51	52	145	191	121	1.86	0.36	0.58	28
0.37	0.11	1.74	0.09	0	127.30	1.17	0.8	26	2.52	71	195	710	4	1.96	0.35	0.78	196
0.12	0.14	1.23	—	—	—	—	15.2	118	4.47	99	214	994	1071	3.45	1.04	—	253
0.17	0.25	2.42	0.36	0	362.90	0.78	3.8	237	6.71	249	624	2528	280	5.4	1.42	3.71	172
0.2	0.13	0.48	0.12	0	36.9	0.17	0.3	258	13.19	118	239	298	17	1.98	0.48	1.49	126
0.1	0.06	0.24	0.06	0	18.6	0.08	0.1	130	6.65	127	120	150	9	1	0.24	0.75	124

Food description; serving; item number	Energy (kcal)	Water (g)	PRO (g)	TFAT (g)	SFAT (g)	PFAT (g)	MFAT (g)	Chol (mg)	CHO (g)	CFib (g)	DFib (g)	Alc (g)	A (RE)
Category 13: Nuts and Seeds													
Almonds, Dried, Blanched; Ounces; #6	166	1.54	5.8	14.92	1.41	3.13	9.69	0	5.26	0.65	—	—	0
Almonds, Oil Roasted, Blanched; Ounces; #8	174	1	5.41	16.06	1.52	3.37	10.43	0	5.12	0.89	3.18	—	0
Brazilnuts, Dried, Unblanched; Ounces; #137	186	0.95	4.07	18.81	4.59	6.85	6.54	0	3.64	0.65	—	—	—
Cashew Nuts, Oil Roasted; Ounces; #254	163	1.11	4.59	13.69	2.7	2.32	8.07	0	8.1	0.36	1.7	—	0
Chestnuts, Chinese, Roasted; Ounces; #311	68	11.42	1.27	0.34	0.05	0.09	0.18	0	14.87	0.5	—	—	0
Coconut Meat, Sweet, Flaked, Pkgd; Cups; #381	351	11.55	2.42	23.79	21.1	0.26	1.01	0	35.22	1.55	—	—	0
Filberts, Dried, Blanched; Ounces; #630	191	0.54	3.61	19.11	1.4	1.83	14.98	0	4.54	0.51	—	—	2
Hazelnuts, Dry Roast, Unblanched; Ounces; #732	188	0.54	2.84	18.83	1.38	1.8	14.76	0	5.08	1.12	—	—	—
Macadamia Nuts, Dried; Ounces; #866	199	0.82	2.36	20.94	3.13	0.36	16.52	0	3.9	1.5	—	—	0
Macadamia Nuts, Oil Roasted; Ounces; #867	204	0.47	2.06	21.73	3.25	0.38	17.15	0	3.66	0.49	—	—	0
Mixed Nuts w/o Peanuts, Oil Rstd; Ounces; #962	175	0.89	4.41	15.95	2.58	3.25	9.41	0	6.33	0.63	—	—	1
Mixed Nuts w/Peanuts, Dry Roasted; Ounces; #963	169	0.5	4.91	14.61	1.96	3.06	8.92	0	7.2	0.26	—	—	0
Pecans, Dry Roasted; Ounces; #1086	187	0.31	2.26	18.35	1.47	4.54	11.44	0	6.34	0.47	—	—	—
Pecans, Oil Roasted; Ounces; #1087	195	1.19	1.97	20.22	1.62	5.01	12.6	0	4.56	0.46	—	—	—
Pine Nuts, Pignolia, Dried; Tbsps; #1125	51	0.67	2.4	5.07	0.78	2.13	1.91	0	1.42	0.08	—	—	—
Pine Nuts, Pinyon, Dried; Ounces; #1126	161	1.68	3.29	17.32	2.66	7.29	6.52	0	5.48	1.34	—	—	1
Pistachio Nuts, Dry Roasted; Ounces; #1132	172	0.59	4.24	15	1.9	2.27	10.13	0	7.82	0.51	—	—	—
Pumpkin/Squash Kernels, Dried; Ounces; #1233	154	1.97	6.97	13.02	2.46	5.94	4.05	0	5.06	0.63	—	—	11
Sesame Seed Kernels, Dried; Tbsps; #1337	47	0.38	2.11	4.38	0.61	1.92	1.65	0	0.75	0.24	—	—	1
Soybean Kernels, Roasted; Ounces; #1415	129	1.2	10.51	6.8	0.9	3.62	1.59	0	8.68	1.01	—	—	6
Sunflower Seed Kernels, Dried; Ounces; #1470	162	1.52	6.47	14.08	1.48	9.3	2.69	0	5.3	1.18	—	—	1
Walnuts, English/Persian Dried; Ounces; #1610	182	1.04	4.06	17.57	1.59	11.11	4.03	0	5.21	1.31	1.36	—	4
Category 14: Pork Products													
Bacon, Cured, Cooked; 3 Slices; #44	109	2.46	5.79	9.36	3.31	1.1	4.5	16	0.11	0	—	—	0
Bologna, Pork, 4" Dia.; Slices; #126	57	13.94	3.52	4.57	1.58	0.49	2.25	14	0.17	0	—	—	—
Braunschweiger, Pork, 2-1/2"; Slices; #136	65	8.64	2.43	5.78	1.96	0.67	2.68	28	0.56	0	—	—	760
Canadian Bacon, Grilled; 2 Slices; #243	86	28.69	11.27	3.92	1.32	0.37	1.88	27	0.63	0	—	—	0
Chorizo, Pork/Beef, Link; Each; #344	265	19.11	14.46	22.96	8.63	2.08	11.04	—	0	—	—	—	—
Frankfurter, Pork/Beef; Each; #655	144	24.24	5.08	13.12	4.84	1.23	6.15	22	1.15	0	—	—	—

B₁ (mg)	B₂ (mg)	NI (mg)	B₆ (mg)	B₁₂ (µg)	Fol (µg)	PA (mg)	C (mg)	Ca (mg)	Fe (mg)	Mg (mg)	P (mg)	K (mg)	Na (mg)	Zn (mg)	Cu (mg)	Mₙ (mg)	Wt (g)
0.05	0.19	0.9	0.03	0	10.9	0.13	0.2	70	1.03	81	151	213	3	0.9	0.3	0.41	28.4
0.02	0.08	1.11	0.03	0	18	0.07	0.3	55	1.51	82	164	197	3	0.4	0.26	0.42	28.4
0.28	0.04	0.46	0.07	0	1.1	0.07	0.2	50	0.97	64	170	170	0	1.3	0.5	0.22	28.4
0.12	0.05	0.51	0.07	0	19.2	0.34	0	12	1.16	72	121	151	5	1.35	0.62	0.23	28.4
0.04	0.03	0.43	—	0	—	—	—	5	0.43	26	29	135	1	0.26	0.11	—	28.4
0.02	0.01	0.22	—	0	—	—	0	10	1.33	36	74	234	189	1.3	0.22	1.77	74
—	—	—	—	0	—	0.34	—	55	0.96	84	92	131	1	0.71	0.44	0.59	28.4
—	—	—	—	0	—	—	—	55	0.96	84	92	131	1	0.71	0.44	0.59	28.4
0.1	0.03	0.61	—	0	—	—	—	20	0.68	33	39	104	1	0.49	0.08	—	28.4
0.06	0.03	0.57	—	0	—	—	0	13	0.51	33	57	94	2	0.31	0.09	—	28.4
0.14	0.14	0.56	0.05	0	16	0.27	0.2	30	0.73	71	127	154	3	1.32	0.51	0.44	28.4
0.06	0.06	1.34	0.08	0	14.3	0.34	0.1	20	1.05	64	124	169	3	1.08	0.36	0.55	28.4
0.09	0.03	—	—	0	11.6	—	—	10	0.62	38	86	105	0	1.61	0.35	1.34	28.4
—	—	—	—	0	—	—	—	10	0.6	37	84	102	0	1.56	0.34	1.29	28.4
0.08	0.02	0.36	—	0	—	—	—	3	0.92	—	51	60	0	0.42	0.1	—	10
0.35	0.06	1.24	—	0	—	—	0.6	2	0.87	67	10	178	20	1.22	1.22	0.29	28.4
0.12	0.07	0.4	—	0	—	—	—	20	0.9	37	135	275	2	0.39	0.34	0.09	28.4
0.06	0.09	0.5	—	0	—	—	—	12	4.25	152	333	229	5	2.12	0.39	—	28.4
0.06	0.01	0.38	—	0	—	0.05	—	10	0.62	28	62	33	3	0.82	—	—	8
0.03	0.04	0.5	0.09	0	64	0.13	0.6	39	1.26	49	103	417	1	1.03	0.3	—	28.4
0.65	0.07	1.28	—	0	—	—	—	33	1.92	100	200	196	1	1.44	0.5	0.57	28.4
0.11	0.04	0.3	0.16	0	18.7	0.18	0.9	27	0.69	48	90	142	3	0.78	0.39	0.82	28.4
0.13	0.05	1.39	0.05	0.33	1	0.2	6.4	2	0.31	5	64	92	303	0.62	0.03	0.01	19
0.12	0.04	0.9	0.06	0.21	1	0.17	8.1	3	0.18	3	32	65	272	0.47	0.02	0.01	23
0.05	0.28	1.51	0.06	3.62	—	0.61	1.7	2	1.68	2	30	36	206	0.51	0.04	0.03	18
0.38	0.09	3.21	0.21	0.36	2	0.24	10	5	0.38	10	138	181	719	0.79	0.03	0.01	46.5
—	—	—	—	—	—	—	—	—	—	—	—	—	—	—	—	—	60
0.09	0.05	1.18	0.06	0.58	2	0.16	12	5	0.52	5	38	75	504	0.83	0.04	0.01	45

Food description; serving; item number	Energy (kcal)	Water (g)	PRO (g)	TFAT (g)	SFAT (g)	PFAT (g)	MFAT (g)	Chol (mg)	CHO (g)	CFib (g)	DFib (g)	Alc (g)	A (RE)
Ham, Boneless, X-Lean Roasted; 3 Ounces; #720	123	57.52	17.79	4.7	1.54	0.46	2.23	45	1.2	0	—	—	0
Ham, Canned, X-Lean/Reg, Roasted; 3 Ounces; #721	142	56.54	17.8	7.16	2.39	0.76	3.45	34	0.41	0	—	—	—
Ham, Center Slice, Unheated; Ounces; #722	57	17.99	5.72	3.66	1.3	0.4	1.73	15	0.01	0	—	—	0
Ham, Cured, Whole, Lean, Roasted; 3 Ounces; #725	133	55.91	21.29	4.67	1.56	0.54	2.15	47	0	0	—	—	—
Ham, Cured, Whole, Roasted; 3 Ounces; #726	207	49.64	18.33	14.25	5.08	1.54	6.7	52	0	0	—	—	—
Ham, Reg, 11% Fat, Roasted; 3 Ounces; #729	151	54.86	19.23	7.66	2.65	1.2	3.78	50	0	0	—	—	0
Hot Dog, Pork/Beef; Each; #761	144	24.24	5.08	13.12	4.84	1.23	6.15	22	1.15	0	—	—	—
Italian Sausage, Pork, Cooked; Links; #780	217	33.47	13.41	17.22	6.05	2.2	8.01	52	1.01	0	—	—	—
Kielbasa, Kolbassy, Pork, Beef; Ounces; #801	88	15.3	3.76	7.7	2.81	0.87	3.67	19	0.61	0	—	—	—
Knockwurst, Pork, Beef, 4" Long; Ounces; #805	87	15.73	3.37	7.87	2.89	0.83	3.63	16	0.5	0	—	—	—
Liverwurst, Pork; Ounces; #859	92	14.8	4	8.1	3	0.74	3.78	45	0.6	—	—	0	—
Lunch Meat, Pork, Canned; Slices; #862	70	10.8	2.6	6.4	2.27	0.75	3	13	0.4	0	—	—	—
Mortadella, Pork/Beef; Ounces; #967	88	14.83	4.64	7.2	2.7	0.89	3.23	16	0.87	—	—	—	—
Pepperoni, Pork/Beef, 1-3/8" Dia.; Slices; # 1092	27	1.49	1.15	2.42	0.89	0.24	1.16	—	0.16	0	—	—	—
Polish Sausage, Pork; Ounces; # 1148	92	15.07	4	8.14	2.93	0.87	3.83	20	0.46	0	—	—	—
Pork, Cured, Arm, Roasted; 3 Oz.; # 1154	238	46.52	17.36	18.15	6.52	1.97	8.62	49	0	0	—	—	0
Pork, Fresh, Blade, Lean, Broiled; 3 Ounces; # 1156	334	37.75	17.56	28.77	10.33	3.27	13.17	83	0	0	—	—	2
Pork, Fresh, Blade, Roasted; 3 Ounces; # 1158	310	41	17.89	25.88	9.3	2.95	11.84	76	0	0	—	—	2
Pork, Fresh, Ctr Loin, Broiled; 3 Ounces; # 1159	269	42.3	23.3	18.78	6.83	2.11	8.63	82	0	0	—	—	2
Pork, Fresh, Ctr Loin, Lean,Broiled; 3 Ounces; # 1160	196	48.25	27.2	8.91	3.07	1.08	4	83	0	0	—	—	2
Pork, Fresh, Ctr Loin, Roasted; 3 Ounces; # 1162	259	43.99	21.6	18.49	6.68	2.11	8.46	78	0	0	—	—	2
Pork, Fresh, Ctr Rib, Lean, Broiled; 3 Ounces; # 1164	219	46.3	24.5	12.7	4.38	1.54	5.71	80	0	0	—	—	2
Pork, Fresh, Ham, Rump, Lean, Rstd; 3 Ounces; # 1167	187	50.37	24.77	9.06	3.12	1.1	4.07	81	0	0	—	—	2
Pork, Fresh, Ham, Shank, Roasted; 3 Ounces; # 1168	258	44.86	20.66	18.8	6.83	2.11	8.64	78	0	0	—	—	2
Pork, Fresh, Ham, Whole, Lean, Rstd; 3 Ounces; # 1169	187	50.75	24.07	9.38	3.23	1.14	4.21	80	0	0	—	—	2
Pork, Fresh, Ham, Whole, Roasted; 3 Ounces; # 1170	250	45.38	21.27	17.59	6.38	1.99	8.06	79	0	0	—	—	2
Pork, Fresh, Shoulder, Whole, Rstd; 3 Ounces; # 1172	277	43.82	18.72	21.83	7.87	2.48	10	81	0	0	—	—	2
Pork, Fresh, Sirloin, Broiled; 3 Ounces; # 1173	281	41.93	20.53	21.47	7.76	2.42	9.85	82	0	0	—	—	2
Pork, Fresh, Sirloin, Lean, Broiled; 3 Ounces; # 1174	207	48.2	24.05	11.54	3.98	1.4	5.19	83	0	0	—	—	2
Pork, Fresh, Sirloin, Lean, Roasted; 3 Ounces; # 1175	201	49.92	23.37	11.2	3.86	1.36	5.03	77	0	0	—	—	2
Pork, Fresh, Spareribs, Braised; 3 Ounces; # 1177	338	34.36	24.7	25.75	10	2.99	12.04	103	0	0	—	—	3
Pork, Fresh, Top Loin, Broiled; 3 Ounces; # 1179	306	39.21	20.18	24.34	8.8	2.74	11.18	79	0	0	—	—	2

B₁ (mg)	B₂ (mg)	NI (mg)	B₆ (mg)	B₁₂ (µg)	Fol (µg)	PA (mg)	C (mg)	Ca (mg)	Fe (mg)	Mg (mg)	P (mg)	K (mg)	Na (mg)	Zn (mg)	Cu (mg)	Mn (mg)	Wt (g)
0.64	0.17	3.42	0.34	0.55	3	0.34	17.9	7	1.26	12	167	244	1023	2.45	0.07	0.05	85
0.82	0.21	4.28	0.34	0.7	4	0.53	19.4	6	0.91	17	188	298	908	1.97	0.07	0.02	85
0.24	0.06	1.36	0.13	0.23	—	0.14	—	2	0.21	5	61	96	393	0.53	0.02	0.01	28.35
0.58	0.22	4.27	0.4	0.6	3	0.42	—	6	0.79	19	193	269	1128	2.19	0.07	0.01	85
0.51	0.19	3.79	0.32	0.55	3	0.39	—	6	0.74	16	181	243	1009	1.97	0.07	0.01	85
0.62	0.28	5.23	0.26	0.59	—	0.61	19.3	7	1.14	18	239	348	1275	2.1	0.12	0.04	85
0.09	0.05	1.18	0.06	0.58	2	0.16	12	5	0.52	5	38	75	504	0.83	0.04	0.01	45
0.42	0.16	2.79	0.22	0.87	—	0.3	1.3	16	1.01	12	114	204	618	1.59	0.05	0.05	67
0.06	0.06	0.82	0.05	0.46	—	0.23	6	12	0.41	5	42	77	305	0.57	0.03	0.01	28.35
0.1	0.04	0.77	0.05	0.33	—	0.09	8	3	0.26	3	28	57	286	0.47	0.02	—	28.35
0.08	0.29	—	0.05	3.81	9	0.84	—	7	1.81	—	65	—	—	—	—	—	28.35
0.08	0.04	0.66	0.04	0.19	1	0.1	0	1	0.15	2	17	45	271	0.31	0.01	0	21
0.03	0.04	0.76	0.04	0.42	—	—	7	5	0.4	3	27	46	353	0.6·	0.02	0.01	28.35
0.02	0.01	0.27	0.01	0.14	—	0.1	—	1	0.08	1	7	19	112	0.14	0	—	5.5
0.14	0.04	0.98	0.05	0.28	—	0.1	0.3	3	0.41	4	39	67	248	0.55	0.02	0.01	28.35
0.16	3	3.51	0.79	3.51	0.24	0.47	0.52	9	0.81	12	188	220	912	2.14	0.1	0.02	85
0.56	0.27	3.55	0.29	0.8	4	0.7	0.2	9	0.77	18	172	283	57	2.59	0.09	0.01	85
0.44	0.25	3.6	0.31	0.64	3	0.51	0.2	10	0.91	12	147	249	52	2.54	0.08	0.01	85
0.85	0.23	4.25	0.34	0.6	4	0.5	0.3	4	0.69	22	179	305	59	1.64	0.06	0.01	85
0.98	0.26	4.71	0.4	0.63	5	0.59	0.3	4	0.78	25	208	357	66	1.89	0.07	0.01	85
0.7	0.2	4.29	0.34	0.51	1	0.66	0.3	5	0.84	16	167	274	54	1.73	0.06	0.01	85
0.76	0.28	4.45	0.34	0.59	7	0.63	0.2	13	0.69	25	226	373	57	2.02	0.07	0.02	85
0.65	0.3	4.27	0.26	0.62	5	0.64	0.2	6	0.96	24	242	332	55	2.56	0.09	0.02	85
0.49	0.26	3.79	0.33	0.59	5	0.5	0.3	5	0.83	18	203	263	50	2.49	0.08	0.02	85
0.59	0.3	4.2	0.38	0.61	10	0.57	0.3	6	0.95	21	239	317	55	2.77	0.09	0.03	85
0.54	0.26	3.88	0.33	0.6	9	0.5	0.3	5	0.85	18	210	280	51	2.43	0.09	0.03	85
0.46	0.27	3.39	0.27	0.71	4	0.42	0.2	6	1.11	15	170	258	58	3.05	0.1	0.02	85
0.76	0.29	3.69	0.37	0.68	4	0.64	0.2	4	0.66	25	192	312	46	1.72	0.08	0.01	85
0.88	0.34	4.05	0.46	0.72	5	0.77	0.3	5	0.75	29	225	369	51	2.01	0.09	0.01	85
0.68	0.28	4.72	0.36	0.66	5	0.54	0.3	8	0.92	20	214	315	53	2.11	0.09	0.02	85
0.35	0.32	4.65	0.3	0.92	4	0.64	—	40	1.58	21	222	272	79	3.91	0.12	0.01	85
0.65	0.23	3.92	0.29	0.57	6	0.51	0.2	10	0.6	21	186	303	51	1.67	0.06	0.01	85

Food description; serving; item number	Energy (kcal)	Water (g)	PRO (g)	TFAT (g)	SFAT (g)	PFAT (g)	MFAT (g)	Chol (mg)	CHO (g)	CFib (g)	DFib (g)	Alc (g)	A (RE)
Pork, Fresh, Top Loin, Lean Broiled; 3 Ounces; # 1180	219	46.3	24.5	12.7	4.38	1.54	5.71	80	0	0	—	—	2
Salami, Hard/Dry, Pork/Beef; Slices; # 1297	42	3.47	2.29	3.44	1.22	0.32	1.71	8	0.2	0	—	—	—
Sausage, Pork, Fresh, Cooked; Links; # 1332	48	5.79	2.55	4.05	1.4	0.5	1.81	11	0.13	0	—	—	—
Smoked Link Sausage, Pork; Links; # 1357	265	26.7	15.1	21.6	7.7	2.56	9.95	46	1.4	0	—	—	—
Smoked Sausage, Pork/Beef; Links; # 1359	229	35.47	9.11	20.62	7.22	2.21	9.65	48	0.97	0	—	—	—
Turkey Pastrami; 2 Slices; # 1556	80	40.05	10.41	3.52	1.03	0.9	1.16	—	0.94	—	—	—	—
Vienna Sausage, Canned, 2" Long; Each; # 1605	45	9.59	1.65	4.03	1.48	0.27	2.01	8	0.33	0	—	—	—

Category 15: Poultry Products

Food description; serving; item number	Energy (kcal)	Water (g)	PRO (g)	TFAT (g)	SFAT (g)	PFAT (g)	MFAT (g)	Chol (mg)	CHO (g)	CFib (g)	DFib (g)	Alc (g)	A (RE)
Bologna, Turkey; Ounces; #127	57	18.45	3.89	4.31	—	—	—	28	0.27	—	—	—	—
Chicken Roll, Light; 2 Slices; #313	90	38.9	11.07	4.18	1.15	0.91	1.68	28	1.39	—	—	—	—
Chicken, Breast w/o Skin, Fried; 1.83 Oz.; #314	97	31.31	17.39	2.45	0.67	0.56	0.89	47	0.27	0	—	—	4
Chicken, Breast w/Skin, Roasted; 2.05 Oz.; #317	115	36.22	17.28	4.51	1.27	0.96	1.76	49	0	0	—	—	16
Chicken, Drumstick w/Sk, Fried/Flr; Each; #321	120	27.8	13.21	6.72	1.79	1.58	2.66	44	0.8	0	—	—	12
Chicken, Thigh w/Skin, Fried Flour; Each; #323	162	33.57	16.59	9.29	2.54	2.11	3.64	60	1.97	0.01	—	—	18
Chicken, w/Skin, Roasted; 6.3 Oz.; #325	426	105.81	48.6	24.21	6.74	5.29	9.5	157	0	0	—	—	83
Chicken, Wing w/Skin, Fried/Flour; Each; #326	103	15.56	8.36	7.09	1.94	1.58	2.84	26	0.76	0	—	—	12
Frankfurter, Chicken; Each; #654	116	25.89	5.82	8.76	2.49	1.82	3.81	45	3.06	—	—	—	—
Frankfurter, Turkey; Each; #656	102	28.35	6.43	7.96	—	—	—	48	0.67	—	—	—	—
Hot Dog, Chicken; Each; #760	116	25.89	5.82	8.76	2.49	1.82	3.81	45	3.06	—	—	—	—
Hot Dog, Turkey; Each; #762	102	28.35	6.43	7.96	—	—	—	48	0.67	—	—	—	—
Turkey Breast, Pre-Basted, w/Skin; 1/2 Each; # 1553	1087	612.63	191.47	29.9	8.47	7.27	9.87	359	0	0	—	—	0
Turkey Ham, Cured, Thigh Meat; 2 Slices; # 1554	73	40.47	10.74	2.88	0.97	0.86	0.65	—	0.21	—	—	—	—
Turkey Roast, Frozen, Seasoned; 1/4 Box; # 1557	304	132.97	41.78	11.33	—	—	—	103	6.02	—	—	—	—
Turkey Roll, Light & Dark; Ounces; # 1558	42	19.89	5.14	1.98	0.58	0.51	0.65	16	0.6	—	—	—	—
Turkey, Breast, w/o Skin, Roasted; 3.1 Oz.; # 1559	117	59.51	26.15	0.64	0.2	0.17	0.11	73	0	0	—	—	0
Turkey, Breast, w/Skin, Roasted; 3.95 Oz.; # 1560	212	70.8	32.16	8.3	2.35	2.02	2.75	83	0	0	—	—	0
Turkey, Leg, w/Skin, Roasted; 2.5 Oz; # 1564	147	43.45	19.78	6.97	2.17	1.93	2.04	61	0	0	—	—	0
Turkey, Light Meat w/Skin, Roasted; 4.8 Oz.; # 1566	268	85.45	38.85	11.32	3.18	2.74	3.86	103	0	0	—	—	0
Turkey, w/Skin, Roasted; 8.47 Oz.; # 1569	498	148.08	67.43	23.34	6.81	5.96	7.66	196	0	0	—	—	0

Category 16: Snacks

Food description; serving; item number	Energy (kcal)	Water (g)	PRO (g)	TFAT (g)	SFAT (g)	PFAT (g)	MFAT (g)	Chol (mg)	CHO (g)	CFib (g)	DFib (g)	Alc (g)	A (RE)
Beef Jerky, Frito-Lay; Pieces; #73	25	—	3	1	—	—	—	10	1	—	—	—	—
Beef Sticks, Frito-Lay; Pieces; #74	80	—	3	7	—	—	—	15	1	—	—	—	—
Cheetos Cheese Flavored Snacks; Ounces; #300	150	—	2	10	—	—	—	0	15	—	—	—	—

B₁ (mg)	B₂ (mg)	NI (mg)	B₆ (mg)	B₁₂ (μg)	Fol (μg)	PA (mg)	C (mg)	Ca (mg)	Fe (mg)	Mg (mg)	P (mg)	K (mg)	Na (mg)	Zn (mg)	Cu (mg)	Mn (mg)	Wt (g)
0.76	0.28	4.45	0.34	0.59	7	0.63	0.2	13	0.69	25	226	373	57	2.02	0.07	0.02	85
0.06	0.03	0.49	0.05	0.19	—	0.11	3	1	0.15	2	14	38	186	0.32	0.01	0	10
0.1	0.03	0.59	0.04	0.22	—	0.09	0.2	4	0.16	2	24	47	168	0.33	0.02	0.01	13
0.48	0.17	3.08	0.24	1.11	—	0.53	1	20	0.79	13	110	228	1020	1.92	0.05	—	68
0.18	0.12	2.19	0.12	1.03	—	0.3	13	7	0.99	8	73	129	642	1.44	0.04	0.03	68
0.03	0.14	2	—	—	—	—	—	5	0.94	8	113	147	593	1.22	0.03	—	56.7
0.01	0.02	0.26	0.02	0.16	—	—	0	2	0.14	1	8	16	152	0.26	0	0	16
0.02	0.05	1	—	—	—	—	—	24	0.43	4	37	56	249	0.49	0.01	—	28.35
0.04	0.07	3	—	—	—	—	—	24	0.55	10	89	129	331	0.41	0.02	—	56.7
0.04	0.06	7.69	0.33	0.19	2	0.54	0	8	0.59	16	128	143	41	0.56	0.03	0.01	52
0.04	0.07	7.37	0.32	0.19	2	0.54	0	8	0.62	16	124	142	41	0.59	0.03	0.01	58
0.04	0.11	2.96	0.17	0.16	4	0.6	0	6	0.66	11	86	112	44	1.42	0.04	0.01	49
0.06	0.15	4.31	0.21	0.19	5	0.74	0	8	0.93	5	116	147	55	1.56	0.05	0.02	62
0.11	0.3	15.11	0.71	0.54	9	1.83	0	27	2.25	42	324	397	146	3.45	0.12	0.04	178
0.02	0.04	2.14	0.13	0.09	1	0.28	0	5	0.4	6	48	57	25	0.56	0.02	0.01	32
0.03	0.05	1.39	—	—	—	—	—	43	0.9	—	—	—	617	—	—	—	45
0.02	0.08	1.86	—	—	—	—	—	48	0.83	—	60	80	642	—	—	—	45
0.03	0.05	1.39	—	—	—	—	—	43	0.9	—	—	—	617	—	—	—	45
0.02	0.08	1.86	—	—	—	—	—	48	0.83	—	60	80	642	—	—	—	45
0.46	1.15	78.34	2.72	2.77	—	—	0	75	5.71	185	1851	2141	3434	13.18	0.35	—	864
0.03	0.14	2	—	—	—	—	—	5	1.57	—	108	184	565	—	—	—	56.7
0.09	0.32	12.29	0.52	2.98	—	1.58	—	10	3.19	43	478	584	1334	4.97	0.12	—	196
0.03	0.08	1.36	—	—	—	—	—	9	0.38	5	48	77	166	0.57	0.02	—	28.35
0.04	0.11	6.52	0.49	0.34	6	0.62	0	11	1.33	25	195	254	45	1.51	0.06	0.02	87
0.06	0.15	7.13	0.54	0.4	7	0.71	0	24	1.56	30	235	323	70	2.27	0.05	0.02	112
0.04	0.17	2.53	0.24	0.26	6	0.86	0	23	1.63	17	141	199	55	3.03	0.11	0.02	71
0.08	0.18	8.55	0.64	0.48	8	0.85	0	29	1.92	36	283	388	85	2.77	0.06	0.03	136
0.14	0.43	12.21	0.97	0.85	17	2.06	0	63	4.29	60	487	673	164	7.11	0.22	0.05	240
—	0.03	0.4	—	—	—	—	—	—	0.36	—	8	40	200	—	—	—	5.95
—	0.07	0.4	0.04	—	—	—	—	—	0.36	—	8	60	300	—	—	—	12.75
0.03	0.03	0.4	—	—	—	—	—	—	0.36	—	0.02	45	280	—	—	—	28.35

Food description; serving; item number	Energy (kcal)	Water (g)	PRO (g)	TFAT (g)	SFAT (g)	PFAT (g)	MFAT (g)	Chol (mg)	CHO (g)	CFib (g)	DFib (g)	Alc (g)	A (RE)
Cheez Curls, Planters; Ounces; #302	160	—	2	11	2	1	—	5	14	—	—	—	—
Corn Chips, Fritos; Ounces; #451	150	—	1	9	—	—	—	0	16	—	—	—	—
Crackers, Cheez-It Snack Crackers; 12 Each; #491	70	—	1	4	—	—	—	0	7	—	—	—	—
Crackers, Sunshine Krispy Saltines; 5 Each; #518	60	—	1	1	—	—	—	0	11	—	—	—	—
Crackers, Sunshine Krispy Unsalted; 5 Each; #519	60	—	1	1	—	—	—	0	11	—	—	—	—
Crackers, Sunshine Oyster/Soup; 16 Each; #520	60	—	1	2	—	—	—	0	10	—	—	—	—
Crackers, Sunshine Wheat Wafers; 8 Each; #521	80	—	1	4	—	—	—	0	10	1	—	—	—
Dip, Kraft Prem., French Onion; 2 Tbsps; #585	45	—	1	4	2	0	—	10	2	—	—	—	—
Dip, Kraft Prem., Jalapeno Cheese; 2 Tbsps; #586	50	—	1	4	3	0	—	15	3	—	—	—	20
Dip, Kraft, Guacamole (Avocado); 2 Tbsps; #588	50	—	1	4	2	1	—	0	3	—	—	—	—
Dip, Kraft, Jalapeno Pepper; 2 Tbsps; #589	50	—	1	4	2	1	—	0	3	—	—	—	—
Grain Cakes, Quaker, Rye; Each; #684	35	0.3	1.4	0.3	0	0.1	0.1	0	6.5	0.2	0.8	—	0
Granola Bar Choc Chip, Quaker Chewy; Each; #686	128	1.5	2	4.7	1.5	0.4	1.2	0.3	19.3	0.3	1.4	—	0
Granola Bar Cin/Raisn, Quaker Chewy; Each; #687	128	1.8	2.2	5	1.1	0.6	1.3	0.3	18.6	0.3	1.2	—	0
Hostess Chocolate Cupcake; Each; #746	170	—	2	6	—	—	—	3	29	—	—	—	0
Hostess Cinnamon Donuts; Each; #748	110	—	1	6	—	—	—	6	15	1	—	—	0
Hostess Ding Dongs; Each; #749	170	—	1	9	—	—	—	6	21	—	—	—	0
Hostess Twinkies; Each; #758	160	—	1	5	—	—	—	20	26	—	—	—	0
Potato Chips; 10 Chips; # 1183	120	0.51	1.28	7.08	1.81	3.63	1.25	0	10.37	0.28	0.96	—	0
Potato Chips, Lay's; Ounces; # 1186	150	—	1	10	—	—	—	0	15	—	—	—	—
Potato Chips, Ruffles; Ounces; # 1188	150	—	1	10	—	—	—	0	15	—	—	—	—
Pretzels, Mister Salty, Minis; 16 Pcs; # 1215	110	—	3	1	—	—	—	—	21	—	—	—	—
Pretzels, Mister Salty, Rings; 22 Pcs; # 1216	110	—	3	2	—	—	—	—	21	—	—	—	—
Pretzels, Mister Salty, Twists; 5 Pcs; # 1217	110	—	3	2	—	—	—	—	21	—	—	—	—
Pretzels, Rods, 7.5" Long; Each; # 1218	55	0.63	1.4	0.6	—	—	—	—	10.6	—	—	—	0
Pretzels, Sticks, 2 1/4" Long; 10 Sticks; # 1220	12	0.14	0.3	0.1	—	—	—	—	2.3	—	—	—	0
Rice Cakes, Quaker, Plain Lite Salt; Each; # 1259	35	0.5	0.8	0.3	0.1	0.1	0.1	0	7.1	0.1	0.3	—	—
Rice Cakes, Quaker, Sesame Lite Sal; Each; # 1261	35	0.5	0.8	0.3	0.1	0.1	0.1	0	7.1	0.1	0.3	—	—
Tortilla Chips, Doritos; Ounces; # 1536	140	—	2	6	—	—	—	0	19	—	—	—	—
Tortilla Chips, Tostitos; Ounces; # 1538	140	—	2	8	—	—	—	0	18	—	—	—	—

B₁ (mg)	B₂ (mg)	NI (mg)	B₆ (mg)	B₁₂ (μg)	Fol (μg)	PA (mg)	C (mg)	Ca (mg)	Fe (mg)	Mg (mg)	P (mg)	K (mg)	Na (mg)	Zn (mg)	Cu (mg)	Mn (mg)	Wt (g)
—	—	—	—	—	—	—	—	—	—	—	—	35	290	—	—	—	28.4
—	—	—	—	—	—	—	—	20	—	16	0.04	50	230	—	—	—	28.35
0.06	0.03	0.4	—	—	—	—	—	20	0.36	—	—	—	135	—	—	—	14.2
0.06	0.03	0.8	—	—	—	—	—	—	0.36	—	—	—	210	—	—	—	14.2
0.06	0.03	0.8	—	—	—	—	—	—	0.36	—	—	—	120	—	—	—	14.2
0.06	0.03	0.4	—	—	—	—	—	—	0.72	—	—	—	190	—	—	—	14.9
0.03	—	0.4	—	—	—	—	—	—	0.36	—	—	—	190	—	—	—	14.2
—	0.03	—	—	—	—	—	—	20	—	—	0.02	40	150	—	—	—	30
—	0.07	—	—	—	—	—	—	40	—	—	0.06	55	160	—	—	—	30
—	0.03	—	—	—	—	—	—	—	—	—	—	25	210	—	—	—	30
—	—	—	—	—	—	—	2.4	—	—	—	—	15	160	—	—	—	30
0.06	0.01	0.37	—	—	—	—	0	6	0.46	15	38	46	52	—	—	—	9
0.05	0.05	0.24	0.03	0.04	6	0.13	0	27	0.7	22	65	94	90	0.43	0.11	0.37	28
0.05	0.06	0.28	0.03	0.05	5	0.12	0	29	0.67	20	62	101	92	0.37	0.08	0.36	28
0.06	0.07	0.4	—	—	—	—	0	20	0.72	—	—	—	250	—	—	—	49.6
0.03	0.03	0.4	—	—	—	—	0	20	0.36	—	—	—	140	—	—	—	28.4
0	0.03	0.4	—	—	—	—	0	20	0.36	—	—	—	130	—	—	—	37.7
0.06	0.07	0.4	—	—	—	—	0	20	0.36	—	—	—	150	—	—	—	42.5
0.03	0	0.84	0.1	0	9	0.08	8.3	5	0.24	12	31	260	94	0.21	0.04	0.09	20
0.03	—	1.2	0.16	—	—	—	6	—	0.36	16	0.04	370	200	—	—	—	28.35
0.03	0.03	1.2	0.2	—	—	—	4.8	—	0.36	16	0.04	360	190	—	—	—	28.35
0.12	0.14	1.6	—	—	—	—	—	—	1.08	—	—	40	450	—	—	—	28.35
0.12	0.14	1.6	—	—	—	—	—	—	1.08	—	—	40	510	—	—	—	28.35
0.12	0.14	1.6	—	—	—	—	—	—	1.08	—	—	40	590	—	—	—	28.35
—	—	0.1	—	—	—	—	0	3	0.2	—	18	18	235	—	—	—	14
—	—	—	—	—	—	—	0	1	—	—	4	4	50	—	—	—	3
0	0.01	0.54	0.01	—	2	0.08	0	1	0.15	12	32	25	36	0.23	0.04	0.55	9
0	0.01	0.51	0.01	—	2	0.08	0	1	0.13	12	33	25	36	0.23	0.04	0.55	9
—	—	—	—	—	—	—	—	20	—	16	0.04	80	230	—	—	—	28.35
—	—	—	—	—	—	—	—	40	—	24	0.04	65	170	—	—	—	28.35

Category 17: Soups, Sauces, Gravies

Food description; serving; item number	Energy (kcal)	Water (g)	PRO (g)	TFAT (g)	SFAT (g)	PFAT (g)	MFAT (g)	Chol (mg)	CHO (g)	CFib (g)	DFib (g)	Alc (g)	A (RE)
Broth, Beef, R-T-S; Cups; #183	16	234.12	2.74	0.53	0.26	0.02	0.22	—	0.1	—	—	—	0
Broth, Chicken, Condensed; Cups; #184	78	230.82	11.09	2.61	0.78	0.55	1.17	3	1.88	—	—	—	0
Gravy, Canned, Beef; Cups; #703	124	203.83	8.74	5.5	2.68	0.19	2.24	7	11.2	—	0.93	—	0
Gravy, Dehy, Brown w/Water; Cups; #706	75	237.03	2.4	1.73	0.84	0.07	0.7	2	13.04	0.01	—	—	—
Gravy, Dehy, Chicken w/Water; Cups; #707	83	237.48	2.62	1.92	0.53	0.45	0.86	3	14.34	0.06	—	—	—
Horseradish, Prepared; Tsps; #745	2	4.36	0.1	—	—	—	—	—	0.5	—	—	—	—
Salsa Picante, Ortega; Ounces; #1303	10	—	0	0	—	—	—	—	2	—	—	—	40
Sauce, Barbecue, Kraft; 2 Tbsps; #1309	45	—	0	1	0	0	—	0	10	—	—	—	40
Sauce, Chili Hot Dog, Gebhardt; 2 Tbsps; #1310	20	—	1	1	—	—	—	—	2	—	—	—	150
Sauce, Horseradish, Kraft; Tbsps; #1321	50	—	0	5	1	3	—	5	2	—	—	—	—
Sauce, Picante, Pace; 2 Tbsps; #1323	3.39	10.84	0.13	0.09	—	—	—	—	0.55	—	—	—	6
Sauce, Soy, R-T-S; Tbsps; #1324	11	12.16	1.56	0	0	0	0	0	1.5	—	—	—	0
Sauce, Tartar, Sauceworks; Tbsps; #1327	50	—	0	5	1	3	—	5	2	—	—	—	—
Sauce, Worcestershire, Heinz; Tbsps; #1329	11	—	—	—	—	—	—	—	—	—	—	—	—
Soup, Bean w/Bacon, w/Water; Cups; #1365	173	212.92	7.89	5.94	1.53	1.82	2.18	3	22.8	1.52	—	—	89
Soup, Beef Noodle, w/Water; Cups; #1366	84	224.45	4.83	3.08	1.15	0.49	1.24	5	8.98	—	—	—	63
Soup, Chicken Noodle, w/Water; Cups; #1369	75	221.7	4.04	2.45	0.65	0.55	1.11	7	9.35	0.24	—	—	72
Soup, Chicken Rice, w/Water; Cups; #1370	60	226.1	3.53	1.91	0.46	0.42	0.91	7	7.15	—	—	—	66
Soup, Chicken Veg., w/Water; Cups; #1372	74	223.26	3.61	2.84	0.85	0.6	1.27	10	8.58	0.12	—	—	266
Soup, Chili Beef, w/Water; Cups; #1374	169	211.72	6.69	6.61	3.34	0.27	2.8	12	21.46	1.45	—	—	151
Soup, Clam Chowder, Manhattan w/Wt; Cups; #1376	77	224.16	2.19	2.21	0.38	1.29	0.38	3	12.23	0.45	—	—	96
Soup, Clam Chowder, New England w/W; Cups; #1377	95	220.91	4.81	2.88	0.41	1.1	1.22	5	12.43	0.27	—	—	1
Soup, Cream of Asparagus, w/Milk; Cups; #1378	161	213.27	6.31	8.18	3.33	2.24	2.07	22	16.4	0.74	—	—	83
Soup, Cream of Celery, w/Milk; Cups; #1380	165	214.41	5.69	9.68	3.95	2.65	2.47	32	14.53	0.38	—	—	68
Soup, Cream of Chicken, Condensed; Cups; #1381	233	205.19	6.86	14.72	4.15	2.98	0.82	20	18.53	0.25	—	—	112
Soup, Cream of Chicken, w/Milk; Cups; #1382	191	210.38	7.46	11.45	4.63	1.64	4.45	27	14.97	0.13	—	—	94
Soup, Cream of Mushroom, w/Milk; Cups; #1384	203	209.72	6.05	13.59	5.12	4.61	2.98	20	15	0.25	—	—	38
Soup, Cream of Potato, w/Milk; Cups; #1385	148	214.95	5.78	6.45	3.76	0.56	1.73	22	17.17	—	—	—	67
Soup, Dehy, Vegetable Beef, w/Water; Cups; #1394	53	237.54	2.93	1.12	0.56	0.05	0.47	1	8.01	0.15	—	—	24
Soup, Lentil w/Ham, R-T-S; Cups; #1395	140	212.65	9.26	2.78	1.12	0.32	1.29	7	20.24	1.4	—	—	36
Soup, Minestrone, w/Water; Cups; #1397	83	220.11	4.26	2.51	0.54	1.11	0.69	2	11.24	0.72	—	—	234
Soup, Onion, Condensed; Cups; #1398	114	212.43	7.53	3.49	0.52	1.31	1.5	0	16.42	0.98	—	—	0

B₁ (mg)	B₂ (mg)	NI (mg)	B₆ (mg)	B₁₂ (µg)	Fol (µg)	PA (mg)	C (mg)	Ca (mg)	Fe (mg)	Mg (mg)	P (mg)	K (mg)	Na (mg)	Zn (mg)	Cu (mg)	Mn (mg)	Wt (g)
0	0.05	1.87	—	—	—	—	0	15	0.41	—	31	130	782	—	—	—	240
0.01	0.12	5.6	0.05	0.5	—	—	0	14	1.03	5	151	427	1571	0.5	0.25	0.5	251
0.08	0.08	1.54	0.02	0.23	—	—	0	14	1.63	—	70	189	1305	2.33	0.23	0.47	233
0.04	0.09	0.81	—	—	—	—	—	66	0.24	10	44	57	1076	0.31	0.06	0.09	258
—	0.14	—	—	—	—	—	—	39	—	—	—	—	1133	0.32	0.03	—	259.7
—	—	—	—	—	—	—	—	3	—	—	2	15	5	—	—	—	5
—	—	0.4	—	—	—	—	9	—	0.36	—	—	60	300	—	—	—	28.4
—	—	—	—	—	—	—	—	—	—	—	—	65	460	—	—	—	33
—	—	—	—	—	—	—	—	—	—	—	—	20	150	—	—	—	40.2
—	—	—	—	—	—	—	—	—	—	—	—	—	100	—	—	—	14
0.01	0	0.2	—	—	—	—	0.78	1.86	0.07	—	—	—	138	—	—	—	12
0.01	0.02	0.61	0.03	0	1.9	0.06	0	3	0.49	8	38	64	1029	0.04	0.02	0	18
—	—	—	—	—	—	—	—	—	—	—	—	5	85	—	—	—	14
—	—	—	—	—	—	—	—	—	—	—	—	—	234	—	—	—	14
0.09	0.03	0.57	0.04	—	31.9	—	1.6	81	2.05	44	132	403	952	1.03	0.4	0.67	253
0.07	0.06	1.07	0.04	0.2	4.4	—	0.3	15	1.1	6	46	99	952	1.54	0.14	0.27	244
0.05	0.06	1.39	0.03	—	2.2	—	0.2	17	0.78	5	36	55	1107	0.4	0.19	0.29	241
0.02	0.02	1.13	0.02	—	1.1	—	0.1	17	0.75	1	21	100	814	0.26	0.12	0.37	241
0.04	0.05	1.23	0.05	—	—	—	1	18	0.87	6	41	154	944	0.37	0.12	0.37	241
0.06	0.08	1.07	0.16	0.32	—	—	4.1	43	2.13	30	148	525	1035	1.4	0.4	1.05	250
0.3	0.04	0.82	0.1	4.06	10	—	4	26	1.64	11	41	188	1029	0.97	0.13	0.38	244
0.02	0.04	0.96	0.08	8.01	3.7	0.32	2	43	1.48	7	54	146	914	0.75	0.12	0.25	244
0.1	0.28	0.88	0.06	—	—	—	3.9	175	0.87	20	153	359	1041	0.93	0.14	0.38	248
0.07	0.25	0.44	0.06	—	8.5	—	1.4	186	0.69	22	151	309	1010	0.2	0.15	0.25	248
0.06	0.12	1.64	0.03	—	3.2	—	0.3	68	1.21	5	75	174	1973	1.25	0.25	0.75	251
0.07	0.26	0.92	0.07	—	7.7	—	1.3	180	0.67	18	152	273	1046	0.68	0.14	0.38	248
0.08	0.28	0.91	0.06	—	—	—	2.3	178	0.59	20	156	270	1076	0.64	0.14	0.25	248
0.08	0.24	0.64	0.09	—	9.2	—	1.1	166	0.54	17	160	323	1060	0.68	0.26	0.38	248
0.03	0.04	0.46	0.05	—	—	—	—	—	0.85	—	37	—	1000	0.27	0.03	—	253.1
0.17	0.11	1.35	0.22	0.3	49.6	0.35	4.2	42	2.64	—	184	356	1318	—	—	—	248
0.05	0.04	0.94	0.1	0	16.1	—	1.1	34	0.92	7	56	312	911	0.74	0.12	0.37	241
0.07	0.05	1.21	0.1	0	30.6	—	2.5	53	1.35	5	22	138	2116	1.23	0.25	0.49	246

Food description; serving; item number	Energy (kcal)	Water (g)	PRO (g)	TFAT (g)	SFAT (g)	PFAT (g)	MFAT (g)	Chol (mg)	CHO (g)	CFib (g)	DFib (g)	Alc (g)	A (RE)
Soup, Oyster Stew, w/Milk; Cups; # 1399	134	217.89	6.14	7.93	5.05	0.31	2.08	32	9.78	—	—	—	45
Soup, Pea, Green, w/Milk; Cups; # 1400	239	197.93	12.63	7.03	4	0.52	2.18	18	32.22	0.66	—	—	58
Soup, Split Pea w/Ham, R-T-S; Cups; # 1401	184	194.29	11.09	3.98	1.59	0.57	1.63	7	26.8	—	—	—	487
Soup, Tomato Rice, w/Water; Cups; # 1404	120	217.63	2.11	2.72	0.52	1.35	0.6	2	21.93	0.64	—	—	76
Soup, Tomato, Condensed; Cups; # 1405	171	203.93	4.12	3.84	0.73	1.92	0.86	0	33.19	1	—	—	139
Soup, Tomato, w/Milk; Cups; # 1406	160	209.75	6.09	6.01	2.91	1.11	1.6	17	22.31	0.5	—	—	108
Soup, Turkey Vegetable, w/Water; Cups; # 1407	74	233.86	3.09	3.02	0.9	0.67	1.33	2	8.64	—	—	—	244
Soup, Vegetable Beef, w/Water; Cups; # 1409	79	223.53	5.58	1.9	0.85	0.11	0.8	5	10.17	0.31	—	—	189
Soup, Vegetarian, w/Water; Cups; # 1412	72	222.52	2.1	1.93	0.29	0.73	0.83	0	11.98	0.49	—	—	300
Spaghetti Sauce, Prego, Meat Flvrd; 4 Oz.; # 1424	140	—	2	6	—	—	—	—	20	—	—	—	200
Spaghetti Sauce, Prego, Mushroom; 4 Oz.; # 1425	130	—	2	5	—	—	—	—	20	—	—	—	200
Spaghetti Sauce, Prego, Regular; 4 Oz.; # 1427	130	—	2	5	—	—	—	—	20	—	—	—	200

Category 18: Sugars and Sweets

Food description; serving; item number	Energy (kcal)	Water (g)	PRO (g)	TFAT (g)	SFAT (g)	PFAT (g)	MFAT (g)	Chol (mg)	CHO (g)	CFib (g)	DFib (g)	Alc (g)	A (RE)
Baby Ruth Candy Bar, Nabisco; 1/2 Pc; #43	130	—	2	6	—	—	—	—	18	—	—	—	—
Butterfinger Candy Bar, Nabisco; 1/2 Pc; #208	130	—	2	6	—	—	—	—	19	—	—	—	—
Cake Icing, Chocolate; Cups; #215	1034	39.33	8.8	38.2	21.3	—	—	—	185.4	—	—	—	116
Candy, Butterscotch; Ounces; #244	113	0.42	—	1	0.5	—	—	—	26.9	—	—	—	8
Chocolate Bar w/Almonds, Nestle; Ounces; #335	160	—	3	10	—	—	—	—	15	—	—	—	—
Chocolate Syrup, Fudge Type; 2 Tbsps; #338	124	9.52	1.9	5.1	2.9	—	—	—	20.3	—	—	—	12
Chocolate, Bittersweet; Ounces; #340	135	0.5	2.2	11.3	6.3	—	—	—	13.3	—	—	—	2
Chocolate, Semi-Sweet, Small Pieces; Cups; #341	862	1.87	7.1	60.7	34	—	—	—	96.9	—	—	—	6
Cocoa, Hershey's; 1/3 Cups; #380	120	—	7	4	—	—	—	0	13	—	—	—	—
Dessert Topping, Cool Whip; Tbsps; #578	11	2.1	0.1	0.8	—	0	—	0	1	—	—	—	—
Fudge, Chocolate, Plain; Ounces; #668	113	2.3	0.8	3.5	1.2	—	—	—	21.3	—	—	—	—
Gelatin, Dessert Made w/Water; Cups; #672	142	202.08	3.6	0	—	—	—	—	33.8	—	—	—	—
Gum Drops; Ounces; #711	98	3.28	—	0.2	—	—	—	—	24.8	—	—	—	0
Hard Candy; Ounces; #730	109	0.39	0	0.3	—	—	—	—	27.6	—	—	—	0
Honey, Strained; Tbsps; #743	64	3.61	0.1	0	—	—	—	—	17.3	—	—	—	0
Jams & Preserves; Tbsps; #781	54	5.8	0.1	—	—	—	—	—	14	—	—	—	—
Jellies; Tbsps; #783	49	5.22	—	—	—	—	—	—	12.7	—	—	—	—
Jelly Beans, Approx. 10; Ounces; #784	104	1.76	—	0.1	—	—	—	—	26.4	—	—	—	0
Life Savers, Most Flavors; Each; #852	8	—	0	0	—	—	—	—	2	—	—	—	—
M & M's Peanut Candies, Mars; 1.74 Oz; #864	250	—	5	13	—	—	—	—	30	—	—	—	—

B₁ (mg)	B₂ (mg)	NI (mg)	B₆ (mg)	B₁₂ (µg)	Fol (µg)	PA (mg)	C (mg)	Ca (mg)	Fe (mg)	Mg (mg)	P (mg)	K (mg)	Na (mg)	Zn (mg)	Cu (mg)	Mn (mg)	Wt (g)
0.07	0.23	0.34	0.06	2.63	—	—	4.3	167	1.04	21	162	235	1040	10.34	1.61	0.37	245
0.16	0.27	1.34	0.1	0.44	7.9	—	2.9	173	2.01	55	238	377	1048	1.75	0.39	0.66	254
0.12	0.09	2.52	—	—	4.7	—	7	33	2.14	—	—	—	965	—	—	—	240
0.06	0.05	1.05	0.08	0	—	—	14.8	23	0.79	5	33	330	815	0.51	0.13	0.38	247
0.18	0.1	2.84	0.23	0	29.5	—	133	27	3.51	15	68	527	1744	0.49	0.5	0.5	251
0.13	0.25	1.52	0.16	0.44	20.9	—	67.7	159	1.82	23	148	450	932	0.29	0.26	0.25	248
0.03	0.04	1	0.05	0.17	—	—	0	17	0.76	4	40	175	905	0.61	0.12	0.25	241
0.04	0.05	1.03	0.08	0.31	10.6	—	2.4	17	1.11	6	40	173	957	1.54	0.18	0.31	244
0.05	0.05	0.92	0.05	0	10.6	—	1.4	21	1.08	7	35	209	823	0.46	0.12	0.46	241
0.03	0.03	1.2	—	—	—	—	15	40	1.08	—	—	—	660	—	—	—	113.6
0.03	0.07	1.2	—	—	—	—	15	40	0.72	—	—	—	630	—	—	—	113.6
0.03	0.03	0.8	—	—	—	—	18	40	1.08	—	—	—	630	—	—	—	113.6
—	0.03	0.8	—	—	—	—	—	—	0.36	—	—	60	60	—	—	—	14.18
—	0.03	0.8	—	—	—	—	—	—	0.36	—	—	60	60	—	—	—	14.18
0.06	0.28	0.6	—	—	—	—	1	165	3.3	—	305	536	168	—	—	—	275
0	—	—	—	—	—	—	0	5	0.4	—	2	1	19	—	—	—	28
—	0.14	—	—	—	—	—	—	60	0.36	—	—	125	15	—	—	—	28.35
0.02	0.08	0.2	—	—	—	—	—	48	0.5	—	60	107	33	—	—	—	37.5
0.01	0.05	0.3	—	—	—	—	0	16	1.4	—	81	174	1	—	—	—	28
0.02	0.14	0.9	—	—	—	—	0	51	4.4	—	255	553	3	—	—	—	170
—	0.14	0.4	—	—	—	—	—	40	4.5	—	—	—	10	—	—	—	28.35
0	0	0	—	0	—	—	0	0	0	0	0	0	1	—	—	—	4
0.01	0.03	0.1	—	—	—	—	—	22	0.3	—	24	42	54	—	—	—	28
—	—	—	—	—	—	—	—	—	—	—	—	—	122	—	—	—	240
0	—	—	—	—	—	—	0	2	0.1	—	—	1	10	—	—	—	28
0	0	0	—	—	—	—	0	6	0.5	—	2	1	9	—	—	—	28
—	0.01	0.1	—	—	—	—	—	1	0.1	—	1	11	1	—	—	—	21
—	0.01	—	—	—	—	—	—	4	0.2	—	2	18	2	—	—	—	20
—	0.01	—	—	—	—	—	1	4	0.3	—	1	14	3	—	—	—	18
0	—	—	—	—	—	—	0	3	0.3	—	1	—	3	—	—	—	28
—	—	—	—	—	—	—	—	—	—	—	—	0	0	—	—	—	2
—	0.07	1.6	—	—	—	—	—	40	0.36	—	—	—	55	—	—	—	49.3

Food description; serving; item number	Energy (kcal)	Water (g)	PRO (g)	TFAT (g)	SFAT (g)	PFAT (g)	MFAT (g)	Chol (mg)	CHO (g)	CFib (g)	DFib (g)	Alc (g)	A (RE)
M & M's Plain Candies, Mars; 1.69 Oz; #865	230	—	3	10	—	—	—	—	35	—	—	—	—
Mars Almond Bar, Mars; Each; #899	240	—	4	11	—	—	—	—	30	—	—	—	—
Marshmallows, Plain, Regular; Each; #902	23	1.25	0.1	—	—	—	—	—	5.8	—	—	—	0
Milk Chocolate, Plain; Ounces; #941	147	0.25	2.2	9.2	5.1	—	—	—	16.1	—	0.78	—	16
Milk Chocolate, w/Almonds; Ounces; #942	151	0.42	2.6	10.1	4.5	—	—	—	14.5	—	—	—	14
Milky Way Bar, Mars; Each; #959	280	—	3	11	—	—	—	—	42	—	—	—	—
Molasses, Cane, Light; Tbsps; #965	50	4.8	—	—	—	—	—	—	13	—	—	—	—
Nestle's Crunch Bar; 1 1/6 Oz.; #1004	160	—	2	8	—	—	—	5	19	—	—	—	—
Peanut Brittle, Kraft; Ounces; #1067	130	—	3	5	1	1	—	0	20	—	—	—	—
Peanut Butter Morsels, Nestle; Ounces; #1068	160	—	5	10	—	—	—	—	12	—	—	—	—
Pudding, Chocolate, From Mix; Cups; #1226	322	182	8.8	7.8	4.3	—	—	—	59.3	—	—	—	68
Pudding, Tapicoa; Cups; #1229	221	118.47	8.3	8.4	3.9	—	—	—	28.2	—	—	—	96
Raisinets, Nestle; Ounces; #1244	120	—	2	4	—	—	—	—	20	—	—	—	—
Reese's Pieces Candy; Serving; #1254	260	—	8	11	—	—	—	5	32	—	—	—	—
Snickers Bar, Mars; Each; #1363	280	—	5	13	—	—	—	—	36	—	—	—	—
Sugar, Brown, Packed; Cups; #1465	821	4.62	0	0	—	—	—	—	212.1	—	—	—	0
Sugar, Powdered, Sifted; Cups; #1466	385	0.5	0	0	—	—	—	—	99.5	—	—	—	0
Sugar, White, Granulated; Tbsps; #1467	46	0.06	0	0	—	—	—	—	11.9	—	—	—	0
Syrup, Maple; Tbsps; #1480	50	6.5	—	—	—	—	—	—	12.8	—	—	—	—
Syrup, Table Blends (Light & Dark); Tbsps; #1481	59	4.92	0	0	—	—	—	—	15.4	—	—	—	0
Three Musketeers Bar, Mars; Each; #1513	260	—	2	9	—	—	—	—	44	—	—	—	—
Twix Caramel Cookie Bar; Each; #1573	140	—	2	7	—	—	—	—	19	—	—	—	—
Whatchamacallit Candy Bar; Serving; #1625	260	—	5	13	—	—	—	10	30	—	—	—	—

Category 19: Vegetables and Vegetable Products

Food description; serving; item number	Energy (kcal)	Water (g)	PRO (g)	TFAT (g)	SFAT (g)	PFAT (g)	MFAT (g)	Chol (mg)	CHO (g)	CFib (g)	DFib (g)	Alc (g)	A (RE)
Alfalfa Seeds, Sprouted; Tbsps; #3	1	2.73	0.12	0.02	0	0.01	0	0	0.11	0.05	—	—	0
Artichokes, Raw, Medium; Each; #38	60	108.72	4.19	0.19	0.04	0.08	0.01	0	13.45	1.5	6.66	—	24
Asparagus, Fresh, Boiled; 4 Spears; #40	15	55.23	1.55	0.19	0.04	0.08	0.01	0	2.64	0.5	—	—	50
Bamboo Shoots, Canned, Sliced; Cups; #53	25	123.56	2.26	0.52	0.12	0.23	0.01	0	4.22	0.87	—	—	1
Beans, Snap, Boiled; Cups; #68	44	111.53	2.36	0.36	0.08	0.18	0.01	0	9.86	1.79	—	—	83
Beet Greens, Boiled, 1/2" Pcs; 1/2 Cups; #115	20	64.17	1.85	0.14	0.02	0.05	0.03	0	3.93	0.76	—	—	367
Beets, Boiled, Sliced; 1/2 Cups; #116	26	77.27	0.9	0.04	0.01	0.01	0.01	0	5.69	0.72	—	—	1
Broccoli Spears, Boiled; Each; #178	51	163.24	5.36	0.63	0.1	0.3	0.04	0	9.11	2	4.68	—	250
Broccoli, Boiled, Chopped; 1/2 Cups; #180	22	70.74	2.32	0.27	0.04	0.13	0.02	0	3.95	0.87	2.03	—	108

B₁ (mg)	B₂ (mg)	NI (mg)	B₆ (mg)	B₁₂ (μg)	Fol (μg)	PA (mg)	C (mg)	Ca (mg)	Fe (mg)	Mg (mg)	P (mg)	K (mg)	Na (mg)	Zn (mg)	Cu (mg)	Mn (mg)	Wt (g)
—	0.07	—	—	—	—	—	—	40	0.36	—	—	—	60	—	—	—	47.9
—	0.14	0.4	—	—	—	—	—	80	0.36	—	—	—	85	—	—	—	50
0	—	—	—	—	—	—	0	1	0.1	—	—	—	3	—	—	—	7.2
0.02	0.1	0.1	—	—	—	—	—	65	0.3	—	65	109	27	—	—	—	28
0.02	0.12	0.2	—	—	—	—	—	65	0.5	—	77	125	23	—	—	—	28
—	0.14	—	—	—	—	—	—	60	0.36	—	—	—	150	—	—	—	60.8
0.01	0.01	—	—	—	—	—	—	33	0.9	—	9	183	3	—	—	—	20
—	0.07	—	—	—	—	—	—	60	—	—	—	110	50	—	—	—	30.1
—	—	1.2	—	—	—	—	—	—	—	—	0.04	75	135	—	—	—	28
—	—	3.2	—	—	—	—	—	—	0.36	—	—	205	60	—	—	—	28.35
0.05	0.39	0.3	—	—	—	—	2	265	0.8	—	247	354	335	—	—	—	260
0.07	0.3	0.2	—	—	—	—	2	173	0.7	—	180	223	257	—	—	—	165
—	0.07	—	—	—	—	—	—	40	0.36	—	—	280	10	—	—	—	28.35
—	0.1	2	—	—	—	—	—	20	0.36	—	—	—	90	—	—	—	51.03
0.03	0.07	1.6	—	—	—	—	—	60	0.36	—	—	—	160	—	—	—	58.7
0.02	0.07	0.4	—	—	—	—	0	187	7.5	—	42	757	66	—	—	—	220
0	0	0	—	—	—	—	0	0	0.1	—	0	3	1	—	—	—	100
0	0	0	—	—	—	—	0	0	—	—	0	—	—	—	—	—	12
—	—	—	—	—	—	—	0	20	0.2	—	2	35	2	—	—	—	19.7
0	0	0	—	—	—	—	0	9	0.8	—	3	1	14	—	—	—	20.5
—	0.07	—	—	—	—	—	—	40	0.36	—	—	—	120	—	—	—	60.4
—	0.03	—	—	—	—	—	—	20	—	—	—	—	60	—	—	—	28.4
—	0.1	0.8	—	—	—	—	—	60	—	—	—	—	130	—	—	—	51.03
0	0	0.01	0	0	1.1	0.02	0.2	1	0.03	1	2	2	0	0.03	0	0.01	3
0.09	0.08	1.34	0.15	0	87	0.43	15	57	1.64	76	115	473	121	0.62	0.3	0.33	128
0.06	0.07	0.63	0.09	0	58.8	0.1	15.7	15	0.4	11	36	186	3	0.29	0.06	0.13	60
0.03	0.03	0.18	—	0	—	—	1.4	10	0.42	6	33	104	9	—	—	—	131
0.09	0.12	0.77	0.07	0	41.6	0.09	12.1	58	1.6	32	48	373	4	0.45	0.13	0.37	125
0.08	0.21	0.36	0.09	0	—	0.24	17.9	82	1.37	49	29	654	173	0.36	0.18	—	72
0.03	0.01	0.23	0.03	0	45.2	0.08	4.7	9	0.53	31	26	266	42	0.21	0.05	0.2	85
0.1	0.2	1.03	0.26	0	89	0.92	134.2	82	1.5	43	107	526	46	0.68	0.08	0.39	180
0.04	0.09	0.45	0.11	0	39	0.4	58.2	36	0.65	19	46	228	20	0.3	0.03	0.17	78

Food description; serving; item number	Energy (kcal)	Water (g)	PRO (g)	TFAT (g)	SFAT (g)	PFAT (g)	MFAT (g)	Chol (mg)	CHO (g)	CFib (g)	DFib (g)	Alc (g)	A (RE)
Brussels Sprouts, Boiled; 1/2 Cups; #187	30	68.11	1.99	0.4	0.08	0.2	0.03	0	6.76	1.07	3.35	—	56
Cabbage, Boiled, Shredded, Drained; 1/2 Cups; #210	16	70.2	0.72	0.18	0.02	0.09	0.01	0	3.57	0.45	—	—	6
Cabbage, Pak-choi, Boiled, Shredded; 1/2 Cups; #212	10	81.22	1.32	0.14	0.02	0.06	0.01	0	1.52	0.51	1.36	—	218
Cabbage, Raw, Shredded; 1/2 Cups; #213	8	32.38	0.42	0.06	0.01	0.03	0	0	1.88	0.28	—	—	4
Cabbage, Red, Raw, Shredded; Cups; #214	19	64.08	0.97	0.18	0.02	0.09	0.01	0	4.29	0.7	1.4	—	3
Carrots, Boiled, Sliced; 1/2 Cups; #251	35	68.15	0.85	0.14	0.03	0.07	0.01	0	8.18	1.15	—	—	1915
Carrots, Raw, 7 1/2" Long; Each; #253	31	63.21	0.74	0.14	0.02	0.05	0.01	0	7.3	0.75	2.3	—	2025
Cauliflower, Boiled, 1" Pieces; 1/2 Cups; #257	15	57.35	1.16	0.11	0.02	0.07	0.01	0	2.87	0.51	1.36	—	1
Cauliflower, Raw, 1" Pieces; 1/2 Cups; #258	12	46.13	0.99	0.09	0.01	0.04	0.01	0	2.46	0.42	1.2	—	1
Celery, Raw, 7 1/2" Stalk; Each; #260	6	37.86	0.3	0.06	0.01	0.03	0.01	0	1.46	0.32	0.64	—	5
Chard, Swiss, Boiled, Drained; 1/2 Cups; #262	18	81.53	1.65	0.07	—	—	—	0	3.64	0.83	—	—	276
Coleslaw, Homemade; 1/2 Cups; #402	42	48.9	0.8	1.6	0.2	0.8	—	5	7.5	—	—	—	49
Collards, Boiled, Chopped; 1/2 Cups; #403	17	58.79	0.87	0.12	—	—	—	0	3.92	0.31	—	—	175
Collards, Raw, Chopped; 1/2 Cups; #404	6	16.3	0.28	0.04	—	—	—	0	1.28	0.1	—	—	60
Corn, Sweet, Boiled; 1/2 Cups; #461	89	57.04	2.72	1.05	0.16	0.49	0.31	0	20.59	0.49	3.03	—	18
Corn, Sweet, Canned; 1/2 Cups; #462	66	63.07	2.15	0.82	0.13	0.39	0.24	0	15.24	—	1.15	—	13
Corn, Sweet, Canned, Creamed; 1/2 Cups; #463	93	100.78	2.23	0.54	0.08	0.25	0.16	0	23.2	0.62	1.54	—	12
Corn, Sweet, Frozen, Boiled; 1/2 Cups; #464	67	62.11	2.47	0.06	0.01	0.03	0.02	0	16.83	0.39	—	—	20
Cowpeas, Boiled, Drained; 1/2 Cups; #475	79	61.89	2.6	0.31	0.08	0.13	0.03	0	16.67	1.59	—	—	65
Cowpeas, Leafy Tips, Boiled/ Chopped; 1/2 Cups; #477	6	23.74	1.21	0.03	0.01	0.01	0	0	0.73	0.68	—	—	15
Cucumber, Sliced; 1/2 Cups; #557	7	49.94	0.28	0.07	0.02	0.03	0	0	1.51	0.31	0.52	—	2
Eggplant, Boiled, 1" Cubes; Cups; #623	27	88.1	0.8	0.22	0.04	0.09	0.02	0	6.37	0.93	—	—	6
Endive, Raw, Chopped; 1/2 Cups; #624	4	23.45	0.31	0.05	0.01	0.02	0	0	0.84	0.23	—	—	51
Garlic, Raw, Cloves; Each; #669	4	1.76	0.19	0.02	0	0.01	0	0	0.99	0.05	—	—	0
Ginger Root, Raw, Sliced; 5 Each; #675	8	8.98	0.19	0.08	0.02	0.02	0.02	0	1.66	0.11	—	—	0
Kale, Boiled, Chopped; 1/2 Cups; #785	21	59.28	1.24	0.26	0.03	0.13	0.02	0	3.66	0.52	—	—	481
Lettuce, Butterhead, Raw; 2 Leaves; #847	2	14.34	0.19	0.03	0	0.02	0	0	0.35	—	0.15	—	15
Lettuce, Cos/Romaine, Shredded; 1/2 Cups; #848	4	26.58	0.45	0.06	0.01	0.03	0	0	0.66	0.2	0.48	—	73
Lettuce, Iceberg, Raw; 1 Leaf; #849	3	19.18	0.2	0.04	0	0.02	0	0	0.42	0.11	0.2	—	7
Lettuce, Looseleaf, Raw; 1 Leaf; #850	2	9.4	0.13	0.03	0	0.02	0	0	0.35	0.07	—	—	19
Mushrooms, Boiled, Pieces; 1/2 Cups; #985	21	71.04	1.69	0.37	0.05	0.14	0.01	0	4.01	0.68	1.72	—	0
Mushrooms, Raw, Pieces; 1/2 Cups; #986	9	32.13	0.73	0.15	0.02	0.06	0	0	1.63	0.26	0.46	—	0

B₁ (mg)	B₂ (mg)	NI (mg)	B₆ (mg)	B₁₂ (µg)	Fol (µg)	PA (mg)	C (mg)	Ca (mg)	Fe (mg)	Mg (mg)	P (mg)	K (mg)	Na (mg)	Zn (mg)	Cu (mg)	Mn (mg)	Wt (g)
0.08	0.06	0.47	0.14	0	46.8	0.2	48.4	28	0.94	16	44	247	17	0.25	0.06	0.18	78
0.04	0.04	0.17	0.05	0	15.2	0.05	18.2	25	0.29	11	18	154	14	0.12	0.02	0.1	75
0.03	0.05	0.36	—	0	—	—	22.1	79	0.88	9	25	315	29	—	—	—	85
0.02	0.01	0.1	0.03	0	19.8	0.05	16.5	16	0.2	5	8	86	6	0.06	0.01	0.06	35
0.04	0.02	0.21	0.15	0	14.5	0.23	39.9	36	0.35	11	29	144	7	0.15	0.07	0.13	70
0.03	0.04	0.4	0.19	0	10.8	0.24	1.8	24	0.48	10	24	177	52	0.23	0.1	0.59	78
0.07	0.04	0.67	0.11	0	10.1	0.14	6.7	19	0.36	11	32	233	25	0.14	0.03	0.1	72
0.04	0.03	0.34	0.13	0	31.7	0.08	34.3	17	0.26	7	22	200	4	0.15	0.06	0.11	62
0.04	0.03	0.32	0.12	0	33.1	0.07	35.8	14	0.29	7	23	178	7	0.09	0.02	0.1	50
0.02	0.02	0.13	0.04	0	11	0.08	2.8	16	0.16	4	10	115	35	0.05	0.01	0.04	40
0.03	0.08	0.32	—	0	—	0.14	15.8	51	1.99	76	29	483	158	—	—	—	88
0.04	0.04	0.2	0.08	0.02	16	0.08	20	27	0.35	6	19	109	14	0.12	0.01	0.06	60
0.01	0.03	0.19	0.03	0	4	0.03	7.7	15	0.1	5	5	84	10	0.07	0.02	0.14	64
0	0.01	0.07	0.01	0	2	0.01	4.2	5	0.03	2	2	30	4	0.02	0.01	0.05	18
0.18	0.06	1.32	0.05	0	38.1	0.72	5.1	2	0.5	26	84	204	14	0.39	0.04	0.16	82
—	—	—	—	0	—	—	—	—	0.7	—	—	—	—	0.32	0.05	0.14	82
0.03	0.07	1.23	0.08	0	57.3	0.23	5.9	4	0.49	22	65	172	365	0.68	0.07	0.05	128
0.06	0.06	1.05	0.08	0	18.7	0.18	2.1	2	0.25	15	39	114	4	0.28	0.03	0.15	82
0.08	0.12	1.15	0.05	0	104	0.13	1.8	105	0.92	42	42	342	3	0.85	0.11	0.47	82
0.07	0.04	0.26	—	0	—	—	4.8	18	0.28	16	11	91	2	—	—	—	26
0.02	0.01	0.16	0.03	0	7.2	0.13	2.4	7	0.14	6	9	78	1	0.12	0.02	0.03	52
0.07	0.02	0.58	0.08	0	13.8	0.07	1.3	5	0.34	13	22	238	3	0.14	0.1	0.13	96
0.02	0.02	0.1	0	0	35.5	0.22	1.6	13	0.21	4	7	79	6	0.2	0.03	0.1	25
0.01	0	0.02	—	0	0.1	—	0.9	5	0.05	1	5	12	1	—	—	—	3
0	0	0.08	0.02	0	—	0.02	0.6	2	0.05	5	3	46	1	—	—	—	11
0.03	0.05	0.32	0.09	0	8.6	0.03	26.7	47	0.59	12	18	148	15	0.15	0.1	0.27	65
0.01	0.01	0.05	—	0	11	—	1.2	—	0.04	—	—	39	1	0.03	0	0.02	15
0.03	0.03	0.14	—	0	38	—	6.7	10	0.31	2	13	81	2	—	—	—	28
0.01	0.01	0.04	0.01	0	11.2	0.01	0.8	4	0.1	2	4	32	2	0.04	0.01	0.03	20
0	0.01	0.04	0.01	0	—	0.02	1.8	7	0.14	1	3	26	1	—	—	—	10
0.06	0.23	3.48	0.07	0	14.2	1.68	3.1	4	1.36	10	68	277	2	0.68	0.39	0.09	78
0.04	0.16	1.44	0.03	0	7.4	0.77	1.2	2	0.43	4	36	130	1	0.17	0.04	0	35

Food description; serving; item number	Energy (kcal)	Water (g)	PRO (g)	TFAT (g)	SFAT (g)	PFAT (g)	MFAT (g)	Chol (mg)	CHO (g)	CFib (g)	DFib (g)	Alc (g)	A (RE)
Mushrooms, Shiitake, Dried; Each; #988	11	0.34	0.34	0.04	0.01	0	0.01	0	2.71	0.41	—	—	0
Mustard Greens, Boiled, Drained; 1/2 Cups; #990	11	66.12	1.58	0.17	0.01	0.03	0.08	0	1.47	0.48	—	—	212
Olives, Green, Canned, Large; 10 Each; #1020	45	78.2	0.5	4.9	—	—	—	—	0.5	—	—	—	—
Olives, Ripe, Greek Style, Medium; 10 Each; #1023	65	43.8	0.4	6.9	—	—	—	—	1.7	—	—	—	—
Onions, Boiled, Chopped; Tbsps; #1025	7	13.18	0.2	0.03	0	0.01	0	0	1.52	0.1	—	—	0
Onions, Raw, Chopped; Tbsps; #1027	4	8.97	0.12	0.02	0	0.01	0	0	0.86	0.04	0.16	—	0
Parsnips, Boiled, Sliced; 1/2 Cups; #1054	63	60.62	1.03	0.23	0.04	0.04	0.09	0	15.23	1.72	—	—	0
Peas and Carrots, Frozen, Boiled; 1/2 Cups; #1077	38	68.64	2.47	0.34	0.06	0.16	0.03	0	8.1	1.11	—	—	621
Peas, Edible-Podded, Boiled; 1/2 Cups; #1079	34	71.13	2.62	0.18	0.04	0.08	0.02	0	5.64	0.83	2.24	—	10
Peas, Green, Canned; 1/2 Cups; #1082	59	69.44	3.76	0.29	0.05	0.14	0.03	0	10.69	1.69	2.89	—	65
Peppers, Green, Boiled, Drained; Each; #1093	20	67.06	0.67	0.14	0.02	0.08	0.01	0	4.89	0.33	—	—	43
Peppers, Green, Raw, 3 3/4"; Each; #1094	20	68.22	0.66	0.14	0.02	0.08	0.01	0	4.76	0.32	1.18	—	47
Peppers, Sweet, Yellow, Large, Raw; 10 Strips; #1097	14	47.85	0.52	0.11	—	—	—	0	3.29	—	—	—	12
Potato Pancakes, Home-Prepared; Each; #1191	495	30.34	4.63	12.61	3.42	2.54	5.35	93	26.36	0.5	—	—	27
Potato Salad, Homemade; 1/2 Cups; #1193	179	95	3.4	10.3	1.8	4.7	—	86	14	—	—	—	41
Potatoes, Baked w/Skin, 4 3/4"; Each; #1196	220	143.83	4.65	0.2	0.05	0.09	0	0	50.97	1.33	—	—	—
Potatoes, Boiled in Skin, Flesh; Each; #1197	119	104.69	2.54	0.14	0.04	0.06	0	0	27.38	0.43	—	—	—
Potatoes, French-Fried, in Veg. Oil; 10 Strips; #1202	158	19	2.01	8.28	2.5	3.78	1.64	0	19.78	0.37	—	—	—
Potatoes, Hashed Brown, Frzn, Prep; 1/2 Cups; #1203	170	43.76	2.46	8.97	3.51	1.03	4.01	—	21.92	0.42	1.56	—	—
Potatoes, Mashed w/Milk, Home Prep.; 1/2 Cups; #1204	81	82.39	2.03	0.62	0.35	0.06	0.15	2	18.43	0.33	—	—	6
Potatoes, Mashed, w/Milk/Marg. Home; Cups; #1206	222	160.15	3.95	8.87	2.17	2.54	3.72	4	35.08	0.64	—	—	41
Potatoes, Scalloped, Dry, Prepared; 1/6 Box; #1210	127	108.46	2.9	5.89	3.61	0.26	1.66	—	17.5	0.37	—	—	—
Radishes, Raw; 10 Each; #1240	7	42.68	0.27	0.24	0.01	0.02	0.01	0	1.61	0.24	—	—	0
Sauerkraut, Valsic Old Fashioned; Ounces; #1330	4	—	0	0	—	—	—	—	1	—	—	—	—
Shallots, Raw, Chopped; Tbsps; #1344	7	7.98	0.25	0.01	0	0	0	0	1.68	0.07	—	—	—
Spinach, Boiled; 1/2 Cups; #1438	21	82.09	2.67	0.23	0.04	0.1	0.01	0	3.38	0.79	1.98	—	737
Spinach, Frozen, Boiled; 1/2 Cups; #1440	27	85.48	2.98	0.2	0.03	0.08	0.01	0	5.08	1.04	—	—	739
Spinach, Raw, Chopped; 1/2 Cups; #1441	6	25.64	0.8	0.1	0.02	0.04	0	0	0.9	0.25	0.73	—	188
Squash, Summer, Boiled, Sliced; 1/2 Cups; #1451	18	84.33	0.82	0.28	0.06	0.12	0.02	0	3.88	0.54	1.26	—	26
Squash, Zucchini, Italian, Canned; 1/2 Cups; #1452	33	103.3	1.17	0.13	0.03	0.05	0.01	0	7.81	0.58	—	—	61
Sweetpotatoes, Boiled w/o Skin; 1/2 Cups; #1474	172	119.45	2.7	0.49	0.1	0.22	0.02	0	39.81	1.39	4.92	—	2797
Tomato Juice, Canned; 6 Fl Oz; #1520	32	170.91	1.38	0.11	0.01	0.04	0.02	0	7.7	0.72	—	—	101

B$_1$ (mg)	B$_2$ (mg)	NI (mg)	B$_6$ (mg)	B$_{12}$ (μg)	Fol (μg)	PA (mg)	C (mg)	Ca (mg)	Fe (mg)	Mg (mg)	P (mg)	K (mg)	Na (mg)	Zn (mg)	Cu (mg)	Mn (mg)	Wt (g)
0.01	0.05	0.51	—	0	—	—	0.1	0	0.06	5	11	55	0	—	—	—	3.6
0.03	0.04	0.3	—	0	—	0.08	17.7	52	0.49	10	29	141	11	—	—	—	70
—	—	—	—	—	—	—	—	24	0.6	—	7	21	926	—	—	—	46
—	—	—	—	—	—	—	—	—	—	—	6	—	631	—	—	—	24
0.01	0	0.03	0.02	0	2	0.02	0.8	3	0.04	2	5	25	0	0.03	0.01	0.02	15
0	0	0	0.01	0	2	0.01	0.6	2	0.02	1	3	16	0	0.02	0.01	0.01	10
0.06	0.04	0.56	0.07	0	45.4	0.46	10.1	29	0.45	23	54	287	8	0.2	0.11	0.23	78
0.18	0.05	0.92	0.07	0	20.8	0.13	6.5	18	0.75	13	39	127	55	0.36	0.06	0.16	80
0.1	0.06	0.43	0.12	0	—	0.54	38.3	33	1.58	21	44	192	3	0.3	0.06	0.13	80
0.1	0.07	0.62	0.05	0	37.7	0.11	8.1	17	0.81	15	57	147	186	0.6	0.07	0.26	85
0.04	0.02	0.35	0.17	0	11	0.06	54.3	7	0.33	7	13	121	1	0.09	0.05	0.08	73
0.05	0.02	0.38	0.18	0	16	0.06	66.1	7	0.34	7	14	131	1	0.09	0.05	0.09	74
0.01	0.01	0.46	0.09	0	14	0.09	95.4	6	—	6	12	110	1	0.09	0.06	0.06	52
0.1	0.09	1.61	0.29	0.22	21.5	0.71	0.4	21	1.21	24	78	538	388	0.68	0.27	0.3	76
0.1	0.08	1.1	0.18	0.19	8	0.67	13	24	0.81	19	65	317	661	0.39	0.15	0.13	125
0.22	0.07	3.32	0.7	0	22.2	1.12	26.1	20	2.75	55	115	844	16	0.65	0.62	0.46	202
0.14	0.03	1.96	0.41	0	13.6	0.71	17.6	7	0.42	30	60	515	6	0.41	0.26	0.19	136
0.09	0.01	1.63	0.12	0	14.5	0.33	5.2	10	0.38	17	47	366	108	0.19	0.07	0.1	50
0.09	0.02	1.89	0.1	0	—	0.35	4.9	12	1.17	13	56	340	27	0.25	0.12	0.17	78
0.09	0.04	1.17	0.25	0.06	8.6	0.5	7	28	0.29	19	50	314	318	0.3	0.15	0.12	105
0.18	0.08	2.27	0.47	0.11	16.7	1.2	12.9	54	0.55	37	97	607	619	0.58	0.29	0.24	210
0.03	0.08	1.41	0.06	—	1.5	0.45	4.5	49	0.52	19	77	278	467	0.34	0.07	—	137
0	0.02	0.14	0.03	0	12.2	0.04	10.3	9	0.13	4	8	104	11	0.13	0.02	0.03	45
—	—	—	—	—	—	—	—	—	0.36	—	—	—	280	—	—	—	28.4
0.01	0	0.02	—	0	—	—	0.8	4	0.12	—	6	33	1	—	—	—	10
0.09	0.21	0.44	0.22	0	131.20	0.13	8.9	122	3.21	79	50	419	63	0.69	0.16	0.84	90
0.06	0.16	0.4	0.14	0	102.10	0.08	11.6	139	1.44	65	46	283	82	0.66	0.13	0.89	95
0.02	0.05	0.2	0.05	0	54.4	0.02	7.9	28	0.76	22	14	156	22	0.15	0.04	0.25	28
0.04	0.04	0.46	0.06	0	18.1	0.12	5	24	0.32	22	35	173	1	0.35	0.09	0.19	90
0.05	0.05	0.6	—	0	—	—	2.6	19	0.78	16	33	312	427	0.29	0.11	—	114
0.09	0.23	1.05	0.4	0	18.2	0.87	28	35	0.92	16	44	301	21	0.43	0.26	0.55	164
0.09	0.06	1.23	0.2	0	36.1	0.46	33.2	16	1.06	20	34	400	658	0.26	0.18	0.14	182

Food description; serving; item number	Energy (kcal)	Water (g)	PRO (g)	TFAT (g)	SFAT (g)	PFAT (g)	MFAT (g)	Chol (mg)	CHO (g)	CFib (g)	DFib (g)	Alc (g)	A (RE)
Tomato Paste, Canned; 1/2 Cups; # 1521	110	97.02	4.95	1.17	0.17	0.47	0.18	0	24.65	1.25	5.63	—	323
Tomato Puree, Canned; Cups; # 1522	102	218.15	4.18	0.29	0.04	0.12	0.04	0	25.05	2.05	5.75	—	340
Tomato Sauce, Canned; 1/2 Cups; # 1523	37	108.67	1.62	0.2	0.03	0.08	0.03	0	8.76	0.87	1.83	—	119
Tomatoes, Green, Raw 2-3/5" Dia.; Each; # 1524	30	114.39	1.48	0.25	0.03	0.1	0.04	0	6.27	0.62	—	—	79
Tomatoes, Red, Canned, Whole; 1/2 Cups; # 1526	24	112.4	1.12	0.29	0.04	0.12	0.04	0	5.15	0.55	—	—	72
Tomatoes, Red, Raw, 2-3/5" Dia.; Each; # 1527	23	115.32	1.04	0.4	0.06	0.17	0.06	0	5.71	0.81	1.6	—	77
Turnip Greens, Boiled, Chopped; 1/2 Cups; # 1572	15	67.1	0.82	0.16	0.04	0.07	0.01	0	3.14	0.44	2.23	—	396
Vegetable Juice Cocktail, Canned; 6 Fl Oz; # 1589	34	170.2	1.14	0.17	0.02	0.07	0.03	0	8.29	0.42	—	—	213
Vegetables, Mixed, Frozen, Boiled; 1/2 Cups; # 1600	54	75.74	2.61	0.14	0.03	0.07	0.01	0	11.91	1.07	3.46	—	389
Waterchestnuts, Chinese, Canned; 4 Each; # 1611	14	24.2	0.25	0.02	—	—	—	0	3.48	0.16	—	—	0
Watercress, Raw, Chopped; 1/2 Cup; # 1612	2	16.17	0.39	0.02	0	0.01	0	0	0.22	0.12	0.39	—	80
Yams, Cooked, Cubed; 1/2 Cups; # 1644	79	47.69	1.01	0.09	0.02	0.04	0	0	18.76	—	—	—	0
Zucchini Squash, Boiled, Sliced; 1/2 Cups; # 1654	14	85.27	0.57	0.05	0.01	0.02	0	0	3.54	0.45	—	—	22

Category 20: Miscellaneous

Food description; serving; item number	Energy (kcal)	Water (g)	PRO (g)	TFAT (g)	SFAT (g)	PFAT (g)	MFAT (g)	Chol (mg)	CHO (g)	CFib (g)	DFib (g)	Alc (g)	A (RE)
Baking Powder, Calumet; Tsps; #51	3	0.2	0	0	0	0	—	0	0.7	—	—	—	0
Baking Soda; Tsps; #52	0	0.2	0	0	—	—	—	0	0	0	—	—	0
Catsup; Tbsps; #256	16	9.99	0.23	0.05	0.01	0.02	0.01	0	4.09	0.16	0.24	—	6
Chili Powder; Tsps; #330	8	0.2	0.32	0.44	—	—	—	0	1.42	0.58	0.89	—	91
Cinnamon, Ground; Tsps; #357	6	0.22	0.09	0.07	0.01	0.01	0.01	0	1.84	0.56	—	—	1
Cloves, Ground; Tsps; #362	7	0.14	0.13	0.42	0.09	—	—	0	1.29	0.2	—	—	1
Cream of Tartar; Tsps; #537	8	0	0	0	—	—	—	0	1.8	—	—	—	0
Curry Powder; Tsps; #560	6	0.19	0.25	0.28	—	—	—	0	1.16	0.33	—	—	2
Dill Weed, Fresh; 5 Sprigs; #581	0	0.86	0.03	0.01	0	0	0.01	0	0.07	—	—	—	A
Ginger, Fresh; 5 Slices; #676	8	8.98	0.19	0.08	0.02	0.02	0.02	0	1.66	0.11	—	—	0
Jell-O, All Flavors; 1/2 Cups; #782	81	118.9	1.6	0	0	0	—	0	18.8	—	—	—	0
Marjoram, Dried; Tsps; #898	2	0.05	0.08	0.04	—	—	—	0	0.36	0.11	—	—	5
Mustard, Brown; Tsps; #993	5	3.9	0.3	0.3	—	—	—	—	0.3	—	—	—	—
Mustard, Prepared, Yellow; Tsps; #994	4	4.01	0.2	0.2	—	—	—	—	0.3	—	—	—	—
Paprika; Tsps; # 1052	6	0.2	0.31	0.27	0.04	0.17	0.03	0	1.17	0.44	—	—	127
Parsley, Fresh; 10 Sprigs; # 1053	4	8.77	0.3	0.08	0.01	0.01	0.03	0	0.63	—	0.44	—	52
Pepper, Black; Tsps; # 1089	5	0.22	0.23	0.07	0.03	0.03	0.03	0	1.36	0.28	—	—	—
Pepper, Red or Cayenne; Tsps; # 1090	6	0.14	0.22	0.31	0.06	0.15	0.05	0	1.02	0.45	—	—	75
Pickles, Cucumber, Dill, Med.; Each; # 1101	12	59.58	0.4	0.12	0.03	0.05	0	0	2.68	0.37	0.78	—	21
Pickles, Cucumber, Sweet, Large; Each; # 1102	41	22.84	0.13	0.09	0.02	0.04	0	0	11.13	0.2	—	—	4
Relish, Hamburger; Tbsps; # 1257	19	9.17	0.09	0.08	0.01	0.02	0.04	0	5.17	0.14	—	—	4
Salt, Table; Tsps; # 1305	0	0.01	0	0	—	—	—	—	0	—	—	—	0
Sauce, Soy, Tamari; Tbsps; # 1325	11	11.88	1.89	0.02	0	0.01	0	0	1	0	—	—	0
Syrup, Karo, Corn, Light; Tbsps; # 1479	60	5.4	0	0	—	—	—	—	14.9	—	—	—	—
Thyme, Ground; Tsps; # 1514	4	0.11	0.13	0.1	0.04	0.02	0.01	0	0.89	0.26	—	—	5

B₁ (mg)	B₂ (mg)	NI (mg)	B₆ (mg)	B₁₂ (μg)	Fol (μg)	PA (mg)	C (mg)	Ca (mg)	Fe (mg)	Mg (mg)	P (mg)	K (mg)	Na (mg)	Zn (mg)	Cu (mg)	Mn (mg)	Wt (g)
0.2	0.25	4.22	0.5	0	—	0.99	55.4	46	3.91	67	104	1221	86	1.05	0.78	—	131
0.18	0.14	4.29	0.38	0	—	1.1	88.2	37	2.32	60	99	1051	49	0.54	0.41	—	250
0.08	0.07	1.4	—	0	—	0.38	16	17	0.94	23	39	452	738	0.3	0.24	—	122
0.07	0.05	0.62	—	0	—	0.62	28.8	16	0.63	13	35	251	16	0.09	0.11	0.12	123
0.05	0.04	0.88	0.11	0	—	0.2	18.2	32	0.73	14	23	265	195	0.19	0.13	—	120
0.07	0.06	0.77	0.1	0	18	0.3	23.5	6	0.55	13	30	273	11	0.11	0.09	0.13	123
0.03	0.05	0.3	0.13	0	85.3	0.2	19.7	99	0.57	16	21	146	21	0.1	0.18	0.24	72
0.08	0.05	1.32	0.25	0	—	—	50.4	20	0.77	20	31	351	664	0.36	0.36	0.18	182
0.06	0.11	0.77	0.07	0	17.3	0.14	2.9	22	0.75	20	46	154	32	0.45	0.08	0.34	91
0	0.01	0.1	—	0	—	—	0.4	1	0.24	1	5	33	2	0.11	0.03	—	28
0.01	0.02	0.03	0.02	0	—	0.01	7.3	20	0.03	4	10	56	7	—	—	—	17
0.06	0.02	0.38	0.16	0	10.9	0.21	8.2	9	0.35	12	33	455	6	0.13	0.1	—	68
0.04	0.04	0.38	0.07	0	15.1	0.1	4.2	12	0.32	19	36	228	2	0.16	0.08	0.16	90
0	0	0	0	0	0	0	0	241	0	0	83	0	426	0	0	—	4
0	0	0	0	0	0	0	0	0	0	0	0	0	1259	0	0	0	4.6
0	0	0.08	0.01	0	1	0.01	0.9	1	0.04	1	2	29	71	0.01	0.01	0.01	15
0.01	0.02	0.2	—	0	—	—	1.67	7	0.37	4	8	50	26	0.07	0.01	0.06	2.6
0	0	0.03	—	0	—	—	0.65	28	0.88	1	1	11	1	0.05	—	—	2.3
0	0.01	0.03	—	0	—	—	1.7	14	0.18	6	2	23	5	0.02	0.01	0.63	2.1
0	0	0	0	0	0	0	0	0	0.11	0	0	495	2	0.01	0.01	0.01	3
0	0.01	0.07	—	0	—	—	0.23	10	0.59	5	7	31	1	0.08	—	—	2
0	0	0.02	0	0	1	0	—	2	—	1	1	7	1	0.01	0	0.01	1
0	0	0.08	0.02	0	—	0.02	0.6	2	0.05	5	3	46	1	—	—	—	11
0	0	0	0	0	0	0	0	0	0.02	0	30	0	54	0	0	—	140
0	0	0.03	—	0	—	—	0.31	12	0.5	2	2	9	—	0.02	0.01	0.03	0.6
—	—	—	—	—	—	—	—	6	0.1	—	7	7	65	—	—	—	5
—	—	—	—	—	—	—	—	4	0.1	—	4	7	63	—	—	—	5
0.01	0.04	0.32	—	0	—	—	1.49	4	0.5	4	7	49	1	0.08	—	—	2.1
0.01	0.01	0.13	0.01	0	15	0.04	13.3	14	0.62	5	6	55	6	0.11	0.01	0.02	10
0	0	0.02	—	0	—	—	—	9	0.61	4	4	26	1	0.03	—	—	2.1
0.01	0.02	0.16	—	0	—	—	1.38	3	0.14	3	5	36	1	0.05	—	—	1.8
0.01	0.02	0.04	0.01	0	1	0.04	1.3	6	0.35	7	14	75	833	0.09	0.05	0.01	65
0	0.01	0.06	0	0	0	0.04	0.4	1	0.21	1	4	11	328	0.03	0.04	0	35
0	0.01	0.09	—	0	—	—	0.3	1	0.17	1	3	11	164	0.02	0.01	—	15
0	0	0	—	—	—	—	0	14	—	—	—	—	2132	—	—	—	5.5
0.01	0.03	0.71	0.04	0	3.3	0.07	0	4	0.43	7	23	38	1005	0.08	0.02	—	18
—	—	—	—	—	—	—	—	—	—	—	—	—	30	—	—	—	21
0.01	0.01	0.07	—	0	—	—	—	26	1.73	3	3	11	1	0.09	—	—	1.4

Food description; serving; item number	Energy (kcal)	Water (g)	PRO (g)	TFAT (g)	SFAT (g)	PFAT (g)	MFAT (g)	Chol (mg)	CHO (g)	CFib (g)	DFib (g)	Alc (g)	A (RE)
Vinegar, Cider; Tbsps; # 1606	2	14.1	0	0	—	—	—	—	0.9	—	—	—	—
Yeast, Bakers, Active, Dry; 1/4 Oz Pkg; # 1647	21	0.5	2.7	0.3	0.04	0	0.18	0	2.7	0	—	—	0

B$_1$ (mg)	B$_2$ (mg)	NI (mg)	B$_6$ (mg)	B$_{12}$ (μg)	Fol (μg)	PA (mg)	C (mg)	Ca (mg)	Fe (mg)	Mg (mg)	P (mg)	K (mg)	Na (mg)	Zn (mg)	Cu (mg)	Mn (mg)	Wt (g)
—	—	—	—	—	—	—	—	1	0.1	—	1	15	0	—	—	—	15
0.17	0.38	2.78	0.11	0	266	0.79	0	5	1.16	7	90	140	3	0.45	0.16	0.04	7

Answers to Progress Checks

Module 1: Introduction to Nutrition

Activity 1: Nutrition Definitions and Concepts

1. F 3. T 5. T 7. b
2. T 4. F 6. a 8. d
9. Nutrition is the process by which food is selected and becomes part of the human body. Culture is the set of beliefs, arts, and customs that make up a way of life for a group of people. Health: a state of complete physical and mental well-being.

Activity 2: Food Selections

1. Individual scoring
2. *See* 1980 RDAs for your age and sex.
3. Watch portion sizes given for more accuracy.
4. Check Dietary Guidelines for Americans for suggestions, if you need to improve your diet.
5. b 7. T 9. T
6. c 8. F

Activity 3: Reliable Nutrition Sources

1. T 5. All are correct.
2. F 6. c
3. T 7. b
4. *See* module text and appendix.

Module 2: Food Habits

Activity 1: Factors Affecting Food Consumption

1–3. Personal responses: Need to include factors that apply to your particular individual situation, such as where you live, your finances, emotions, traditions, seasonal considerations, and the like.

4. F 9. F 14. b 18. a, b, c, d
5. T 10. F 15. d 19. d
6. T 11. F 16. b 20. b
7. F 12. T 17. b 21. a, b, c, d
8. F 13. F

Activity 2: Some Effects of Culture, Religion, and Geography on Food Behaviors

The student is responsible for submitting the answers. The instructor may wish to have the student discuss a client's diet plan, or give a grade for this assignment.

Module 3: Meeting Energy Needs

Activity 1: Energy Balance

1. (a) The basal metabolic rate. (b) Activity or voluntary energy expenditures. (c) The thermic effect of food.
2. 89 kcal.
   $4 \times 4 = 16$ kcal protein
   $5 \times 9 = 45$ kcal fat
   $7 \times 4 = \underline{28 \text{ kcal}}$ carbohydrate
   Total 89 kcal
3. Your caloric intake is in balance with your energy needs when you maintain the same weight. Excess calories are converted to fat and stored in adipose tissue (fat cells).
4. Potatoes are grouped with bread and pasta (rich in carbohydrates) and as such contain only four calories per gram.
5. a. Present intake:
   12,600 calories per week ($1,800 \times 7 = 12,600$)
   3,500 cal = 1 lb. body fat $\times$ 3 (desired weight loss)
   = 10,500 cal

     12,600 cal
   $-\underline{10,500}$ cal
      2,100 cal per week ÷ 7 days = 300 calories per day

   b. No. 300 calories per day are inadequate and represent semi-starvation.
6. a. 1 c. skim milk
   b. $\frac{1}{2}$ c. unsweetened fruit
   c. 1 slice bread
   d. $\frac{1}{2}$ c. cooked vegetables
   e. 1 tsp. solid fat or oil
   f. 1 oz. lean meat
7. 1. c
   2. a
   3. b

Activity 2: The Effects of Energy Imbalance

1. F 9. F 17. c
2. T 10. T 18. a
3. T 11. T 19. e
4. F 12. T 20. a, b
5. F 13. F 21. b
6. F 14. a, b, c, d 22. c
7. T 15. b 23. a
8. T 16. b 24. c
25. a 700 calorie reduction plus 300 calories used in activity = 1,000 kcal per daily reduction;

1,000 kcal per day × 7 days per week = 7,000 kcal deficit
per week;
7,000 ÷ 3,500 (kcal in 1 lb. body fat) = 2 lb. per week.
  b. 20 lb. ÷ 2 lb. per week = 10 weeks;
October 1 to December 7 = 10 weeks.
The answer is yes.
  c. 300 kcal burned × 7 days per week = 2,100 calories per
week deficit;
2,100 ÷ 3,500 = .6 lb. per week
  d. October 1 to December 7 = 10 weeks;
10 weeks × 0.6 lb. per week = 6.0 lb. loss in 10 weeks.
No; it would take 33 $1/_3$ weeks to lose 20 lb. at 0.6 lb. per
week (20 lb. ÷ 0.6 = 33$1/_3$).

Activity 3: Weight Control and Dieting

1. d
2. c
3. c
4. (a) altered metabolism; (b) fluid and electrolyte imbalance; (c) nutrient deficits.

5. F
6. F
7. T
8. T

Module 4: Carbohydrates and Fats: Implications for Health

Activity 1: Carbohydrates: Characteristics and Effects on Health

1. __4__ 1 orange
   __2__ 1 c. whole kernel corn
   __1__ $1/_{10}$ of a devil's food cake with icing (from a mix)
   __3__ 1 slice wheat bread
   __5__ $1/_2$ c. zucchini squash
   __3__ $1/_3$ c. cooked oatmeal
2. Vegetables:
   __3__ $1/_2$ c. green beans, cooked
   __3__ $1/_2$ c. cooked carrots
   __2__ 1 baked potato
   __1__ 1 sweet potato
   __4__ 1 stalk broccoli
   __5__ $1/_2$ c. lettuce, chopped
3. It is converted to fat and stored in adipose tissue.
4. Fiber promotes normal functioning of the lower intestinal tract (helps to prevent constipation, possibly
colon cancer).
5. Good sources include raw fruits and vegetables, bran,
and whole grains.
6. (1) Dental caries; and (2) diets of poor nutritional
quality that are high in calories can result in obesity.
7. Because they increase the risk of ketosis, dehydration,
diarrhea, and loss of muscle mass.
8. c (1000 ÷ 4 = 250)

9. b	15. a	21. b	27. c
10. b	16. b	22. c	28. a
11. b and d	17. c	23. a	29. b
12. b	18. d	24. c	30. a
13. b	19. e	25. b	
14. a	20. d	26. a	

Activity 2: Fats: Characteristics and Effects on Health

1. 50 g
2. S lamb chops
   S nondairy whipped topping
   S mayonnaise
   M olive oil
   S regular margarine
   S scrambled eggs
   P safflower oil
3. __2__ 3 oz. sirloin steak (15 g)
   __1__ $1/_2$ c. ice cream (10 g)
   __2__ 1 c. whole milk (10 g)
   __2__ 20 potato chips (10 g)
   __2__ 1 glazed doughnut (10 g)
   __3__ 2 oz. white turkey meat (6 g)
4. Cholesterol is involved in the production of body cells,
vitamin D (with aid of sunlight), and hormones.
5. b   10. b (2,000 × .42 ÷ 9)
6. a   11. a
7. c   12. b
8. c   13. a
9. c   14. b

Module 5: Proteins and Health

Activity 1: Protein as a Nutrient

1. If you are uncertain about your answers, look at the tables
provided and/or discuss with your teachers.
2. Because all essential amino acids (present in good quality
protein) must be present at one time in the body or the body
cannot utilize them to build body proteins.
3. No. (However, it is relatively more common among low-
income groups.)
4. c   6. b   8. d   10. T
5. b   7. c   9. T

Activity 2: Meeting Protein Needs and Vegetarianism

1. a	5. b	9. a	13. d
2. b	6. a	10. b	14. T
3. a	7. a	11. b	
4. a	8. c	12. a	

15. A diet history with as much detail as possible. List of food
likes, dislikes, and allergies. Mary's present knowledge of
nutritional needs and of food composition, especially protein. Her knowledge of complementary proteins and methods of food preparation. Type of vegetarianism practiced.
History of pre-pregnancy eating and exercise habits.
16. Protein: 30 g extra daily; must be high quality. There is also
need for 300 more kcal per day as well as extra vitamins and
minerals. *See* RDA chart.
17. 40 g (110 lb. ÷ 2.2 = 50 kg × 0.8 = 40.0).

18. Mary is underweight for her height, even if she is of small frame and very athletic. It will depend upon her physician's decision, of course, but she probably needs to gain extra weight.
19. It will be more difficult, because plant proteins have lower biological values than animal. It will also be difficult to get enough calcium and fat-soluble vitamins as well as other essential nutrients contained in animal foods. Extra soy milk, fortified with vitamin B_{12}, should be consumed with each meal. Leafy green vegetables (without oxalates), sunflower seeds, and fortified soy milk for calcium should be part of the diet.

Module 6: Vitamins and Health
Activity 1: The Water-Soluble Vitamins

1. a	6. b	11. a and b	16. d
2. b	7. d	12. d	17. a
3. a	8. c	13. a	18. a
4. b	9. c	14. b	
5. b	10. d	15. d	

Activity 2: The Fat-Soluble Vitamins

1. b	5. d	9. c	13. d
2. c	6. a	10. a	14. c
3. d	7. d	11. b	
4. c	8. d	12. a	

Module 6

1. c	9. c	17. b	25. c
2. a	10. b	18. a	26. d
3. d	11. T	19. a	27. d
4. e	12. T	20. b	28. a
5. b	13. T	21. a	29. b
6. d	14. T	22. b	30. b
7. e	15. T	23. b	
8. a	16. T	24. a	

Module 7: Minerals, Water, and Body Processes
Module 7

1. b	17. a	33. b	49. F
2. c	18. d	34. c	50. T
3. d	19. c	35. b	51. F
4. b	20. b	36. b	52. T
5. c	21. b	37. a	53. T
6. d	22. a	38. c	54. T
7. b	23. b	39. a	55. T
8. d	24. b	40. a	56. T
9. c	25. c	41. a	57. T
10. b	26. c	42. c	58. T
11. a	27. b	43. b	59. T
12. c	28. a	44. d	60. e
13. d	29. b	45. T	61. a
14. b	30. c	46. F	62. c
15. c	31. c	47. T	63. b
16. c	32. a	48. T	64. d

Module 8: Nutritional Assessment and Health Care Model
Activity 1: Assessment of Nutritional Status

1. Physical, anthropometric, laboratory, and historical data.
2. The health education areas needed will depend on the problems you identified with your client in the Practices.
3. See Table 8-1.
4. See Table 8-3.
5. a 7. b 9. b
6. a 8. a 10. b

Activity 2: Health Care Model: The Problem-Solving Process

1. Any 3 of these dietary changes will lower your client's fat intake to 35%.
   a. cut butter servings to 3 servings a day—saves 15 g fat
   b. use skim milk—will delete 10 g fat from diet
   c. bake or broil fish fillet—deletes 10 g fat
   d. omit chocolate chip cookies
   This diet barely meets the percentage recommended for protein. For a female this age, the higher range of 20% would be desirable from a health standpoint. To increase protein, suggest adding 1 cup skim milk and/or 1 to 2 oz. good quality protein to her lunch. To increase complex carbohydrates and nutrients:
   a. omit cookies and add fruit to the diet
   b. omit doughnuts and add fruit to the diet
   c. omit sugar and add 1 serving from grain group
   d. add vegetables, including 1 potato and 3 other vegetable servings
2. See the listing in number 5 for potassium sources.
3. No. A 2 g (2,000 mg) sodium diet is considered moderately restricted. This diet is in the moderate range. We need more information before we can answer this fully. For example, does your client use additional salt in food preparation? Is her usual intake from more salty foods such as bacon, ham, pretzels, etc.?
4. Vitamins: A, C, B_6; minerals: calcium, iron, magnesium, potassium.
5. Food sources for the nutrients your client is low in are listed below:
   Vitamin A (IUs): apricot, broccoli, cantaloupe, carrots, liver, mixed vegetables, nectarine, peach, spinach, sweet potatoes, tomato products, tossed salad, vegetable/vegetable beef soup, winter squash.
   Vitamin C (mg): asparagus, broccoli, cabbage, cantaloupe, cauliflower, grapefruit (and juice), honeydew melon, orange (and juice), potatoes, spinach, strawberries, summer squash or zucchini, sweet green pepper, tomato products.
   Vitamin B_6 (mg): banana, beef, cabbage, chicken, corn, fortified ready-to-eat cereals, halibut, ham, liver, milk, potato, salmon, tuna, turkey.
   Calcium: cheese, cottage cheese, cream soup, enchilada, ice cream, macaroni and cheese, milk, milkshake, pizza (cheese), pudding, salmon, spinach, whole grain and enriched breads and cereals, yogurt.
   Iron: beans (dried), beef, dried fruit, egg yolks, fortified

ready-to-eat cereals, kidney, lamb, liver, liverwurst, oysters, peas, pork, spinach, turkey.

Magnesium: asparagus, beef, broccoli, cauliflower, chocolate, dried beans, hulled sunflower seeds, lima beans, peanuts and other nuts, spinach, sweet green pepper, tomato products, tossed salad, whole wheat breads and cereals.

Potassium: avocado, banana, cantaloupe, dates, figs, flounder, grapefruit (and juice), halibut, honeydew melon, nectarine, orange (and juice), potato, prunes (and juice), soybeans.

6. As stated, energy requirements are based on sex, weight, height, age, and activity level. Generally, for a sedentary individual, 24 kcal/kg of body weight for BMR and 400 calories for activity are allowed. The computer printout is somewhat more precise but in the above range.

7. 2,226 calories needed per day
    −1,279 calories consumed (see total in Idaho diet analysis)
       947 kcal
    or
    100.0%
    − 57.5
     42.5%

8. a No. The 287 calories above the 1,200 could be easily reduced by omitting the lemon meringue pie. The student will recall, however, that a major criterion for a safe weight loss is that the diet be balanced. This diet is inadequate in the Basic Four food groups and seven of the essential nutrients listed in the RDAs.

   b. To lose 1 lb. of body fat, your client will need to eat 3,500 calories less than her body needs. If she decreases her calorie intake by 500 calories per day, she will lose 1 lb. per week. If she decreases her calorie intake by 1,000 calories per day, she will lose 2 lb. per week. At her intended level or daily calorie intake (1,200 calories), she should reach her desired or ideal weight in about 10 weeks.

9. For a 1,200 calorie reduction diet, made up of 50% carbohydrates, 20% protein, and 30% fat, your client should be adhering to the menu pattern on the right (above).

10. Objectives for teaching plans: The client will be able to:
    a. Plan a 1,200 calorie reduction diet using the exchange system.
    b. State five each of foods high in vitamin C, calcium, and iron.
    c. Identify three acceptable preparation methods.
    d. List several behavior techniques useful in changing diet habits.
    e. Commit to a regular exercise program.

Module 9: Nutrition and the Life Cycle

Activity 1: Maternal and Infant Nutrition

1. c	9. d	17. c	25. F
2. c	10. a	18. a	26. T
3. b	11. b	19. d	27. F
4. c	12. a	20. c	28. F
5. b	13. b	21. b	29. F
6. a	14. a	22. d	30. F
7. b	15. a	23. c	
8. b	16. c	24. T	

Menu Pattern*

	Carbo-hydrate	Protein	Fat	Kcal	Sample Menu
Breakfast					
1 milk exchange	12	8	Trace	80	1 c. skim milk
1 fruit exchange	15	—	—	60	½ banana
2 bread exchanges	30	6	—	140	¾ c. wheat flakes
1 fat exchange	—	—	5	45	1 tbsp. cream cheese
1 free item	—	—	—	—	hot beverage
Lunch					
2 lean meat exchanges	—	14	6	110	2 oz. tuna
1 fat exchange	—	—	5	45	5 olives
1 bread exchange	15	3	—	70	5 wheat crackers
1 vegetable exchange	5	2	—	25	½ c. raw carrot
1 fruit	10	—	—	40	1 apple
free item(s)	—	—	—	—	ice tea/lemon
Snack					
1 skim milk, 1 bread	27	10	—	150	
1 fruit	10	—	—	40	
Dinner					
2 lean meat exchanges	—	14	6	110	2 oz. broiled fish
1 bread exchange	15	2	—	70	1 baked potato
2 vegetable exchanges	10	4	—	50	½ c. green beans/coleslaw
2 fat exchanges	—	—	10	90	2 tbsp. sour cream
1 fruit	10	—	—	40	½ c. peaches
Totals	158	58	32	1165	

*This menu pattern may vary slightly and still be within the parameters. There is an infinite number of menu combinations possible within the exchange system.

Activity 2: Childhood and Adolescent Nutrition

1. b	9. a	17. d	25. F
2. a	10. a	18. d	26. T
3. d	11. b	19. T	27. T
4. b	12. d	20. T	28. F
5. d	13. b	21. F	29. F
6. c	14. c	22. F	
7. c	15. a	23. T	
8. d	16. b	24. T	

30. Any four of these: milk, wheat, seafood, chocolate, egg white, citrus, nuts.

Activity 3: Adulthood and Nutrition

1. b	8. d	15. a	22. F
2. c	9. a	16. a	23. T
3. a	10. c	17. d	24. T
4. d	11. d	18. a	25. F
5. a	12. d	19. b	26. T
6. c	13. c	20. T	27. T
7. c	14. d	21. T	28. F

29. They may not have transportation or the stamina for lengthy shopping trips.

30. Reduced BMR; reduced activity level.

31. Remain the same.

32. a. complication of existing or developing health problems;
    b. interference with movement; and
    c. increased risk of injurious falls.

33. Decreased consumption of meat (perhaps due to high cost or difficulty in eating) and other iron-rich foods.

34. Vitamin A, ascorbic acid (vitamin C), and calcium.

35. Food is provided in group social setting; some nutrition education is provided.

Activity 4: Exercise, Fitness, and Stress Reduction Principles

1. Duration, intensity, frequency, type.
2. Predicted rate that won't cause chest pain.
3. Any three if these increased strength, flexibility, endurance. Weight control. Lower blood pressure, lower cholesterol, increase cardiovascular strength.
4. Warm up, endurance, competition, cool down.
5. Optimal nutrition, RDAs or above, adequate calories, low in fat, high in complex carbohydrates.
6. c. 365 × 100 = 36,500 ÷ 3500 = 10 lb. (app.)
7. Depression, heart disease, hypertension, angina.
8. Any of these: exercise, relaxation techniques, proper diet, socialization, enough rest/sleep, counseling.
9. Scientific data only may be used to evaluate the product.
10. Those measures that enable a person to stay young and healthy in body and mind.

Module 10: Drugs and Nutrition

Background Information

Answers 1–8 found in glossary at the beginning of the module.

9. Any five of these:
   a. Damage intestinal walls
   b. Lower absorption
   c. Destruction of accessory organs
   d. Destroy or displace nutrients
   e. Change the nutrient
   f. Render nutrients incapable of acting
   g. Cause nutrient excretion
10. a. diarrhea/constipation
    b. nausea/vomiting
    c. altered taste/smell
11. a. drug
    b. dosage
    c. time
    d. frequency
    e. health status
12. a. Drug interference
    b. Drug-induced antagonists
13. Any five: niacin, riboflavin, pantothenic acid, ascorbic acid, folic acid, B_{12}, protein, fat, glucose, iron, copper, calcium, zinc, magnesium
14. Reabsorption/transport
15. Change in urine pH/Increase in precipitation of some

Activity 1: Food and Drug Interaction

1. a. Change absorption rate
   b. Neutralize effects
   c. Interact
   d. Influence excretion rate
2. Alcohol
   Various amines
3. Hypertensive crisis
4. a. Drug dose
   b. Amount of food
   c. Interval between drug and food ingestion
   d. Patient susceptibility
   e. Condition of the food
5. Decrease taste sensitivity

6. Causing dry mouth, constipation, and urinary retention
7. c
8. d   11. a   14. T
9. d   12. F   15. T
10. b   13. T

Activity 2: Drugs and the Life Cycle

1. Renal anomalies
   CNS malformation
   Cleft palate
   Severe defects
2. a. Type of drug
   b. Concentration of drug
   c. Time lapse between drug ingestion and breast-feeding
3. Anomalies of eyes, ears, heart, CNS, mental retardation
   Male: enlargement of the mammary glands (gynecomastia)
   Female: overgrowth of vaginal lining
4. High rate of abortions
   Abruptio placenta
   Low birth weight babies
5. a. Length of time used
   b. Nutritional status
   c. Nutritional intake
   d. Susceptibility
6. a. Decreased ability to digest, absorb, and metabolize food
   b. Decreased ability to metabolize and excrete drugs
   c. Interaction of multiple drug use
7. Aspirin—bleeding (GI)
   Laxatives—inhibit vitamin absorption
   Diuretics—decreased K and Ca+
   Alcohol—decreased folate, thiamin
8. e   11. F   14. T
9. c   12. F   15. F
10. b   13. F   16. T

Module 11: Food Ecology

Activity 1: Food Safety

1. All of the answers below are correct:
   a. failing to wash hands after going to the bathroom
   b. not washing hands after handling meat, fish, poultry, or eggs before handling other foods
   c. failing to clean counters, cutting boards, and cooking equipment
   d. failing to wash fresh food products thoroughly before preparation
   e. failing to use clean cloths, sponges, or hand towels
   f. handling food if you have upper respiratory infections (URIs)
   g. working with sores, boils, etc., on hands, face
   h. failing to wash after touching hair, face, or other body parts before returning to food preparation
   i. talking, laughing, sneezing during food preparation
   j. poor personal hygiene: dirty clothing, body, hair, etc.
2. b
3. Bacteria—the spores themselves and/or the toxins produced from them.
4. A warm moist place is a perfect environment for bacteria to

multiply. With these favorable conditions, they quickly increase by geometric progression (1-2-4-8-16-32-64, etc.).

5. All of the answers below are correct:
   a. use of pure drinking water
   b. adequate sewage disposal
   c. adequate cooking of foods
   d. proper storage of foods
   e. thorough cleaning of foods
   f. sanitary handling of all foods
   g. areas free of pests, rodents, vermin, etc.
6. Nausea, vomiting, diarrhea, flatulence, abdominal distention.
7. F
8. T
9. T
10. T
11. This soup may make the residents ill. It was at room temperature overnight and reheating will not destroy any microorganism, especially if contaminated by staph.
12. She should throw the cans away. Even if not bulged, there is an opening at the seam which allows for contamination.
13. Leaving ingredients such as mayonnaise and eggs out of the refrigerator to stand at room temperature for extended periods of time is a dangerous practice.
14. Handling food in this manner is dangerous because
    a. the cutting board is not washed before using and is stored near pipes
    b. the cutting board is not washed before chopping of different foodstuffs, making cross contamination possible
    c. the practice of cutting fruits and vegetables ahead of time and leaving uncovered causes excessive nutrient loss

Activity 2: Nutrient Conservation

1. a. When a nutrient is added.
   b. When a nutrition claim is made.
2. a. It identifies the nutrients.
   b. It aids in balancing diets.
   c. It may enhance the nutritive value of food.
3. *See* Table 11-1.
4. *See* Table 11-1.
5. *See* glossary for this module.
6. *See* glossary for this module.
7. *See* glossary for this module.
8. a. Enrichment: addition of iron to bread
   b. Fortification: addition of vitamin D to milk

Module 12: Overview of Therapeutic Nutrition

Background Information

1. Therapeutic nutrition is based on modifications of the nutrients in a normal diet.
2. The purpose of diet therapy is to restore or maintain good nutritional status.
3. The diet should be altered to the specific disease (pathophysiology).
4. a. Altering basic nutrients.

b. Altering energy value.
   c. Altering texture or consistency.
   d. Altering seasonings.
5. a. Anxiety and fear about an illness can change attitudes and personality.
   b. Immobilization compounds nutritional problems.
   c. Drug therapy may affect intake and utilization of nutrients.
   d. The disease process modifies food acceptance.
6. The nurse has a key role. He or she assists the patient at mealtimes and explains, interprets, and supports both the physician's orders and the efforts of the dietary staff. The nurse observes and charts pertinent information and coordinates the team. The nurse also involves the patient in his or her own care and provides a care plan for other staff members to follow. And, finally, the nurse plans for discharge teaching of the patient and follow-up care.

Activity 1: Principles and Objectives of Diet Therapy

1. a. Cultural aspects
   b. Socioeconomic background
   c. Psychological factors
   d. Physiological factors
2. a. The patient is often fearful and rejects hospital food.
   b. Immobilization brings about nutritional stress.
   c. The disease process alters food acceptance.
   d. Medications may interfere with nutrient utilization.
3. Diet therapy focuses on the patient's identified needs and problem.
4. Therapeutic nutrition is based upon modifications of the nutrients in a normal diet.
5. The purpose of diet therapy is to restore or maintain good nutritional status.

Activity 2: Routine Hospital Diets

1.	a	5.	b	9.	c	13.	c
2.	c	6.	b	10.	d		
3.	d	7.	a	11.	b		
4.	c	8.	b	12.	c		

14. Canned fruit cup; oatmeal with milk and sugar; toast with butter (tea with sugar, if desired)
15. a. N
    b. Y
    c. Y
    d. N
    e. Y
    f. Y
    g. N
    h. Y
    i. N
    J. N

Activity 3: Diet Modifications for Therapeutic Care

1. Modify basic nutrients; modify energy value; modify texture; and modify seasoning.
2. There are numerous examples that would be correct. For

instance, the diet restricted in simple carbohydrates used for the diabetic whose pancreas does not produce enough insulin. Calories are not nutrients, so a low calorie diet is not appropriate here.

3. a. When the diet imposes severe restrictions.
   b. When the patient's appetite is poor.
   c. When digestion, absorption, or metabolism is impaired.
4. Within the framework of the correctly modified diet, the individual's likes, dislikes, and tolerances should be built in. Foods of equal value should be substituted to meet the patient's ethnic and cultural desires. Participation by the patient in choosing foods within the specified diet is desirable.

Activity 4: Alterations in Feeding Methods

1. c	4. F	7. T	10. a
2. a	5. F	8. F	11. b
3. c	6. T	9. c	

12. A nutritionally adequate diet of liquified foods administered through a tube into the stomach or duodenum.
13. One advantage is that it is safer to feed enterally. Other answers may be found in the activity.
14. a. When the GI tract cannot be used.
    b. When the patient is severely depleted nutritionally.
15. a. Assist the patient's adjustment to an alternate feeding method.
    b. Monitor glucose levels.
    c. Be alert for signs of contaminated solutions and discard them.
16. a. Milk-based formula: milk and cream are primary ingredients.
    b. Blenderized formula: adds strained meats, vegetables, and fruits to the milk base.
    c. Meat-based formula: milk and cream are omitted.

Module 13: Diet Therapy for Surgical Conditions

Background Information

1. a
2. a
3. Effective wound healing
4. Increased resistance to infection
5. Lowered mortality rate
6. Shortened convalescent period (decreased probability of complications arising during and after surgery)

7. e	11. c	15. c	19. F
8. d	12. d	16. a	20. F
9. a	13. e	17. T	
10. f	14. b	18. T	

Activity 1: Pre- and Postoperative Nutrition

1. b and d	5. T
2. c	6. F
3. a	7. F
4. F	

8.

	Pro	CHo	Thia	Nia	Ribo	Fe	VitC
Oyster stew	X	X	X	_	X	X	_
Whole wheat garlic toast	X	X	X	X	X	X	_
Green pepper and cabbage slaw	X	X	_	_	_	_	X
Raisin rice pudding with orange sauce	X	X	_	_	_	X	X

Activity 2: The Postoperative Diet Regime

1. Regain normal body weight.
2. a. Correct fluid and electrolyte balance.
   b. Carefully plan dietary and nutritional support.
   c. Monitor food intake.
3. a. Prevent shock/edema.
   b. Provide for synthesis of albumin, antibodies, etc.
   c. Accelerate wound healing.
4. a. Blood.
   b. Fluids and electrolytes.
   c. 5% dextrose.
   d. Protein-sparing solutions.
   e. Vitamin supplement.
   f. Intralipids single or in any combination.
5. Clear liquid—24 hours (after bowel sounds return).
   Full liquid—1–2 days, should be supplemented with commercial formula if used longer.
   Soft Regular—remainder of hospital stay. May need supplements.
6. 150/2.2 = 68 × 0.45 = 30.6 × 100 = 3060.
7. 3060 × 0.15 = 459 kcal/4 = 115 g protein (rounded).
8. 3060 × 30 = 1009.8 kcal/9 = 112 g fat (rounded).
9. 3060 × 0.55 = 1683 kcal/4 = 420 g carbohydrate (rounded).
10. Your choice. Use exchange lists as needed.

Module 14: Diet Therapy for Cardiovascular Disorders

Activity 1: The Lipid Disorders

1. See Tables 14-1 and 14-2.	4. c	9. F
2. Elevated serum cholesterol, obesity, hypertension, lifestyle	5. b	10. F
	6. b	11. T
3. d	7. F	12. T
	8. F	

Activity 2: Heart Disease and Sodium Restriction

1. See the Low-Sodium Diet, Activity 2.
2. Example of menu for a 500 mg sodium diet.

Breakfast
Puffed wheat cereal
½ cup skim milk
1 sliced banana
Sugar
2 slices low-sodium toast with unsalted soft margarine and honey
Coffee or decaffeinated beverage

Mid morning
½ cup orange juice
Unsalted crackers

Lunch
2 oz. baked chicken*
½ cup rice*
½ cup green peas*
1 slice unsalted bread with special margarine
Sliced peaches
½ cup skim milk

Mid afternoon
½ cup skim milk
1 cupcake*

Dinner
3 oz. roast beef
Baked potato
½ cup glazed carrots*
Lettuce with special dress-ing*

1 slice unsalted bread with
  special margarine
Canned pineapple
Coffee, tea, or decaffeinated
  beverage

Bedtime
Fruit cup
½ cup skim milk

*All food prepared without seasonings that contain so-dium.

3. a. lemon juice/slices; orange juice/slices
   b. thyme, basil, marjoram, oregano, sage, bay leaf
   c. onion, garlic (fresh or powdered, not salt)
   d. chives, dill, mint, parsley, rosemary
   e. unsalted chopped nuts
   f. green pepper, pimiento
   g. cinnamon, nutmeg, brown sugar, ginger
   h. vinegar, tarragon, curry, black pepper
   i. mushrooms, cranberry sauce, dry mustard
   j. fresh tomatoes; unsalted juice

Progress Check on Nursing Implications

1. a. Reducing the workload of the heart.
   b. Improving cardiac output; promoting patient comfort.
   c. Restoring and maintaining adequate nutrition.
   d. Controlling any existing conditions such as hyperlipoproteinemia or hypertension.
2. a. Position the patient for maximal benefit; for example, allow the patient to sit up with the tray on his or her unaffected side.
   b. Place food in unaffected side of the patient's mouth.
   c. Gently stroke the patient's throat, and teach the patient to do so to relieve fear of choking (patient feels the food going down).
   d. Provide feeding devices when necessary.
   e. Protect the patient from spillage. Preserve the patient's dignity. Change linens as necessary.
   f. Take plenty of time to feed or assist self-feeding.
   g. Cut food into small bites. Open all packages and cartons.
   h. Emphasize all successes; praise attempts at self-feeding.
   i. Talk to the patient whether or not the patient can answer.
   j. Try to find out from the family what foods the patient dislikes and do not feed the patient those foods.

Activity 3: Dietary Care after Heart Attack and Stroke

1. Baking powder, baking soda, patent medicines, prescribed drugs, commercial mixes, most convenience foods, frozen and canned vegetables, softened water, cured and dried meats, and vegetables.
2. *See* list of acceptable alternatives to salt.
3. *See* Nursing Implications.
4. To rest the heart and reduce or prevent edema.
5. c
6. b

Module 15: Diet and Disorders of Ingestion, Digestion, and Absorption

Activity 1: Disorders of the Mouth, Esophagus, and Stomach

Diet	Disease or Condition	Foods Allowed	Foods Limited	Foods Forbidden	Nursing Implications
Low-Residue Diet	Hiatal hernia Diverticulitis Hemorrhoidectomy Ostomies Ulcerative Colitis (U.C.)		See Table 4-2 for guidance		See Nursing Implications, this module
Bland Diets a. Traditional bland b. Liberal bland	Ulcers: a. severe pain or bleeding b. convalescing Also used for gastritis, stomach cancer		See Table 4-3 for guidance		See Nursing Implications, this module
Bland #2 Diet	Severe ulcers, i.e., perforation, etc.	See a clinical agency diet manual for guidance in writing menu			

Activity 2: Disorders of the Intestines

1. a. N   e. N   i. N
   b. Y   f. N   j. Y
   c. N   g. Y
   d. N   h. Y
2. a   6. a   10. d
3. a   7. c   11. d
4. b   8. c
5. d   9. c
12. Choose from this group:
    a. any whole grain breads/cereals
    b. any fresh fruits
    c. any fresh vegetables
    d. cooked fruits and vegetables may be used in some cases; i.e., broccoli, spinach
    e. prunes, figs, raisins
    f. nuts
13. a. correct nutrient deficits
    b. restore adequate intake
    c. prevent further losses
    d. promote repair and maintenance of body tissue
    e. promote healing
    f. control substances that are not absorbed easily
14. *See* nursing implications for ileostomy, colostomy.

Module 16: Diet Therapy for Diabetes Mellitus

Activity 1: Diet Therapy and Diabetes Mellitus

1. *See* Answer Sheet for Exercise 16-1 and 16-2 following question #34.
2. d   9. d   16. F   23. d
3. a   10. c   17. F   24. b
4. c   11. a   18. F   25. c
5. b   12. b   19. T   26. a
6. d   13. d   20. T
7. a   14. F   21. T
8. d   15. F   22. e

27. *See* Nursing Implications.
28. *See* Patient Education: What the diabetic patient must know.
29.

	Carbo- hydrate (grams)	Protein (grams)	Fat (grams)
Milk, 2 exchanges	24	16	8
Vegetables, 3 exchanges	15	6	—
Fruit, 3 exchanges	60	—	—
Lean meat, 6 exchanges	—	42	18
Medium fat meat, 2 exchanges	—	14	10
Fat, 5 exchanges	—	—	25
Bread, 5 exchanges	75	15	=
Total	174 g	93 g	61 g

30. Your choice. Be sure to use all exchanges, but no more than the number specified.

31. c
$$174 \times 4 = 696 \text{ calories}$$
$$93 \times 4 = 372 \text{ calories}$$
$$61 \times 9 = 549 \text{ calories}$$
1617 calories (Total). Round to 1600.

32. b   7,000 calories = 2 lb. body fat
33. b, c   Potatoes and bread have 70 calories each; meat, though lean, has 55 calories per oz.; 8 oz. whole milk has 150 calories.
34. *See* Answer Sheet for Exercise 16-1 and 16-2.

Answer Sheet for Exercises 16-1 and 16-2

Diet	Disease or Condition	Foods Allowed	Foods Limited	Foods Forbidden	Nursing Implications
Calculated	Diabetes mellitus	All of those listed in the 6 food exchanges (*see* exchange list in appendix D)	Foods are limited by *amount*: larger amounts for higher caloric allowances; smaller amounts for lower caloric allowances	Sugar, sweets and desserts containing sugar; any foods with unacceptable levels of sugar	*See* section: Nursing Implications. Also see section on Juvenile Diabetes Mellitus.
	Weight control	Same as diabetes	Same as diabetes	Same as diabetes	*See* Module 3, Part 1 for responsibilities of the health team.

Module 17: Diet and Disorders of the Gallbladder and Pancreas

Activity 1: Diet and Gallbladder Disorders

1. *See* Table 17-1, for guidance; *also see* Nursing Implications.
2. Menu alterations for low-fat diet:

Breakfast
Orange juice
Oatmeal, skim milk, sugar
Poached egg (1)
Toast, 1 tsp. butter, jelly
Coffee

Lunch
Baked chicken; no skin
Mashed potato
Green beans with pimiento
Roll; 1 tsp. butter

Skim milk
Tea/sugar

Dinner
Lean broiled hamburger patty
Parsley carrots
Tossed green salad/vinegar or lemon
French bread/1 tsp. butter
Sherbet
Red wine
Coffee

Activity 2: Diet Therapy for Pancreatitis

Example only; other foods of similar type and value may be used.

Breakfast
Orange juice
Oatmeal/brown sugar/butter
Toast, butter, jelly
Skim milk

Mid-morning
Fruit
Sugar cookies
Skim milk

Lunch
Baked chicken
Mashed potato
Green beans
Roll/butter
Tapioca pudding
Skim milk

Mid-afternoon
Milkshake made with skim milk, sherbet, and fruit

Dinner
Broiled lean hamburger patty
Parsley carrots
Wild rice/mushrooms
French bread/butter
Sherbet
Fruit juice

Pre-bed Snack
Low-fat yogurt with fruit or cottage cheese and fruit
Crackers
Juice or skim milk

Module 18: Diet Therapy for Disorders of the Liver

Activities 1 and 2: Diet Therapy for Hepatitis and Cirrhosis

1. *See* Tables 18-1 and 18-2, and Nursing Implications.
2. Example: (whole day's menu)

Breakfast
Orange juice, 8 oz.
Cream of Wheat, 1 cup with sugar and milk
Poached egg, 1, on whole wheat buttered toast
Milk/coffee

Mid-morning
English muffin with 2 tbsp. cream cheese
Milk, 8 oz.

Lunch
Chicken noodle soup

Tuna salad sandwich (3 oz. tuna, 2 slices bread, 1 tbsp. mayonnaise, lettuce)
Carrot/raisin salad
Assorted crackers
Fruit juice, 8 oz.
Milk, 8 oz.
Sherbet with sugar cookies

Mid-afternoon
Hardboiled egg
Cottage cheese with fruit
Toast with 1 tsp. butter
Juice, 8 oz.

Dinner
Lean roast beef, 4 oz.
Mashed potatoes, 1 cup with butter, 1 tsp.
Green beans
Fruited gelatin salad
Rolls, 1 tsp. butter

Angel food cake
Milk, 8 oz.

Pre-bed Snack
1 cup buckwheats
1 cup milk
1 banana

3. Example: (menu altered to reduce protein and sodium levels)

Breakfast
Orange juice, 4 oz.
Cereal, ½ cup with sugar and milk
Whole wheat toast, 1 slice with butter and jelly
Coffee with 2 tbsp. cream
Milk, ½ cup

Mid-morning
English muffin with jelly
Fruit juice
Coffee with sugar

Lunch
Small baked potato
Green peas, ½ cup
Carrot/raisin salad
Bread, 1 slice with butter
Sliced peaches
Milk, ½ cup

Tea with lemon and sugar
Fruit juice, 8 oz.

Mid-afternoon
Fresh fruit
Sugar cookies
Tea

Dinner
Lean beef, 2½ oz.
Potato, ½ cup with butter
Green beans
Tossed salad with low-sodium dressing
Roll, 1
Fruit cocktail, ½ cup
Coffee with sugar
Juice, 4 oz.

Snack
Buttered toast with jelly
Banana

Note: ½ regular amount salt in cooking; no added salt at table.

4. a. 2,700 calories
    b. To cover the extra energy needs from fever, infection, and stress.
    c. For an adult, nonpregnant woman, the 1989 RDA for protein is 46 grams + 54 grams to bring the total to 100 grams as stated in the diet prescription.
    d. To repair and regenerate liver tissue.
    e. To spare protein for its primary functions and to furnish fiber, vitamins, and minerals.
    f. The vitamins are coenzymes for proper utilization of foods, especially carbohydrates. Extra vitamins replace vitamins lost through the disease process and improve overall well-being.
    g. Fatty meats, desserts high in fat content or chocolate, hard-to-digest fats, fried foods, and any foods or spices that cause discomfort or upset the patient. Alcohol is strictly forbidden.
    h. Sodium, both in products and salt at table.
    i. Isolation techniques vary somewhat from hospital to hospital, but, in general, disposable items are used. There is some problem with food getting cold unless care is taken. The nurse should visit with the patient while he or she eats, if possible, as eating in isolation usually results in decreased consumption. Consult protocol manual at institution.
    j. Cancer, severe malnutrition (marasmus), and early cirrhosis (this diet regime also is suitable for postoperative patients with no complications).

Module 19: Diet Therapy for Renal Disorders

Background Information and Activity 1: Kidney Function and Disease

1.	c	3.	d	5.	d
2.	a	4.	c	6.	c

7–12. *See* Background Information.
13–17. *See* Activity 1.
18. A proteolytic enzyme secreted by the kidney
19. Condition of soft bones with Ca deposited in tissues
20. High biological value of protein—especially animal protein, milk, and eggs

Activity 2: Chronic Renal Failure

1.	a	3.	a	5.	a
2.	b	4.	c		

6–11. *See* Nursing Implications (any two from each category).
12–15. *See* section on dietary management.

Activity 3: Kidney Dialysis

1. Diffusion of solutes from one side of a semipermeable membrane to another.
2. Use of an artificial "kidney" outside the body to clear waste from blood.
3. Use of a catheter placed in the abdominal cavity to clear waste from blood.
4. Solution into which the blood waste products diffuse.
5. Continuous ambulatory peritoneal dialysis.
6. Nitrogenous wastes, sodium, potassium, and fluids.

7.	d	10.	c	13.	b
8.	c	11.	d	14.	c
9.	a	12.	a	15.	e

Activity 4: Diet Therapy for Renal Calculi

1. c
2. b

Check your answers to Questions 3 through 10 by referring to Table 19-3, acid-based foods.

3.	c	6.	c	9.	c
4.	b	7.	a	10.	c
5.	a	8.	b		

Module 20: Diet Therapy for Burns, Cancer, Anorexia Nervosa, and Acquired Immune Deficiency Syndrome

Activity 1: Diet and the Burn Patient

1.	T	4.	F	7.	c
2.	F	5.	F	8.	a
3.	T	6.	d	9.	d

10. Anorexia, pain, inability to move head, swallow, chew
11. Body protein, fat, water
12. a. 77 lb. = 35 kg
     b. 35 kg × 1 g protein/kg/bw. = 35 g

c. 40% body surface burned × 3 g/% surface burned = 120 g

d. 35 g + 120 g = 155 g protein required

13. *See* list of 14 nursing implications.

Activity 2: Diet and the Cancer Patient

1. Anorexia, depression, pain, anxiety, hyperactivity
2. Anemia, fluid electrolyte imbalance, dysglusia, negative nitrogen balance, edema, altered metabolic rate
3. Any of the eight from Table 20-1
4. Sweet, sour, salty, bitter
5. *See* p. 271.
6. b
7. d
8. a
9. d
10. c
11. a–f. Any cold foods such as carbonated drinks, iced tea, jello, watermelon, and meat substitutes. *See* Nursing Implications.

Activity 3: Anorexia Nervosa

1. a 3. c 5. a
2. d 4. b
6–10. Any of the nine listed under *feeding routines*.
7–15. Any of the eight listed under *nursing implications*.

Activity 4: Acquired Immune Deficiency Syndrome

1. High caloric, small frequent feedings. Supplements as desired.
2. Encourage consumption of HBV protein in whatever form and quantity is effective.
3. Use easily digested fats such as cream, butter, egg yolk, oils, and medium chain triglycerides (MCT). Keep fiber content low. Limit refined sugars.
4. a. Serve attractive, appealing foods. Cold usually better. Invite guests, friends, family to socialize. Encourage food from "outside" that's well liked.
   b. Antiemetics administered before mealtimes. Far enough ahead to be effective, change schedule if necessary. Rearrange eating times if needed.
   c. Use whatever method and type of feeding that is most effective. Supply HBV protein, vitamin mineral supplements as necessary. Assist with eating if patient is fatigued.
   d. Serve cold or chilled soft bland and liquid foods in small quantities 6–8 times daily.
   e. Parenteral feedings, drug therapy as necessary, protection from others, protection of others.
5. *See* nursing implications.
6. All standard sanitation procedures that are implemented by the facility must be complied with. In addition, particular attention and compliance with stringent sanitation of food preparation areas, storage, and service must be adhered to. Nursing and dietary employees should have joint inservice to make sure all applicable measures are being implemented.

Module 21: Principles of Feeding a Sick Child

Background Information

1. Any five of these: fatigue, vomiting, diarrhea, anorexia, pain, lethargy, confusion, effects of medication, fear, anxiety.
2. a. Anthropometric measures
   b. Physical assessment
   c. Laboratory tests
3. T 5. F 7. d
4. T 6. c

Activity 1: The Child, the Parents, and the Health Team

1. Any of these: fatigue, nausea, vomiting, pain, fear, anxiety, anorexia, medications, separation from parents, treatments.
2. The nurse's primary role is that of liaison and child advocate. She coordinates and provides optimal dietary care.
3. *See* Nursing Implications.

Activity 2: Special Considerations and Diet Therapy

1. Height, weight, allergies, likes, dislikes, food and fluid intake at home, culture, and/or ethnic group.
2. Since burns cause stress to the body and require greatly increased nutrient intake, the major nutrients for wound healing as described in Module 12 apply. The RDAs for children are in the appendix. In general, normal requirements will double or triple, depending on the extent of the burn. Example: protein RDA for 5-year-old = 30 grams; protein requirement for Allen = 80 to 90 grams.
3. The diet should be increased in all essential nutrients. Total calories needed are high. Fats remain in the moderate range. In general, the diet prescription would read high-protein, high-carbohydrate, and moderate-fat, with supplemental vitamins and minerals as condition requires. The increases aid wound healing, restore nutrient losses, return the child to a positive nutritional status, and maintain growth and development.
4. Your choice: protein should be high quality; snacks included as part of the caloric/nutrient allowance.
5. Allow favorite foods, serve familiar food, observe likes/dislikes as diet permits, encourage group eating (if child is allowed up), establish a pleasant environment, allow food selection, provide companionship, encourage eating (take a snack with each visit to the room, unless treatment or therapy will interfere), relieve pain ahead of mealtimes, and furnish caregivers with list of acceptable foods they can bring from home.

Module 22: Diet Therapy and Cystic Fibrosis

Background Information

1. Any five of these: frequent, large, foul-smelling stools; substandard weight gain; abdominal bloating; steatorrhea; excessive crying; sodium deficiency; circulatory collapse; frequent pneumonia.
2. b

3. b
4. c

Activity 1: Dietary Management of Cystic Fibrosis

1. No. She is undersized. The range for children seven to ten years old to the RDAs is approximately 52 inches height and 62 pounds. Susie is 8 to 10 inches shorter than average, and about 12 pounds underweight.
2. a. Diarrhea: undigested food in the stools.
   b. Lethargy: general malnutrition/fever.
3. High-calorie diet for growth and compensation for food lost in stools. High-protein diet for growth and compensation for food lost in stools. High- to moderate-carbohydrate diet to spare protein and compensate for food lost in stools (simple carbohydrates are better tolerated than starches). Low- to moderate-fat diet because fats are not tolerated well; altered types of fat such as medium-chain triglycerides may be used. High-vitamin and mineral diet: double doses of multiple vitamins in water-soluble form. Salt added generously. Pancreatic enzymes are given by mouth with meals and snacks.
4. Food from home, fast food favorites, group eating, socializing occasions, cheerful atmosphere, frequent meals, some favorite foods added, compromises.
5. Your choice. Diet should contain 90 to 100 grams protein and at least 2,500 calories—3,000 to 3,500 calories would be better. Calories can be increased as appetite improves. Use exchange lists for figuring protein and calories, plus any caloric chart available for items not listed in exchanges.

Module 23: Diet Therapy and Celiac Disease

Activity 1: Dietary Management of Celiac Disease

1. a
2. b
3. a
4. Gluten is the protein fraction found in wheat, rye, oats, and barley to which some people are intolerant. It may be due to an immune reaction or an inherited defect, but it has a toxic effect on the intestine. Inform Mrs. Jones of products containing gluten that must be omitted from her diet to prevent changes in the jejunum. Explain that these changes will prevent absorption of nutrients into the cell, causing acute symptoms and malnutrition.
5. Advise Mrs. Jones to pack a lunch, as most restaurants use mixes, thickeners, and other products containing gluten. She might pack: baked chicken, potato chips, celery and carrot sticks, fruit gelatin, olives, fruit or tomato juice, vanilla tapioca pudding (homemade), crisped rice cookies (made with marshmallows), etc.
6. Pasta, breads, cereals, all breaded products, commercial mixes, thickeners, commercial candies, some salad dressings, canned cream soups, etc. (also *see* Table 23-1).
7. Rice and corn.
8. Any creamed, thickened and filled products, including candies, gravies, sauces, puddings, casseroles, stuffings, and meat loaf.

9. Milk in all forms: fresh, dry, evaporated, fermented or malted. All foods containing milk: cocoa, chocolate, all breads, rolls, waffles, cakes made with milk. Desserts made with milk: cookies, custard, ice cream, puddings, sherbets, cream pies. Margarine that contains milk or cream. Meats: franks, any luncheon meats containing milk powder. Candy: caramel or chocolate. Vegetables in cream sauces.
10. Yes. Medium-chain triglycerides are better tolerated than regular fats and the need for calories is high. The typical client is usually underweight.

Module 24: Diet Therapy and Congenital Heart Disease

Activity 1: Dietary Management of Congenital Heart Disease

1. b	4. c	7. d	10. c
2. a	5. b	8. b	
3. d	6. d	9. a	

11. *Breakfast*
    Fruit juice, 3 oz.
    Salt-free cereal, 2 tbsp.
    Toast, ½ slice

    Lunch and Dinner
    Pureed or mashed vegetables, 2 tbsp.
    Pureed meat (prepared without salt), 1 oz.

    Pureed fruit, 2–3 tbsp.
    Mashed potatoes, 1 tbsp.

    Snacks:
    High-calorie, low-protein, low-sodium beverages as appropriate to age. This will assist in meeting fluid requirements.
12. *See* Managing Feeding Problems.
13. *See* Managing Feeding Problems *and* Nursing Implications.
14. *See* Discharge Procedures.

Module 25: Diet Therapy and Food Allergy

Background Information and Activity 1: Food Allergy and Children

1. Excess sensitivity to certain substances or conditions.
2. Allergens or antigens.
3. First exposure to antigen produces no overt symptoms, causes the body to form these immunoglobulins.
4. When an allergic reaction does not manifest quickly or in the usual ways, but rather over a period of time, the child shows the tension-fatigue syndrome.
5. A food allergy triggers the immunological system of the body, whereas a food intolerance is a direct result of maldigestion or malabsorption.
6. a. Amount of allergen consumed.
   b. Whether it is cooked or raw.
   c. Cumulative effects.
   d. Allergic to inhalable as well as ingestible items.
   e. Allergic at one time but not at another.
   f. Reacts to allergen when physical or emotional problems occur. Also, may be another food chemical, not protein.
7. a. Offending substances must be identified and removed.
   b. Monitors the antiallergenic diet to ensure adequate nutrient intake.

8. Breast milk does not contain beta lactoglobulins, the substance in cow's milk that may trigger reactions.
9. Skin testing and elimination diets.

Activity 2: Common Offenders

1. b	4. T	7. F	10. F
2. a	5. F	8. F	
3. c	6. T	9. T	

Module 26: Diet Therapy and Phenylketonuria

Background Information

1. b	3. a	5. b	7. F
2. c	4. d	6. F	

Activity 1: Phenylketonuria and Dietary Management

1. a	5. b	9. d	13. F
2. c	6. a	10. T	
3. b	7. c	11. T	
4. b	8. d	12. T	

14. a. determine age, weight, and activity level of the child;
    b. determine the client's daily requirement for phenylalanine;
    c. determine the contribution of protein from Lofenalac evaporated milk;
    d. determine calories from formula, milk, and any other food consumed; and
    e. determine total phenylalanine from formula, milk, and any other food consumed.
15. *See* Table 26-3. Also: the use of special, low-protein products: cookies, bread, pasta, drinks, and desserts made primarily from free foods; and the increased use of flavorings and spices as tolerated.

Module 27: Therapy for Constipation, Diarrhea, and High-Risk Infants

Activity 1: Constipation

1. b	3. d	5. c
2. a	4. b	

6. No regular schedule for elimination (not taking time for bathroom).
7. a. Clean out the colon with enema.
   b. Continue use until a regular defecation pattern is established.
   c. Put the child on a conditioning schedule.
   d. Reduce milk to approximately 60–80 percent of normal and increase other fluids and fiber until goal is attained. Keep on maintenance dosage of fiber and other fluids. Return milk to normal amount.
8. *See* Nursing Implications.

Activity 2: Diarrhea

1. a. Stool profile.
   b. Cause.
   c. Site of defect.
2. a. Clinical disorder.
   b. Bacteria in food/formula.
   c. Reactions to certain foods.
3. a. Restore fluid and electrolyte balance.
   b. Restore adequate nutrition.
4, 5, 6. *See* Table 27-2.
7. a. Add corn syrup to formula.
   b. Feed strained cereals, strained fruits.
   c. Provide extra feedings.

Activity 3: High-Risk Infants

1. c	3. a	5. b
2. d	4. a	

6. a. Child can suck.
   b. Child weighs more than 2,000 grams.
7. a. Manual expression.
   b. Give by tube, bottle, or dropper.
   c. Milk less than 8 hours old, unrefrigerated.
8. a. 100–130 kcal/kg/b.w.
   b. 3–4 g pro/kg/b.w.
   c. fluid = to output.
   d. Supplement calcium, iron, vitamin K, tyrosine, and cystine as needed.
9. One containing specific amounts of essential nutrients necessary for the growth of the infant.

Introduction to Nutrition

Multiple Choice

Circle the letter of the correct answer.

1. The components that supply energy, promote growth and repair, and regulate body processes are termed
   a. chemicals.
   b. nutrients.
   c. metabolism.
   d. nutrition.

2. The healthy body requires
   a. specific foods to control specific functions.
   b. certain food combinations to achieve specific physiological effects.
   c. "natural" foods to prevent disease.
   d. specific nutrients in a number of different foods to perform specific body functions.

3. To which of these does the term *essentials of an adequate diet* refer?
   a. the food groups commonly called the basic food groups
   b. an abridged version of USDA Handbook #8
   c. the recommendations published by the National Academy of Science
   d. the macronutrients grouped collectively

4. The leading causes of death in the United States are
   a. iron and zinc deficiencies.
   b. scurvy and pellagra.
   c. degenerative diseases.
   d. infectious diseases.

5. Malnutrition
   a. is an inadequate supply of nutrients.
   b. is an excessive supply of nutrients.
   c. may have a permanent effect on the body.
   d. all of the above

6. Which of the following does not describe the U.S. Dietary Guidelines?
   a. It is published by USDA and DHEW.
   b It establishes recommended sodium intake.
   c. It suggests moderating fat and salt intake.
   d. It is directed toward all healthy Americans.
   e. It is intended to reduce risk of degenerative diseases.

7. The dietary guide specifically designed for nutritional labeling is the
   a. essentials of an adequate diet.
   b. daily food guide.
   c. exchange system.
   d. U.S. RDA.
   e. RDA.

8. Which of the following claims is reliable?
   a. Eating foods lower in cholesterol can decrease the risk of heart disease.
   b. "Super-vitamins" with minerals give you all the vitamins and minerals that are absent in the food supply.
   c. You can lose 5 pounds while you sleep.
   d. Vitamin B_{14} gives extra energy, builds muscle, and cures fever blisters

9. Which of the following is *not* a responsibility of health personnel?
   a. providing accurate nutrition education to clients
   b. prescribing dietary supplements as needed
   c. recommending an appropriate diet
   d. evaluating advertising

10. Which of these agencies provides reliable information to a consumer?
    a. Federal Drug Administration
    b. Federal Trade Commission
    c. U.S. Department of Agriculture
    d. all of the above

Matching

Match the definitions in the right column to the term they define in the left column.

11. nutrition
12. malnutrition
13. daily food guide
14. U.S. RDA
15. the exchange system

a. lists of food by nutrients, calories, and serving sizes
b. the Basic Four plus a fifth group which includes fats, sweets, and alcohol
c. a condition in which the body receives too much or too little of a nutrient or energy
d. levels of nutrients used as standards for food labels
e. the total process of food utilization and the factors affecting food choices

True/False

Circle T for True and F for False.

16. (T) F Everyone needs the same nutrients throughout life, but in differing amounts.

17. (T) F Quackery implies a false claim about a product that may have harmful effects.

18. (T) F The U.S. RDA serves as a standard for nutritional labeling.

19. (T) F Nutrition is the science of food and the processes that act on food once it is consumed.

20. (T) F Nutrition is concerned with the biochemical and physiological processes and economic, social, and cultural implications that act on food.

21. T (F) Mary is interested in finding out what foods she should eat in order to meet the RDA for her sex and age group. If she looks at the RDA table, she will find these foods listed.

22. (T) F The basic food groups is a food guide that groups foods with similar nutrient content together.

23. (T) F Nutrition labels must list percentages of U.S. RDA for carbohydrate, fat, and protein.

24. T (F) The exchange system is a listing of recipe substitutes.

25. (T) F The U.S. Dietary Guidelines make specific recommendations aimed at reducing the incidence of degenerative diseases.

Situation

As you stand in the grocery line, you notice your neighbors, one in front, the other in back of you. You automatically check the contents of their carts. Answer the following questions regarding this situation:

Mary's cart contains lettuce, frozen peas, orange juice, rye bread, margarine, macaroni, and peanut butter.

26. Which of the four food groups is missing from Mary's cart? _Milk_

27. Which of these foods would complete the required number of servings for an adult in one of the groups?
    a. cornflakes
    b. apples
    c. ice cream
    d. cooking oil

Jane's cart contains frozen shrimp, fresh tomatoes, whole milk, sausage links, butter, waffle mix, and syrup.

28. Which of the four food groups is missing from Jane's cart? _None_

29. The cart containing the most expensive foods is
    a. Mary's.
    b. Jane's.

30. The cart containing foods highest in saturated fat content is
    a. Mary's.
    b. Jane's.

Food Habits

Multiple Choice

Circle the letter of the correct answer.

1. Which of the following mechanisms stimulates the appetite?
   a. the central nervous system
   b. the body's biological needs
   c. the sight, smell, and taste of food
   d. the time of day

2. Lack of money affects eating patterns by
   a. curtailing the kind of food bought.
   b. curtailing the amount of food bought.
   c. increasing the amount of starchy foods bought.
   d. all of the above.

3. Hunger is a mechanism controlled by
   a. the central nervous system.
   b. the body's biological needs.
   c. the sight, smell, and taste of food.
   d. the time of day.

4. The one requirement that the biological food needs of an individual must provide is
   a. adaptation to the culture and traditions of the people.
   b. essential nutrients which the body can digest, absorb, and utilize.
   c. pleasant taste, smell, and appearance of food.
   d. adequate intake.

5. Which of the following provides the best framework for changing eating behaviors?
   a. scientific knowledge
   b. relating the changes to the culture and habits
   c. teaching in a group where others have the same problem
   d. sending a home health aide out to check

6. Which of the following nutrients tend to be deficient in the diet of the American Indian?
   a. calcium and riboflavin
   b. vitamins A and C
   c. protein
   d. all of these

7. The typical Chinese diet may be low in which of the following nutrients?
   a. protein, calcium, vitamin D
   b. carbohydrates, fats, fiber
   c. thiamin, niacin, riboflavin
   d. carbohydrates, iron, vitamin K

8. Which of the following meats are avoided by Muslims, Jews, and Seventh Day Adventists?
   a. beef
   b. poultry
   c. pork
   d. seafood

9. What is the condition that results when children have diets inadequate in protein?
   a. pellagra
   b. kwashiorkor
   c. PEM
   d. galactosemia

10. The diet of the Mexican American tends to be high in
    a. fats and sodium.
    b. calcium and folacin.
    c. protein and carbohydrate.
    d. vitamins A and D.

11. Blacks, American Indians, and Orientals have a high incidence of
    a. diabetes.
    b. heart disease.
    c. lactose intolerance.
    d. marasmus.

12. Yin and yang foods refer to
    a. the soul food of Cheech and Chong.
    b. the number 1 and 2 foods used in China.
    c. hot and cold foods, not related to temperature.
    d. hot, spicy foods.

Matching

Match the statement in the left column to the type of food symbolism in the right column.

13. "I take 500 mg of organic vitamin C three times per day to keep from getting a cold"

14. "I want the best steaks you have; my boss is coming to dinner"

15. "I ate a pound of chocolate fudge after that awful day I had at the office"

16. The food symbolism most likely to change

a. sociological
b. biological
c. emotional

True/False

Circle T for True and F for False.

17. T F Diseases of malnutrition are a problem in most countries except the United States.
18. T F A hospitalized vegetarian should not have difficulty selecting from a hospital menu.
19. T F The Jewish diet is usually high in saturated fats and cholesterol.
20. T F Hot red and green peppers, which are used liberally in the Mexican diet, contain good sources of vitamins A and C.
21. T F The practice of using lime-soaked tortillas should be discouraged.
22. T F Obesity is not a problem in United States culture.
23. T F All of the different cultures in the United States have substandard diets.
24. T F Eating behaviors develop from cultural conditioning, not from an instinct to choose adequate foods.
25. T F The economic status of an individual often changes his or her food habits.
26. T F Food has hidden meanings and may become an outlet for stress.
27. T F Poverty is a subculture in the United States.

Situation

Billy is a five-year-old who is admitted to the hospital for the first time. He will be hospitalized for approximately a week for diagnostic tests and possible surgery. When his food is not being withheld, he receives a regular diet. From this brief situation, answer the following questions by circling the letter of the best answer.

28. The breakfast tray, which has been held until 10 a.m. because of tests, has an egg, bacon, juice, and toast on it. Billy refuses it, though he has stated he was hungry. You could assume that his refusal is due to which of the following?
    a. He has lost his appetite by 10 a.m.
    b. The foods are unfamiliar.
    c. He wants to be fed.
    d. He wants his mother.

29. Billy's roommate is a one-year-old who receives a supplemental bottle feeding. When this child receives a bottle, Billy cries for one also. You could assume that this behavior is
    a. a bid for attention.
    b. regression to an earlier developmental stage.
    c. because he still takes a bottle when he is home.
    d. due to hunger.

30. You place Billy's supper tray on the bedside table and encourage him to take a few bites. He shoves the tray to the floor and starts crying loudly. The reason for this hostility is probably due to
    a. being a spoiled brat.
    b. anxiety and fear.
    c. dislike of hospital food.
    d. all of the above.

Meeting Energy Needs

Multiple Choice

Circle the letter of the correct answer.

1. The most successful and healthful way to lose weight is to
   a. eat less but still choose a variety of foods.
   b. exercise regularly.
   c. follow an 800 kcal diet until goal weight is reached.
   d. a and b.

2. How many kcalories are in a food if it contains 10 grams of carbohydrate, 8 grams of fat, 7 grams of protein, 5 milligrams of thiamin, and 40 grams of water?
   a. 138 kcalories
   b. 140 kcalories
   c. 142 kcalories
   d. 145 kcalories

3. All of the following affect the basal metabolic rate (BMR) except
   a. muscle tone.
   b. gender.
   c. body composition.
   d. emotional state.

4. Which of the following factors is directly responsible for controlling basal metabolic energy expenditure?
   a. amount of daily physical activity
   b. thyroid hormone secretion
   c. daily caloric intake
   d. percent of body weight that is fat

5. Which of the following would influence the number of kcalories burned in a given physical activity?
   a. a person's body weight
   b. number of muscles used
   c. length of time the activity is performed
   d. all of the above

6. Which of the following are characteristics of a fad diet?
   a. It does not provide adequate carbohydrate.
   b. It severely restricts food choices.
   c. It emphasizes one or two foods.
   d. all of the above

7. In human nutrition, the kilocalorie (calorie) is used
   a. to measure heat energy.
   b. to provide nutrients.
   c. as a measure of electrical energy.
   d. to control energy reactions.

8. Which of the following foods has the highest energy value per unit of weight?
   a. potato
   b. bread
   c. meat
   d. butter

9. The basal metabolic rate indicates the energy necessary for
   a. digestion of food.
   b. maintaining basal standard test conditions.
   c. sleep.
   d. maintaining vital life functions.

10. Growth, fever, and food intake
    a. decrease basal metabolic rate.
    b. increase basal metabolic rate.
    c. provide nitrogen equilibrium.
    d. cause basal metabolic rate to cease.

Matching

Match the statements in the left column to their equivalents in the right column. Answers may be used more than once.

11. calories per g of carbohydrate   a. 9
12. calories per oz. of carbohydrate   b. 270
13. calories per g of protein   c. 120
14. calories per oz. of protein   d. 4
15. calories per g of fat
16. calories per oz. of fat

True/False

Circle T for True and F for False.

17. T F Ketosis is an abnormal metabolic condition resulting from low-carbohydrate and semi-starvation diets.

18. T F The body has an unlimited capacity to store fat.

19. T F Altering your physical activity level is usually the easiest way to change your energy expenditure.

20. T F A 20 calorie raw carrot and a 20 calorie mint candy both supply the same amount of food energy.

21. T F A hamburger probably contains more calories from fat than from protein.

22. T F   A diet containing 75 g carbohydrate, 100 g protein, and 50 g fat yields 1,000 calories of energy.
23. T F   Mental effort requires a large output of energy.
24. T F   The body is more efficient than an auto in its use of fuel.
25. T F   Energy is neither created nor destroyed.

Situation

Mary is a student nurse in her first semester of college. She has been very busy and usually studies late at night. Many times she and her roommate go for a snack before bedtime. She skips breakfast a lot because she gets up too late. She figures she gets enough exercise going to clinical, but she thinks wistfully of the long bicycle rides she used to take. Lately, she has been feeling sluggish and her clothes are tight. She thinks she's "holding water." Mary is 5' 2" and weighs 130 pounds. She is 21 years old. Answer the following questions.

26. Mary keeps a record of her intake for 24 hours. When she totals it, she finds she has consumed 300 grams of carbohydrate, 50 grams of protein and 150 grams of fat. What is the total caloric value of her diet?
    a. 2,750 calories
    b. 500 calories
    c. 1,800 calories
    d. 1,250 calories

27. Based on the estimated RDA range of 1,700–2,300 calories per day for a female 21–25 years of age, estimate how much weight Mary is likely to gain or lose by the end of the school year (6 months).

    _____

28. Which of the following statements is true concerning Mary's present weight?
    a. She is obese.
    b. She is average weight for her height.
    c. More information is needed.
    d. She has extra muscle tissue.

29. Mary decides to go on a diet. She comes to you for advice. List five important principles for weight reduction that you would give her.

    a. _____
    b. _____
    c. _____
    d. _____
    e. _____

Carbohydrates and Fats: Implications for Health

Multiple Choice

Circle the letter of the correct answer.

1. Which of the following is not a rich source of polysaccharides?
   a. poultry
   b. vegetables
   c. cereals
   d. potatoes

2. What organ of the body relies primarily on glucose for energy?
   a. heart
   b. lungs
   c. muscles
   d. brain

3. Which of these substances is necessary for the uptake of glucose by the cells?
   a. insulin
   b. epinephrine
   c. adrenalin
   d. thyroxin

4. Which of the following is a function of sugars?
   a. They enhance the flavor of some foods.
   b. They add kcalories to a diet.
   c. They prevent microbial growth in jams and jellies.
   d. all of the above

5. The incidence of dental caries is most influenced by
   a. the total amount of sugar consumed.
   b. the number of times a sugar food is consumed.
   c. the length of time sugar is in contact with the teeth.
   d. the type of sugar consumed.

6. A steady blood glucose level is best achieved by consuming which of the following types of diets?
   a. high-sugar foods like candy and soft drinks
   b. no fluids with meals
   c. small meals containing complex carbohydrate, protein, and fat
   d. meals high in protein, fat, and water but low in carbohydrate

7. A high-fiber diet has proven to be an effective treatment for
   a. varicose veins.
   b. coronary heart disease.
   c. appendicitis.
   d. diverticulosis.

8. A therapeutic diet frequently used in the treatment of heart disease is the *low-saturated fat* diet. Which of the following foods would *not* be allowed?
   a. whole milk
   b. corn oil
   c. special soft margarine
   d. whole grains

9. Fats provide the body with its main stored energy source. Another function of fat in the body is
   a. furnishing essential fatty acids required by the body.
   b. regulating body temperature through insulation.
   c. preventing shock to vital organs by padding.
   d. all of the above

10. The function of cholesterol in the body is to serve in the formation of
    a. hormones, bile, and vitamin D.
    b. enzymes, antibodies, and vitamin B_{12}.
    c. central nervous system tissue.
    d. vitamins, enzymes, and fats.

11. From which of these sources is cholesterol obtained?
    a. animal foods containing fat
    b. plant foods rich in polyunsaturated fats
    c. synthesis in the liver
    d. a and c

12. Which of the foods listed below contains predominantly saturated fats?
    a. fruits
    b. vegetables
    c. meats
    d. breads

13. Select the food item from the list below that does *not* contain cholesterol.
    a. liver
    b. cheddar cheese
    c. shrimp
    d. peanut butter

Matching

Match the phrases on the right to the terms on the left that they best describe.

14. hydrogenation
15. bile salts
16. linoleic
17. hypoglycemia
18. glycogen and lactose

a. blood sugar level below normal
b. an essential fatty acid
c. animal sources of carbohydrates
d. substance that breaks fat into small particles
e. conversion of unsaturated oil to a saturated fat

True/False

Circle T for True and F for False.

19. T F Low-density lipoproteins are thought to protect against cardiovascular disease.
20. T F Distribution of carbohydrate in the diet should range between 50 and 60 percent.
21. T F Fat should constitute approximately 40 percent of our food intake for healthful eating according to dietary guidelines.
22. T F Athletes need the same basic nutrients as all other people.
23. T F Carbohydrates are the most efficient energy source for athletes and nonathletes.
24. T F Athletes and nonathletes need some fat on their bodies.

Situation

Stacy is a sixteen-year-old high school student who is on the wrestling team. He is 5'8" tall and weighs 150 lbs. Recently his coach told him he had to lose 10 lbs. to wrestle in a lower weight division. He has 10 days before the next meet.

25. Stacy tells his mother the coach told him to eat only 1 meal a day and to increase his workouts by 1 hour.

Which of the following responses is most appropriate?
a. "No son of mine is going to starve like that."
b. "You will lose weight but it will be muscle loss, not fat loss."
c. "You should lose the required amount of weight if you don't cheat on the diet."
d. "I need to lose 10 lbs. I'll go on the diet with you."

26. The foods that Stacy is allowed to eat are meats of all kinds and green salads. He gets no milk or cheese. The coach also recommends that his mother buy him a megavitamin/mineral supplement and a buddy recommends bee pollen. What is the most likely response of Stacy's body to this diet regime?
a. The extra protein and vitamins will increase his endurance and stamina.
b. The bee pollen will cause him to have an allergic reaction.
c. He will get diarrhea, dehydration, and ketosis.
d. He will improve his performance by 30 percent.

27. By decreasing his water intake the day before the match and using no salt, Stacy manages to make the 140 lb. weight. Ten minutes into the match he collapses and has to be seen by a physician. The probable reason for this happening is
a. he was coming down with the flu.
b. he should have had carbohydrate loading the night before to get more energy.
c. he was dehydrated, weakened, and debilitated from the diet regime.
d. he had been to a big party and had not gotten enough rest.

28. List at least three dietary principles you would have recommended for Stacy if you had been his coach.

a. _____

b. _____

c. _____

Proteins and Health

Multiple Choice

Circle the letter of the correct answer.

1. Of the twenty-two amino acids involved in total body metabolism, building and rebuilding various tissues, eight are termed *essential* amino acids. This means
   a. the body cannot synthesize these eight amino acids and must obtain them in the diet.
   b. these eight amino acids are essential in body processes, and the remaining fourteen are not.
   c. these eight amino acids can be made by the body because they are essential to life.
   d. after synthesizing these eight amino acids, the body uses them in key processes essential for growth.

2. A complete food protein of high biologic value would be one that contains
   a. all 22 of the amino acids in sufficient quantity to meet human requirements.
   b. the eight essential amino acids in any proportion, since the body can always fill in the difference needed.
   c. most of the 22 amino acids from which the body will make additional amounts of the eight essential amino acids needed.
   d. all eight of the essential amino acids in correct proportion to human needs.

3. Besides carbon, hydrogen, and oxygen, what other element is found in all proteins?
   a. calcium
   b. nitrogen
   c. glycogen
   d. carbon dioxide

4. The basic building blocks of proteins are
   a. fatty acids.
   b. keto acids.
   c. amino acids.
   d. nucleic acids.

5. Sufficient carbohydrate in the diet allows a major portion of protein to be used for building tissue. This is known as
   a. digestion, absorption, and metabolism.
   b. the halo effect of carbohydrate regulation.
   c. the protein-sparing action of carbohydrate.
   d. carbohydrate loading.

6. Which of the following foods contain the largest amounts of essential amino acids?
   a. soybeans and peanuts
   b. milk and eggs
   c. meat and whole wheat bread
   d. poultry and fish

7. Which two foods contain proteins that are so incomplete they will not support life if eaten alone with no other added source of protein?
   a. meat, eggs
   b. fish, cheese
   c. gelatin, corn
   d. rice, dried beans

8. Protein complementation is
   a. combining foods that taste good.
   b. combining foods with mutually supplemental amino acid patterns.
   c. combining similar protein foods.
   d. combining carbohydrates and fats with proteins.

9. Joe is a lacto-vegetarian. Which of the following would he be most likely to consume?
   a. cheese omelette
   b. strawberry yogurt
   c. tuna noodle casserole
   d. boiled egg and toast

10. The essential amino acid present in a food in the smallest amount in relation to human need is termed
   a. nonessential amino acid.
   b. limiting amino acid.
   c. target amino acid.
   d. missing amino acid.

11. Kcalories provided by excess dietary protein can be
   a. converted to muscle tissue.
   b. converted to fat.
   c. used for energy.
   d. b and c.

12. Anemia results from a deficiency of hemoglobin and/or red blood cells in the circulating blood. Can protein deficiency cause anemia?
   a. yes
   b. no
   c. only if vitamin B_{12} is also deficient
   d. only if folacin is not present

Matching

Match the protein part of the food listed in the left column to its type in the right column. (Answers can be used more than once.)

13. nuts
14. fish
15. whole wheat bread
16. cheese
17. legumes

a. complete protein
b. incomplete protein

True/False

Circle T for True and F for False.

18. T F All enzymes and hormones are protein substances.
19. T F Lipoproteins are transport forms of fat, produced mainly in the intestinal wall and in the liver.
20. T F Complete proteins of high biologic value are found in whole grains, dried beans and peas, and nuts.
21. T F Protein is best absorbed and utilized when complementary protein foods are eaten in the same meal.
22. T F 30 grams of protein yields 270 calories.
23. T F Enzymes are proteins involved in metabolic processes.
24. T F The RDA for protein for an adult is figured on 0.8 gram per kg of body weight.
25. T F Kwashiorkor is a type of malnutrition resulting from a very low-calorie diet.

Situation

Five-year-old Lisa lives in a strict vegetarian family. Lately, her mother has been concerned because Lisa has been tired, cross, and withdrawn, so she takes her to the doctor.

The pediatrician who examines her tells her mother that Lisa has several nutritional deficiencies and sends her to a dietitian for a consultation. Answer the following questions regarding this situation.

26. Which of the following nutrients are likely to be low in Lisa's diet?
    a. calcium, iron, iodine
    b. vitamins B_{12}, D, riboflavin
    c. essential amino acids
    d. all of the above

Lisa eats the following foods in a 24-hour period:

Breakfast: whole wheat toast, applesauce, grape juice

Lunch: steamed rice with honey and cinnamon, carrot and raisin salad, canned pears, sweetened instant drink

Dinner: alfalfa sprouts, mushroom and tomato sandwich on whole wheat bread, vegetrian vegetable soup, apple, peach nectar

Snacks: homemade raised doughnut, applesauce

27. Based upon the foods listed above, what would you expect to happen to Lisa if the eating pattern continues?
    a. Her growth will slow or stop.
    b. She will grow up very healthy.
    c. She will become overweight.
    d. She will get scurvy.

28. List at least five foods that should be added to Lisa's diet and indicate the proper combinations.

    a. _____

    b. _____

    c. _____

    d. _____

    e. _____

Vitamins and Health

Multiple Choice

Circle the letter of the correct answer.

1. A dietary deficiency of vitamin A can produce
   a. xerophthalmia.
   b. a prolonged blood-clotting time.
   c. osteomalacia.
   d. all of the above.

2. Vitamin A toxicity is likely to occur from
   a. consuming too many dark green and deep orange vegetables.
   b. eating liver twice a week.
   c. consuming high dosage vitamin A supplements.
   d. drinking too much vitamin A-fortified milk.

3. The most reliable source of vitamin D in the diet is
   a. meat.
   b. fruits and vegetables.
   c. fortified milk.
   d. enriched breads and cereals.

4. Rickets is most likely to be caused by deficiencies of
   a. iron and phosphorus.
   b. calcium and vitamin D.
   c. magnesium and vitamin D.
   d. phosphorus and fluoride.

5. Major sources of vitamin E in the diet are
   a. meats.
   b. milk and dairy products.
   c. citrus fruits.
   d. vegetable oils.

6. Vitamin K deficiency is most often observed in
   a. newborns.
   b. children.
   c. teenagers.
   d. adults.

7. The vitamin that is synthesized in the intestines by bacteria is
   a. vitamin A.
   b. vitamin C.
   c. vitamin D.
   d. vitamin K.

8. Factors that may cause a deficiency of water soluble vitamins include
   a. taking no vitamin supplement.
   b. fad diets.
   c. an 1,800 calorie diet from the four food groups.
   d. a regular pregnancy.

9. B complex vitamins
   a. function as coenzymes.
   b. are best supplied by supplements.
   c. include vitamin C.
   d. include laetrile.

10. A deficiency of vitamin C
    a. causes delayed wound healing.
    b. decreases iron absorption.
    c. increases capillary bleeding.
    d. all of the above

Matching

Match the statements on the left side with the letter of the corresponding vitamins listed on the right side.

11. inadequate intake causes osteomalacia and rickets
12. inadequate intake causes poor night vision and skin infection
13. promotes normal blood clotting
14. prevents destruction of unsaturated fatty acids

   a. vitamin A
   b. vitamin D
   c. vitamin E
   d. vitamin K

Match the statements on the left side with the letter of the corresponding vitamins listed on the right side.

15. deficiency causes cracked skin around the mouth, inflamed lips, and sore tongue
16. helps change one amino acid into another
17. a cobalt-containing vitamin needed for red blood cell formation
18. promotes the formation of collagen

   a. ascorbic acid
   b. pyridoxine
   c. vitamin B_{12}
   d. riboflavin

True/False

Circle T for True and F for False.

19. T F Natural and synthetic vitamins are used by the body in the same way.
20. T F Vitamin K is required for the synthesis of blood clotting factors.
21. T F B-vitamins serve as coenzymes in metabolic reactions in the body.

439

22. T F Natural vitamin supplements are more efficiently utilized by the body than synthetic vitamins because they are in a form the body prefers.

23. T F Vitamins are a good source of food energy.

24. T F There is no RDA for vitamin K because it is produced by the body.

25. T F A deficiency of vitamin B_{12} produces sickle cell anemia.

26. T F Niacin is found in abundance in meats, poultry, and fish.

27. T F Pyridoxine (B_6) is found in wheat, corn, meats, and liver.

28. T F Riboflavin is found abundantly in milk and cheese.

Situation

Mrs. A. is preparing dinner for visitors. She decides to do as much preparation ahead of time as she can in order to spend more time with her guests. The day before the dinner, she chops greens for a salad, puts them in a large, shallow container and refrigerates them uncovered so that they will stay crisp. The afternoon prior to the dinner she slices tomatoes and peppers and refrigerates. She peels, dices, and puts potatoes on to boil to make mashed potatoes later and reheat. She also puts green beans on about two hours prior to dinner in a large quantity of water so that they can cook slowly. She has cooked a roast which she will slice and reheat at the appropriate time. Answer the following questions.

29. Identify the practices that contribute to a loss of vitamins in the preparation and storage of this meal.

   _____

   _____

   _____

30. Identify the vitamins that are lost.

   _____

   _____

   _____

31. List at least three things you would teach Mrs. A. regarding conservation of nutrients.

   a. _____

   b. _____

   c. _____

Minerals, Water, and Body Processes

Multiple Choice

Circle the letter of the correct answer.

1. Minerals most often deficient in the diet in the United States are
   a. iodine and fluorine.
   b. phosphorus and calcium.
   c. calcium and iron.
   d. potassium and sodium.

2. Iron deficiency anemia
   a. is not a major problem until age 25.
   b. is a problem for male teenagers.
   c. is a problem for young children and menstruating women.
   d. is a problem in the geriatric adult.

3. Calcium is widely involved in body processes. Among the best known functions are all except
   a. nerve transmission.
   b. muscle contraction.
   c. maintenance of heartbeat.
   d. coenzyme action.

4. The disease of later years that is primarily due to an inadequate calcium intake during younger years is
   a. osteoporosis
   b. rickets.
   c. xerophthalmia.
   d. marasmus.

5. The body survives the shortest time when _____ is lacking.
   a. protein
   b. carbohydrate
   c. fat
   d. water

6. Which of these nutrients contributes the most weight to the human body?
   a. calcium
   b. zinc
   c. water
   d. iron

7. Water functions in the body as all of these except
   a. a participant in chemical reactions.
   b. a solvent.
   c. a lubricant.
   d. a source of energy.

8. Excess consumption of meat, fish, and poultry could
   a. cause iron deficiency.
   b. increase calcium excretion.
   c. favor calcium absorption.
   d. prevent iron toxicity.

9. Fluoride deficiency is best known to cause
   a. mottling of teeth.
   b. osteoporosis.
   c. nutritional muscular dystrophy.
   d. dental decay.

10. Which of these foods provides the best source of iron?
    a. egg white
    b. oranges
    c. bananas
    d. prunes

Matching

Match the function in the left column with the letter of the mineral in the right column. (Answers may be used more than once.)

11. promotes bone calcification
12. deficiency causes endemic goiter
13. found in some proteins
14. part of hemoglobin molecule
15. necessary for hemoglobin formation combined with another mineral

a. iron
b. phosphorus
c. copper
d. iodine
e. sulfur

True/False

Circle T for True and F for False.

16. T F Most of the dietary iron ingested is absorbed.
17. T F The best food source of iron is milk.
18. T F The person constantly taking baking soda for his "acid stomach" may develop iron deficiency anemia and/or calcium deficiency.
19. T F Acid fruits, particularly citrus and tomato, make the blood acid.
20. T F "Softened" water is usually high in sodium.
21. T F Minerals involved in maintaining the water balance of the cells are in the special form of ions.
22. T F The best source of calcium available to people who need to increase their calcium intake is calcium pills.
23. T F The major minerals are more important than the trace minerals.

24. T F The major minerals are found in larger quantities in the body than the trace minerals.
25. T F Fluoride actually forms part of the growing tooth crystal.
26. T F Manganese facilitates bone development.
27. T F Sulfur performs a structural role in the proteins of the hair, nails, and skin.

Situation

The following 24-hour intake was consumed by a 25-year-old female married graduate student.

Breakfast: coffee, cream and sugar
Lunch: green salad with blue cheese dressing
               6 crackers
               Jello with fruit cocktail
               tea with lemon and sugar
Dinner: 4 oz. broiled chicken
               ½ c. rice with gravy
               apple and celery salad
               roll with butter
               coffee, cream and sugar

Assuming that this is her typical eating pattern, answer the following questions regarding her diet:

28. Which of the following minerals would you expect to be deficient in her diet?

a. sodium and potassium
b. calcium and iron
c. magnesium and zinc
d. fluoride and iodine

29. For the minerals you identified as deficient in this diet (#28) list three good food sources and the daily amount needed according to the RDAs.

Daily Amount   *Foods*

Mineral #1

_____   a. _____

                    b. _____

                    c. _____

Mineral #2

_____   a. _____

                    b. _____

                    c. _____

30. If this person's diet remains unchanged, what nutritionally based diseases would you expect her to develop?

a. iron deficiency anemia and osteoporosis
b. hypertension and xerophthalmia
c. skin lesions and dwarfism
d. dental caries and goiter

POST-TEST FOR MODULE 8

Nutritional Assessment and Health Care Model

Multiple Choice

Circle the letter of the correct answer.

1. The major techniques used for assessing nutritional status are
   a. physical findings and measurements.
   b. blood tests and data collection.
   c. the problem-solving process.
   d. a and b.

2. Depletion of subcutaneous fat may be a result of
   a. dieting.
   b. undernutrition.
   c. illness.
   d. all of the above.

3. The components of the health care model consist of
   a. interviewing, testing, diagnosing, and planning health care.
   b. assessing, planning, implementing, and evaluating.
   c. testing, measuring, interviewing, and teaching.
   d. goal-setting, care plan, implementation, and follow-up care.

4. The most common biochemical tests measure
   a. creatinine clearance.
   b. hemoglobin and hematocrit.
   c. nitrogen balance.
   d. all of the above.

5. Evaluation is possible for which of the following learning objectives?
   a. Understand the rationale for a modified diet.
   b. State four foods allowed and four omitted on a modified diet.
   c. Appreciate the difference between old and new diet patterns.
   d. Tell the dietitian the diet plan will be followed.

6. Responsibilities of health personnel for community health education include all but
   a. teaching.
   b. preparing menus.
   c. acting as a liaison.
   d. providing referrals.

7. A balanced diet should contain _____ percent carbohydrate, _____ percent protein, and _____ percent fat:
   a. 50–60, 14–20, 20–30
   b. 42.5–48.9, 30.5–35.7, 30.2–35.6
   c. 60–70, 10–12, 30–35
   d. 30–35, 40–50, 10–20

8. If you decrease your food intake by 500 calories per day, you will lose
   a. 2 pounds per week.
   b. 1 pound per week.
   c. 0.5 pound per week.
   d. no weight.

9. A test useful in determining if there is a normal amount of sugar in the blood is known as a
   a. serum folate test.
   b. blood urea nitrogen test.
   c. plasma glucose test.
   d. blood transaminase test.

10. Pale nail beds, brittle nails, stomatitis, and anemia indicate a deficiency in which of the following minerals?
    a. calcium
    b. iron
    c. iodine
    d. magnesium

Matching

Match the physical indicators of nutritional status listed on the left to the type of status listed at the right.

11. thin, fine, sparse hair
12. bloodshot eyes
13. weakness and tenderness in muscles
14. dry, flaky, sandpaper skin
15. deep pink tongue, slightly rough

   a. good nutritional status
   b. malnutrition
   c. not a positive sign of nutritional status

True/False

Circle T for True and F for False.

16. T F   Approximately one-half the fat in our bodies is directly below the skin.
17. T F   Assessment provides a baseline for identifying problems.
18. T F   Assessment provides a baseline for later evaluation.
19. T F   Nutritional needs remain the same throughout life even though people change.

20. T F All physical findings that are indicators of health are directly related to good or poor nutrition.

21. T F Subjective data are not considered helpful to the health practitioner.

22. T F Lab tests for assessing vitamins, minerals, and trace elements are routinely performed in most hospitals.

23. T F Interviewing skills affect the data obtained from a client.

24. T F Malnutrition can describe an excess of calories as well as a deficit of calories.

25. T F A health care professional's role is defined by law.

Situation

Mr. Lewis, a long distance truck driver, goes for a physical examination because he has been having indigestion and headaches lately. The physical and history reveal the following:

Age: 34. Height: 5' 10". Weight: 205 lb. Blood pressure: 190/100. Eats in restaurants "anything that appeals to him." Drinks approximately 12 cups of coffee per day to "stay awake" and 6–8 beers at night to "unwind." Has not had his eyes checked in 5 years. No history of heart disease in immediate family, but grandfather died suddenly of undiagnosed illness at age 62.

Based on the information given, answer the following questions:

26. Identify at least four major problems presented in the data collected.

   a. _____

   b. _____

   c. _____

   d. _____

27. List the planning steps that would assist the client in solving the identified problems.

   a. _____

   b. _____

   c. _____

   d. _____

28. List the major objectives to be implemented in order to assist the client to attain his goals.

   _____

   _____

   _____

   _____

   _____

   _____

29. Describe how you would evaluate this client for compliance. _____

   _____

   _____

   _____

   _____

   _____

30. The only sure sign that learning has occurred is when there is _____

   _____

   _____

Nutrition and the Life Cycle

Multiple Choice

Circle the letter of the correct answer.

1. An expectant mother's protein intake
   a. may be related to clinical risk.
   b. affects the height of the child.
   c. may provide the child passive immunity.
   d. all of the above

2. Toxemia during pregnancy may be due to
   a. excessive sodium intake.
   b. excessive water intake.
   c. a low-protein diet.
   d. a high-protein diet.

3. Nausea and vomiting during pregnancy
   a. are uncommon.
   b. go away in the third trimester.
   c. can be counteracted to some extent by a dry, high-carbohydrate, low-fat diet.
   d. should be countered with vitamin B_{12}.

4. Advantages of breast-feeding include
   a. psychological benefits for the mother.
   b. anti-infective factors in human milk.
   c. establishing a maternal bond with the child.
   d. all of the above.

5. Advantages of bottle-feeding include
   a. greater calcium absorption by the infant.
   b. greater weight gain by the infant.
   c. a low incidence of diarrhea.
   d. all of the above.

6. The most important factor in establishing a healthy diet in children is
   a. teaching children to make adaptive food choices.
   b. withholding "junk" food so they do not acquire a taste for it.
   c. rewarding a wise choice with a special treat.
   d. requiring them to eat all food served to them.

7. Eating habits of teenagers
   a. usually demonstrate a lack of sound nutrition information.
   b. may be tied to peer acceptance.
   c. cause concern among health professionals.
   d. all of the above

8. Nutrient needs during adulthood
   a. are the same as any other age except for different calorie needs.
   b. may require modification, dependent upon health status.

c. affect the quality of the rest of life.
   d. all of the above

9. The nutritional status of a female on the "Pill" may be worsened with respect to
   a. B vitamins and vitamin C.
   b. vitamin A and iron.
   c. calcium and magnesium.
   d. protein and sodium.

10. The major nutritionally related clinical conditions of old age include
    a. risk of heart disease.
    b. bone disease.
    c. weight imbalance.
    d. all of the above.

Matching

Match the description listed on the left with the infant's age listed on the right:

11. able to digest starch after this age
12. solids usually introduced at this age
13. colostrum is the food the baby is receiving at this age
14. egg white usually withheld until this age

    a. one day old
    b. 3 months old
    c. 4–6 months old
    d. one year old

Match the items in the left-hand column with the conditions in the right-hand column.

15. body fat
16. periodontal disease
17. basal metabolism
18. intestinal motility
19. saliva production

    a. increased in the elderly
    b. decreased in the elderly

True/False

Circle T for True and F for False.

20. T F Aerobic exercise can increase the risk of cardiovascular disease.

21. T F Nutrition-related cancers are more prevalent during the adult years.

22. T F Elderly persons and alcoholics are at high risk for developing drug-induced nutritional deficiencies.

23. **T F** The nutrients most often low in the adolescent's diet are protein, iron, and vitamin D.
24. **T F** Iron deficiency anemia is often a problem in childhood.
25. **T F** Breast-fed babies may need a fluoride supplement.
26. **T F** Excessive use of alcohol during a pregnancy can cause the infant to be mentally retarded.

Situation

Lisa is a 2½-year-old who is brought to a well-child clinic by her grandmother, who is her guardian. Lisa says no to everything and has eaten only peanut butter sandwiches for a week. Her grandmother says her appetite has decreased since last year and she lingers over food for hours. Grandmother states that her own children were not allowed to do this. Answer the following questions in relation to this situation.

27. What developmental problem is Lisa facing and how is this affecting her eating behavior?

_____

_____

_____

28. What other information do you need in order to assess Lisa's nutritional status? _____

_____

_____

_____

29. What would you say regarding Lisa's decreased appetite? _____

_____

_____

_____

30. How would you counsel the grandmother in regard to the peanut butter sandwiches and the difference in two generations of child-rearing practices?

_____

_____

_____

Drugs and Nutrition

Multiple Choice

Circle the letter of the correct answer.

1. Drug and food interactions that compromise nutritional status include
   a. altered taste.
   b. slowed or accelerated intestinal motility.
   c. decreased or increased appetite.
   d. all of the above.

2. Foods may compromise drug actions by which of the following methods?
   a. delayed absorption
   b. altered metabolism
   c. inhibited drug response
   d. altered drug excretion
   e. all of the above

3. Drug therapy can alter which of these functions?
   a. intestinal absorption
   b. utilization of nutrients
   c. storage of nutrients
   d. synthesis of nutrients
   e. all of these

4. Absorption of drugs is accomplished by all except
   a. enzymes.
   b. gastrointestinal pH.
   c. fat solubility.
   d. particle size.

5. Persons who are malnourished are likely to respond to a drug in all except which of these ways?
   a. They respond more profoundly to the drug.
   b. They require a higher dose of the drug.
   c. They require a smaller dose of the drug.
   d. They will not exhibit toxic effects to the drug.

6. Diarrhea, steatorrhea, and weight loss are usually the result of
   a. malabsorption of drugs.
   b. poor excretory function.
   c. intolerance to foods ingested.
   d. malnutrition.

7. Foods can increase or decrease
   a. acidity.
   b. digestive juices.
   c. intestinal motility.
   d. all of the above.

8. Fatty low-fiber meals given with oral medications
   a. decrease drug absorption.
   b. slow drug action.
   c. increase drug absorption.
   d. form a neutral base for absorption.

9. High protein meals given with medications
   a. increase gastric blood flow.
   b. increase drug absorption.
   c. decrease gastric blood flow.
   d. a and b
   e. a and c

10. People who use mineral oil for a laxative should be taught that mineral oil
    a. depletes fat-soluble vitamins.
    b. depletes water-soluble vitamins.
    c. may cause rickets.
    d. a and b
    e. a and c

11. Oral contraceptives result in a deficiency of which of these vitamins?
    a. tocopherol
    b. niacin
    c. B_6
    d. B_{12}

12. Aspirin will decrease the absorption and utilization of which of these vitamins?
    a. ascorbic acid
    b. folacin
    c. B_6
    d. a and b
    e. a, b, and c

13. The drug and food components that have been identified as causing harmful effects on the course and outcome of pregnancy include
    a. alcohol.
    b. food additives.
    c. food contaminants.
    d. all of these.

14. If a nursing mother is taking a prescribed drug that carries potential risk that passes to the infant, what should be the doctor's recommendation?
    a. Change to another drug.
    b. Warn the mother and let her decide.
    c. Stop breast-feeding.
    d. Alert her to report all signs and symptoms.

15. Administering drugs with foods is a common practice used for all except which of these reasons?
    a. reduce GI side effects
    b. disguise taste
    c. chelate the drug
    d. All of these are reasons.

16. Pregnant women who are carriers, or who have phenylketonuria, should avoid aspartame ingestion because it
    a. makes the infant hyperactive.
    b. causes birth defects.
    c. contains phenylalanine.
    d. contains caffeine.

True/False

Circle T for True and F for False.

17. T F Drug-induced malnutrition is not a problem since so many supplements are available.
18. T F Overmedicating means the person takes a larger dose than prescribed.
19. T F Prescription medications are safer than OTC medications.
20. T F OTCs and prescribed medicines usually enhance the effects of both drugs so are safer taken together.
21. T F Alcohol and OTCs are safe taken together, but prescribed medicine with alcohol is contraindicated.
22. T F Pregnant women may drink unlimited amounts of caffeine-containing beverages.
23. T F Mercury poisoning leads to permanent brain damage in the fetus.
24. T F Nicotine ingestion will cause fetal growth retardation.

Fill-in

25. Name the most common side effects of medication.

    _____

    _____

26. Name three drugs that increase appetite.
    a. _____
    b. _____
    c. _____

27. Name three drugs that decrease appetite.
    a. _____
    b. _____
    c. _____

28. Name three drugs that affect taste sensation.
    a. _____
    b. _____
    c. _____

29. Name two drugs that contain a large amount of glucose.
    a. _____
    b. _____

30. Name two drugs that contain large amounts of sodium.
    a. _____
    b. _____

Food Ecology

Multiple Choice

Circle the letter of the correct answer.

1. Custards and cream fillings should be eaten soon after preparation and properly refrigerated when stored because
   a. bacteria such as staphylococci multiply rapidly in these foods unless they are kept at low temperatures.
   b. the fat in these foods is poisonous if it becomes rancid.
   c. all minerals and vitamins are lost if these foods are cooked at temperatures high enough to destroy the bacteria in them.
   d. cooling these foods alters their taste and destroys the vitamins.

2. If several persons become ill from food poisoning while at a picnic, which of the following foods would *most* likely be the cause?
   a. tuna salad
   b. Jello salad
   c. bean salad (kidney, wax, and green beans in oil and vinegar dressing)
   d. baked beans

3. Whenever possible, *raw* fruits and vegetables should be included in the menu because
   a. cooking destroys flavor.
   b. excessive heat destroys minerals.
   c. cooking removes the cellulose in plants.
   d. cooking destroys some of the minerals and vitamins.

4. The nutritive value, color, and flavor of cooked vegetables will be retained if they are prepared
   a. in an open kettle, in boiling salted water, until they are tender.
   b. in a large amount of rapidly boiling unsalted water until done.
   c. in cold water and cooked just until tender.
   d. in a covered container, in a small amount of boiling salted water just until tender.

5. The nutrients most susceptible to destruction from improper handling, processing, and cooking are
   a. niacin and iron.
   b. folacin and niacin.
   c. vitamin C and iron.
   d. vitamin C and folacin.
   e. folacin and iron.

6. Raw meats should not be stored in the refrigerator for more than _____ days, while poultry or fish can be safely stored for _____ days.
   a. 2, 2
   b. 5, 2
   c. 7, 5
   d. 9, 7

7. Which of the following temperature ranges for holding food may make it unsafe to eat?
   a. 60°–125°F
   b. 130°–140°F
   c. 160°–175°F
   d. 10°–32°F

8. The most common biological illnesses transmitted from the food supply to people are from
   a. bacteria.
   b. viruses.
   c. parasites.
   d. all of these are common

9. What is the meaning of the phrase "illness transmission by the oral-fecal route"?
   a. transmitted from beast, to human, to food
   b. transmitted from unwashed hands, to food, to mouth
   c. transmitted by improper storage methods, to food, to human
   d. transmitted by a contaminated water supply to food and liquids

10. The toxin produced by staphylococcus
    a. is seldom found in food.
    b. is anaerobic under ideal conditions.
    c. is the most common foodborne illness.
    d. will grow even in frozen foods.

Matching

Match the procedures in the left column to the statements in the right column.

11. Peel potatoes before cooking.
12. Store fresh vegetables in air-tight containers.
13. Add baking soda to cooking water of vegetables.
14. Use as little water as possible when cooking.
15. Keep freezer at constant temperature below 0° F.

a. The procedure will help to conserve nutrients.
b. The procedure will increase nutrient losses.
c. The procedure is unrelated to conservation of nutrients.

True/False

Circle T for True and F for False.

16. T F Anaerobic bacteria thrive when food is stored in open containers.
17. T F Food should be cooled before being refrigerated; otherwise the temperature in the refrigerator will get too high.
18. T F Bacteria is the major cause of foodborne illness.
19. T F Foods high in protein are the group that most commonly causes food poisoning.
20. T F Boiling a food for five minutes will make it safe to eat.
21. T F A can opener not washed after each use can cause food poisoning.
22. T F Bulging ends of a can indicate the food has spoiled.
23. T F The bacteria that thrives in low acid conditions is called perfringins.
24. T F A person who has a sore on his hand should not prepare or serve food.
25. T F Food tasting with fingers or cooking utensils during preparation is acceptable practice only at home.

Situation

Dana is a newlywed whose closest encounter with a kitchen has been to find the cook and tell her what to prepare. Her lifestyle has changed and now she is doing her own shopping and food preparation. On Wednesday afternoon she shops for fresh produce because her local market is having a sale.

26. The peaches are very pretty but she finds that the least expensive ones are not fresh. Even though they are very soft and contain some bruises, they could be used when peeled and cut up. Which of the following will happen with the peaches?
    a. They will be very sweet because they are so ripe.
    b. The vitamin content will be much lower because the produce is not fresh.
    c. They will be fine because they will be cut and chilled ahead of time.
    d. all of the above

27. While she is shopping she buys some dry cereal and cooking oil, which she forgets and leaves in her car trunk. The result of this may be
    a. she will have to buy more the next time because she forgot she had them.
    b. nothing will happen; this kind of food keeps for a long time.
    c. the cooking oil will get rancid and the cereal will get weevils.
    d. since they are stored in a dry dark place they will probably last longer than otherwise.

28. Dana is in a hurry to fix the potatoes she bought, so she puts them on to cook without peeling them. A likely outcome of this is
    a. she will get food poisoning.
    b. the nutrients will be conserved.
    c. she will have to change her menu as these will be unusable.
    d. the caloric content will be less.

29. Dana notices that the bread she bought was labeled "enriched." This means that
    a. nutrients were added that were not originally present.
    b. thiamin, niacin, riboflavin, and iron were added.
    c. substances were added to preserve the food from spoilage.

30. Dana should know that nutrition labeling after 1992 is mandatory
    a. at all times.
    b. when a nutrient is added.
    c. when a claim is made.
    d. b and c

Overview of Therapeutic Nutrition

Multiple Choice

Circle the letter of the correct answer.

1. The purpose of diet therapy is
   a. to modify texture and energy values.
   b. to restore and maintain good nutritional status.
   c. to interpret the diet in terms of the disease.
   d. to involve the patient in his or her care.

2. The basis of therapeutic nutrition is
   a. assisting a patient to identify his or her malnutrition.
   b. removing excess modifications.
   c. modifying the nutrients in a normal balanced diet.
   d. modifying the patient's behavior to gain appropriate acceptance.

3. Which of the following conditions is not a result of poor nutrition in the recovery to health?
   a. delayed convalescence
   b. overeating
   c. delayed wound healing
   d. anemia

4. The stress of illness may negatively affect
   a. personality.
   b. nutritional balance.
   c. developmental tasks.
   d. all of the above.

5. When planning modified diets, the *major* factors to be observed include altering the diet to the specific pathophysiology and
   a. considering the patient's attitude toward hospitalization.
   b. considering emotional interferences with diet.
   c. individualizing the diet to the patient's total acculturation.
   d. focusing on patient's development of a trust relationship.

6. What factor will determine a patient's nutritional requirements?
   a. nature and severity of the disease or injury
   b. functioning capacity of the hypothalamus
   c. previous nutritional state and duration of the disease
   d. a and c

7. Nutritional requirements during disease, injury, and hospitalization include
   a. increased calories and protein.
   b. increased vitamins and minerals.
   c. decreased fluids and exercise.
   d. a and b.

8. Routine hospital diets include all of these except
   a. clear- and full-liquid.
   b. low-residue.
   c. mechanical- and medical-soft.
   d. regular.

9. Blocks to nutritional adequacy that the nurse may encounter when counseling a patient on a modified diet include
   a. cultural differences.
   b. ignorance.
   c. environmental stressors.
   d. all of the above.

Matching

Match the terms listed on the left to their descriptions listed on the right.

10. ascites
11. edema
12. gastritis
13. peritoneum

a. inflammation of the stomach
b. membrane lining the walls of the abdominal and pelvic cavity
c. abnormal accumulation of fluid in the peritoneal cavity
d. abnormal accumulation of fluid in intercellular spaces

Match the diets listed on the left to their descriptions listed on the right.

14. regular
15. medical-soft
16. mechanical-soft
17. clear-liquid
18. full-liquid

a. reduced fiber, texture, and seasonings
b. used for people who have chewing difficulty
c. the most frequently used of all diets
d. the most nutritionally inadequate of the standard hospital diets
e. consists of liquids and foods that liquefy at body temperature

True/False

Circle T for True and F for False.

19. T F A modified diet is an asset rather than a stressor.
20. T F The focus of diet therapy is based upon the patient's identified needs and problems.
21. T F The regular or house diet restricts foods to the basic food groups.
22. T F A modified diet is successful only if it is accurate.
23. T F Environment and attitude affect a patient's acceptance of a modified diet.

Situation

James, age 19, is admitted to the hospital following a motorcycle accident. He has compound fractures of both legs. He is 6' tall, weighs 130 lb., and has a past history of drug abuse.

24. Therapeutic nutrition for James would focus upon
    a. measures to restore optimal nutrition.
    b. measures to reduce liver damage.
    c. measures to increase his self-esteem.
    d. allowing him to select as he chooses.

25. Diet modification will include
    a. increasing all basic nutrients.
    b. increasing energy value.
    c. decreasing fiber content.
    d. a and b.

26. The goals of the diet therapy used for James would center upon his specific needs. These needs would include
    a. restoration of weight and nutrient reserves.
    b. promotion of bone formation.
    c. regulation of methadone dosage.
    d. a and b.

27. The nurse's role in adapting a client to a modified-diet regime includes all except
    a. diffusion of responsibility.
    b. explanation of the diet to the patient.
    c. interpretation, follow-through.
    d. discharge planning.

28. List the four most common diet modifications. Based upon your knowledge of these modifications, write the diet prescription for James.

    a. _____

    b. _____

    c. _____

    d. _____

    James's prescription: _____

    _____

    _____

    _____

29. State the rationale for the diet prescription you just wrote for James. _____

    _____

    _____

    _____

30. The greatest amount of calcium for bone healing can be provided to James through
    a. 1 egg.
    b. 2 tbsp. cream cheese.
    c. 1 oz. cheddar cheese.
    d. ½ c. orange sherbet.

Diet Therapy for Surgical Conditions

Multiple Choice

Circle the letter of the correct answer.

1. Complete dietary protein of high biologic value is essential to tissue building and wound healing after surgery because it
   a. supplies all the essential amino acids needed for tissue synthesis.
   b. spares carbohydrate to supply the necessary energy.
   c. is easily digested and does not cause gastrointestinal upsets.
   d. provides the most concentrated source of calories.

2. Mrs. Jones is two days postoperative following a hysterectomy and tells you she wants to be on a 1,000 calorie reduction diet when she is allowed to eat again. Your most appropriate response would be to
   a. ask her doctor to prescribe it.
   b. explain that a reduction diet should be at least 1,200 calories.
   c. explain that tissue repair requires more nutrients.
   d. tell her a 1,000 calorie high-protein diet will be okay.

3. Fluids given after surgery should
   a. be increased to replace losses.
   b. be decreased to prevent edema.
   c. be kept at maintenance levels to counteract overhydration.
   d. be withheld to prevent nausea.

4. A minimum of _____ calories per day is needed after surgery to spare protein for tissue repair.
   a. 1,000
   b. 1,200
   c. 1,800
   d. 2,800

5. Both pre- and postoperative patients need proteins of high biological value. These include
   a. milk, eggs, cheese, meats.
   b. grains, legumes, nuts, vegetables.
   c. a and b.
   d. none of the above.

6. Increased ascorbic acid is essential for wound healing. Which of these foods is highest in ascorbic acid?
   a. creamed cottage cheese.
   b. egg whites.
   c. peanut butter.
   d. coleslaw.

7. For which of the following would total parenteral nutrition be inappropriate diet therapy?
   a. a patient with 50 percent of his body surface burned
   b. a patient with a cholecystectomy
   c. a patient with advanced stomach cancer
   d. a patient admitted for surgery who has not eaten in a week

8. The most common nutrient deficiency related to surgery is that of
   a. iron.
   b. vitamin C.
   c. protein.
   d. zinc.

9. All kinds of stress related to surgery may
   a. reduce the function of the GI tract.
   b. interfere with the desire to eat.
   c. deplete liver glycogen.
   d. all of the above.

10. Good nutrition prior to surgery can
    a. shorten convalescence.
    b. increase resistance to infection.
    c. increase the mortality rate.
    d. a and b.

Matching

Match the vitamins listed on the left to their function in wound healing listed on the right.

11. vitamin C
12. folic acid
13. vitamin K
14. thiamin

   a. coenzyme in carbohydrate metabolism
   b. cementing material for connective tissue
   c. formation of hemoglobin
   d. essential for blood clotting

True/False

Circle T for True and F for False.

15. T F Usually nothing is given by mouth for at least eight hours prior to surgery to avoid food aspiration during anesthesia.

16. T F Oral liquid feedings usually provide little nourishment regardless of the type.

17. T F Tube feedings can only be made successfully from commercial preparations.

18. T F As much as one pound of muscle tissue per day may be lost following surgery.

19. T F Vitamin D is essential to wound healing, since it provides a cementing substance to build strong connective tissue.

20. T F Most patients are at optimum nutritional status before they go to surgery.

21. T F Obese patients are high surgical risks but underweight patients are no greater risks than those of normal weight.

22. T F An inadequate protein intake will delay the healing of a fractured bone.

23. T F Inadequate diet may depress pulmonary and cardiac functions in a patient who has no history of respiratory or cardiac disease.

Situation

Mrs. H., a 40-year-old woman, was involved in an auto accident. She suffered multiple broken bones and underwent emergency surgery for a ruptured spleen. The following questions pertain to this situation.

24. The surgical team is considering placing her on total parenteral nutrition (TPN). What is the rationale for their decision? _____

_____

_____

25. Mrs. H. finds breathing difficult because of several broken ribs. She is also 20 pounds overweight. Should she be placed on a reduction diet to ease this situation? Explain your answer. _____

_____

_____

26. List four important nutrients necessary for Mrs. H.'s speedy recovery and two foods that are good sources for each nutrient.

a. _____

b. _____

c. _____

d. _____

27. List three nutritional nursing measures appropriate to this situation.

a. _____

b. _____

c. _____

Diet Therapy for Cardiovascular Disorders

Multiple Choice

Circle the letter of the correct answer.

1. A low-cholesterol diet would restrict all of the following foods except
   a. shellfish.
   b. liver.
   c. eggs.
   d. skimmed milk.

2. Which of these seasonings may be used on a 1 gram sodium-restricted diet?
   a. lemon juice, herbs, spices
   b. soy sauce, m.s.g. (*Accent*)
   c. butter or margarine
   d. garlic or celery salt

3. Which of the following foods may be used freely on a 500 mg sodium diet?
   a. fruits
   b. milk
   c. meat
   d. spinach

4. Lipid disorders are classified as to the type of lipid that is elevated. Of the five types identified, which two are the most common?
   a. Types I and III
   b. Types II and IV
   c. Types III and V
   d. Types I and V

5. The fat-controlled diet is used with many of the lipid disorders. This diet reduces
   a. unsaturated fats.
   b. saturated fats.
   c. weight.
   d. stress.

6. Which of the following meals would be most appropriate for a person on a fat-controlled diet?
   a. macaroni and cheese, avocado/grapefruit salad, Jello, tea
   b. roast beef, baked potato with sour cream, coconut cookie, skim milk
   c. broiled chicken breast with wild rice, tossed salad with French dressing, baked apple with walnuts and raisins, tea
   d. tuna salad on lettuce, crackers, sliced cheese, lemon pudding, skim milk

7. Poor eating habits that can increase risk of heart disease include all except
   a. consumption of large amounts of alcohol.
   b. consumption of large amounts of beef, pork, butter, ice cream.
   c. excess total daily calories.
   d. daily consumption of peanut butter, chicken, fish.

8. Which of these would be the diet therapy of choice for a patient following a myocardial infarction?
   a. clear-liquid first 24 hours
   b. regular low-residue first 24 hours
   c. limited in sodium, caffeine-restricted, soft
   d. caffeine and sodium restricted, clear-liquid

9. Following a cerebrovascular accident, the diet therapy
   a. will be an I.V. line for the first 24 hours.
   b. may be a tube feeding or oral liquids.
   c. may be semi-solid.
   d. may be any of these, or any combination.

10. Diet therapy appropriate for a patient on a Type II hyperlipoproteinemia diet should include instructions for
    a. omitting foods containing cholesterol.
    b. restricting use of commercially prepared foods.
    c. increasing use of safflower, sunflower, and corn oil.
    d. all of the above.

Matching

Match the factors involved in heart disease listed on the left with the recommended measures to prevent or lessen the effects listed on the right.

11. hypertension
12. elevated cholesterol
13. elevated triglycerides
14. obesity
15. sedentary lifestyle

a. regular program of exercise
b. limiting sodium intake
c. limiting sugar intake
d. limiting saturated fats in diet
e. limiting total energy value of diet

True/False

Circle T for True and F for False.

16. T F About two-thirds of the total fat in the United States diet is of animal origin and therefore mainly saturated.

17. T F Coconut oil is a polyunsaturated vegetable oil, used in low-saturated-fat diets.

18. T F Sodium restriction is effective therapy in congestive heart failure and hypertension.

19. T F Regular cheese may be used on a low-sodium diet.

20. T F Tea, coffee, and alcohol are not used in the diet of cardiac patients.

21. T F Spices such as cinnamon, nutmeg, and garlic are high in sodium content.

22. T F HDL carries cholesterol from the arteries to the liver.

23. T F Low-potassium serum levels are not a problem for persons who are taking antihypertensive medicine.

24. T F An objective of diet therapy for a patient who has had a myocardial infarction is to reduce the workload of the heart.

25. T F Persons who must limit their intake of foods containing cholesterol should be able to eat lunchmeat and lean hamburgers.

Situation

26. Mr. J., age 45, is in the hospital recovering from a myocardial infarction. He is on a 1,500 calorie diet, low in saturated fats and high in polyunsaturated fats.

The chief purpose of the diet ordered for Mr. J. is to reduce weight and
   a. prevent development of edema.
   b. lower the blood cholesterol level.
   c. decrease blood clotting time.
   d. provide for ease of digestion.

27. Which of these food choices, as ordinarily prepared, would be most suitable for Mr. J.?
   a. roast turkey, baked trout, breaded veal cutlet
   b. lean roast beef, breaded veal cutlet, cheese soufflé
   c. baked trout, lean roast beef, roast turkey
   d. roast turkey, baked trout, broiled calves' liver

28. Which of these foods would be most suitable for Mr. J.'s meal?
   a. baked potato, tossed salad with French dressing, grapefruit
   b. cauliflower with cheese sauce, sliced tomato, orange sherbet
   c. hash brown potatoes, tomato salad, Jello with whipped cream
   d. broccoli, Waldorf salad, custard

29. In counseling Mr. J. regarding diet management, the nurse would
   a. discuss food preparation methods.
   b. need more information regarding the patient's usual habits.
   c. explain the importance of weight control.
   d. all of the above

30. The diet for Mr. J. should be
   a. restricted only in carbohydrates.
   b. a basic pattern within the limitations imposed by the diet orders.
   c. a list of foods to be eaten at the same time each day.
   d. a weighed diet.

Diet and Disorders of Ingestion, Digestion, and Absorption

Multiple Choice

Circle the letter of the correct answer.

1. Which of these factors is most important to the healthy functioning of the gastrointestinal tract?
   a. specific food combinations
   b. physiological and psychological conditions
   c. a regular exercise program
   d. few environmental pollutants

2. Which of the following statements is true regarding the treatment of infants with cleft palate?
   a. The nutritional requirements are higher than those of unaffected infants.
   b. Surgery is performed after the age of one year.
   c. Lack of essential nutrients is the most likely cause of cleft palate.
   d. all of the above

3. Mr. H. received a fractured mandible in an auto accident and is in the hospital. He will go home before the wires are removed. Which of the following instructions for eating will you give him?
   a. His diet, though liquid, must be high in all nutrients.
   b. He must learn to pass the tube down.
   c. He will need water and mouthwash before and after each feeding.
   d. a and c

4. Which of the following is a major cause of the high incidence of dental caries?
   a. lack of essential nutrients in the diet
   b. Vincents' disease
   c. high use of concentrated sweets
   d. pregnancy

5. The disadvantages of wearing dentures include
   a. the need for frequent realignment.
   b. lowered self-esteem.
   c. the fact that everyone knows you wear them.
   d. halitosis.

6. Which of the following are appropriate dietary measures for a person with a hiatal hernia?
   a. a low-fiber, bland diet in six feedings
   b. antacids and fluids between meals
   c. no spices, no alcohol, limited fat intake
   d. all of the above

7. The diet containing a minimum amount of residue will be deficient in which of these nutrients?
   a. calcium, iron, and vitamins
   b. carbohydrates, proteins, and fats
   c. water, sodium, and potassium
   d. cellulose, glycogen, and glucose

8. The low-residue diet would be the diet of choice for all but which of the following disorders?
   a. diverticulosis
   b. diarrhea
   c. cancer of the colon
   d. ulcerative colitis

9. Foods allowed on the very low-(minimal) residue diet include
   a. cheddar cheese, fruits, milk, creamed soup.
   b. green beans, carrots, butter, broiled steak.
   c. roast turkey, mashed potatoes, butter, tomato juice.
   d. bouillon, whole wheat toast, jelly, orange sherbet.

10. Nutrients that frequently will be deficient in the traditional ulcer diet include
    a. calcium, phosphorus, vitamin D.
    b. iron, ascorbic acid, protein.
    c. riboflavin, fat, vitamin A.
    d. thiamin, niacin, and phenylalanine.

11. Foods recommended to be avoided in the liberal bland diet include
    a. alcohol, coffee, tea, cola, broth.
    b. cinnamon, paprika, nutmeg, garlic.
    c. olives, spinach, lettuce, tomatoes.
    d. all of the above.

12. A patient had a gastrectomy and developed a "dumping syndrome." His diet must be modified. Which of these modifications would be appropriate?
    a. Lower the fat content of the diet.
    b. Avoid sugars, restrict starches.
    c. Decrease protein content of diet.
    d. all of the above

13. Diverticulitis is best treated with a _____ diet.
    a. bland
    b. low-fiber
    c. high-fiber
    d. full-liquid

14. The dietary changes that help to reduce the incidence of constipation include
    a. using laxatives and stool softeners.
    b. increasing fiber and fluid intake.
    c. increasing protein and fat intake.
    d. all of the above.

15. The most serious consequence of functional diarrhea is
    a. weight loss.
    b. hemorrhoids.
    c. dehydration.
    d. pain and fever.

Matching

Match the guidelines listed on the right that would best restore nutritional status of the cancer patient who has the depleted nutritional conditions listed on the left.

16. reduced G.I. motility, sore mouth
17. elevation in tolerance for sweet and salty tastes
18. anorexia due to depression, malnutrition, and chemotherapy
19. malabsorption of milk carbohydrates
20. decreased tolerance for bitter taste of meats

  a. provide extra seasonings for food
  b. use low-lactose foods and supplements
  c. use cool, smooth-bland liquids, semi-solids
  d. use beans, cheese, and peanut butter as protein sources
  e. use high-density liquid formulas or total parenteral nutrition

True/False

Circle T for True and F for False

21. T F The state of the body system determines how food is digested and absorbed.
22. T F Cleft lip or palate is a congenital birth defect.
23. T F The G.I. tract consists of stomach, small and large intestine, and colon.
24. T F All of the teeth a person will ever have are formed before birth.
25. T F Poorly fitting dentures can lead to malnutrition.

Situation

Carmen is a twenty-year-old female college student, hospitalized with ulcerative colitis. She has many food intolerances; she does not like raw fruits or vegetables, and does not drink milk. She is fond of soda pop and tacos. She will be going home soon and back to school, but is very anxious and apprehensive because she feels she will not be able to maintain her diet. The doctor has ordered a 150 gram protein, 3,000 calorie diet for her. The following questions pertain to this situation.

26. Carmen has been in negative nitrogen balance. This means that she
    a. was dehydrated.
    b. was losing more tissue protein than she was replacing.
    c. was gaining tissue protein, so, therefore, excreted nitrogen.
    d. had an electrolyte imbalance.

27. Which of the following nutritional problems would the nurse *not* encounter in Carmen?
    a. skin lesions and inflammation
    b. anorexia and weight loss
    c. avitaminosis and anemia
    d. esophageal varices and pulmonary edema

28. If Carmen wanted tacos as part of her meals, the nurse would
    a. tell her firmly "no."
    b. tell her she will try to get them for her.
    c. explain the situation to dietary aides.
    d. compromise: if Carmen agrees to eat them with less seasoning, the nurse will ask the dietitian to include them occasionally.

29. In counseling Carmen so that she will comply with the diet, the nurse explains the rationale. List three of these reasons.

    a. _____

    b. _____

    c. _____

30. The nurse asks Carmen to keep very careful daily records. List three important records she would need in order to evaluate her progress.

    a. _____

    b. _____

    c. _____

Diet Therapy for Diabetes Mellitus

Multiple Choice

Circle the letter of the correct answer.

Mr. G., a 40-year-old man, is a newly diagnosed diabetic. He weighs 160 lb., and is 5' 10" tall. The diet prescribed contains 250 g carbohydrate, 100 g protein, and 70 g fat.

Answer the following questions relating to this patient.

1. Mr. G's daily caloric intake is
   a. 1,230 calories.
   b. 1,530 calories.
   c. 1,830 calories.
   d. 2,030 calories.

2. This caloric allowance should
   a. prevent hypoglycemia.
   b. decrease body weight.
   c. maintain body weight.
   d. promote normal potassium balance.

3. Emphasis is placed on using polyunsaturated fats and limiting foods high in cholesterol in the diet of the diabetic. This will
   a. aid in preventing cardiovascular diseases.
   b. aid in the digestive process.
   c. prevent skin breakdown.
   d. control blood sugar.

4. In counseling Mr. G. regarding diet management, the nurse should
   a. explain the importance of weight control.
   b. interpret food exchanges to him.
   c. discuss food preparation methods.
   d. all of the above.

5. Mr. G. should know that factors which can trigger hyperglycemia in a diabetic include
   a. decreased exercise.
   b. increased food intake.
   c. decreased insulin.
   d. all of the above.

6. The daily intake of foods for the diabetic is spaced at regular intervals throughout the day. This should
   a. prevent hunger pangs.
   b. avoid symptoms of hypoglycemia or hyperglycemia.
   c. modify eating habits.
   d. prevent obesity.

7. Although diabetics are taught to omit foods containing sugar, exception can be made to that rule when
   a. vigorous exercise is undertaken.
   b. there is fever.
   c. gangrene has developed.
   d. there are no exceptions.

8. The caloric value of a diabetic diet should be
   a. increased above normal requirements to meet the increased metabolic demand.
   b. decreased below normal requirements to prevent glucose formation.
   c. the same as normal energy requirements to maintain ideal weight.
   d. contributed mainly by fat to spare carbohydrate.

9. The diabetic diet is designed for long-term use and contains a balance of
   a. energy.
   b. nutrients.
   c. distribution.
   d. all of the above.

10. Sources of blood glucose include
    a. carbohydrates, proteins, and fats.
    b. amino acids, cellulose, and polysaccharides.
    c. water and vitamin and mineral compounds.
    d. by-products of metabolism.

Matching

Match the terms listed on the left to the descriptions listed on the right.

11. insulin
12. hypoglycemia
13. glucagon
14. hyperglycemia
15. glycogen
16. ketosis
17. high biological value

a. a complete protein containing large amounts of essential amino acids
b. glucose in blood exceeds the normal range
c. glucose in blood below the normal range
d. a hormone that raises blood sugar levels
e. a hormone that lowers blood sugar levels
f. one result of poor utilization of carbohydrate
g. emergency supply of (stored) glucose

True/False

Circle T for True and F for False.

18. T F Group teaching of diabetics is more useful than one-on-one teaching.
19. T F The exchange lists may be successfully used whenever nutrients in a diet need to be calculated.
20. T F The milk exchange list contains cheddar and cottage cheese.
21. T F Diabetic and dietetic foods are the same thing.
22. T F Large doses of vitamin C give a false urinary glucose test.

Situation

Jane is a newly diagnosed ten-year-old diabetic. She weighs 70 lb. and is placed on a 150 g carbohydrate, 80 g protein, 50 g fat diet with afternoon and bedtime feedings. Answer the following questions by circling the letter of the correct answer.

23. The diet prescribed for Jane furnishes
    a. 1,370 calories and 1.5 g protein per kg body weight.
    b. 1,370 calories and 2.5 g protein per kg body weight.
    c. 1,110 calories and 1.5 g protein per kg body weight.
    d. 1,110 calories and 2.5 g protein per kg body weight.

24. The night feeding, consisting of milk, crackers, and butter will provide
    a. high-carbohydrate nourishment for immediate utilization.
    b. nourishment with latent effect to counteract late insulin activity.
    c. encouragement for Jane to stay on her diet.
    d. added calories to help her gain weight.

25. In planning menus for this child, one should
    a. limit calories to encourage weight loss.
    b. allow for normal growth needs.
    c. avoid using potatoes, bread, and cereal.
    d. discourage substitutions in the menu pattern.

26. The diet should be
    a. restricted only in carbohydrates.
    b. a detailed pattern of special food and insulin.
    c. a list of foods to be eaten at some time each day.
    d. a basic pattern that can be varied by substituting foods of equal nutrient content.

27. Jane's mother should know that
    a. all of her food must be weighed.
    b. she needs a snack before she exercises.
    c. she should always carry hard candy with her.
    d. she can liberalize the diet in a few years.

Diet and Disorders of the Gallbladder and Pancreas

Multiple Choice

Circle the letter of the correct answer.

1. The gallbladder stores
    a. fats.
    b. bile.
    c. cholecystokinin.
    d. cholesterol.

2. Bile functions in the digestion of food in which of the following ways?
    a. breaks fat into fatty acids and glycerol
    b. forms lipoproteins for transport to bloodstream
    c. breaks fats into very small particles for enzyme action
    d. prevents cholesterol from entering the bloodstream

3. The function of the hormone cholecystokinin is
    a. to convert fats to cholesterol.
    b. to stimulate the gallbladder to contract.
    c. to provide the necessary enzyme for fat digestion.
    d. to prevent cholesterol from crystallizing.

4. Symptoms of cholecystitis that interfere with nutrient intake include all except
    a. distention.
    b. pain.
    c. internal bleeding.
    d. nausea and vomiting.

5. Gallstones are primarily composed of
    a. calcium.
    b. chloride.
    c. cholesterol.
    d. cholecystokinin.

6. The initial diet for acute pancreatitis is
    a. I.V. therapy.
    b. low-protein, high-carbohydrate, soft.
    c. low-fat.
    d. full-liquid.

7. The diet therapy for chronic pancreatitis is
    a. bland in six feedings.
    b. low-residue every hour.

    c. liquids via tube.
    d. I.V. therapy.

Matching

Match the nursing measures appropriate to diet therapy for gallbladder disease listed on the left with the rationale for the action listed on the right.

8. Evaluate diet for vitamins A, D, E and K.
9. Provide recipes for broiling and baking foods.
10. Ask dietary personnel to remove raw apple and baked beans.
11. Ask for canned peaches and cottage cheese as a replacement for foods omitted in #10.

a. Substitute alternate sources of nutrients.
b. Fat-soluble vitamins are often inadequate.
c. Discourage use of fried foods.
d. Individual intolerance to foods requires omitting them.

True/False

Circle T for True and F for False.

12. T F Pancreatitis is a complication of cirrhosis but would not occur as a result of cholelithiasis.
13. T F Cholesterol is normally found in solution in bile.
14. T F Heredity is an important factor in gallbladder disease.
15. T F Excess polyunsaturated fats increase the risk of cholelithiasis.
16. T F Obesity is not significant in contributing to gallbladder disease.

Situation

Mrs. O., age 58, 5'1" tall, 165 lb., is admitted to the hospital with a diagnosis of acute cholecystitis. Further tests confirm the presence of cholelithiasis. The doctor tells her that surgery will be necessary, but that she will be dismissed with a modified-diet plan and return for surgery at a later date. The following questions pertain to this situation.

17. From the information given, which of the following diet prescriptions would be appropriate for Mrs. O.?
    a. 500 calorie high-protein (100 g) soft diet
    b. 1,000 calorie moderate-fat (100 g) diet
    c. 1,200 calorie, 60 g protein, 50 g fat, regular diet
    d. low-cholesterol, regular diet

Mrs. O.'s diet history reveals the following information:

Breakfast:	2 fried eggs, sausage or bacon, 2 pieces buttered toast, 1 glass milk, coffee with cream and sugar
Mid-morning snack:	1 cup dry cereal with sugar and half-and-half cream
Lunch:	sandwich (2 slices lunch meat, 1 tbsp. mayonnaise, lettuce, 2 slices bread), 1 glass milk, 1 cup canned fruit in sugar syrup
Dinner:	fried pork chop or hamburger steak with gravy, 1 c. mashed potatoes with butter, avocado salad, pie, cake or ice cream for dessert, coffee with cream and sugar
Bedtime snack:	leftover dessert or cheese and crackers or handful of peanuts, glass of cola beverage

18. This diet pattern
    a. contains adequate amounts of all the basic food groups.
    b. is short in the bread-cereal group.
    c. is short in the meat group.
    d. is short in the milk group.
    e. is short in the fruit-vegetable group.

19. In order to modify her diet to prepare for surgery, which of the following adjustments will she need to make?
    a. change methods of preparation
    b. decrease total quantity
    c. omit all snacks
    d. change type of foods consumed
    e. a, b, and d

Alter the following items from Mrs. O.'s diet history to make them suitable for her present modified diet requirements (substitutes may be made if necessary):

20. fried eggs: _____

21. fruit in sugar syrup: _____

22. lunch meat: _____

23. pie or cake: _____

24. cheese: _____

25. avocado salad: _____

26. ice cream: _____

27. lettuce: _____

Mrs. O. returns to the hospital after a few months for a cholecystectomy and an uneventful recovery.

28. The diet she was on prior to surgery will be
    a. suitable for her convalescence.
    b. changed to meet her recovery needs.
    c. permanent to maintain her weight.
    d. discontinued and TPN used.

29. While in surgery, Mrs. O. was given an injection of vitamin K. The purpose of this was to
    a. counteract bleeding tendencies present following a cholecystectomy.
    b. prevent rapid blood clotting.
    c. prevent anemia.
    d. follow routine postoperative orders.

30. A diet very low in fat may also be low in
    a. thiamin.
    b. vitamin C.
    c. vitamin A.
    d. calcium.

Diet Therapy for Disorders of the Liver

Multiple Choice

Circle the letter of the correct answer.

1. The liver stores
    a. glycogen and vitamins.
    b. ACTH and cholecystokinin.
    c. bile and cholesterol.
    d. calcium and chlorides.

2. The symptoms of hepatitis that interfere with food intake include
    a. anorexia.
    b. confusion.
    c. constipation.
    d. internal bleeding.

3. Which of the following foods may be restricted in the diet of the hepatitis patient?
    a. milk
    b. butter
    c. noodles
    d. chocolate

4. The symptom of cirrhosis that may interfere with nutrient intake is
    a. anorexia.
    b. distention.
    c. pain.
    d. all of the above.

5. Which of the following meals would best fit the needs of a cirrhotic patient with esophageal varices who is on a 350 g carbohydrate, 80 g protein, 100 g fat diet?
    a. chicken soup, beef patty, mashed potato, stewed tomatoes, cantaloupe
    b. cranberry juice, meat loaf, hash brown potato, orange slices
    c. tuna noodle casserole, lima beans, apple juice, pineapple slice
    d. peach nectar, scrambled eggs, cooked spinach, applesauce

6. The purpose of the low-protein diet (15–20 g) is to help prevent the development of hepatic coma by
    a. decreasing ammonia production.
    b. increasing sodium excretion.

    c. decreasing serum potassium.
    d. increasing the utilization of carbohydrates.

7. Which of the following meals would be appropriate for a person on a 15 g protein diet?
    a. baked potato, green beans, fruit salad, coffee with cream
    b. sliced cheese, crackers, tossed salad, Jello with whipped cream
    c. meat patty, mashed potato, steamed carrots, peach half
    d. tomato stuffed with tuna fish, crackers with butter, ice cream, tea

8. Hepatic coma results from increased blood levels of
    a. glucose.
    b. fatty acids.
    c. ammonia.
    d. sodium.

9. Diet treatment for hepatic coma includes
    a. high protein tube feedings.
    b. increased fluids.
    c. N.P.O. to rest the liver.
    d. controlled I.V. fluids.

Matching

Diet therapy for hepatitis is a major part of the treatment. Match the diet modifications on the left with the rationale for their use on the right.

10. high-protein diet
11. high-carbohydrate diet
12. high-calorie diet
13. high-fluid diet
14. moderate-fat diet

a. improves total intake
b. regenerates liver cells
c. meets increased energy demands
d. restores glycogen reserves
e. compensates for losses from fever, diarrhea

Match the actions listed on the left that apply to the nutrition and elimination needs of the patient with cirrhosis with the rationale for the action listed on the right.

15. support, encouragement, small feedings, nutrition education
16. careful monitoring of patient's mental/physical status
17. individualizing the diet
18. careful measurement of all foods/fluids ingested and excreted
19. accurate charting

a. to record the patient's condition and measures taken to restore homeostasis
b. to combat anorexia, low self-esteem
c. to watch for signs of impending coma
d. to achieve adequate nutrition and changes in diet as condition indicates
e. to prevent excess accumulation of fluids in the tissues

True/False

Circle T for True and F for False.

20. T F The diet modifications for early cirrhosis are the same ones used for hepatitis.
21. T F The diet modifications for late stages of cirrhosis are the same as for hepatitis.
22. T F Optimum nutrition can help damaged liver cells regenerate.
23. T F Ascites is accumulation of fluid in the chest cavity.
24. T F The diet for a client with liver cancer is high in carbohydrates, protein, fluid, vitamins, and calories.
25. T F Diet therapy for a patient with liver disease is individualized.

Situation

Mr. L. was admitted to the hospital complaining of abdominal pain, fatigue, and anorexia. His skin showed a yellow tinge as did the sclera of his eyes. Laboratory tests and assessments revealed evidence of liver dysfunction, fluid retention, and portal hypertension. Macrocytic anemia, thiamin and zinc deficiency were also identified. The following questions pertain to this situation.

26. From the presenting symptoms, identify the probable diagnosis.
    a. hepatitis
    b. jaundice
    c. cirrhosis
    d. cancer

27. Which of the following diet modifications would be appropriate for Mr. L.?
    a. 250 mg sodium
    b. 60 g protein
    c. fluid restriction to 1,000 ml
    d. all of the above

28. What daily measurements are appropriate for Mr. L.'s condition?
    a. intake and output
    b. weight and abdominal girth
    c. skinfold thickness
    d. all of the above

Four days after admission, Mr. L.'s condition seemed to worsen. He appeared confused, forgetful, and lethargic. His blood levels of ammonia were elevated and his skin color had deepened.

29. Given these symptoms, the most probable cause of his worsening condition is
    a. allergic reaction.
    b. impending hepatic coma.
    c. esophageal varices.
    d. advanced cirrhosis.

30. All except which of the following foods should be omitted from Mr. L.'s diet while he is in this stage of his illness?
    a. milk and meat
    b. vegetables and fruits
    c. butter and honey
    d. grains and legumes

Diet Therapy for Renal Disorders

Multiple Choice

Circle the letter of the correct answer.

1. Antiotensin II, which is secreted by the kidneys, is a(an)
   a. proteolytic enzyme.
   b. vasoconstrictor.
   c. precursor to erythropoietin.
   d. indicator of kidney disease.

2. Lack of erythropoietin results in
   a. anemia.
   b. albuminuria.
   c. hematuria.
   d. hypertension.

3. Lack of active vitamin D hormone will
   a. result in high blood pressure.
   b. cause an imbalance of calcium and phosphorus.
   c. cause metabolic acidosis.
   d. result in oliguria.

4. Acute glomerulonephritis is the result of
   a. hereditary defects.
   b. hypertensive crisis.
   c. acute malnutrition.
   d. streptococci infection.

5. Dietary management of renal disease requires correction of imbalances in which of these?
   a. fluids and electrolytes
   b. acidosis or alkalosis
   c. blood pressure and weight
   d. all of these

6. Blood protein loss is _____ in hemodialysis than in peritoneal dialysis.
   a. greater
   b. lesser
   c. the same
   d. not lost in either

7. A major disruption in renal functioning affects the metabolism of which of these nutrients?
   a. carbohydrates, fats, and vitamins
   b. protein, minerals, and water
   c. blood, acids, and alkalines
   d. cellulose, chlorides, and calcium

8. Hemodialysis treatments for a person in renal failure will
   a. increase the protein requirement.
   b. decrease the protein requirement.
   c. maintain the protein synthesis.
   d. not affect the protein requirement.

9. The principles of dietary treatment for urinary calculi center around which of the following?
   a. diet therapy based on stone chemistry
   b. an attempt to change urinary pH
   c. a large fluid intake
   d. all of the above

10. The most common type of kidney stone is that composed of
    a. calcium.
    b. uric acid.
    c. cystine.
    d. magnesium.

11. The type of diet recommended for a calcium stone would be
    a. alkaline ash.
    b. acid ash.
    c. protein restricted.
    d. protein increased.

12. Which of the following foods would you expect to be prohibited on an acid-ash diet?
    a. bread, macaroni, eggs, cranberries
    b. oranges, bananas, lima beans, olives
    c. meat, cheese, eggs, plums
    d. spaghetti, prunes, eggs, meat

13. Which of the following foods would you expect to find on an alkaline-ash diet?
    a. meat, cheese, eggs, corn
    b. milk, coconut, chestnuts, oranges
    c. prunes, cranberries, plums, honey
    d. peanuts, walnuts, bacon, rice

True/False

Circle T for True and F for False

14. T F Each kidney contains over a million nephrons.
15. T F Vitamin D activity is maintained by the kidney.

16. T F   Hyperphosphaturia lowers serum calcium.
17. T F   Dietary management of CRF is more moderate than the diet for acute glomerulonephritis.
18. T F   Deterioration of the nephrons can cause anemia.
19. T F   Diet therapy for renal disease is a standard prescription of 500 mg sodium 25 gm protein.
20. T F   500 ml of water to cover insensible loss is added to the amount of urine excreted.

Matching

Match the terms on the left with their definitions listed on the right.

21. diaphoresis
22. glomerulus
23. nephron
24. antigen
25. antibody

a. a foreign invader of the body
b. cluster of capillaries in a capsule
c. destroyer of foreign invaders
d. profuse perspiration
e. basic unit of the kidney

Situation

Mrs. J. has a diagnosis of uremia. After an individualized assessment of her status, she is placed on a 2,000-calorie, 1,000-mg sodium, 2,500-mg potassium, 60-g protein diet. Her fluid intake is restricted to 500 ml plus the amount excreted the prior 24 hours.

26. This diet regime will fulfill which of the following treatment objectives?
    a. correct electrolyte imbalance
    b. minimize protein catabolism
    c. avoid dehydration/overhydration
    d. all of the above

27. If Mrs. J. is still hungry after eating all of her meal, which of the following snacks would you suggest to comply with her restrictions?
    a. banana and sugar wafers
    b. arrowroot cookies with whipped topping
    c. cottage cheese and fruit cocktail
    d. puffed wheat with milk and sugar

28. Mrs. J.'s usual eating pattern includes many protein foods with low biological value, which must be avoided. Which of the following foods would you restrict?
    a. cereal grains and vegetables
    b. milk and eggs
    c. cream, honey, and most fruits
    d. meat, fish, and poultry

29. Mrs. J.'s output for the previous 24 hours is 500 ml, so she receives 1,000 ml of fluids the next 24 hours. This fluid intake
    a. should come from water and be consumed all at once.
    b. should come from foods, water, and other fluids and be divided equally throughout the day.
    c. should be given by I.V. drip.
    d. should be a saline/dextrose solution.

30. Mrs. J. develops a fever and diarrhea. Her fluid intake should
    a. remain the same.
    b. be further restricted to curtail the diarrhea.
    c. be increased to compensate for the fluid loss.
    d. be administered via tube feeding.

Diet Therapy for Burns, Cancer, Anorexia Nervosa, and AIDS

Multiple Choice

Circle the letter of the correct answer.

1. Interferences to successful feeding of burn patients include all except which of these?
   a. food brought from home
   b. difficulty swallowing or chewing
   c. psychological trauma
   d. anorexia

2. Aggressive nutritional therapy aims to keep weight loss at less than _____ percent of preburn body weight.
   a. 35
   b. 25
   c. 15
   d. 10

3. Fluid and electrolyte replacement are crucial to recovery from burns. Which of these two electrolytes are most likely to be deficient?
   a. iron and zinc
   b. glucose and calcium
   c. sodium and potassium
   d. phosphorus and magnesium

4. Immediate replacement of fluid and electrolytes is necessary to prevent
   a. edema and ascites.
   b. hypovolemic shock.
   c. hyperphosphatemia.
   d. anaphylactic shock.

5. Daily caloric need for a patient with a burn injury is calculated at _____ kcal/kg of normal body weight and _____ kcal/kg percent of body surface burned.
   a. 25, 40
   b. 10, 30
   c. 40, 40
   d. 25, 50

6. Daily protein need for a patient with a burn injury is calculated at _____ gm/kg normal body weight and _____ g/kg percent of body surface burned.
   a. 2, 4
   b. 1, 3
   c. 0.8, 1.2
   d. 2, 2.5

7. The amount of vitamin C given to a burn patient is usually
   a. 2–10 times RDA.
   b. 10–20 times RDA.
   c. 20–30 times RDA.
   d. 1,000 mg daily.

8. A food high in zinc includes
   a. seafood.
   b. liver.
   c. eggs.
   d. all of the above.

9. The burn patient with edema and/or ascites may also be
   a. fatigued.
   b. nervous.
   c. thirsty.
   d. confused.

10. What method(s) is/are used to combat renal calculi in an immobilized patient?
    a. provide a low-calcium diet
    b. increase fluids
    c. assist early ambulation
    d. all of these

11. The nutritional changes that are characteristic of nearly all cancer patients include all except which of these?
    a. altered metabolic rate
    b. increased drug absorption
    c. negative nitrogen balance
    d. susceptibility

12. After surgical correction of a problem that once caused abdominal pain, the patient continues to experience pain. This is known as
    a. avoidance.
    b. aversion.
    c. conditioned response.
    d. referred pain.

13. The most negative effects on nutritional status occurring from radiation therapy include
    a. reduced food intake.
    b. impaired taste acuity.
    c. intestinal obstruction.
    d. all of these.

14. The most negative effects of chemotherapy include all except which of these?
    a. esophageal varices
    b. fluid and electrolyte imbalance
    c. impaired taste acuity
    d. diarrhea

15. A "rule of thumb" guideline for feeding cancer patients is which of these?
    a. Serve the foods known to be acceptable to most patients.
    b. There are no "rules" for feeding cancer patients.
    c. Most cancer patients should be on TPN.
    d. Verbal reminders at frequent intervals of the importance of eating.

Matching

For each nutritional intervention for an AIDS patient listed at the left, supply the rationale.

16. Stop weight loss
17. Preserve or rebuild lean body mass
18. Use nutritional supplements with an adequate diet
19. Minimize malabsorption
20. Deal with specific diet problems

a. Provide nutrition education
b. Assess nutritional status regularly
c. Supply HBV protein
d. Ask for vitamin/mineral supplements in high concentration
e. Provide easily assimilated fats

True or False

21. T F An AIDS patient may exhibit symptoms of mental disorders.

22. T F Parenteral feedings may be ordered for an AIDS patient with varying degrees of sepsis.

23. T F An AIDS patient may have respiratory problems resembling those of COPD (chronic obstructive pulmonary disease).

24. T F Foodborne infections occur no more frequently in AIDS patients than in any other sick person.

25. T F Food safety and sanitation practices, as prescribed by the state, should be enough protection for an AIDS patient.

26. T F Radiation therapy effects depend upon the site of radiation.

27. T F Insulin deficiency may occur after surgical therapy, especially gastric or pancreatic resection.

28. T F While anorexia may occur with radiation therapy, tooth decay and gum disease are symptoms of intestinal obstruction.

29. T F Different combinations of chemotherapy may cause exacerbations of existing nutritional problems.

30. T F The likelihood of mortality from second and third degree burns decreases with age.

Principles of Feeding a Sick Child

Multiple Choice

Circle the letter of the correct answer.

1. Which of these factors decrease the probability of adequately feeding a sick child?
   a. fear, anxiety, anorexia
   b. pain, fatigue, lethargy
   c. vomiting, nausea, medications
   d. all of the above

2. Which of the following is not a factor in planning nutritional care for a hospitalized child?
   a. individual likes and dislikes
   b. personal eating patterns
   c. home feeding environment
   d. type of disease

3. Which of these considerations has little influence on the dietary care of a sick child?
   a. nutritional status of the child before hospitalization
   b. the onset and duration of symptoms
   c. rehabilitation measures needed
   d. the presence of others at mealtime

4. From which of these factors are feeding problems unlikely to develop?
   a. child's past experience with food
   b. child's nutritional status when admitted
   c. child's unreasonable demands
   d. child's fear and anxiety

5. Which of these functions would not be appropriate for the pediatric nurse to perform?
   a. Suggest changes in diet orders to the physician when deemed necessary.
   b. Request supplemental fluids/foods as needed.
   c. Ask the parents to refrain from being present at feeding time and upsetting the child.
   d. Record incidences of feeding tantrums and/or manipulation.

6. If a child must have a modified diet, which of the following guidelines will be likely to increase acceptance?
   a. Start the new regime immediately in order to teach the child to comply.
   b. Move into the new diet gradually in order to give the child time to adjust.
   c. Put the new diet in writing and let the mother start the child on the diet when they get home.
   d. Use different kinds of utensils and foods to spark interest in the new diet.

7. Which of these responses would be the most appropriate for the hospitalized child who is not eating?
   a. "If you don't eat better than this, the doctor will stick a tube down your throat."
   b. "You can't have your dessert unless you clean your plate."
   c. "Would you help me select your food for the next meal?"
   d. "Do you want to upset your mother by refusing to eat?"

8. A child's food intake may be improved by using all of the following measures except
   a. allowing self-selection.
   b. serving familiar foods.
   c. providing a cheerful environment.
   d. requiring a child to "clean the plate."

9. Instructions given to children on modified diets should be
   a. given to both parent and child.
   b. given slowly, repeated, and responses noted.
   c. based on the child's readiness to learn.
   d. all of the above.

10. The hospitalized child who is allowed freedom in choosing the foods he or she eats
    a. may become malnourished.
    b. may eat more food.
    c. may get diarrhea.
    d. may become unmanageable.

11. Sick children fail to receive adequate intake for which of the following reasons?
    a. Their gastrointestinal tract malfunctions.
    b. They have high metabolic demands.
    c. They have neurological and psychological disturbances.
    d. all of the above

12. Diarrhea in very young children
    a. is often caused by overfeeding.
    b. causes fluid and electrolyte imbalances.
    c. requires hospitalization.
    d. causes colic.

Matching

Match the assessment data listed on the left to the type of assessment it represents at the right. (Terms may be used more than once.)

13. hemoglobin/hematocrit
14. head circumference
15. distended abdomen
16. x-rays
17. skinfold thickness

a. anthropometric
b. physical
c. laboratory

True/False

Circle T for True and F for False

18. T F The same diet principles used for feeding a well child apply to feeding a sick child.
19. T F A diet that meets the RDAs and is based on the basic food groups satisfies the needs of all growing children.
20. T F Children of different ethnic origins should be fed the same foods in order to not discriminate.
21. T F The food choices for sick children should not be limited regardless of the disease process.
22. T F Children like to eat in groups rather than alone.
23. T F Psychosocial problems may contribute to a child's failure to eat adequately.
24. T F Children like to try new and different foods.
25. T F It is not unusual for a five-year-old to want to be fed.

Situation

Johnny, age six, was hospitalized for tests, due to weight loss, irritability, diarrhea, and a low-grade fever.

26. Which of the following statements is most accurate regarding Johnny's nutritional status?
    a. He probably has pneumonia.
    b. He has extensive nutrient and fluid loss.
    c. He has lactose intolerance.
    d. His condition may be due to neglect by his mother.

27. Johnny has food and fluids withheld for tests. When he is allowed to eat again, which of these interventions is most appropriate?
    a. Make up missed meals with supplements.
    b. Provide six small meals instead of three large ones.
    c. Ask for soft solids instead of regular food.
    d. all of the above

28. Johnny does not seem to care for hospital food. The nurse should allow
    a. food brought in from home or a fast food outlet.
    b. him to skip meals he doesn't like.
    c. only what the diet order calls for.
    d. none of the above.

Diet Therapy and Cystic Fibrosis

Multiple Choice

Circle the letter of the correct answer.

1. Cystic fibrosis is an inherited disease that primarily affects the
   a. mucous and sweat glands.
   b. lungs and liver.
   c. pancreas and mucous and sweat glands.
   d. digestive system.

2. Malnutrition in the child with cystic fibrosis is caused primarily by
   a. lack of digestive enzymes.
   b. excessive electrolytes in sweat.
   c. lung infections.
   d. vomiting and diarrhea.

3. Failure to thrive, which is a manifestation of cystic fibrosis, describes the child who
   a. is small for gestational age.
   b. shows reduced weight gain or height appropriate for age.
   c. is malnourished.
   d. dies before reaching maturity.

4. The proper diagnosis of a child with cystic fibrosis is determined from
   a. x-rays of the chest.
   b. clinical symptoms.
   c. sodium chloride in sweat.
   d. all of the above.

5. Lack of which of the following secretions creates the malabsorption syndrome in cystic fibrosis children?
   a. lipase, trypsin, amylase
   b. sodium, potassium, iron
   c. antibodies
   d. fat-soluble vitamins

6. Early diagnosis and treatment of cystic fibrosis
   a. can restore normal body size and appearance.
   b. cannot prevent mental retardation.
   c. prevents delayed sexual development.
   d. all of the above

7. The goals of diet therapy for cystic fibrosis include which of the following?
   a. increase body weight
   b. control or prevent rectum prolapse
   c. control or improve emotional problems associated with the disease
   d. all of the above

8. Which of these statements is correct regarding the use of pancreatic enzymes?
   a. Infants and small children are given injections of enzymes.
   b. Enzymes are given at least one hour before mealtimes.
   c. Prolonged use of enzymes can cause psychological problems.
   d. Enzymes may cause ulceration.

9. Which of the following statements is true regarding use of medium chain triglycerides?
   a. They increase energy intake.
   b. They promote fat absorption.
   c. They reduce malabsorption.
   d. all of the above

10. Nutrient dense supplements useful in diet therapy for cystic fibrosis include all except which of these products?
    a. protein hydrolysate solutions
    b. beef serum, commercial supplements
    c. medium-chain triglycerides and glucose solutions
    d. fat polymers

Matching

Match the principles of dietary management listed on the left with the rationale listed on the right.

11. high-calorie diet
12. high-protein diet
13. low- to moderate-fat diet
14. generous salt in diet
15. vitamin supplements
16. pancreatic enzymes

a. to compensate for pancreatic deficiency
b. to compensate for fecal losses
c. to meet high energy demands
d. to limit steatorrhea
e. to replace electrolyte losses
f. to meet need for three times the RDA

True/False

Circle T for True and F for False.

17. T F Children with cystic fibrosis produce heavy viscid mucus.
18. T F Children with cystic fibrosis digest very little of their protein.

471

19. T F Up to 12 percent of cystic fibrosis patients are diagnosed at birth because of a bowel obstruction.
20. T F The child with cystic fibrosis usually is anorexic.
21. T F General feeding techniques used for all children cannot be applied to cystic fibrosis children.
22. T F Use of pancreatic enzymes definitely improves the nutritional status of the child with cystic fibrosis.
23. T F A child with cystic fibrosis may have deficient linoleic acid.
24. T F The caloric need for children with cystic fibrosis may be 80–110 percent above normal requirements.
25. T F Lactose deficiency is sometimes a complication in cystic fibrosis.

Situation

José is a fourteen-year-old male with cystic fibrosis admitted to the hospital with pneumonia. He is short of breath, is coughing, and has a temperature of 102°. His appetite is poor and he is approximately 20 lb. underweight for his age and height. The orders are for a 3,500 calorie high-protein, low-fat, soft diet. He also is prescribed pancreatic enzymes, water-miscible fat-soluble vitamin supplements, medium-chain triglyceride supplements, and extra fluid.

26. In order to increase calories, he receives a chocolate milk shake between meals, which he likes. The most probable outcome of this kind of supplement is that
   a. he will regain some lost weight.
   b. he will get diarrhea.
   c. he will receive excessive amounts of cholesterol.
   d. he will get acne.

27. Briefly explain the reason for each of the following diet orders:

a. fat-soluble, water-miscible vitamin supplements

_____

_____

b. pancreatic enzymes

_____

_____

c. medium-chain triglyceride supplements

_____

_____

d. extra fluids

_____

_____

28. List four important instructions to be given to José and his family regarding his diet when he returns home.
   a. _____
   b. _____
   c. _____
   d. _____

29. List the four major nursing implications required to adequately implement nutrition principles for a cystic fibrosis patient.
   a. _____
   b. _____
   c. _____
   d. _____

Diet Therapy and Celiac Disease

Multiple Choice

Circle the letter of the correct answer.

1. The protein to which patients are intolerant when they have celiac disease is
   a. phenylalanine.
   b. casein.
   c. gluten.
   d. glycogen.

2. Celiac patients have mucosal atrophy of the small intestine. This means that
   a. villi are lacking.
   b. the villi are flat instead of round.
   c. only small amounts of digestive enzymes are secreted.
   d. all of the above.

3. Which of the following are presenting symptoms of celiac disease?
   a. diarrhea, steatorrhea, irritability
   b. irregular heartbeat, fever, lethargy
   c. anorexia, eczema, dehydration
   d. hyperactivity, infections, weight loss

4. Which of these symptoms indicate malnutrition in the celiac patient?
   a. cheilosis, glossitis, anemia, tetany
   b. hyperosmolarity, arrhythmias, acidosis
   c. hypoglycemia, flatulence, cramps
   d. all of the above

5. The basic principle of diet therapy for celiac disease is to
   a. exclude all sources of glycogen.
   b. exclude all sources of gluten.
   c. exclude all sources of lactose.
   d. exclude all sources of casein.

6. Celiac disease in children can be cured in which of the following time frames?
   a. 1–2 weeks
   b. 1–5 years
   c. time varies with each child
   d. celiac disease is never cured

7. Which of the following foods must be excluded from the diet of the person with celiac disease?
   a. rye, wheat, barley, and oats
   b. potatoes, corn, rice, malt
   c. arrowroot, soybean, tapioca
   d. all of these

8. Which of the following foods would be suitable for a celiac patient?
   a. chicken fried steak, breaded veal cutlet, fish sticks
   b. roast beef, baked chicken, broiled salmon
   c. fried chicken, meat loaf, lobster thermidor
   d. marinated herring, chili con carne, lamb chops

9. Which of the following statements is appropriate when teaching a celiac patient regarding his diet therapy?
   a. "You must read all labels carefully."
   b. "Let's talk about ways to prevent infections."
   c. "These substitutes are needed to help you balance your diet."
   d. a, b, and c are all appropriate

10. When the offending foods have been removed from the diet of the celiac patient, which of these nutrients are most likely to be deficient?
    a. vitamins A, D, E, and K
    b. thiamin, niacin, and iron
    c. sodium, protein, and carbohydrates
    d. all of these

Matching

Match the food in the left column to its appropriate use in the right column.

11. crisped rice cereal
12. ice cream cone
13. pancakes
14. fruit
15. potatoes
16. chocolate candy
17. peanut butter
18. malted milk shake
19. cornbread and butter
20. catsup

a. permitted
b. prohibited
c. limited

True/False

Circle T for True and F for False.

21. T F Children are the only population group to have celiac disease.

22. T F A lowered prothrombin time indicates that the blood clots too quickly.

23. T F Adult patients seem to recover from celiac disease better than children.

24. T F Celiac diet therapy usually requires vitamin supplements.
25. T F The symptoms of celiac disease and cystic fibrosis are very similar.

Situation

Bonnie is an 18-month-old infant brought to the clinic after her mother called the nurse there to ask what she might do to alleviate the problem of 3 or 4 foul smelling, foamy stools per day. The mother had been offering Bonnie lots of fluids but she refused them. A diagnosis of celiac disease was made.

26. What additional information would you need in order to plan diet therapy?

    _____

    _____

    _____

27. Loss of which of the following nutrients would be of greatest concern for Bonnie?
    a. water, sodium, potassium
    b. fat-soluble and water-soluble vitamins
    c. fats, calcium, carbohydrates
    d. all of the above

28. Plan a one-day menu pattern that could be used as a teaching tool for Bonnie's mother.

    _____

    _____

    _____

    _____

    _____

29. List three commercial products useful in supplementing the diet of the child with celiac disease.

    a. _____

    b. _____

    c. _____

30. Bonnie's mother asks how long she will have to be on this diet. Your most appropriate answer would be
    a. to recommend the diet be continued indefinitely.
    b. three to six months.
    c. until she is at least six years old.
    d. until she is a teenager.

Diet Therapy and Congenital Heart Disease

Multiple Choice

Circle the letter of the correct answer.

1. Which of the following manifestations, in a child with congenital heart disease, affects nutritional status?
   a. malabsorption of nutrients
   b. elevated body temperature
   c. excessive urinary output
   d. all of the above

2. Caloric need is higher for children with congenital heart disease than for healthy children because
   a. the metabolic rate is higher.
   b. the antibody production is low.
   c. the kidneys are malfunctioning.
   d. all of these

3. Which of these nutrients are primarily responsible for renal overload?
   a. water, oxygen
   b. sodium, potassium
   c. calcium, iron
   d. phosphates, chlorides

4. Which of these foods are not tolerated well by children with congenital heart disease?
   a. fats and sugar in quantity
   b. proteins
   c. fluids in quantity
   d. vitamin supplements

5. Which of these factors result in vitamin/mineral deficiencies in children with congenital heart disease?
   a. amount of food consumed is too small to be adequate
   b. allergy to foods containing vitamins
   c. nonprescription vitamins do not contain all the child needs
   d. a and c

6. The introduction of solid foods to a child with congenital heart disease is delayed in order to
   a. keep the sodium content in the diet low.
   b. avoid the problem of diarrhea.
   c. reduce the workload on the heart.
   d. prevent dehydration.

7. Caretakers of children with congenital heart disease should be taught
   a. to omit sodium from the diet.
   b. principles of a balanced diet.
   c. to read labels.
   d. all of these

8. Which of these discharge procedures should the nurse follow when a child with congenital heart disease is going home?
   a. Provide teaching and referrals for follow up.
   b. Provide psychiatric counseling.
   c. Provide special products.
   d. all of these

9. Which of these guidelines provides appropriate distribution of nutrients for the child with congenital heart disease?
   a. 40% carbohydrates, 20% proteins, 30% fat
   b. 35–65% carbohydrates, 10% proteins, 30–50% fat
   c. 30% carbohydrates, 30% protein, 40% fat
   d. none of these

10. Which of the following statements best describes a milliequivalent?
    a. a metric unit of volume
    b. amount of solute dissolved in a milliliter of solution
    c. concentration of an ion in solution
    d. amount of solution in a metric unit

Matching

Match the dietary alteration at the left to the correct rationale at right.

11. MCT oil
12. folic acid
13. extra juices, water
14. extra energy supplements
15. limited sodium, potassium

a. prevent dehydration
b. prevent renal overload
c. prevent vitamin deficiency
d. provide adequate fat absorption
e. increase caloric intake

True/False

Circle T for True and F for False.

16. **T F** A child with congenital heart disease may voluntarily reduce food intake.
17. **T F** The only cure for congenital heart disease is successful surgery.
18. **T F** The child should weigh at least 30 pounds before surgery is performed.
19. **T F** Regular foods are not used at all for children with congenital heart disease.
20. **T F** A congenital disease means that it is inherited.
21. **T F** Heart disease in children is readily identified at birth.
22. **T F** The cause of congenital heart disease is unknown.
23. **T F** The mortality rate for children with congenital heart disease is not as high for small children as for larger ones.
24. **T F** Children with congenital heart disease tend to be overdependent.
25. **T F** Children with congenital heart disease and parents may need counseling for psychological problems as well as dietary ones.

Situation

Teresa is eight months old and has a ventricular septal defect (V.S.D., a common congenital heart defect). She needs to gain a minimum of 10 pounds before she can have surgery to close the hole in the septum.

26. The major nutritional management for this child is to
   a. provide essential nutrients that are easily digested.
   b. provide high calorie food and fluids without overloading the kidneys.
   c. provide small, frequent feedings rather than three large meals.
   d. all of these.

27. List three suitable energy supplements for Teresa that should assist in weight gain.

   a. _____

   b. _____

   c. _____

28. Provide a one-day menu pattern that Teresa's mother may use to plan her food intake.

   _____

   _____

   _____

29. Describe four feeding problems Teresa's mother may encounter and solutions to each.

   a. _____

   b. _____

   c. _____

   d. _____

30. List four important dietary principles Teresa's mother should learn.

   a. _____

   b. _____

   c. _____

   d. _____

Diet Therapy and Food Allergy

Multiple Choice

Circle the letter of the correct answer.

1. Maldigestion or malabsorption of food may be termed
   a. a food allergy.
   b. malnutrition.
   c. a food intolerance.
   d. an immunological reaction.

2. Substances that trigger allergic reactions are
   a. allergens.
   b. enzymes.
   c. antigens.
   d. a or c.

3. Less than _____ of all people in the United States have some form of food allergy.
   a. 8 percent
   b. 25 percent
   c. 50 percent
   d. 1 percent

4. Allergens are usually
   a. food additives.
   b. proteins.
   c. sugars.
   d. food preservatives

5. Food allergies are more prevalent in
   a. adolescence.
   b. childhood.
   c. adulthood.
   d. both b and c.

6. The most common food allergy in children is an allergy to
   a. nuts.
   b. wheat.
   c. soy.
   d. cow's milk.

7. The milk of choice for an infant from a family prone to allergies is
   a. cow's milk.
   b. soy formula.
   c. breast milk.
   d. evaporated milk.

Matching

Match the potential offender on the right with the food source on the left. Answers may be listed more than once.

8. mayonnaise
9. tartrazine
10. chocolate
11. tangerine
12. pumpkin pie
13. custard
14. licorice
15. corn syrup

a. legumes
b. corn
c. milk
d. eggs
e. kola nuts
f. citrus fruits
g. spices
h. artificial food colors

True/False

Circle T for True and F for False.

16. T F Most people exhibit symptoms of a food allergy, but are unaware that these symptoms are the result of a food allergy.

17. T F Skin testing is an accurate method of detecting food allergies.

18. T F An infant with a risk for developing allergies should receive solid foods as early as possible.

19. T F Depending on the number of foods eliminated, an antiallergic diet may be nutritionally inadequate.

20. T F Food allergies are relatively easy to diagnose and confirm.

21. T F Once the offending food has been determined, it should never be reintroduced into the patient's diet.

22. T F Raw foods are more likely to be allergens than the cooked form.

Situation

Bobby is exhibiting the following symptoms: skin rash, diarrhea, and nasal congestion. His mother is concerned that he may be allergic to something he is eating.

23. What would be your first course of action in determining whether a food allergy is actually the cause of the symptoms?

24. You notice that Bobby is routinely eating some of the foods listed among the top ten offenders for children. These are cow's milk, wheat, eggs, and corn. What would you suggest to Bobby's mother at this point?

_____

_____

_____

_____

_____

25. From close monitoring of Bobby's diet, it has been determined that Bobby is allergic to cow's milk and wheat. Besides fluid milk, name five sources of cow's milk that Bobby may also be allergic to.

a. _____

b. _____

c. _____

d. _____

e. _____

Name five sources of wheat Bobby may need to avoid.

f. _____

g. _____

h. _____

i. _____

j. _____

26. As Bobby grows older, should he try to reintroduce milk or wheat products back into his diet? Why or why not? _____

_____

_____

Diet Therapy and Phenylketonuria

Multiple Choice

Circle the letter of the correct answer.

1. Which of the following statements most accurately describes the etiology of PKU (phenylketonuria)?
   a. There is an inability to convert phenylalanine into tyrosine.
   b. There is a lack of synthesis of phenylalanine.
   c. There is a lack of the essential amino acids.
   d. There is a lack of leucine conversion to lysine.

2. The most serious effect of untreated PKU is
   a. behavior disturbances.
   b. convulsive seizures.
   c. mental retardation.
   d. reticulosarcoma.

3. Children with PKU usually have lighter complexions, hair, and eyes than normal children because of
   a. their genetic makeup.
   b. lack of tyrosine.
   c. failure to thrive.
   d. lack of amino acid metabolism.

4. Which of the following statements expresses the dietary management of PKU children?
   a. Rigidly restrict phenylalanine intake.
   b. Make the diet very low in tyrosine.
   c. Make the diet very low in galactose.
   d. Omit phenylalanine and tyrosine entirely.

5. If treatment is started after retardation has occurred, which of the following outcomes may be expected?
   a. Normal ability will return completely.
   b. Retardation will continue, as the process is irreversible.
   c. Growth and development will slow or stop.
   d. Normal ability will not return but the retardation will not proceed any further.

6. An infant should be provided with enough phenylalanine to maintain a serum level of
   a. 3–10 mg per 100 ml.
   b. 10–29 mg per 100 ml.
   c. 20–25 mg per 100 ml.
   d. PKU infants should not have a serum phenylalanine.

7. After the clinical condition of a one-year-old child with PKU stabilizes, what information concerning blood tests is most appropriate?

   a. The blood should be tested twice weekly.
   b. The blood should be tested daily.
   c. The blood should be tested weekly.
   d. The blood should be tested monthly.

8. The diet for PKU children must meet which of these criteria?
   a. Provide for normal growth and development.
   b. Maintain phenylalanine within safe limits.
   c. Permit liberalization to conform to culture.
   d. a and b

9. The steps necessary for planning the diet for a PKU child include which of these?
   a. Determine age, weight, activity level.
   b. Determine daily phenylalanine required and amount of protein to be given.
   c. Determine calories received from formula, milk, and food.
   d. All of these steps are necessary.

10. Which of these techniques would promote dietary compliance in a PKU child?
    a. Remove all desserts until the child eats other food.
    b. Vary taste, texture, and variety within limits of diet.
    c. Increase the amount of milk in the diet.
    d. Omit all snacks.

Matching

Match the foods at the left with their use in the PKU diet at right.

11. meats
12. Lofenalac
13. fruits
14. vegetables
15. cheese

a. permitted
b. prohibited
c. limited

True/False

Circle T for True and F for False.

16. T F The only treatment for PKU is diet therapy.
17. T F Babies born with PKU can now be diagnosed early enough to prevent serious side effects.
18. T F Once PKU has been diagnosed, all offending substances must be omitted entirely from the diet.

19. T F Emotional support for the family is an important part of the management of PKU children.
20. T F The symptoms of PKU and cystic fibrosis are very similar.
21. T F A baby with PKU can be successfully breast-fed if the mother is willing to try.
22. T F PKU is self-limiting; the child will outgrow it.
23. T F Insufficient phenylalanine will result in mental retardation.
24. T F Excessive phenylalanine will result in mental retardation.
25. T F It is recommended that the special diet be discontinued by age four.

Situation

Terry is a three-year-old male who is seen in the pediatrician's office for a routine checkup. He has PKU but no other problems. He is 40 inches tall and weighs 36 pounds. His mother asks for a consultation with a dietitian because she believes it is time to liberalize Terry's diet. He still drinks Lofenalac and his mother monitors all the food he eats, but lately he has been crying for the hamburgers and hot dogs his father and older brothers eat. He will also start nursery school soon. His phenylalanine level is 9mg/100 ml of blood.

Circle the correct response.

26. a. Is the phenylalanine level acceptable? Yes No
    b. Is Terry's weight and height in normal range? Yes No

27. What response would be appropriate regarding liberalizing Terry's diet?
    a. "Yes, I agree it's time he got other foods."
    b. "You may ask for a second opinion, but specialists agree that three years is too early."
    c. "Why don't you stop feeding the others what Terry can't eat?"
    d. "Do you think this is just a phase he's going through?"

28. Plan a one-day menu suitable for Terry. _____
    _____
    _____
    _____
    _____
    _____
    _____
    _____
    _____

29. What substances must be calculated in this diet to make sure it is adequate and safe?
    a. carbohydrate, protein, fat
    b. phenylalanine, protein, calories
    c. calcium, magnesium, iron
    d. phenylalanine, vitamins, calories

Diet Therapy for Constipation, Diarrhea, and High-Risk Infants

Multiple Choice

Circle the letter of the correct answer.

1. Safe food(s) that may be used to combat constipation in infants include
   a. prune juice.
   b. 1 teaspoon sugar/4 ounces formula.
   c. strained apricots.
   d. all of the above.

2. Recommended treatment for dry, hard stools in an infant is to
   a. increase formula feedings.
   b. increase fluids.
   c. increase laxative intake.
   d. increase activity level.

3. Two types of constipation common in children under five years old are
   a. physiological and psychological.
   b. anatomical and environmental.
   c. psychological and anatomical.
   d. environmental and physiological.

4. Parents may initiate a regular pattern of elimination by which of these methods?
   a. Put the child on a regular schedule.
   b. Increase foods with fluids and fiber.
   c. Decrease formula to 80 percent of normal.
   d. all of the above

5. If a child has diarrhea for several weeks, but continues to grow at a normal rate, the problem is classified as
   a. celiac disease.
   b. chronic diarrhea.
   c. acute diarrhea.
   d. allergy diarrhea.

6. Which of these beverages contain high amounts of both sodium and potassium?
   a. orange juice
   b. Pepsi Cola
   c. skim milk
   d. grape juice

7. The dietary management of diarrhea in children includes all except which of these steps?
   a. Restore fluid and electrolyte balance.
   b. Use an elimination diet.
   c. Restore adequate nutrition.
   d. Increase the kcal content of the diet.

8. Added foods that will increase a one year old's kcal content when the child is recovering from diarrhea include
   a. eggnog.
   b. milkshakes.
   c. strained cereal.
   d. all of these.

9. Caloric needs of the high-risk infant are
   a. twice those of a normal infant.
   b. three to four times those of a normal infant.
   c. approximately six times those of a normal infant.
   d. the same as those of a normal infant; they have little movement.

10. High-risk infants need large amounts of fluid for all except which of these reasons?
    a. They require extra essential amino acids.
    b. They have a larger body water content than normal infants.
    c. Their kidneys can't concentrate urine.
    d. They have increased water evaporation.

11. First feedings for high-risk infants include
    a. TPN.
    b. fluid with extra calories.
    c. 10 percent glucose IVs.
    d. no feeding until stabilized.

12. A mother can breast feed her premature infant when
    a. the baby weighs more than 4 pounds.
    b. the baby has sucking reflexes.
    c. the baby gets additional supplements.
    d. all of the above.

True/False

Circle T for True and F for False.

13. T F Diarrhea is an infrequent occurrence among infants and young children.
14. T F Infants and young children with diarrhea can be managed at home unless dehydration occurs.
15. T F Milk is high in sodium.
16. T F A hypotonic solution contains excess electrolytes and glucose.
17. T F Low-residue diets are used after diarrhea has subsided.
18. T F Tyrosine and cystine are essential amino acids.

481

19. **T F** Lytren is an essential amino acid especially for children.
20. **T F** High-risk infants may be able to breast feed.

Matching

Match the term on the left to the definition that best defines it.

21. Meconium
22. Mucilage
23. Benign
24. Electrolyte
25. Prematurity

   a. substance that dissolves in water into ions
   b. interrupted before maturity
   c. not recurrent
   d. dark green substance in fetal intestine
   e. aqueous gummy substance

Match the characteristics of normal fecal material on the right to the most likely type of feeding.

26. Commercial formula
27. Breast milk, 3 months
28. Regular foods, 10 months
29. Whole milk, 10 months
30. Mixed diet (liquid, solid), 1 year

   a. similar to adult
   b. intense yellow, firm
   c. highly variable
   d. golden, creamy texture
   e. compressed, pale yellow

Module 1

1.	b	8.	a	15.	a	22.	T
2.	d	9.	b	16.	T	23.	T
3.	a	10.	d	17.	T	24.	F
4.	c	11.	e	18.	T	25.	T
5.	d	12.	c	19.	T		
6.	a	13.	b	20.	T		
7.	b	14.	d	21.	F		

26. Milk and milk products (margarine is a fat, and does not contain the nutrients of milk).
27. b. This would make four servings of fruit and vegetables, the required amount daily for an adult.
28. None—there is at least one food from each group in Jane's cart.
29. b. Meats, fresh vegetables, butter, fluid milk, mixes, and sweets cost more.
30. b. Shrimp, sausage, butter, and the cream in whole milk contain saturated fats.

Module 2

1.	c	9.	b	17.	F	25.	T
2.	d	10.	a	18.	T	26.	T
3.	a	11.	c	19.	T	27.	T
4.	b	12.	c	20.	T	28.	b
5.	b	13.	b	21.	F	29.	b
6.	d	14.	a	22.	F	30.	b
7.	a	15.	c	23.	F		
8.	c	16.	b	24.	T		

Module 3

1.	d	8.	d	15.	a	22.	F
2.	b	9.	d	16.	b	23.	F
3.	d	10.	b	17.	T	24.	T
4.	b	11.	d	18.	T	25.	T
5.	d	12.	c	19.	T	26.	a
6.	d	13.	d	20.	T		
7.	a	14.	c	21.	T		

27. 2,750 = present consumption. Using the mid-range of 2,000 calories, Mary's intake is 750 kcal per day in excess of output. 750 kcal × 7 days per week = 5,250 extra kcal per week. This is roughly 1½ lbs. per week weight gain. Estimate 6–7 lbs. per month × 6 months. Mary will gain 36 to 42 lbs. by the end of school.
28. c
29. While there are 22 items listed under responsibilities of health personnel, 5 that are especially important in Mary's case are:
    a. Do not use any fad diets: a low-calorie diet that contains essential nutrients is to be used. (#18)
    b. Become familiar with behavior modification techniques and use them to gain control of eating patterns. (#22)

c. Adopt a more healthful diet instead of giving up certain foods (#20)
d. Use a balanced diet, proper food preparation, portion control, sound food guides. (#9)
e. Encourage regular exercise (daily), at the same time as reducing quantity of food. (#15)
Note: #16, 19, and 21 are also important, so if you listed any of those you may count them.

Module 4

1.	a	8.	a	15.	d	22.	T
2.	d	9.	d	16.	b	23.	T
3.	a	10.	a	17.	a	24.	T
4.	d	11.	d	18.	c	25.	b
5.	c	12.	c	19.	F	26.	c
6.	c	13.	d	20.	T	27.	c
7.	d	14.	e	21.	F		

28. Any of these:
    1. Use the recommended distribution of nutrients.
        a. 50–60 percent of total calories from carbohydrates—mainly from grains, fruits, and vegetables.
        b. Protein for a teenage athlete at 1–1.5 g/kg of body weight.
        c. Remainder of total calories from fat.
    2. No reduced caloric intake at all unless percent of body fat exceeded normal range.
    3. No vitamin/mineral supplements, no electrolyte solutions, no bee pollen.
    4. No carbohydrate loading for a teenager.
    5. High-fluid intake, especially water, at all times before, during, and after a match. If sweet drinks are used, they should be diluted.

Module 5

1.	a	8.	b	15.	b	22.	F
2.	d	9.	b	16.	a	23.	T
3.	b	10.	b	17.	b	24.	T
4.	c	11.	d	18.	T	25.	F
5.	c	12.	a	19.	T	26.	d
6.	b	13.	b	20.	F	27.	a
7.	c	14.	a	21.	T		

28. The missing nutrients in Lisa's diet are all of those listed in question #26. Therefore, any and all of these foods need to be added to her diet:
    Soy milk fortified with calcium and vitamin D, rice and bean combinations, legumes, nuts, seeds (i.e., date-nut breads), peanut butter sandwiches and peanut butter cookies, corn and beans, meat analogs, combined cereals and legumes, dark green leafy vegetables such as kale, turnip greens, mustard greens, oranges and orange juice.

Suggest: Vitamin B_{12} supplements, perhaps iron and use of iodized salt. As fiber content is high, small frequent meals may be indicated.

Module 6

1.	a	8.	b	15.	d	22.	F
2.	c	9.	a	16.	b	23.	F
3.	c	10.	d	17.	c	24.	F
4.	b	11.	b	18.	a	25.	F
5.	d	12.	a	19.	T	26.	T
6.	a	13.	d	20.	T	27.	T
7.	d	14.	c	21.	T	28.	T

29. Storing uncovered and 24-hour advance salad preparation accelerates vitamin loss due to oxidation. Dicing potatoes and cooking ahead destroys vitamins. The smaller the cut, the greater the loss. Cooking foods in large amounts of water over long periods of time increases vitamin loss by leaching and oxidation.
30. The water-soluble vitamins, especially vitamin C which is the least stable of the vitamins, were lost.
31. Ways to conserve nutrients include:
    a. cook vegetables whole and unpared
    b. use cooking methods that shorten cooking time
    c. use the smallest amount of water
    d. cook covered to use shortest cooking time possible
    e. slice or cut fruits and vegetables just before use to prevent oxidation

Module 7

1.	c	8.	b	15.	c	22.	F
2.	c	9.	d	16.	F	23.	F
3.	d	10.	d	17.	F	24.	T
4.	a	11.	b	18.	T	25.	T
5.	d	12.	d	19.	F	26.	T
6.	c	13.	e	20.	T	27.	T
7.	d	14.	a	21.	T	28.	b

29. calcium   800 mg   See calcium table for food sources.
    iron   18 mg   See iron table for food sources.
30. a

Module 8

1.	d	8.	b	15.	a	22.	F
2.	d	9.	c	16.	T	23.	T
3.	b	10.	b	17.	T	24.	T
4.	b	11.	b	18.	T	25.	T
5.	b	12.	c	19.	F		
6.	b	13.	b	20.	F		
7.	a	14.	b	21.	F		

26. a. overweight to obese depending on further fatfold measurements
    b. hypertension
    c. excess caffeine and alcohol consumption
    d. excess sodium (indiscriminate restaurant eating)
    e. lack of nutrition information and desirable eating behaviors
27. a. Explain significance of findings to client.

b. Set up realistic goals with client; set specific objectives.
c. Find resources and materials as needed.
d. Plan at his level of education and understanding.
e. Use as many methods of teaching as necessary for understanding.
f. Set up evaluation criteria.

28. a. The client will be able to choose from a restaurant menu those foods that will comply with his diet plan.
    b. The client will be able to modify his eating behaviors to moderate his intake of caffeine, alcohol, and calories.
    c. The client will be able to list foods high in sodium to be omitted when choosing food.
    d. The client will be able to manage his diet plan while traveling.
    e. The client will recognize the importance of regular checkups and follow up on his plan.
29. Measure progress by
    a. evaluating each objective and subobjective separately through questioning, written tests, verbal tests, observation of client's behavior and attitude.
    b. evaluating teaching by team conference, peer evaluation, etc.
    c. revising objectives as needed.
    d. requesting return for follow up evaluation at regular intervals; successful progress may be observed by weight loss and lower blood pressure in follow up tests.
30. Changed behavior.

Module 9

1.	d	8.	d	15.	a	22.	T
2.	c	9.	a	16.	a	23.	F
3.	c	10.	d	17.	b	24.	T
4.	d	11.	b	18.	b	25.	T
5.	b	12.	c	19.	b	26.	T
6.	a	13.	a	20.	F		
7.	d	14.	d	21.	T		

27. Lisa is striving for autonomy and it is reflected in the eating behavior. As she struggles for control she wants to do everything her way. It is a phase that will pass.
28. a. What and how much food does the child eat per day?
    b. Is her weight normal for her height/age?
    c. Is she gaining at a regular, slow, steady rate?
    d. Do other physical characteristics appear normal (hair, eyes, teeth, etc.)?
    e. Does she appear to be a happy child?
29. The growth rate has slowed since last year and her appetite has diminished. Accordingly, she does not need as much food as during her first year of life.
30. a. "Food jags" are common at this age. As long as the food is nutritious, the grandmother should not be concerned.
    b. Children are no longer forced to "finish everything" because obesity is a problem to be avoided at any age, but especially early childhood. After a reasonable time, remove the food from the table without comment.

Module 10

1.	d	7.	d	13.	d	19.	F
2.	e	8.	a	14.	c	20.	F
3.	e	9.	d	15.	b	21.	F
4.	a	10.	e	16.	c	22.	F
5.	c	11.	c	17.	F	23.	T
6.	a	12.	d	18.	F	24.	T

25. Anorexia, increase or decrease intestinal motility, change absorption and metabolism of nutrients, nausea, vomiting, damage intestinal walls.
26. Antidepressants, antihistamines, oral contraceptives and alcohol (small amounts only)
27. Amphetamines, Cholinergic agents, some expectorants and narcotic analgesics (Elderly: tranquilizers)
28. Penacillamine, streptomycin, KCL, Vitamin B complex in liquid form and some chemotherapies
29. Cough syrup, expectorants, elixirs
30. Antibiotics and parenteral drug solutions

Module 11

1.	a	9.	b	17.	F	25.	F
2.	a	10.	c	18.	T	26.	b
3.	d	11.	b	19.	T	27.	c
4.	d	12.	a	20.	F	28.	b
5.	d	13.	b	21.	T	29.	b
6.	b	14.	a	22.	T	30.	a
7.	a	15.	a	23.	F		
8.	a	16.	F	24.	T		

Module 12

1.	b	8.	b	15.	a	22.	F
2.	c	9.	d	16.	b	23.	T
3.	b	10.	c	17.	d	24.	a
4.	d	11.	d	18.	e	25.	d
5.	c	12.	a	19.	F	26.	d
6.	d	13.	b	20.	T	27.	a
7.	d	14.	c	21.	F		

28. The most common diet modifications are alterations in basic nutrients, energy value, texture, and seasonings. James needs an alteration in basic nutrients and energy value. Unless further assessment reveals a need for additional adjustments, the diet prescription should be a high carbohydrate, high protein, high vitamin, moderate fat, regular diet containing approximately 3,500 calories.
29. Rationale: to restore and maintain nutritional status: James is underweight, apparently malnourished, and injured.
30. c

Module 13

1.	a	7.	b	13.	d	19.	F
2.	c	8.	c	14.	a	20.	F
3.	a	9.	d	15.	T	21.	F
4.	d	10.	d	16.	F	22.	T
5.	a	11.	b	17.	F	23.	T
6.	d	12.	c	18.	T		

24. Because of extensive injuries and surgery, this patient is in a hypermetabolic state. She needs to be maintained at the high rate of TPN.
25. No. Patients are never placed on reduction diets until after healing has taken place. Other measures to relieve breathing must be considered.
26. *See* Table 13–1.
27. *See* Nursing Implications, Module 13.

Module 14

1.	d	9.	d	17.	F	25.	F
2.	a	10.	d	18.	T	26.	b
3.	a	11.	b	19.	F	27.	c
4.	b	12.	d	20.	T	28.	a
5.	b	13.	c	21.	F	29.	d
6.	c	14.	e	22.	T	30.	b
7.	d	15.	a	23.	F		
8.	d	16.	T	24.	T		

Module 15

1.	b	8.	a	15.	c	22.	T
2.	a	9.	c	16.	c	23.	F
3.	d	10.	b	17.	a	24.	T
4.	c	11.	a	18.	e	25.	T
5.	a	12.	b	19.	b	26.	b
6.	d	13.	b	20.	d	27.	d
7.	a	14.	b	21.	T	28.	d

29. Any three of these: restore nutritional deficits, prevent further losses, promote healing, repair and maintain body tissue, improve chances for recovery.
30. a. fluid intake and output
    b. nutrient intake (amount of protein especially important, and vitamins)
    c. caloric intake and weight changes

Module 16

1.	d*	8.	c	15.	g	22.	T
2.	c	9.	d	16.	f	23.	b**
3.	a	10.	a	17.	a	24.	b
4.	d	11.	e	18.	F	25.	b
5.	d	12.	c	19.	T	26.	d
6.	b	13.	d	20.	F	27.	c
7.	a	14.	b	21.	F		

*(250 × 4) + (100 × 4) + (70 × 9) = 2,030
**70 lb. ÷ 2.2 = 32 kg (rounded)
80 g protein ÷ 32 kg = 2.5 g/kg body weight
(150 × 4) + (80 × 4) + (50 × 9) = 1,370 calories

Module 17

1.	b	6.	a	11.	a	16.	F
2.	c	7.	a	12.	F	17.	c
3.	b	8.	b	13.	T	18.	e
4.	c	9.	c	14.	T	19.	e
5.	c	10.	d	15.	T		

20. boiled or poached, three times a week
21. fruit, fresh or in natural juice

22. omit, substitute chicken or tuna
23. omit, substitute fruit
24. use low-fat cottage cheese only
25. omit, use a fresh spinach or other dark green salad
26. substitute sherbet within the caloric allowance
27. no alteration necessary
28. b
29. a
30. c

Module 18

1.	a	9.	d	17.	d	25.	T
2.	a	10.	b	18.	e	26.	c
3.	d	11.	d	19.	a	27.	d
4.	d	12.	c	20.	T	28.	d
5.	d	13.	e	21.	F	29.	b
6.	a	14.	a	22.	T	30.	c
7.	a	15.	b	23.	F		
8.	c	16.	c	24.	T		

Module 19

1.	b	9.	d	17.	F	25.	c
2.	b	10.	a	18.	T	26.	d
3.	b	11.	b	19.	F	27.	b
4.	d	12.	b	20.	T	28.	a
5.	d	13.	b	21.	d	29.	b
6.	b	14.	T	22.	b	30.	c
7.	b	15.	T	23.	e		
8.	a	16.	T	24.	a		

Module 20

1.	a	9.	c	17.	c	25.	F
2.	d	10.	d	18.	d	26.	T
3.	c	11.	b	19.	e	27.	T
4.	b	12.	c	20.	a	28.	F
5.	a	13.	d	21.	T	29.	T
6.	b	14.	a	22.	T	30.	F
7.	a	15.	b	23.	T		
8.	d	16.	b	24.	F		

Module 21

1.	d	8.	d	15.	b	22.	T
2.	c	9.	d	16.	c	23.	T
3.	d	10.	b	17.	a	24.	F
4.	c	11.	d	18.	T	25.	T
5.	c	12.	b	19.	T	26.	b
6.	b	13.	c	20.	F	27.	d
7.	c	14.	a	21.	F	28.	a

Module 22

1.	c	8.	c	15.	f	22.	T
2.	a	9.	d	16.	a	23.	T
3.	b	10.	d	17.	T	24.	T
4.	d	11.	c	18.	F	25.	T
5.	a	12.	b	19.	T	26.	b
6.	a	13.	d	20.	F		
7.	d	14.	e	21.	F		

27. a. He cannot absorb the fat-soluble vitamins until they are made water-miscible.
    b. These are effective in assisting the patient to utilize more of his ingested food.
    c. Medium-chain triglyceride supplements are better tolerated than regular fats and therefore increase caloric intake.
    d. He has a fever; also extra fluids help dissolve the mucus collection. *Note:* Extra salt may also be needed.
28. a. The essentials of the daily food guide.
    b. How to make appropriate substitutions for high-fat and poorly tolerated foods.
    c. How to keep an accurate food record for assessment and follow up care.
    d. The essentials of low-fat cookery and cooking with medium-chain triglycerides.
29. a. Maintain adequate nutrition (*see* Nursing Implications #1, a–e).
    b. Promote growth and development through adequate nutrition.
    c. Provide support to the family.
    d. Educate the child and its family (*see* Nursing Implications, #4, a–e).

Module 23

1.	c	8.	b	15.	a	22.	F
2.	d	9.	d	16.	b	23.	F
3.	a	10.	b	17.	a	24.	T
4.	a	11.	a	18.	b	25.	T
5.	b	12.	b	19.	a		
6.	c	13.	b	20.	a		
7.	a	14.	a	21.	F		

26. Weight at present. Signs of dehydration, social behavior at present. Deviations (loss) of weight. Eating behaviors (anorexia, hunger, etc.). Any physical signs of malnutrition.
27. d
28. Breakfast meal pattern (amounts and textures appropriate for 18-month-old child): Juice or fruit; rice or corn cereal; milk; egg, special bread, margarine.
    Lunch and dinner meal pattern (amounts and textures appropriate for 18-month-old child): Meat, fish, poultry or meat substitute; potato, rice, grits, sweet potatoes; vegetables (any appropriate for age); fruit (any appropriate for age); special low gluten bread or cornbread, margarine; milk.
    Between-meal snacks: Chocolate, Kool-Aid, cornstarch, rice or tapioca pudding; fruits or juices, sherbet, gelatin, cheese (no cheese foods); cookies/cakes from low gluten, rice or arrowroot flour.
29. a. low protein (gluten) flour, cookies, pastas
    b. MCT.
    c. water-miscible vitamins
30. a

Module 24

1.	d	3.	b	5.	d	7.	d
2.	a	4.	a	6.	c	8.	a

9.	b	14.	e	19.	F	24.	T
10.	b	15.	b	20.	F	25.	T
11.	d	16.	T	21.	F	26.	d
12.	c	17.	T	22.	T		
13.	a	18.	T	23.	T		

27. **a.** Extra carbohydrate: karo syrup or polycose
   b. Extra fats: MCT and corn oil
   c. Extra low protein, low electrolyte formula in addition to solids

28. Breakfast: 3 oz. juice; 2 tbsp. salt-free cereal; 1 slice toast
   Lunch and dinner: 2 tbsp. mashed or junior vegetables; 1 oz. chopped or ground meat; 2–3 tbsp. soft mashed or pureed fruit; 1 tbsp. mashed potato
   Snacks: Any high calorie, low protein, low sodium beverages or formulas, such as SMA.

29. Problems: Crying; refusing to eat; using food to get their way; becoming too tired to eat; turning blue.
   Coping: Stay calm; avoid overconcern; do not "invalidize"; be consistent; don't feed when the child is tired; divide food into small feedings; foster independence as soon as possible.

30. All nursing implications should be reinforced for the mother to assist her in competently caring for Teresa at home. *See also* Nursing Implications, Module 24.

Module 25

1.	c	7.	c	13.	c, d	19.	T
2.	d	8.	b*	14.	a	20.	F
3.	a	9.	h	15.	b	21.	F
4.	b	10.	e	16.	F	22.	T
5.	b	11.	f	17.	F		
6.	d	12.	c, d, g	18.	F		

*(if made from corn oil, d)

23. Have Bobby's mother keep a detailed food record of everything Bobby eats for a certain time period.

24. Although diagnosing food allergies is difficult, the elimination diet is probably the most successful. Bobby's mother should try eliminating the four foods one at a time. When symptoms disappear, try reintroducing one food at a time until symptoms reappear, the food causing the reappearance of symptoms may be the offender. Make sure Bobby receives substitutes for the foods removed from his diet, i.e., soy milk for cow's milk, rice products for wheat products, to avoid nutritional inadequacies.

25. a. ice cream
   b. cheese
   c. custard
   d. cream and cream foods
   e. yogurt
   f–j. any of the following: most baked goods, cream sauce, macaroni, noodles, pie crust, cereals, chili, breaded foods

26. Bobby should try to reintroduce these foods into his diet occasionally because allergies may fade over time.

Module 26

1.	a	8.	d	15.	b	22.	F
2.	c	9.	d	16.	T	23.	T
3.	b	10.	b	17.	T	24.	T
4.	a	11.	b	18.	F	25.	F
5.	d	12.	a	19.	T		
6.	a	13.	a	20.	F		
7.	c	14.	c	21.	F		

26. **a.** Yes   **b.** Yes
27. b
28. Your choice; however, the menu pattern will follow these guidelines.
   Breakfast: fruit, 1 serving; allowed cereal, ½ cup; Lofenalac, 8 oz.
   Lunch: fruit, 1 serving; green vegetable, 1 serving; starchy vegetable, 1 serving; crackers (4); butter or margarine; 2 tbsp. allowed dessert; Lofenalac, 4 oz.
   Snacks at 10, 2 and bedtime: fruit; arrowroot cookies (5); Lofenalac, 4 oz.
   Dinner: green vegetable, 1 serving; vegetable soup, ¼ cup; potato, ½ cup; butter or margarine; 2 tbsp. allowed dessert; Lofenalac, 8 oz.

29. b

Module 27

1.	d	9.	b	17.	T	25.	b
2.	b	10.	a	18.	T	26.	e
3.	c	11.	c	19.	F	27.	d
4.	d	12.	d	20.	T	28.	a
5.	b	13.	F	21.	d	29.	b
6.	c	14.	T	22.	e	30.	c
7.	b	15.	T	23.	c		
8.	c	16.	F	24.	a		